Arthroscopy of the Temporomandibular Joint

Arthroscopy of the Temporomandibular Joint

Mohan Thomas, D.D.S., F.A.C.D.

Chief – Division of Oral and Maxillofacial Surgery
Director – Center for Corrective Jaw Surgery
and Temporomandibular Disorders
Hospital for Joint Diseases Orthopaedic Institute
New York, New York
Assistant Clinical Professor
Mount Sinai School of Medicine
Attending Staff, Oral/Maxillofacial Surgery
Mt. Sinai Medical Center
New York, New York

Sidney L. Bronstein, D.D.S., M.Sc.D., F.A.C.D.

Associate Professor and Chairman
Division of Oral and Maxillofacial Surgery
School of Dentistry
University of Colorado
Denver, Colorado

W.B. SAUNDERS COMPANY
Harcourt Brace Jovanovich, Inc.

Philadelphia   London   Toronto
Montreal   Sydney   Tokyo

W. B. SAUNDERS COMPANY
Harcourt Brace Jovanovich, Inc.

The Curtis Center
Independence Square West
Philadelphia, PA 19106

Library of Congress Cataloging-in-Publication Data

Arthroscopy of the temporomandibular joint / [edited by] Mohan Thomas, Sidney L. Bronstein.
    p. cm.

  ISBN 0-7216-3119-3

  1. Temporomandibular joint—Examination. 2. Arthroscopy.
3. Temporomandibular joint—Diseases—Treatment. I. Thomas, Mohan.
II. Bronstein, Sidney L.
    [DNLM: 1. Arthroscopy. 2. Postoperative Care. 3. Temporomandibular Joint—pathology. 4. Temporomandibular Joint Diseases—diagnosis.
5. Temporomandibular Joint Diseases—surgery.

WU 140 A787] RK470.A77 1991 617.5'22—dc20
DNLM/DLC
                                                                             91-4860

Editor: John Dyson
Developmental Editor: David Kilmer
Designer: Joan Wendt
Production Manager: Peter Faber
Manuscript Editor: Kathleen G. Mason
Illustration Specialist: Walt Verbitski
Indexer: Norman Duren
Cover Designer: Dorothy Chattin

Arthroscopy of the Temporomandibular Joint   ISBN 0-7216-3119-3

Copyright © 1991 by W. B. Saunders Company.

All rights reserved. No part of this publication may be reproduced or transmitted in any form or by any means, electronic or mechanical, including photocopy, recording, or any information storage and retrieval system, without permission in writing from the publisher.

Printed in the United States of America.

Last digit is the print number: 9 8 7 6 5 4 3 2 1

DEDICATIONS

*This book is dedicated to my parents,
Mr. and Mrs. K. T. Thomas,
for giving me the education they could not have
and for being supportive of my academic endeavors.*

MOHAN THOMAS, D.D.S., F.A.C.D.

*To those who provided me the opportunity to become
an educated man:
my parents and teachers;
to those who have always supported my efforts in life:
my brother, sister, friends, and colleagues;
and to those brilliant, extraordinary, far-sighted individuals,
temporomandibular joint "explorers," who really opened this
frontier—
Flemming Norgaard, Clyde Wilkes, and William Farrar—
I dedicate this work.*

SIDNEY L. BRONSTEIN, D.D.S., M.SC.D., F.A.C.D.

Contributors

GEERT BOERING, D.D.S., Ph.D.
Professor, University of Groningen; Professor and Head, Department of Oral and Maxillofacial Surgery, University Hospital, Groningen, The Netherlands.

JON P. BRADRICK, D.D.S.
Assistant Professor of Surgery, Case Western Reserve University; Fulltime Staff, Oral and Maxillofacial Surgeon, Department of Surgery, MetroHealth Medical Center, Cleveland, Ohio.

SIDNEY L. BRONSTEIN, D.D.S., M.Sc.D., F.A.C.D.
Associate Professor and Chairman, Division of Oral and Maxillofacial Surgery, School of Dentistry, University of Colorado, Denver, Colorado.

DANIEL BUCHBINDER, D.M.D.
Assistant Professor, Mount Sinai School of Medicine; Director, Residency Training Program in Oral and Maxillofacial Surgery, Mount Sinai Medical Center; Chief, Division of Oral and Maxillofacial Surgery, Mount Sinai Medical Center, New York, New York.

JEFFREY B. CARTER, M.D., D.M.D.
Director, Oral Surgical Institute: Clinical Assistant Professor, Department of Oral and Maxillofacial Surgery; Vanderbilt University School of Medicine: Staff Oral and Maxillofacial Surgeon at Baptist Hospital, St. Thomas Hospital, Centennial Medical Center, and Vanderbilt University Medical Center, Nashville, Tennessee.

CHRISTOPHER L. DAVIS, D.D.S., M.D.
Assistant Clinical Professor, University of Southern California, Los Angeles; Active Staff, Memorial Medical Center, Long Beach, California.

LAMBERT G.M. de BONT, D.D.S., Ph.D.
Associate Professor, University of Groningen; Staff Member, Department of Oral and Maxillofacial Surgery, University Hospital, Groningen, The Netherlands.

THOMAS M. EGGLETON, M.S., P.T.
Clinical Instructor, Clinical Research Foundation, San Diego, California.

RICHARD H. HAUG, D.D.S.
Assistant Professor of Surgery, Case Western Reserve University School of Medicine; Metro Health Medical Center, Cleveland, Ohio.

DAVID C. HOFFMAN, D.D.S.
Assistant Clinical Professor, University of Medicine and Dentistry of New Jersey, New Jersey Medical School, Newark, New Jersey; Attending Staten Island Hospital.

ANDERS HOLMLUND, D.D.S., Ph.D.
Associate Professor, Department of Oral Surgery, Karolinska Institute, Stockholm; Associate Professor, Department of Oral Surgery, Huddinge University Hospital, Huddinge, Sweden.

THOMAS A. INDRESANO, D.M.D.
Associate Professor of Surgery, Case Western Reserve University School of Medicine. Associate Clinical Professor, Oral and Maxillofacial Surgery, Case Western Reserve School of Dentistry; Director of Oral and Maxillofacial Surgery, MetroHealth Medical Center, Cleveland, Ohio.

RONALD M. KAMINISHI, D.D.S.
Associate Clinical Professor, University of Southern California, Los Angeles; Assistant Clinical Professor, University of California, Irvine; Assistant Professor of Oral Surgery, Loma Linda University, Loma Linda; Active Staff, Memorial Medical Center, Long Beach, California.

ANDREW S. KAPLAN, D.M.D., F.A.C.D., F.I.C.D.
Assistant Clinical Professor, The Mount Sinai School of Medicine; Director, TMD/Facial Pain Clinic; Coordinator, Dental Department; Assistant Attending at The Mount Sinai Hospital, New York, New York.

RICHARD W. KATZBERG, M.D.
Professor and Chairman, Department of Radiology, Oregon Health Services University Hospital, Portland, Oregon.

MICHAEL G. KOSLIN, D.M.D.
Subspecialty Chief, Oral and Maxillofacial Surgery, Brookwood Medical Center. Active Staff, Health South Medical Center, Birmingham, Alabama.

CHRISTOPHER LANE, D.D.S.
Chief Resident, Department of Oral and Maxillofacial Surgery, The Mount Sinai Hospital, New York, New York.

DENNIS P. LANGTON, B.S., P.T.
Clinical Instructor, Clinical Research Foundation, San Diego, California.

DENNIS C. LEINER, Ph.D.
President, Leiner Associates, Jaffrey, New Hampshire.

HÅKAN LUNDH, D.D.S., Ph.D.
Research Associate, School of Dentistry, University of Lund, Sweden.

RALPH G. MERRILL, D.D.S., M.Sc.D.
Professor and Chairman, Department of Oral and Maxillofacial Surgery, Oregon Health Sciences University Hospital, Portland, Oregon.

JEFFREY J. MOSES, D.D.S.
Chief, Division of Oral and Maxillofacial Surgery, Tri-City Medical Center, Oceanside; Director, Pacific Clinical Research Foundation, Encinitas, California.

KEN-ICHIRO MURAKAMI, D.D.S., Ph.D.
Assistant Professor, Department of Oral and Maxillofacial Surgery, Faculty of Medicine, Kyoto University, Sakyoku, Kyoto, Japan.

J. SERGE PARISIEN, M.D., F.A.C.S.
Associate Clinical Professor of Orthopaedic Surgery, New York University School of Medicine; Chief of Arthroscopic Surgery, Hospital for Joint Diseases Orthopaedic Institute, New York, New York.

ROBERT D. SCHWARTZ, D.M.D.
Clinical Assistant Professor, Department of Dentistry and Oral and Maxillofacial Surgery, University of Illinois and Northwestern University. Attending, Michael Reese Hospital and Medical Center and Northwestern Memorial Hospital, Chicago, Illinois.

HARRY SHEN, M.D.
Assistant Professor of Medicine, Mount Sinai School of Medicine; Associate Attending Physician, Hospital for Joint Diseases and Beth Israel Medical Center, New York, New York.

BOUDEWIJN STEGENGA, D.D.S.
Research Worker, Department of Oral and Maxillofacial Surgery, University Hospital, Groningen, The Netherlands.

TERRY T. TANAKA, D.D.S.
Associate Clinical Professor, University of Southern California School of Dentistry, Los Angeles, California.

ALLEN W. TARRO, D.M.D.
Director, TMJ/Facial Pain Clinic and Assistant Clinical Professor, Department of Oral and Maxillofacial Surgery, Boston University School of Graduate Dentistry, Boston, Massachusetts; Director, TMJ/Facial Pain Clinic, Northeast Rehabilitation Hospital, Salem, New Hampshire.

MOHAN THOMAS, D.D.S., F.A.C.D.
Assistant Clinical Professor, Mount Sinai School of Medicine; Chief, Division of Oral/Maxillofacial Surgery; Director, Center for Corrective Jaw Surgery and Temporomandibular Disorders, Hospital for Joint Diseases Orthopaedic Institute; Attending Staff, Oral/Maxillofacial Surgery, Mount Sinai Medical Center, New York, New York.

CHARLES WEISS, M.D.
Miami Beach, Florida.

PER-LENNART WESTESSON, D.D.S., Ph.D.
Associate Professor of Radiology and Clinical Dentistry, University of Rochester School of Medicine and Dentistry; Senior Research Associate of Orthodontics, Eastman Dental Center, Rochester, New York.

DAVID ZELOUF, M.D.
Chief Resident, Department of Orthopaedics, Hospital for Joint Diseases, New York, New York.

Foreword

Arthroscopy at the Hospital for Joint Diseases Orthopaedic Insitute dates back to 1931 when Dr. Michael Burman devised a clinically useful method of investigating joint pathology through an early arthroscope. Following his pioneering work, there was a hiatus until modern electronics made it possible to match an optical system to a miniature television camera and made arthroscopic surgery a practical reality.

The temporomandibular joint has been the "lost joint" in the human body. The disorders of this joint are seen by dentists; oral maxillofacial surgeons; ear, nose, and throat surgeons; and others, who in the past had very few diagnostic modalities, other than radiography, in the study of disorders of this joint. A correlation of pathology with clinical symptomatology has now been made possible. Through the use of the instrumentation developed for surgery in other joints, it is now possible to perform arthroscopic surgery on a temporomandibular joint.

This book is the result of several collaborators, who have excelled in their areas of research and interest with Drs. Mohan Thomas and Sidney L. Bronstein as contributing editors.

Dr. Stuart Springer set the tone at the Hospital for Joint Diseases Orthopaedic Institute with the formation of the International Arthroscopy Center and inclusion of the temporomandibular joint into the curriculum.

I am particularly delighted with Dr. Thomas's participation in this book. He started his career with a residency at the Hospital for Joint Diseases Orthopaedic Institute.

VICTOR H. FRANKEL, M.D., PH.D.
Director of Orthopaedic Surgery,
Hospital for Joint Diseases Orthopaedic
Institute: Professor of Orthopaedic Surgery,
New York University School of Medicine;
New York, New York

Preface

Surgical therapy of the internally deranged temporomandibular joint has existed for more than a century. Since the report by Annandale in 1887, a plethora of techniques and modalities have been initiated to address the pathoses of the deranged temporomandibular joint, with varying degrees of satisfaction and disappointment. Disc removal was described in the early 1900s as a surgical treatment for a number of painful temporomandibular joint afflictions. During the 1950s the high condylar shave and condylectomy were introduced, with varying levels of research to support clinical findings. The approach during the late 1960s and early 1970s was directed at biomaterials and anatomic reconstruction. During this era as well, disc repair and repositioning were introduced to approach joint reconstruction from an anatomic standpoint. It was not until the 1980s, with clinical applications derived from orthopaedic research, that arthroscopy developed as an indicated surgical modality for the temporomandibular joint.

The advent of small joint arthroscopy and its application to therapy of the diseased temporomandibular joint introduced profound changes in the practice of oral and maxillofacial surgery. Literally dozens of clinical and research publications appeared in the international oral and maxillofacial surgical literature during the 1980s, describing the applications, findings, and clinical efficacy of temporomandibular joint arthroscopy. New terminology, pathologic diagnoses, instrumentation, techniques, and therapy have been the result. It is the aim of this text to provide the practicing oral and maxillofacial surgeon with a complete guide to the clinical practice of arthroscopy of the temporomandibular joint.

Arthroscopy of the Temporomandibular Joint comprises the work of more than 30 contributors, providing a state-of-the-art compendium for the practicing surgeon. The text describes the evolution and development of arthroscopy and its application to the temporomandibular joint. The optics of arthroscopy and arthroscopic instrumentation are described in detail to provide insight into clinical applications. The normal physiology of synovial joints is discussed, as are the functional anatomy and pathophysiology. The clinical diagnosis of temporomandibular joint disorders and their supporting imaging techniques is presented from a preoperative standpoint.

Specific techniques and modalities are described for clinical application to synovitis, adhesions, chondromalacia, osteoarthrosis, and arthritides. Nuances of arthroscopic instrumentation for the more advanced practitioner, postoperative therapy, and complications are reviewed to complete the treatise. From the preoperative work-up to directions of future research, a complete guide is now available for the oral and maxillofacial surgeon. With it go our hopes that all phases of arthroscopy will be detailed for its clinical application.

MOHAN THOMAS, D.D.S., F.A.C.D.
SIDNEY L. BRONSTEIN, D.D.S., M.SC.D., F.A.C.D.

Acknowledgments

This is a good time to remember and thank all of my teachers and colleagues who helped me in my professional career.

I would like to thank all the researchers and educators—the late Dr. Bill Farrar, Drs. Frank Dolwick, Bill McCarty, Ken-Ichiro Murakami, Bruce Sanders, Per-Lennart Westesson, Doran Ryan, and Terry Tanaka, to mention a few—who sparked my interest in the evaluation and treatment of temporomandibular joint disorders. To the Hospital for Joint Diseases Orthopaedic Institute and particularly Dr. Victor H. Frankel, who believed in me and supported me in all of my academic endeavors; Dr. J. Serge Parisien, a good friend who provided the idea for this book; Mr. Abe Moshel, who drove me to "publish"; Dr. Arthur Elias, my mentor and friend for the last 17 years; Drs. Stuart Springer, Jack Katell, Daniel Buchbinder, and Andrew Kaplan for their encouragement and support; and to Dr. Richard H. Haug, a friend I could always count on—to all I am truly grateful.

I would like to thank all of my colleagues at the Hospital for Joint Diseases Orthopaedic Institute for teaching me sound orthopaedic principles and to Dr. Joseph P. McCain for introducing me to the art and science of temporomandibular joint arthroscopy. His technical ability, attention to detail, and willingness to teach have been inspiring.

I would like to thank all my collaborators whose contributions are noteworthy and made this book possible—particularly Dr. Sidney L. Bronstein, Dr. Allen Tarro, and Dr. Robert D. Schwartz, a true "mensch"—for their encouragement and assistance; Mr. Dan Benevento for the photographic assistance; Mr. Hugh Nachamie for the illustrations; Ms. Laura Tritto of Sony Medical Corporation for all of the technical support and assistance that made possible many of the superb color reproductions in this book; and to my office staff, for bringing this book to fruition.

The so-called unsung heroes are truly the wonderful staff at W.B. Saunders Company—David Kilmer, Mary Anne Folcher, Kathleen G. Mason, Jean Kenworthy, Peter Faber, Faith Voit, and others—headed by senior medical editor, John Dyson.

MOHAN THOMAS, D.D.S., F.A.C.D.

Acknowledgments

For the past 11 years my primary interest has been the diagnosis and treatment of temporomandibular joint arthropathy.

There are many to whom I want to offer sincere thanks for their teaching, their support, and their friendship: to my earliest mentors, Doran Ryan and Frank Dolwick, both of whom early on whetted my appetite and stimulated my efforts in this field of study; to Bruce Sanders, who expanded my horizons in temporomandibular joint treatment by suggesting I journey to Minneapolis to meet and learn from Clyde Wilkes—Clyde's inspiration was and still is a tremendous incentive to me; to count him as my friend is a real honor—and later Bruce welcomed me to arthroscopy; to Per-Lennart Westesson, researcher extraordinaire, with whom I was most fortunate to spend my sabbatical and from whom I learned so very much; to Lars Eriksson, a singular human being, a good friend, and an accomplished surgeon; to Ken-Ichiro Murakami, a truly unique individual, who piqued my interest in arthroscopy and assisted me with my very first case; and to Joe McCain, whose example of diligent practice, attention to detail, and precise investigation in arthroscopy set the tone for me—he has never wavered in his support and interest, offering me unique opportunities. To all of these individuals I owe a tremendous debt of gratitude.

Many, many others, close friends all, have influenced my professional direction immensely. To them also, I offer my thanks—Ralph Merrill, Ken Rotskoff, Ron Kaminishi, Chris Davis, Jeff Moses, Bob Schwartz, Lou Mercuri, and Annika Isberg.

SIDNEY L. BRONSTEIN, D.D.S., M.SC.D., F.A.C.D.

Introduction

The use of arthroscopy to diagnose and treat disorders of the temporomandibular joint is still in its infancy. In youth, there is a tremendous capacity for learning, and knowledge can be accumulated rapidly. In time, the bank of information must be assimilated and be put to practical use. This outstanding text organizes this data through multiple collaborators and opens our eyes to a new and an exciting view of the temporomandibular joint via arthroscopy.

Section I offers insight into the development of the small joint arthroscope and utilizes the experience of orthopaedic surgeons and the years of development and refinement of the principles and practice of large joint arthroscopy. Before applying this new information to the understanding of the temporomandibular joint, we must first distinguish between normal and abnormal anatomy not only on gross examination but also on a cellular level.

The editors, Drs. Thomas and Bronstein, have assembled an international cast of outstanding scientists and practitioners who, in sections II and IV, discuss the various elements of normal and pathologic synovial joints. By understanding how diseases affect larger joints of the body, we are able to extrapolate a plethora of information and save years of basic research. Fortunately, from our previous experience with arthrotomy of the temporomandibular joint, we have learned to scrutinize the literature with a keen eye. Differences in joints do exist! The composition of fibrocartilage is not the same as that of hyaline cartilage. Their healing capabilities are also at a different rate and have a different end result. The shape and structure of the knee meniscus are dissimilar from those of the temporomandibular joint disc. These and other differences presuppose dissimilar functions. When transferring information from the orthopaedic literature to the clinical application in the temporomandibular joint, these and other distinctions must be recognized. Function, be it normal or abnormal, begets form.

In section III, abnormal function and form as they exist in the temporomandibular joint are well illustrated by individuals who deal with these problems on a daily basis. These clinical scientists are willing to share their years of education and experience so that the profession can offer better care to the patient.

The progression of the text is well ordered. Only after thoroughly understanding the physiology and pathophysiology of the temporomandibular joint and learning the mechanics of the arthroscope should techniques be discussed. A definite learning curve occurs with arthroscopy. Section III will allow the practitioner to shift that curve to the left. An atraumatic entry into the joint and a recognition of the joint landmarks enhance successes and diminish complications. Lyses of adhesions and lavage of the joint have been extremely helpful by increasing range of motion and decreasing painful symptoms. This technique has a well-documented success rate. Advanced techniques in temporomandibular joint arthroscopy should be done by the experienced surgeon only after adequate training with cadaveric or animal models. These advanced techniques should not be attempted by the clinician until scientific evidence has demonstrated an increase in success rate or an advantage over present techniques.

Postoperative management is as important as the procedure itself. Chronic, limited range of motion secondary to mechanical interference leads to muscle guarding and muscle fiber shortening. Arthroscopy by its very nature institutes inflammation, joint effusion, and extra-articular edema—all predisposing the patient to joint adhesions. Complications can occur even in the hands of the most experienced arthroscopist. Proper postoperative management following normal arthroscopic procedures or complications is well documented in this text.

When temporomandibular joint disease adversely affects the quality of life, the goal is to properly diagnose and treat the patient to a successful conclusion, thereby returning him or her to a happy, normal, and functional life style. In the past, arthrotomy was the treatment of choice if adequate nonsurgical therapy failed. Obviously, these instances included the difficult cases and failures were inevitable in a certain percentage.

Arthrotomy will remain a viable treatment modality, but arthroscopy offers a less aggressive, more cost-effective alternative in many cases, while maintaining a high degree of success. The editors have successfully organized the knowledge of multiple contributors and systematically presented a very logical and practical approach to the utilization of arthroscopy for the treatment of temporomandibular joint arthropathy. All health care providers who treat this malady should read this text and have it available for reference.

DORAN RYAN, D.D.S., M.S.

Contents

Section I

Evolution of Arthroscopy 1

Chapter 1

DEVELOPMENT OF ORTHOPEDIC ARTHROSCOPY 1
J. SERGE PARISIEN, M.D., F.A.C.S., DAVID ZELOUF, M.D.

Chapter 2

DEVELOPMENT OF TEMPOROMANDIBULAR JOINT
ARTHROSCOPY 6
SIDNEY L. BRONSTEIN, D.D.S., M.Sc.D., F.A.C.D.

Chapter 3

PRINCIPLES OF THE ARTHROSCOPE 12
DENNIS C. LEINER, PH.D.

Section II

Temporomandibular Joint Arthropathy.......... 20

Chapter 4

NORMAL PHYSIOLOGY OF SYNOVIAL JOINTS 20

   A. Synovium 20
     CHARLES WEISS, M.D.

   B. Articular Cartilage 28
     *LAMBERT G.M. DE BONT, D.D.S., PH.D., BOUDEWIJN
     STEGENGA, D.D.S., and GEERT BOERING, D.D.S., PH.D.*

Chapter 5

PATHOPHYSIOLOGY OF TEMPOROMANDIBULAR
JOINT DISORDERS 36
ROBERT D. SCHWARTZ, D.M.D.

Chapter 6

FUNCTIONAL ANATOMY OF THE
TEMPOROMANDIBULAR JOINT 56
    SIDNEY L. BRONSTEIN, D.D.S., M.Sc.D., F.A.C.D.

Chapter 7

NATURAL HISTORY OF INTERNAL DERANGEMENT
OF THE TEMPOROMANDIBULAR JOINT 70
    ANDREW S. KAPLAN, D.M.D., F.A.C.D., F.I.C.D.

Chapter 8

CLINICAL DIAGNOSIS OF TEMPOROMANDIBULAR
JOINT ARTHROPATHY 81
    MOHAN THOMAS, D.D.S., F.A.C.D., RICHARD H.
    HAUG, D.D.S.

Chapter 9

NONSURGICAL MANAGEMENT OF
TEMPOROMANDIBULAR JOINT DISORDERS 89

    A. Occlusal Diagnosis and Splint Therapy 89
    TERRY T. TANAKA, D.D.S.

    B. Splint Treatment of Patients with Disc
    Displacement with Reduction: A Research
    Perspective 96
    HÅKAN LUNDH, D.D.S., PH.D., PER-LENNART
    WESTESSON, D.D.S., PH.D.

Chapter 10

IMAGING OF THE TEMPOROMANDIBULAR JOINT 115
    PER-LENNART WESTESSON, D.D.S., PH.D., RICHARD
    W. KATZBERG, M.D.

■ Section III

Arthroscopy of the Temporomandibular
Joint 140

Chapter 11

ARTHROSCOPIC ANATOMY, HISTOLOGY, AND
VISUAL FIELDS IN THE TEMPOROMANDIBULAR
JOINT 140
    KEN-ICHIRO MURAKAMI, D.D.S., PH.D.

Chapter 12

DIAGNOSTIC AND OPERATIVE ARTHROSCOPY OF
THE TEMPOROMANDIBULAR JOINT 154

    A. Operating Room Protocol 154
    MOHAN THOMAS, D.D.S., F.A.C.D.

    B. Instrumentation (Optical and Surgical) 157
    *MOHAN THOMAS, D.D.S., F.A.C.D., CHRISTOPHER
LANE, D.D.S.*

    C. Documentation 162
    *MOHAN THOMAS, D.D.S., F.A.C.D., CHRISTOPHER
LANE, D.D.S.*

    D. Surgical Procedures and Techniques................. 165
    SIDNEY L. BRONSTEIN, D.D.S., M.Sc.D., F.A.C.D.

Chapter 13

SPECIAL APPLICATIONS 188

    A. Arthroscopic Procedures to Increase Disc Mobility 188
    ALLEN W. TARRO, D.M.D.

    B. Endaural Arthroscopic Approach 192
    JEFFREY J. MOSES, D.D.S.

    C. Arthroscopic Biopsy of the Temporomandibular
Joint 199
    RALPH G. MERRILL, D.D.S., M.Sc.D.

    D. Electrocautery and Fluid Mediums 202
    *MOHAN THOMAS, D.D.S., F.A.C.D., CHRISTOPHER
LANE, D.D.S., and MICHAEL G. KOSLIN, D.M.D.*

    E. Disc-Stabilizing Techniques......................... 206
    ALLEN W. TARRO, D.M.D.

    F. Temporomandibular Joint Arthroscopy for
Post-Arthrotomy Patients 213
    DAVID C. HOFFMAN, D.D.S.

Chapter 14

GUIDELINES FOR TEMPOROMANDIBULAR JOINT
ARTHROSCOPY 228
    SIDNEY L. BRONSTEIN, D.D.S., M.Sc.D., F.A.C.D.

■ **Section IV**

Arthroscopic Pathology of the Temporomandibular Joint 235

Chapter 15

SOFT TISSUE PATHOLOGY 235

    A. Intracapsular Fibrosis of the Superior
       Compartment of the Temporomandibular Joint 235
       RONALD M. KAMINISHI, D.D.S., CHRISTOPHER L.
       DAVIS, D.D.S., M.D.

    B. Synovial Chondromatosis 243
       MOHAN THOMAS, D.D.S., F.A.C.D., DANIEL
       BUCHBINDER, D.M.D.

Chapter 16

ARTICULAR PATHOLOGY: DISC DISPLACEMENT
AND LATERAL IMPINGEMENT SYNDROME 249
    JEFFREY J. MOSES, D.D.S.

Chapter 17

HARD TISSUE PATHOLOGY 258

    A. Osteoarthrosis 258
       LAMBERT G.M. DE BONT, D.D.S., PH.D., BOUDEWIJN
       STEGENGA, D.D.S., and GEERT BOERING, D.D.S., PH.D.

    B. Chondromalacia 269
       MOHAN THOMAS, D.D.S., F.A.C.D., CHRISTOPHER
       LANE, D.D.S.

Chapter 18

CONNECTIVE TISSUE PATHOLOGY: ARTHRITIDES 276

    A. Rheumatoid Arthritis 276
       ANDERS HOLMLUND, D.D.S., PH.D.

    B. Systemic Inflammatory Arthritides with
       Temporomandibular Joint Involvement 282
       HARRY SHEN, M.D., MOHAN THOMAS, D.D.S.,
       F.A.C.D.

■ **Section V**

Postoperative Management 294

Chapter 19

POST-ARTHROSCOPIC PHYSICAL REHABILITATION
OF THE TEMPOROMANDIBULAR JOINT 294
    THOMAS M. EGGLETON, M.S., P.T., DENNIS P.
    LANGTON, B.S., P.T.

Chapter 20

PHARMACOLOGIC MANAGEMENT FOLLOWING
ARTHROSCOPY 305
*RICHARD H. HAUG, D.D.S., MOHAN THOMAS, D.D.S.,
F.A.C.D.*

Chapter 21

COMPLICATIONS OF TEMPOROMANDIBULAR JOINT
ARTHROSCOPY 310
JEFFREY B. CARTER, M.D., D.M.D.

Chapter 22

FUTURE DIRECTIONS IN TEMPOROMANDIBULAR
JOINT ARTHROSCOPY 323

  A. The Future 323
  *MOHAN THOMAS, D.D.S., F.A.C.D., CHRISTOPHER
  LANE, D.D.S.*

  B. Laser-Assisted Arthroscopy of the
  Temporomandibular Joint 327
  *JON P. BRADRICK, D.D.S., THOMAS A. INDRESANO
  D.M.D.*

  C. Role of Viscosurgery in Arthroscopy. 335
  CHARLES WEISS, M.D.

■ **Section VI**

Case Reports of Arthroscopic Pathology 338

Chapter 23

CASE REPORTS OF ARTHROSCOPIC PATHOLOGY

  A. Osteoarthritis 338
  KEN-ICHIRO MURAKAMI, D.D.S., Ph.D.

  B. Diagnosis and Lavage: Joint Degeneration by
  "Hyalinization" 339
  SIDNEY L. BRONSTEIN, D.D.S., M.Sc.D.

  C. Lysis, Lavage, and Debridement: Proliferative
  Fibrosis and Synovitis 341
  SIDNEY L. BRONSTEIN, D.D.S., M.Sc.D.

  D. Lysis, Lavage, and Disc Manipulation: Painful
  Hypomobility with Disc Displacement and
  Chondromalacia 342
  SIDNEY L. BRONSTEIN, D.D.S, M.Sc.D.

E. Diagnostic Arthroscopy: Severe Adhesions and
Disc Perforation 344
SIDNEY L. BRONSTEIN, D.D.S., M.Sc.D.

APPENDICES

Appendix A
American Association of Oral and Maxillofacial
Surgeons Statement on Temporomandibular Joint
Arthroscopy 347

Appendix B
Patient Consent Form 351

Appendix C
Diagram of Operating Room Showing Positions of
Surgeon and Assisting Personnel and Placement of
Equipment Needed for Performing Arthroscopic
Procedures 352

Appendix D
Example of Insurance Claim Form to Be Completed
After Providing Therapy for Temporomandibular Joint
Disorders 353

Appendix E
Example of Questionnaire to Be Completed by Patient
with Temporomandibular Joint Problems 355

Appendix F
Temporomandibular Joint Clinical Examination Form 358

Appendix G
Patient Information Sheet Regarding
Temporomandibular Joint Disease 363

Appendix H
Letter of Pre-determination for Temporomandibular
Joint Insurance Coverage 365

Appendix I
TMJ Treatment Follow-Up Questionnaire 367

Appendix J
Postoperative Instructions Following TMJ
Arthroscopy 369

Appendix K
Arthroscopic Examination of the TMJ Suggested
Recording Sheet 373

INDEX 375

■ Section I
Evolution of Arthroscopy

■ Chapter 1
DEVELOPMENT OF ORTHOPEDIC ARTHROSCOPY

*J. SERGE PARISIEN, M.D., F.A.C.S.,
DAVID ZELOUF, M.D.*

HISTORICAL OVERVIEW

In 1918, Kenji Tagaki of Japan made the first endoscopic examination of a knee joint, using a cystoscope. An arthroscope with a diameter of 7.3 mm, which he designed in 1920, was found generally impractical for clinical use because of its large size. In the early 1930s, Tagaki developed an arthroscope with a diameter of 3.5 mm that enabled considerably better vizualization of the interior of the knee joint.[1, 2]

In 1921, independent of Tagaki, Eugene Bircher published the results of his arthroscopic studies of the knee joint, using a Jacobeus laparoscope.[3] In these studies, oxygen or carbon dioxide was used for the first time to distend the joint cavity.

The *Illinois Medical Journal* published the first English-language report on arthroscopy in 1925.[4] The author of the report, Phillip Kreuscher, predicted that arthroscopy not only would be useful for physical examination but also would become a definitive diagnostic modality in the management of meniscal and other internal derangements of the knee.

Another noteworthy contribution to arthroscopy was made by Michael Burman in 1931,[5] who reported the results of direct visualization, using an arthroscope of his own design, of cadaveric knees, shoulders, elbows, hips, and ankles (Fig. 1–1). Three years later, in collaboration with Finkelstein and Mayer,[6] colleagues at the Hospital for Joint Diseases in New York City, he published his clinical experience with 30 cases.

A turning point in the advancement in this field was the No. 21 arthroscope designed by Watanabe.[2] This instrument had an outside diameter of 6.5 mm and a 100-degree field of vision. Illumination was accomplished with a tungsten light bulb, and color illustrations could be made using a 35-mm camera attached to the eyepiece of the arthroscope. The noteworthy studies by Casscells[7] and Jackson[8] in the 1970s were made possible by the availability of this instrument. Subsequently the design of arthroscopes with even smaller diameters allowed the examination of smaller joints.

Pioneering work in the field of arthroscopic surgery was done by Watanabe in the

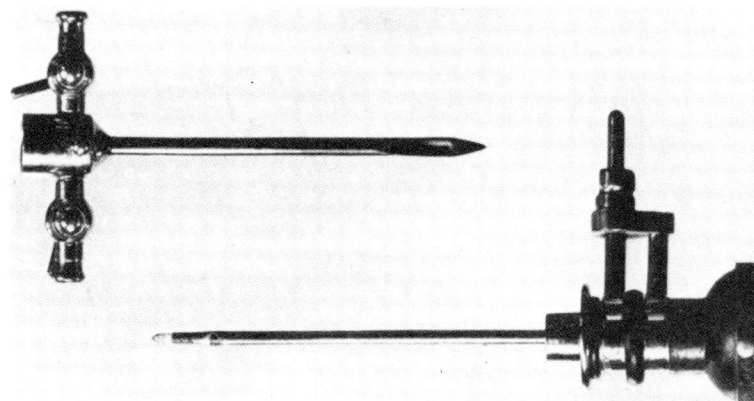

Figure 1–1. Arthroscope designed by M. Burman.

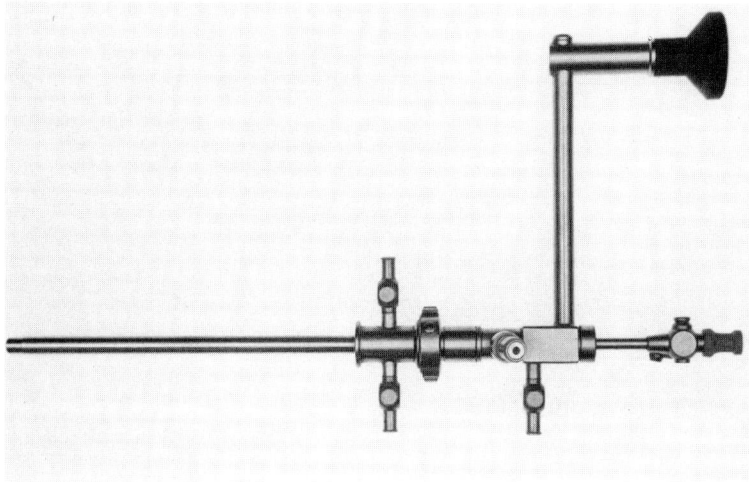

Figure 1–2. Operating arthroscope designed by Richard O'Connor, M.D.

1950s.[1] He is credited with performing the first arthroscopic surgical procedure on a knee in 1955 when he removed a xanthomatous tumor from the suprapatellar pouch. Richard O'Connor, after a trip to Japan in 1970, became interested in arthroscopic surgery. In 1974, he developed the operative arthroscope that allowed him to perform meniscal resection through a single articular incision (Fig. 1–2).[1, 9]

The availability of the intra-articular shaver, along with microinstruments and the video camera system, accelerated further development of modern surgical arthroscopic techniques (Figs. 1–3, 1–4, and 1–5).

PRESENT APPLICATIONS OF ARTHROSCOPIC SURGERY

In the knee joint,[10, 11] many surgical procedures in the menisci, the articular cartilage, the synovium, the joint capsule, and the cruciate ligaments that in the past were done with an arthrotomy incision are now done by closed means, with the obvious advantages of a quicker recovery time, a smaller incision for the patient, and a lower morbidity rate (Figs. 1–6, 1–7, and 1–8). Usually these procedures are done on an outpatient basis; in some situations, a short hospitalization is advisable.

The shoulder joint[10, 11] also has had many useful applications of arthroscopic techniques. Procedures such as the removal of chondral and loose osteochondral bodies, synovectomy and joint debridement, excision of torn glenohumeral labrum, stabilization in selected cases of anterior dislocation of the shoulder, debridement of rotator cuff tears in selected cases, and subacromial space decompression are being done with increasing frequency.

Many ankle disorders have been found to be increasingly amenable to arthroscopic surgery.[10–12] Common indications are (1) loose

1 Development of Orthopedic Arthroscopy

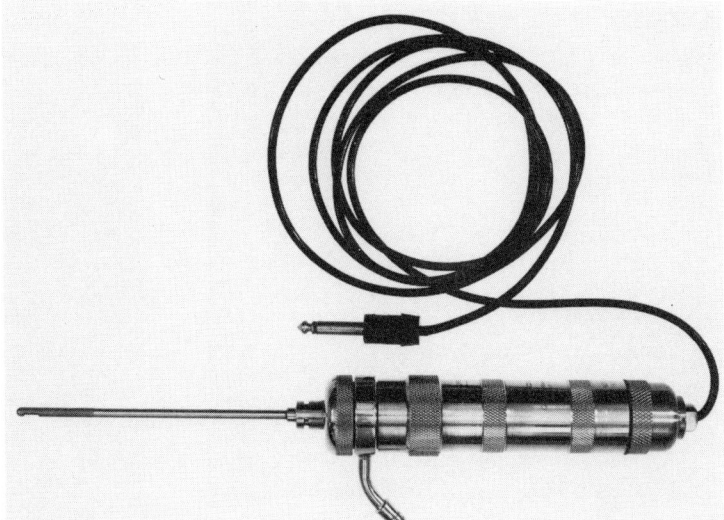

Figure 1-3. First motorized instrument: Dyonics Shaver designed by Lanny Johnson, M.D.

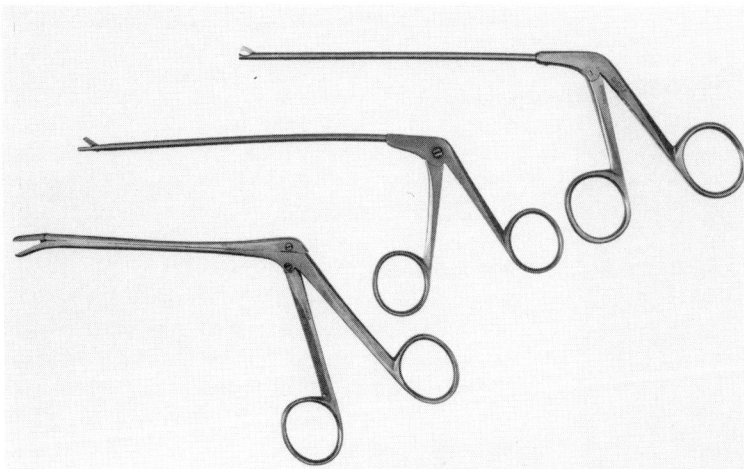

Figure 1-4. Scissors, basket forceps, and pituitary forceps now used in arthroscopic meniscectomy of the knee.

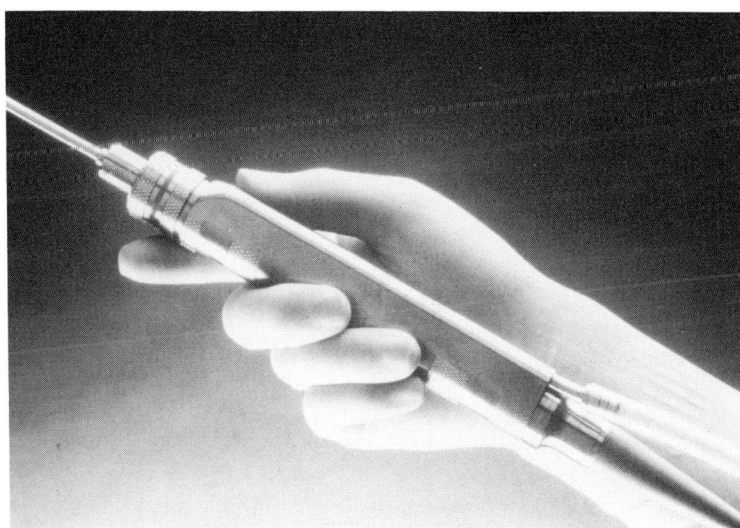

Figure 1-5. A high-speed motorized instrument for arthroscopic surgery.

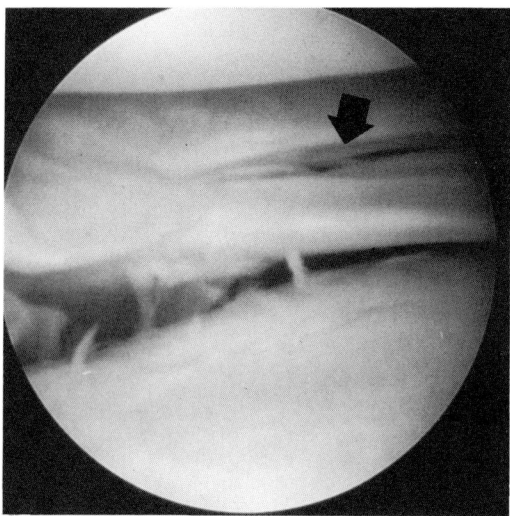

Figure 1–6. Arthroscopic view of a tear *(arrow)* of lateral meniscus amenable to arthroscopic surgery.

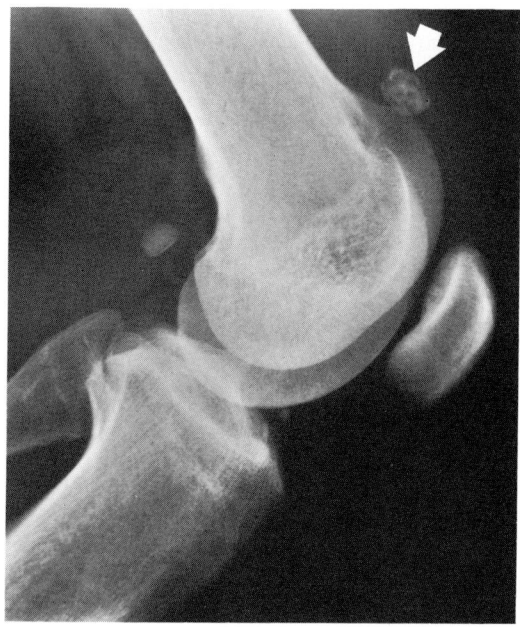

Figure 1–8. Radiograph of a loose osteochondral body of the suprapatellar area *(arrow)*, amenable to arthroscopic surgery.

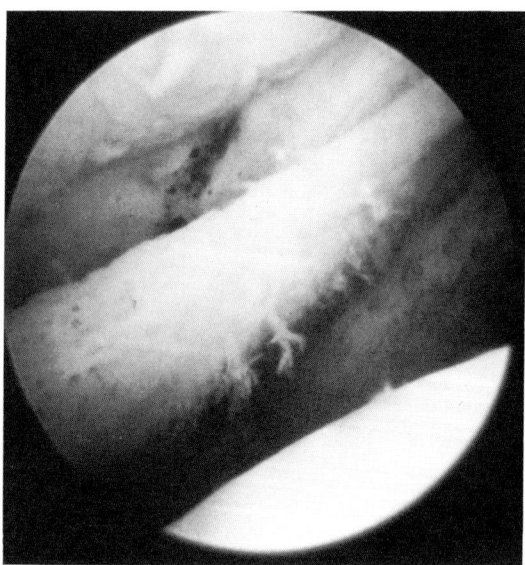

Figure 1–7. Arthroscopic view of a thick medial synovial plica, causing impingement in the patellofemoral joint of a left knee amenable to arthroscopic excision.

body removal, (2) treatment of osteochondritis dissecans of the talus, (3) synovitis, (4) adhesions, (5) impingement exostoses, (6) chronic sprain, and (7) selected cases of osteoarthritis of the ankle.

In cases involving the elbow joint, debridement and lavage have been used successfully in some cases of early rheumatoid synovitis and early post-traumatic arthritis of the elbow. Excision of loose bodies from the anterior joint compartment and the olecranon fossa can be accomplished easily with proper techniques, and lesions of osteochondritis dissecans can be drilled or excised. Arthroscopic surgical techniques, at the present time, are being used successfully in other joints such as the hip and the wrist.[10–13]

CONCLUSION

Thanks to the contributions of many pioneers, the growth and development of arthroscopy has been tremendous over the past few years. Arthroscopy has revolutionized the surgical management of intra-articular lesions. The development of sophisticated instruments has permitted the application of this technique in almost every joint of the body. However, arthroscopic surgery is not without complications. A recent prospective 19-month multicenter collaborative study of 10,262 procedures performed by 21 experienced arthroscopic surgeons yielded a complication rate greater than 1%; some procedures were associated with higher complication rates than others.[14]

References

1. Watanabe M, Bechtol R, Nottage W: History of arthroscopic surgery. In Shahriaree H (ed): O'Connor's Textbook of Arthroscopic Surgery. Philadelphia: Lippincott, 1984, pp 1–6.
2. Watanabe M, Takeda S, Ikeuchi H: Atlas of Arthroscopy. Tokyo: Igaku Shoin, 1969.
3. Bircher E: Die Arthroendoskopie. Zentralbl Chir 48:1460, 1921.
4. Kreuscher PH: Semilunar cartilage disease: A plea for early recognition by means of the arthroscope and early treatment of this condition. IMJ 47:290, 1925.
5. Burman MS: Arthroscopy or direct visualization of joint: An experimental cadaver study. J Bone Joint Surg 13:669, 1931.
6. Burman MS, Finkelstein H, Mayer L: Arthroscopy of the knee Joint. J Bone Joint Surg 16:225, 1934.
7. Casscells SW: Arthroscopy of the knee joint. J Bone Joint Surg 53A:287, 1971.
8. Jackson RW, Abe I: The role of arthroscopy in the management of disorders of the knee: An analysis of 200 consecutive examinations. J Bone Joint Surg 54B:310, 1972.
9. O'Connor RL: Arthroscopy. Philadelphia: Lippincott, 1977.
10. Johnson LI: Arthroscopic Surgery: Principles and Practice. St. Louis: Mosby, 1986.
11. Parisien J.S.: Arthroscopic Surgery. New York: McGraw-Hill, 1988.
12. Parisien JS: Arthroscopic treatment of osteochondral lesions of the talus. Am J Sports Med 14:211, 1986.
13. Parisien JS: Hip arthroscopy: State of the art. Bull Hosp Jt Dis Orthop Inst 45:127, 1985.
14. Small NC: Complications in arthroscopic surgery performed by experienced arthroscopists. Arthroscopy 4(3):215, 1988.

Chapter 2

DEVELOPMENT OF TEMPOROMANDIBULAR JOINT ARTHROSCOPY

SIDNEY L. BRONSTEIN, D.D.S., M.Sc.D., F.A.C.D.

The development of temporomandibular joint (TMJ) arthroscopy was pursued in its early years both as a treatment modality[1-4] and as a new method for researching and studying this joint.[5,6] By 1980, Masatoshi Ohnishi had developed a puncture technique for entering the joint with a small arthroscope, studying its movements, observing its articular surfaces, and obtaining tissue samples to aid in diagnosis. Later, other researchers and clinicians also developed techniques by which the TMJ could be entered repeatedly using identifiable anatomic landmarks.[7,8]

In the more recent past, TMJ arthroscopy has undergone rapid development to fulfill a need for a treatment modality that would be less debilitating than arthrotomy, that has a more predictable postsurgical course, and that can restore optimal joint function more rapidly.[9-11] Although the operative morbidity of arthrotomy in the treatment of TMJ disease has steadily decreased because of improved diagnostic and surgical skills, it is still significant. This unwanted morbidity has provided an additional impetus in the search for a surgical treatment enhancing the rapid return of the TMJ to normal biologic form and function.

The refinement of large joint arthroscopy has been of considerable benefit to TMJ researchers and clinicians. A vast amount of knowledge has been collected regarding synovial joints, and this information is applicable to the TMJ. Investigations have focused especially on the synovial membrane and its diseases and its response to traumatic and/or surgical insult;[12] articular cartilage characteristics and the effect of joint disease on subchondral bone also have been the subject of considerable study during the refinement of large joint arthroscopy.[13,14]

Following the introduction of routine diagnostic TMJ arthrography and the identification of internal joint derangement as the most common dysfunctional disorder of this joint, treatment has been directed at (1) restoring the normal functional anatomy of the articulation itself and (2) management of auxiliary joint components such as the muscles of mastication. Surgical treatment up to the present has involved arthrotomy procedures characterized by lengthy recuperative periods and, in some cases, development of more extensive degenerative pathology.

The concept of internal joint derangement has expanded from that of primarily a disc-fossa-eminence positional disorder to one that includes the pathophysiology of the articulating surfaces and their contribution or response to positional changes. Investigations into the underlying basis and clinical course of osteoarthrosis have played a major role in expanding this concept.[15] Sophisticated magnetic resonance imaging has greatly enhanced our understanding and diagnosis of the tissue changes within the TMJ and how they can affect treatment.

Through the development and improvement of TMJ arthroscopy, detailed anatomic knowledge of the TMJ has been enhanced, its pathophysiology is much better understood, and the side effects of surgical treatment have been reduced.

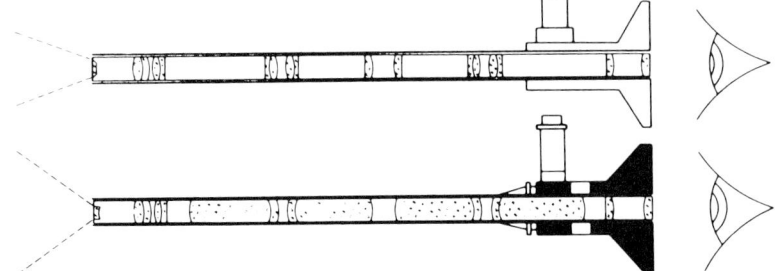

Figure 2–1. Hopkins rod lens system *(below)* compared with traditional lens system *(above)*. (Reprinted with permission from Heffez L, Blaustein D: Diagnostic arthroscopy of the temporomandibular joint. Oral Surg 64(6):654, 1987.)

The involvement of instrument designers, engineers, and manufacturers in providing more sophisticated equipment at the arthroscopist's behest has allowed the development of more effective techniques and has opened a new era in operative arthroscopy. Development of the Hopkins rod lens has been an extremely important contribution in this regard (Fig. 2–1).[16, 17] This invention improved image transmission significantly by decreasing light absorption by the lens and improving color reproduction.

Enhanced instrumentation and techniques have allowed arthroscopists to produce surgical results showing improved ranges of motion postsurgically, decreased pain and dysfunction, and maintenance of more physiologic articulating surfaces.[11]

ORTHOPEDIC PIONEERS

Temporomandibular joint instrumentation essentially has followed large joint arthroscopic development resulting from the early work of many orthopedic pioneers. The general availability of the No. 21 arthroscope designed by Masaki Watanabe in 1959, culminating in the development of the No. 24 arthroscope[18] (Fig. 2–2), was a turning point in the development of arthroscopic techniques as they are known today. This instrument system offered direct viewing as well as fore-oblique viewing telescopes, with relatively little difference in the visual angle between them when used in fluid (Fig. 2–3). By 1962 Dr. Watanabe was considered an expert in diagnostic arthroscopy and had turned his attention to operative arthroscopy. In the early 1970s the technique of diagnostic arthroscopy was introduced into the United States and, indeed, Dr. Watanabe himself instructed, guided, and oversaw many of the early efforts in this country at orthopedic arthroscopic surgery.[13] As discussed in Chapter 1, Dr. Richard O'Conner studied with Dr. Watanabe and in 1971 first performed arthroscopic surgery of the knee. In 1974, Dr. O'Conner continued his innovative approach, using an operating arthroscope which he had de-

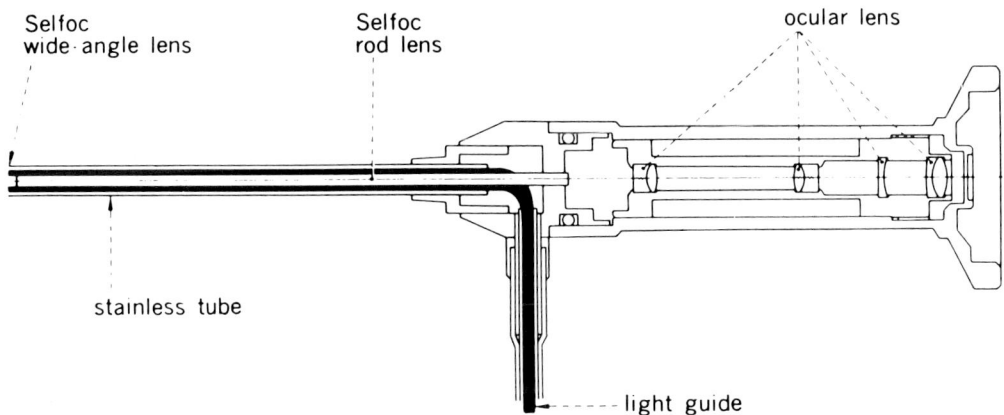

Figure 2–2. Structure of the No. 24 arthroscope (Selfoscope). (Reprinted with permission from Watanabe M: Arthroscopy of Small Joints. New York: Igaku-Shoin, 1985.)

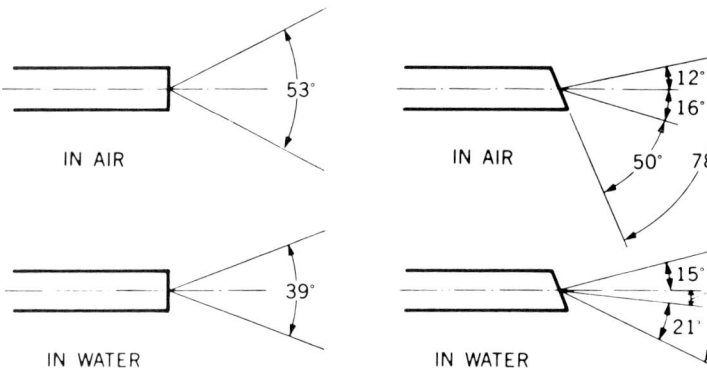

Figure 2–3. Fields of vision of No. 24 arthroscope. *A*, Direct viewing; *B*, fore-oblique viewing. (Reprinted with permission from Watanabe M: Arthroscopy of Small Joints. New York: Igaku-Shoin, 1985.)

signed,[19] publishing his results in 1977. At this time Dr. Lanny Johnson developed a motorized instrument that allowed a significant increase in what could be accomplished through arthroscopic surgery.[20]

The earliest work in knee endoscopy was attempted by Kenji Takagi in 1918, using a pediatric cystoscope. Two years later he developed an instrument with a lens system similar to the cystoscope, an instrument that he continued perfecting until, in 1931, he had developed a suitable 3.5-mm arthroscope. During this same period, Dr. Bircher used a laparoscope in a gas medium to perform diagnostic knee arthroscopy.[21]

The first contributions in American arthroscopic literature were by Kreuscher and coworkers[20, 21] and by Burmann,[23] who described arthroscopic cadaver studies of all the joints excepting the TMJ, toes, and fingers.

Realizing that arthroscopic techniques would have to be taught in courses particularly designed for this purpose, the first hands-on course in arthroscopy in the United States was organized in 1973 in Philadelphia by John Joyce III and by Michael Hardy, an anatomist. The following year the International Arthroscopy Association was founded, and in 1975 the American Academy of Orthopaedic Surgeons organized instructional courses on arthroscopy. Knee models and the use of video equipment as teaching aids were introduced in these courses.[19]

The educational objectives of TMJ arthroscopy have followed this line of development closely, and there are now many workshops that utilize models and human fresh cadaver specimens, allowing surgeons to avail themselves of hands-on instruction in this specialized skill and knowledge (Figs. 2–4 and 2–5). In this way they may learn in a laboratory setting the techniques required for diagnostic and operative TMJ arthroscopy.

TMJ ARTHROSCOPY PIONEERS

TMJ arthroscopy was first reported in the oral and maxillofacial surgical literature by Masatoshi Ohnishi in 1975. Using a No. 24 Watanabe arthroscope 1.7 mm in diameter

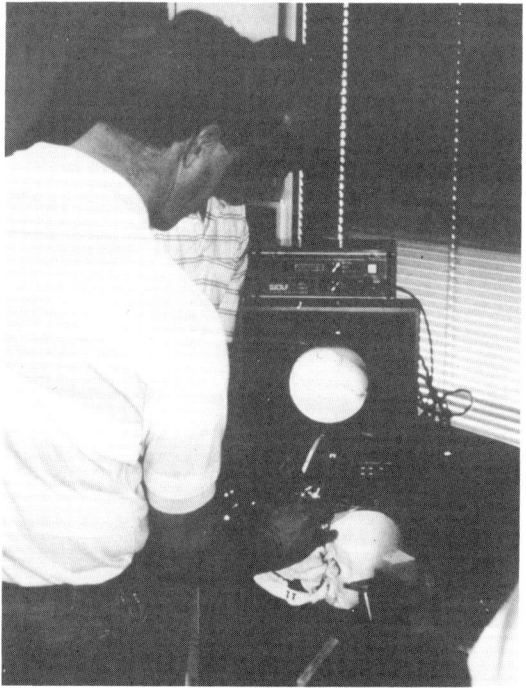

Figure 2–4. Scene from a hands-on cadaver laboratory workshop utilizing model temporomandibular joints for initial experience with the arthroscope.

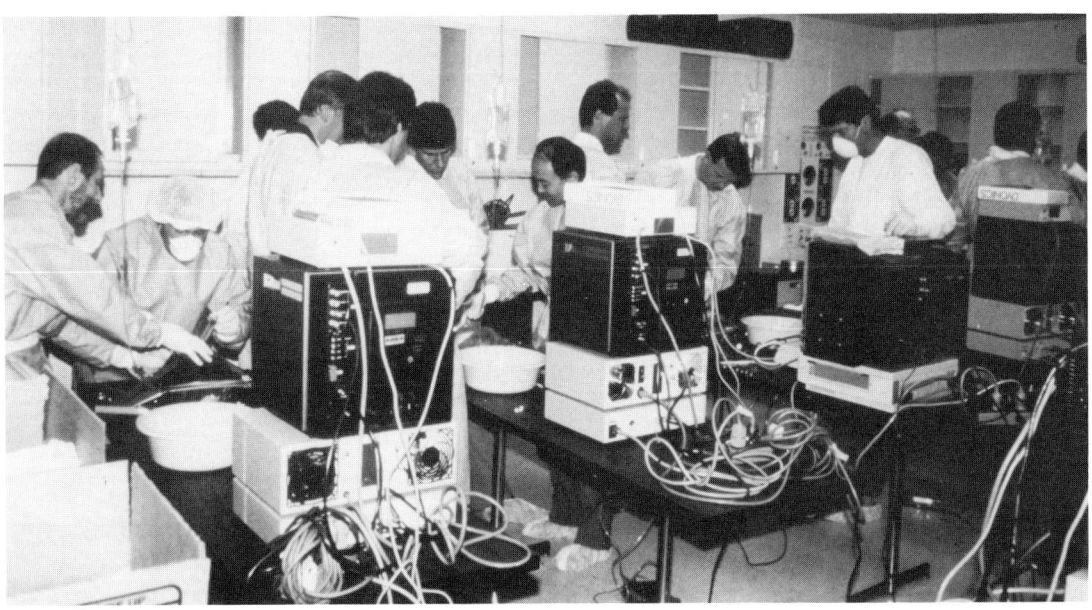

Figure 2–5. Students learning arthroscopic skills at a hands-on cadaver laboratory workshop. (Reprinted with permission from Bronstein SL: Diagnostic and operative arthroscopy. Historical perspectives and indications. Oral Maxillofac Clin North Am. 1(1):59–68, 1989.)

and with a fiberoptic light source (Olympus Selfoscope), developed in 1970, Dr. Ohnishi described the arthroscopic anatomy and articular tissue appearances of several TMJs. This was made possible by the invention of the Selfoc laser beam–transmitting material in Japan, which was introduced as a glass rod in a small-diameter arthroscope. Previous rigid fiberscopes could not focus less than 3.0 mm from the tip of the scope.[18]

Publishing in English, in the Bulletin of the Tokyo Medical Dental University, Ohnishi reported the clinical application of arthroscopy in TMJ diseases.[4] In this article he presented the methodology and findings of arthroscopic examination of the TMJ, utilizing a method that he had pioneered. This involved the tandem insertion of a puncture needle and a sheathed needle into the joint cavity for intra-articular examination under perfusion of physiologic saline solution. The advantages of his method were listed as (1) direct observation of the articular cavity, (2) observation of joint movement, (3) biopsy of tissues for histopathologic diagnosis, and (4) still and dynamic photography of findings.

Ohnishi applied his technique and knowledge clinically and judged it very effective, especially in diagnosis and selection of further therapy. In his writings he described the normal configuration and characteristics of the joint components as seen in the superior compartment. He provided many of the early descriptions of traumatic pathology and results of joint fibrosis.

Ken-Ichiro Murakami, in collaboration with Kazumasa Hoshino, reported in 1982 on regional anatomic features, nomenclature, and arthroscopic terminology in human TMJs.[24] This article, which standardized much of this information, was profusely illustrated with excellent color photographs of cadaver specimens and clinical arthroscopic findings. In 1984, exploring further the possibilities of TMJ arthroscopy, Murakami and co-workers Matsuki, Iizuka, Ono, and Hoshino reported from the Seventh Congress of the European Association for Maxillofacial Surgery on arthroscopic differential diagnosis and treatment of locking of the TMJ. This group further expanded therapeutic application with an exceptionally well-illustrated article on the differential diagnosis of limited jaw opening via arthroscopy.[25]

The histology of the inner surfaces of the articular cavities of the TMJ, with special reference to arthroscopic observations, was reported in 1985 by Murakami and Hoshino, who described in detail the various cellular characteristics of the articular surfaces of the joint.[26] In 1985, in a landmark article, Anders Holmlund and Gustaf Hellsing of the Karolinska Institutet published a cadaver study on TMJ arthroscopy in which they described readily identifiable and repeatable puncture sites correlated with the tragal-lateral canthus line. These landmarks were recommended as guides for placement of arthroscopic trocars. This description has now found its way into the everyday practice of TMJ arthroscopy and represents a guideline upon which joint entry may be based. This investigation represented a significant technical refinement of the procedure.[7, 27]

Meanwhile, Murakami and Ono were continuing their efforts to improve the technique of placing instrumentation within the joint. In 1986, they described the inferolateral approach to joint entry and provided drawings of the visual fields that could be inspected.[8]

In the United States, Joseph McCain presented an abstract at the 1985 annual meeting of the American Association of Oral and Maxillofacial Surgery on his meticulous investigations into TMJ arthroscopic technique. This was followed in 1987 by a report of the pioneering work done by Bruce Sanders.[11] His description of the clinical efficacy of arthroscopic surgical techniques in the treatment of persistent closed lock was a breakthrough in applying arthroscopy to treatment of common TMJ disorders.

CONTINUING EDUCATION

The first major symposium on TMJ diagnostic and operative arthroscopic surgery was convened in Long Beach, California, in 1986, sponsored by the Southern California Society of Oral and Maxillofacial Surgeons and guided by Drs. Kamanishi and Davis. This meeting provided an impetus to continuing education in this field, which was embraced by many academic and health-care institutions and research and clinical investigators.

Following the Long Beach Symposium, in July of 1986, under the leadership of Dr. McCain, the First Annual International Symposium on Arthroscopy of the Temporomandibular Joint gathered in New York, sponsored by the Hospital for Joint Diseases. At that time the International Study Group (ISG) for the Advancement of TMJ Arthroscopy was organized, collecting the skills of many dedicated American, Japanese, Scandinavian, and European TMJ investigators. This group developed into the faculty for the annual symposium. The second annual symposium convened in December of 1987; in December of 1988 the Third Annual Symposium met and included abstracts presented by members and non-members of the study group.

REFINEMENT AND RESEARCH

As a result of these various meetings and symposia and through the actions of the ISG, a rationale for TMJ arthroscopy was evolving and was seen as providing the following advantages:[28]

1. A new step in diagnostic and treatment schema prior to arthrotomy.
2. A procedure that is less invasive than open surgery.
3. The ability to visualize detail in certain areas of the joint much better than with arthrotomy.
4. The ability to witness motion of the surgically undisturbed joint structures.
5. Inspection of joint structures in a more natural environment, so that the arthropathy could be classified by direct visualization and/or by biopsy.
6. More rapid recovery and shorter healing time because of the decreased trauma as compared with arthrotomy.

The ISG has been extremely active, and through the combined interests and efforts of its members certain diagnostic and therapeutic indications have been developed and promulgated. Other guidelines adopted by this organization addressed the following considerations:

1. The importance of hospital-approved credentials for performing arthroscopic procedures.
2. The development of standards in technique.
3. The development of laboratory workshops to teach and acquire arthroscopic skills.
4. The importance of recording complications and clinical results.
5. Participation in compiling information clarifying criteria for insurance coverage.

In response to these deliberations, the American Association of Oral and Maxillofacial Surgeons (AAOMS) convened an ad hoc committee that developed an official organizational statement regarding TMJ arthroscopy.[1] During the latter part of 1988 an insurance task force was appointed by the AAOMS to advise third-party carriers regarding coverage of this procedure.

Important research based on sound scientific principles has developed rapidly, and much of it is currently directed at clarifying and describing the pathology and pathophysiology of TMJ disorders. Prominent among ongoing research at this time is identification and description of pain mediators within the joint, use of the laser for arthroscopic surgery, joint responses to the application of electrocoagulation and electrosurgery, and use of specially developed hyaluronic acid polymers to aid arthroscopic procedures.

References

1. Ohnishi M: Clinical studies on the intra-articular puncture of the temporomandibular joint [in Japanese]. J Jpn Stomat 37:14, 1970.
2. Ohnishi M: Arthroscopy of the temporomandibular joint [in Japanese]. J Jpn Stomat 42:207, 1975.
3. Ohnishi M: Diagnostic application of arthroscope to ankylosis of the temporomandibular joint [in Japanese]. Jpn J Oral Surg 22:436, 1976.
4. Ohnishi M: Clinical application of arthroscopy in temporomandibular joint diseases. Bull Tokyo Med Dent Univ 27:141, 1980.
5. Hilsabeck RB, Laskin DM: Arthroscopy of the temporomandibular joint of the rabbit. J Oral Surg 36:938, 1978.
6. Williams RA, Laskin DM: Arthroscopic examination of experimentally induced pathologic conditions of the rabbit temporomandibular joint. J Oral Surg 38:652, 1980.
7. Holmlund A, Hellsing G: Arthroscopy of the temporomandibular joint. Int J Oral Surg 14:169, 1985.
8. Murakami K-I, Ono T: Temporomandibular joint arthroscopy by inferolateral approach. Int J Oral Maxillofac Surg 15:410, 1986.
9. McCain JP: Proceedings, American Association of Maxillofacial Surgery Abstract Sessions, Annual Meeting, 1985.
10. Sanders B: Arthroscopic surgery of the temporomandibular joint: Treatment of internal derangement with persistent closed lock. Oral Surg 62:361, 1986.
11. Sanders B: Diagnostic and surgical arthroscopy of the temporomandibular joint: Clinical experience with 137 procedures over a 2-year period. J Craniomandib Disord Facial Oral Pain 1(3):202, 1987.
12. Weiss, C.: Basic structures of diarthrodial joints. In Parisien S (ed): Arthroscopic Surgery. New York: McGraw-Hill, 1988, p 3.
13. Shahriaree H: O'Connor's Textbook of Arthroscopic Surgery. Philadelphia: JB Lippincott, 1984, p xi.
14. Whipple TL: Osteoarthrosis and Chondromalacia. In Parisien S (ed): Arthroscopic Surgery, New York: McGraw-Hill, 1988, p 135.
15. DeBont LGM: The Temporomandibular Joint: Articular Cartilage Structure and Function (Thesis). Rijksuniversiteit Groningen, 1985.
16. Heffez L, Blaustein D: Diagnostic arthroscopy of the temporomandibular joint. Oral Surg 64(6):653, 1987.
17. Hopkins H: Optical principles of the endoscope. In Berci G (ed): Endoscopy. New York: Appleton-Century-Crofts, 1976, pp 3–26.
18. Watanabe M: Arthroscopy of Small Joints. Tokyo–New York: Igaku-Shoin, 1985.
19. Bechtol RC: History of arthroscopic surgery. In Shahriaree H (ed): O'Connor's Textbook of Arthroscopic Surgery. Philadelphia: JB Lippincott, 1984, p 4.
20. Bechtol RC: History of arthroscopic surgery. In Shahriaree H (ed): O'Connor's Textbook of Arthroscopic Surgery. Philadelphia: JB Lippincott, 1984, p 5.
21. Shahriaree H (ed): O'Connor's Textbook of Arthroscopic Surgery. Philadelphia: JB Lippincott, 1984, p 1.
22. Kreusher PH: Semilunar cartilage disease: A plea for early recognition by means of the arthroscope and early treatment of this condition. Ill Med J 47:290, 1925.
23. Burmann MS: Arthroscopy, the direct visualization of joints: An experimental cadaver study. J Bone Joint Surg [Am] 13(4):669, 1931.
24. Murakami K-I, Hoshino K: Regional anatomical nomenclature and arthroscopic terminology in human temporomandibular joints. Okajimas Folia Anat Jpn 58:4–6, 1982.
25. Murakami K-I, Matsuki M, Iizuka T, et al: Arthroscopic differential diagnoses and treatments of the locking symptoms of the temporomandibular joint and their regional anatomical interpretations. Proceedings, European Association for Maxillo-Facial Surgery, 1985.
26. Murakami K-I, Hoshino K: Histological studies on the inner surfaces of the articular cavities of human temporomandibular joints with special reference to arthroscopic observations. Anat Anz [Jena] 160:167, 1985.
27. McCain JP: An Illustrated Guide to Temporomandibular Joint Arthroscopy. Dyonics, Inc., 1987.
28. Bronstein SL: Proceedings, Second Annual International Symposium on TMJ Arthroscopy, New York, 1987.

Chapter 3

PRINCIPLES OF THE ARTHROSCOPE

DENNIS C. LEINER, PH.D.

The engineering of the arthroscope represents one of the greatest challenges to an optical designer. The usual design parameters of an optical system such as resolution, brightness, and field of view cannot be optimized without consideration of the biomechanical requirements of the surgical procedure (diameter, insertion depth, direction of view).

Optical parameters that ultimately determine the view in an arthroscope vary greatly, particularly with the small diameter arthroscopes used in TMJ surgery. A knowledge of the optical characteristics found in an arthroscope will enable the prospective arthroscopist to evaluate which type of endoscope is most suitable for the particular procedure. This chapter also serves as a reference guide for the prospective consumer for intelligent comparison of instruments from the multitude of available vendors.

TYPES OF ARTHROSCOPES

Conventional Lens Systems

Arthroscope optical systems using conventional lenses are similar in design to periscopes. In order to transfer an image from inside the joint to the outside of the body, and then to a video system or the eye, a multitude of lenses must be used. The optical designer employs two basic strategies in choosing the type of relay lens type for this image transfer (Fig. 3–1).

In the classic endoscope system, lenses have a thickness on the same order of magnitude as their diameters and are made up of two types of glass, which enables all of the colors from the object to be focused simultaneously. These lens systems are known as *achromatic* (i.e., without color).

In 1966, a professor of applied optics, H. H. Hopkins, patented an endoscope system in which the relay lenses were made much longer than their diameter.[1] Hopkins referred to these optical components as cylindric rod-like lenses, later called *rod lenses*. The advantage of the rod lens design is that the light ray bundles from the object are confined more closely to the center of the relay lenses. This gives a brighter image for a given lens diameter, especially at the edge of the field. The image is brightened further because the separation of the intermediate relay images is greater, reducing the number of air-to-glass interfaces in the system. Like achromatic lenses, rod lenses are made up of at least two different types of glass to correct for color errors.

The mounting of rod lenses is simpler for the manufacturer than mounting of the thinner achromatic lenses. The rod lenses tend to tilt less when they are assembled into the inner lens tube. Also, since the spacers separating the rod lenses are shorter, they can be made thinner, which increases the clear aperture. Rod lenses are typically finely ground on their outer surface to reduce stray reflections. There are now many variations of the rod lens concept, including a design that combines achromatic lenses with long, plane-parallel cylinders. Because there is less glass in achromatic lens endoscopes, they are said to be less sensitive to breakage from flexing than are rod lens systems.

Gradient-Index Optics

A unique type of glass material with a non-uniform refractive index has enabled the development of extremely small-diameter arthroscopes. Developed primarily for use in

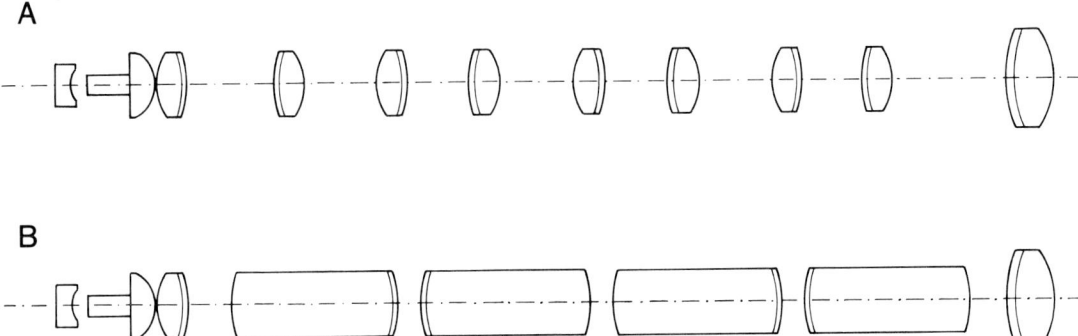

Figure 3–1. *A*, Achromat system; *B*, rod lens system.

table-top copiers, Selfoc (manufactured by the Japanese company Nippon Sheet Glass) was first used in endoscopes in 1970, only 2 years after the material was developed. At diameters much below 2 mm, the difficulty in optical fabrication and assembly increases greatly. The advantage of Selfoc is that curved surfaces are not needed; the glass structure itself provides the focusing power of the system. Like conventional lens systems, a gradient-index endoscope is made up of objective and relay sections (Fig. 3–2). Unlike a conventional lens system, however, the gradient-index objectives and relay are simply long cylinders that are cemented end-to-end with an optical adhesive. Thus, these systems can be manufactured with less than 1-mm diameter optics, giving an outside diameter of 2.5 mm or less for the arthroscope. Compared with conventional systems of the same diameter, gradient-index systems yield a much brighter image. Resolution is comparable to that of conventional systems with arthroscope diameters of 2.5 mm or less. With larger diameters than this, the increased design flexibility of conventional systems tends to produce a superior instrument.

Fiberoptic Relay

Fiberoptics can be used in conjunction with a lens system at the tip of the endoscope to transmit an image to a position outside of the body, to be re-imaged with still another lens system. The image transfer works by bundling several thousand individual optical fibers in a two-dimensional array and maintaining a one-to-one correspondence of the fiber positons at each end of the bundle (Fig. 3–3). These arrays historically are known as coherent fiber bundles but must, of course, be distinguished from our current reference to single-mode telecommunication devices.

Each fiber in the bundle effectively receives one pixel of information about the

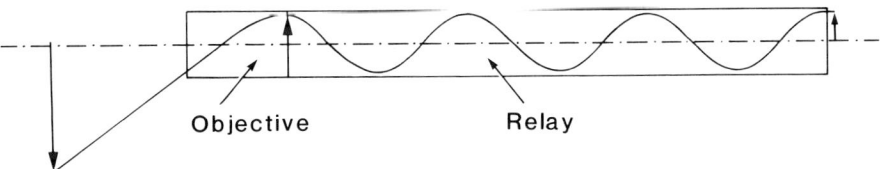

Figure 3–2. Gradient-index endoscope.

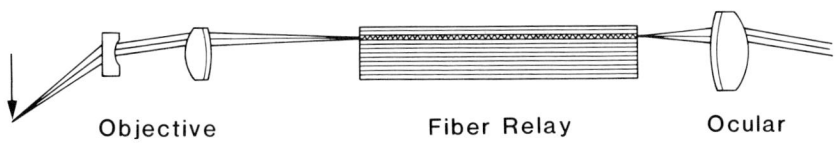

Figure 3–3. Fiberoptic endoscope.

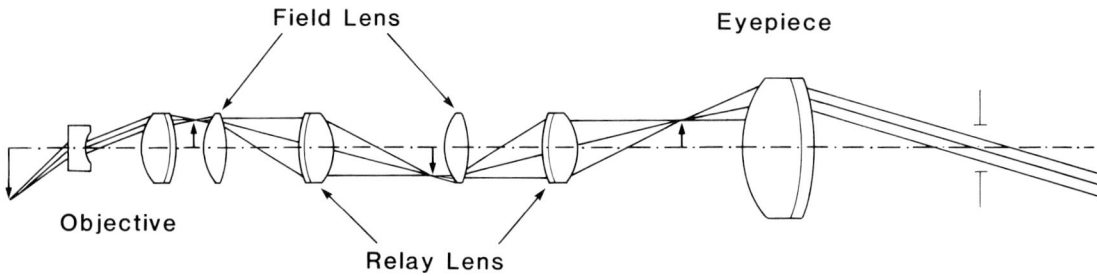

Figure 3–4. Endoscope optics.

image, which is relayed to the opposite end of the bundle outside of the body. Since the fibers need to be fixed only at the ends, most of the length of the endoscope can be flexed to allow passage deep into the body. The image at the proximal, or observer's, end of the fiber bundle is viewed with a simple ocular that presents a magnified view to the eye. Since resolution is limited by the fiber diameter, fiberoptic endoscopes have their greatest use in larger-diameter scopes, where more fibers can be present, and in endoscopes used to probe blood vessels, where flexibility is an absolute requirement.

None of the popular arthroscopes manufactured today utilizes fiberoptics to transmit an image. However, both the fiberoptic system design and the manufacturing processes in making these fiber bundles are progressing rapidly. It is possible that arthroscope systems will one day be built with image-transmitting fibers that not only will yield brighter images but also will be significantly less expensive than the current instruments.

DESIGN OF ENDOSCOPE OPTICS

All conventional lens endoscope systems follow a similar strategy for transferring an image from inside of the body to the physician's eye or to a video camera. With reference to Figure 3–4, the objective lens system forms an inverted image of the internal organ to be observed. A field lens placed near that image redirects the light ray bundle toward the center of the relay lens. Another field lens keeps the ray bundle confined to the small diameter of the endoscope tube. This succession of relay lenses and field lenses is repeated as often as necessary for the required insertion depth of the instrument.

The objective lens system consists of the lenses at the tip of the endoscope for gathering the light from the object under investigation and focusing that light to its first image inside the endoscope. The objective system also usually includes a prism to direct the field of view at an angle to the axis of the endoscope. This prism and the objective lens components are designed in tandem to optimize the image for the desired field of view and direction of view. As can be seen in Figure 3–5, the prism can be replaced conceptually with a simple block of glass of approximate thickness to allow the efficient calculation of these complex systems.

The optics designer uses a concept known as the *entrance pupil* to accomplish the optimization of the lens systems. The entrance pupil is the position in the endoscope optical train where the diameter of the bundle of

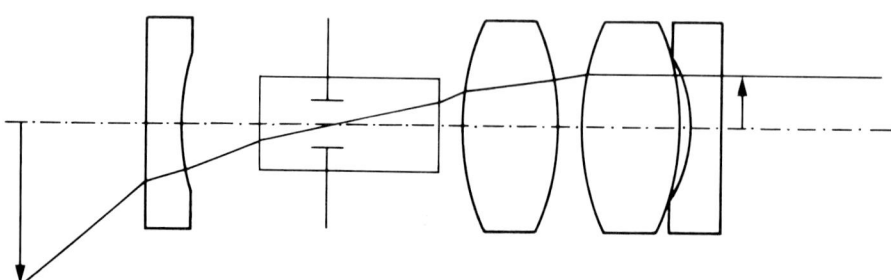

Figure 3–5. Arthroscope objective.

light rays from the object field is at a minimum. In order to maximize the brightness of the image, this diameter should be large, meaning that more light is gathered by the endoscope system. However, several factors place a limit on the diameter of the entrance pupil. In the objective lens system it is usually the direction-of-view prism which limits the brightness. The lens designer must very carefully position the entrance pupil so that it coincides with the restrictions imposed by the finite size of the prism. The other main factor that limits the entrance pupil diameter is the relay system, discussed later.

It is important to remember that the objective lens is the *only* part of the endoscope that controls the ultimate field of view. Thus, if the objective lens is designed to cover a field angle of, say, 80 degrees, no amount of modification of the camera coupler or even of the relay optics will give a field of view greater than 80 degrees. The size of the image on the video screen may be altered, but the actual extent of the object that appears on the screen will be unchanged.

The objective lens is also primarily responsible for distortion in the endoscope (the degree to which the image is compressed at the edge of the field of view). Much of the distortion is produced by the lens component that is actually seen when looking at the tip of an endoscope. This is known as the field-widening lens and is flat on the outer surface but concave on the inside. Sometimes the field-widening lens is placed in back of a protective window at the tip of the endoscope; sometimes the protective window is omitted entirely, with the field-widening lens serving that purpose.

The relay optics are responsible for transferring image-forming light down the endoscope axis, while maintaining or even improving the quality of the first image from the objective lens. The relay optics comprise the majority of lenses in an endoscope and determine the ultimate theoretical brightness of the system. The quality of the relay optics' design and manufacture are what "make or break" an endoscope.

In designing the relay, the designer tries to maximize the size of the light bundle coming from the objective that is able to pass through the entire relay system. This condition is achieved by making the system "telecentric" between the relay and objective systems. Violations of this condition result in a "spillover" of the light bundle at the edge of the field, known as vignetting. As a general rule, therefore, in a properly designed and manufactured endoscope, the field of view is determined by the objective lens and the brightness is determined by the relay optics.

Once the image-forming light exits the body, the system becomes much easier to manufacture, because the designer is not confined to using difficult and expensive tiny lenses. The ocular lens can be thought of as a simple magnifying glass used to enlarge the last small image created by the relay optics. A field stop is usually added at this last image to define sharply the edge of the field.

In most instances, the endoscope image is viewed on a video monitor. An additional lens is required inside the video camera coupler to relay the image to the camera chip. The size of the image on the monitor is directly proportional to the focal length of the camera coupler lens.

It is becoming increasingly popular to combine the action of the video camera coupler with the main endoscope system in order to completely eliminate the possibility of fogging of optical components. When the coupler is integrated into the endoscope, the size of the image can be optimized, the final quality of the video image is better assured, and any questions about the compatibility of the focal adjustments of the endoscope and the camera coupler are eliminated. An accessory eyepiece is often available to check out the endoscope optics before the procedure begins, without having to first attach a camera.

OPTICAL CHARACTERISTICS OF ARTHROSCOPES

The field of view is the maximum angle at the tip of the endoscope that is subtended by the edges of the viewable object (Fig. 3–6). This is sometimes called the *real* field of view, to differentiate it from the size of the circle seen through the ocular, known as the *apparent* field of view.

The apparent field of view should be of sufficient size so that any detail resolved by the objective and relay is large enough to be resolved by the eye. Since the eye can only resolve detail greater than about 1 minute of arc, increasing the magnification too much

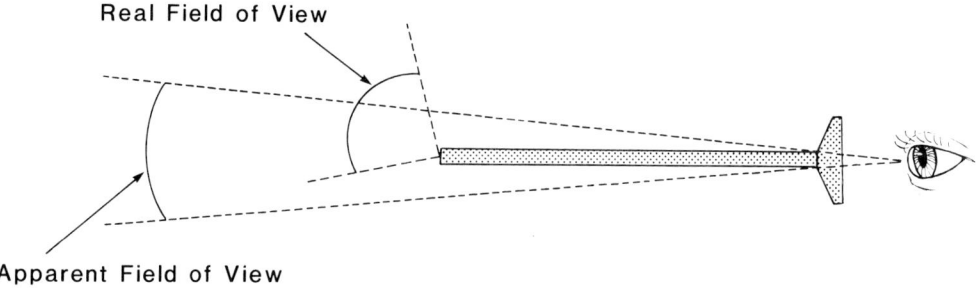

Figure 3-6. Apparent and real field of view.

will dim the image without providing any increased resolution. For larger arthroscopes of approximately 4 mm in diameter, an apparent field of view of about 9 degrees is typical. Small-diameter arthroscopes used in TMJ surgery tend to have smaller apparent fields of view, because the light transmission is less and because the resolution is inadequate to necessitate a larger value.

This nonstandardization of the apparent field of view must be considered when connecting the arthroscope to a video camera coupler. A coupler designed for a 4-mm arthroscope will often produce an image that is too small to be used comfortably with a small-diameter arthroscope. This problem can be circumvented with integrated video arthroscope systems or with zoom camera couplers.

As discussed in the section on the objective lens, the field of view is often inclined by the use of a prism at the distal end of the arthroscope. With a fore-oblique prism, the view angle effectively can be increased by rotating the arthroscope in the joint. As long as the incline is no more than half the field of view, objects along the axis of the endoscope will always be visible.

All popular large-diameter arthroscopes that have inclined views employ two-reflection direction-of-view prisms (Fig. 3-7). An even number of reflections are necessary so that the image has the proper reversion and will not be seen backward.

Because these prisms are difficult to make in small diameters, some manufacturers use a different technique to produce the inclined view. *A* and *B* in Figure 3-7 are cylindric refracting prisms; these are the simplest to manufacture and, unfortunately, the least effective. These prisms typically are epoxied to the end of the objective lens system as a thick window and are ground and polished at an angle after the endoscope needle has been assembled. The prism in Figure 3-7A depicts the maximum prism wedge that is usable in air for a typical small-diameter endoscope. Since endoscopes are invariably used with the tip of the endoscope immersed in fluid, the direction of view is reduced to only about 5 degrees. In this instance the prism wedge angle can be increased to the maximum usable in liquid, which produces an incline at the center of the apparent field of view of about 10 degrees. Asymmetric distortion is particularly severe when using these types of prisms.

The newer, small-diameter arthroscopes employ reflection prisms, as depicted in Figure 3-7C-E. The prism shown in Figure 3-7E allows a particularly bright image to be transmitted through the arthroscope. This prism has one of its internal surfaces silvered

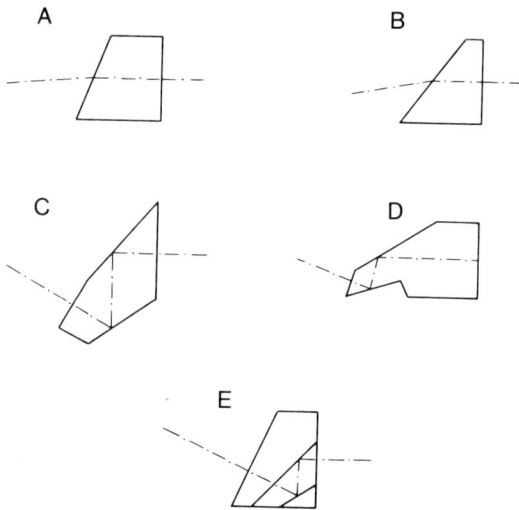

Figure 3-7. Arthroscope prisms. *A* and *B*, Cylindrical refracting prisms. *C-E*, reflection prisms.

over only half of its clear aperture and is fabricated from three long wedges that are coated, bonded, and diced to size. These prisms have been successfully fabricated with outer diameters of 1 mm.

Depth of field refers to the range of object distances that are in acceptable focus at any given time. It is obviously advantageous to maximize an arthroscope's depth of field. However, from theoretical considerations the depth of field can be shown to be completely dependent on the maximal cone of light that is accepted by the tip of the arthroscope. Thus, the designer must face the unfortunate fact that the only way to improve the depth of field of an arthroscope is to reduce its brightness, a prospect rarely desirable.

In use, the arthroscopist will note that the depth of field improves as the object distance increases. Therefore, during diagnostic arthroscopic scans at relatively longer object distances, the depth of field will be improved. When viewing an object up close for a detailed observation, the reduced depth of field may not be as serious a problem, because the focus will remain constant. Depth of field usually is most relevant when observing with a video system, since the camera coupler must be repeatedly refocused when viewing objects very close to the arthroscope tip.

If we were able to trace the light beams emanating from the entrance pupil (discussed above) through the relay system and out of the ocular, we would find that the bundle of light again achieves a minimum diameter a finite distance from the last ocular lens. This position is called the *exit pupil*, and its distance from the eyepiece is called the *eye relief* (Fig. 3–8). The exit pupil position is important because it is the best place to position one's eye when looking through the endoscope. Eye relief is particularly important to consider if one wears eyeglasses.

If the eye relief is too small, the observer may have difficulty seeing the complete field of view without moving his or her eye back and forth. The observer may feel as though he or she is looking through a "knothole" and it may be necessary to circle his or her eye to see the edge of the field of view. If the exit pupil is too far from the last ocular lens, the operator will have difficulty maintaining his or her eye at the best lateral position. (Eye relief is seldom a problem when video systems are employed.)

After resolution, image brightness is probably the most important characteristic of an arthroscope. Since the brightness usually decreases by approximately the square of the arthroscope diameter, this parameter is especially significant in small-diameter arthroscopes.

Image brightness is also determined by the apparent field of view in visual instruments or the image size on the monitor in video systems. It does not make sense to magnify an image to such a large size that the eye is able to resolve more detail than the arthroscope can render; any additional magnification serves only to darken the image.

The exit pupil diameter is an important

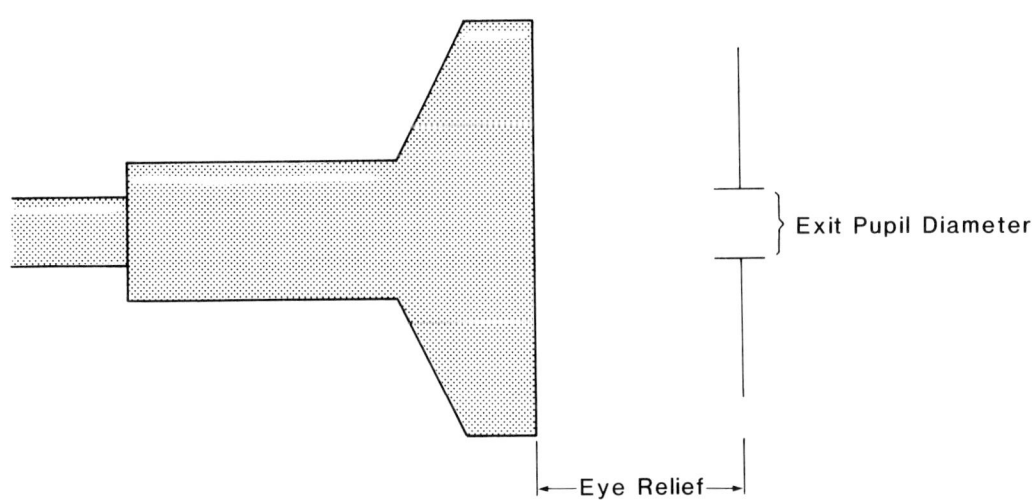

Figure 3–8. Eye relief.

factor in determining the endoscope image brightness and is particularly useful in comparing small-diameter arthroscopes in which brightness can be of paramount importance. It should be noted that it is the combination of the exit pupil and the apparent field of view that determines the brightness of the image.

A particularly troubling problem with many arthroscopes is a non-uniform image brightness over the field of view. Especially in video systems, this non-uniform brightness, or vignetting, contributes to "white-out" of the image, whereby the center of the field is completely saturated with light, whereas the edge of the field has insufficient illumination. This phenomenon is a characteristic of arthroscope optical design and varies significantly from manufacturer to manufacturer. Because the eye can tolerate a much greater variation in light level than can video systems, vignetting is difficult to assess by visual means.

The image brightness may also vary with the color of the light being transmitted through the arthroscope. When the transmission in the blue part of the spectrum is reduced, as is most common, the image will have a decidedly yellow appearance compared with the object under investigation. Image coloration is determined primarily by the types of glass that the optical designer uses in the system and by their antireflection coatings.

ARTHROSCOPE ILLUMINATION

The arthroscopist can choose between two types of light sources: the quartz-halogen bulb and the xenon or mercury-xenon arc lamp. Although quartz-halogen sources are much less expensive than arc sources, the serious user will always choose an arc lamp because of its higher color temperature and much greater light intensity. For strictly visual work in small joints, a quartz-halogen lamp is often sufficient, but for video work an arc lamp is a necessity.

Modern arc lamp systems are often fitted with automatic light level adjustments for use with video camera systems. This is particularly useful during diagnostic arthroscopies when the object distance and thus brightness is constantly varying.

Present-day arthroscopes are always illuminated through fiberoptic light guides connected to the sidearm of the instrument. Each light guide is made up of a bundle of individual optical fibers composed of the light-carrying central core and a thin outer cladding to isolate the fiber from its neighbors.

The total diameter of the bundle should be matched to the diameter of the fiber bundle in the arthroscope sidearm. Increasing the light guide diameter beyond that needed to match the fibers in the arthroscope will not increase the light output of the scope but will only generate excess heat at the sidearm junction. Various adaptors are available for interconnecting different types of arthroscopes and light guides.

The optical glass used in the light guide fibers is designed to possess excellent transmittance across the entire visible spectrum. However, this requires that the cone angle of the output light beam must be reduced. This reduced cone angle is insufficient to illuminate the entire field of view for wide-angle arthroscopes. Therefore, a glass cone (Fig. 3–9) is inserted into the sidearm by the manufacturer to increase the cone angle of the transmitted light rays. These glass cones may be made from a solid piece of glass or may be composed of individual optical fibers, each having a conical cross section.

SELECTION OF AN ARTHROSCOPE

Comparison of arthroscopes available from various vendors is complicated by the lack of complete instrument specifications and of measurement standards. However, several relatively simple measurements that can be performed with minimal equipment will allow an objective comparison of the primary optical characteristics of the various arthroscopes. For multiple arthroscope purchases, it may be desirable to obtain a more complete evaluation from a commercial optical measurement company. The principal optical measurements that characterize an arthroscope are outlined as follows.

Real Field of View

There are several ways to measure the real field of view of an arthroscope. The simplest is to place the instrument on a piece of paper on a table with the sidearm parallel to the

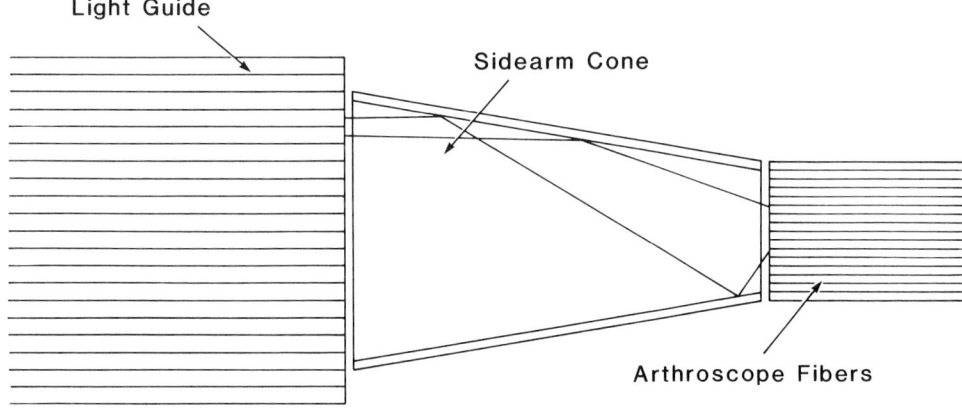

Figure 3–9. Arthroscope sidearm illumination coupling.

table top. Mark the position of the arthroscope tip with a pencil. Then, without moving the scope, view the opposite edges of the field and mark these two positions on the paper at a distance of 6 inches or so from the scope tip. The field of view can then be measured easily with a protractor (Fig. 3–10).

Direction of View

This measurement is similar to the measurement of the real field of view and is often performed at the same time. When marking the position of the tip of the arthroscope, also trace along the edges of the scope needle to define the endoscope axis. It is not difficult when viewing the edges of the field to note the center of the field of view. The angle of the center of the field of view with respect to the arthroscope axis is the direction of view.

ACKNOWLEDGMENT

The author would like to thank Concept, Inc. for their support in the preparation of this chapter.

Reference

1. Hopkins H: Optical principles of the endoscope. *In* Berci G (ed.): Endoscopy. New York: Appleton-Century-Crofts, 1976, pp. 3–26.

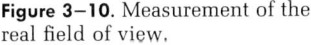

Figure 3–10. Measurement of the real field of view.

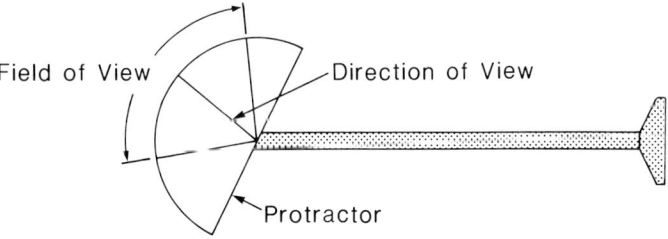

Section II
Temporomandibular Joint Arthropathy

Chapter 4
NORMAL PHYSIOLOGY OF SYNOVIAL JOINTS
A. Synovium

CHARLES WEISS, M.D.

For the dentist, oral surgeon, and arthroscopist who treat patients with disorders of the temporomandibular joint (TMJ), an understanding of its physiology and biochemistry is essential in order to make rational treatment decisions. The availability of increasingly sophisticated prosthetic devices, surgical instrumentation, viscosurgical tools, and medications mandates that mechanical considerations alone are no longer sufficient to restore optimal TMJ function and comfort. This chapter describes the structure, composition, physiology, and interactions of those tissues that compose the TMJ.

Much has been made of the differences between the TMJ, the ginglymoarthrodial joint, and the more common diarthrodial joints; however, from a biologic and functional standpoint, these joints share more similarities than differences. All consist of mesenchymal cells (fibrocytes, chondrocytes, and synovial cells) embedded in solid (collagen, proteoglycan) and liquid (synovial fluid) matrices. The liquid matrix bathes all solid and cellular joint components without any intervening cellular or basement membrane.[1] In mature individuals (Fig. 4–1), the TMJ is surrounded by a loose, well-vascularized capsule that encases the articulating ends of adjacent bones. The TMJ forms as a remnant of the periosteum or perichondrium in embryonic life. The enclosed bones are covered by articular cartilage. This is a composite tissue similar to that found in other joints[2–6] (Fig. 4–2), attached to bone by a calcified zone that supports a layer of hyalin cartilage, which in turn is covered by a dense, collagenous, fibrous tissue layer anchored at the periphery of the joint to the capsule and its continuum with the periosteum of bone. The inner layer of the capsule is lined by synovial cells (Fig. 4–3), and fibrous condensates of the capsular mesenchyme form the articular disc that lies between the articulating ends of bone. All these tissues are bathed and permeated by synovial fluid.[1]

The intimal layer of the synovial membrane (see Fig. 4–3) that lines the inner surface of the joint capsule consists of a loose arrangement of synovial cells (one to four cells deep) bathed in a concentrated synovial fluid that extends from the joint cavity to the subintimal tissues.[7] The subintimal tissues

A. Synovium

arthritic states, such as rheumatoid arthritis, there is a large increase in the number of Type B cells, which likely accounts for the increase in protein-bound HA found in this condition.[8, 13]

SYNOVIAL FLUID

Normal synovial fluid is a dialysate of blood plasma (free of large molecules such as fibrinogen) to which has been added the sodium salt of HA[14-16] (a glycosaminoglycan containing equimolar amounts of glucuronic

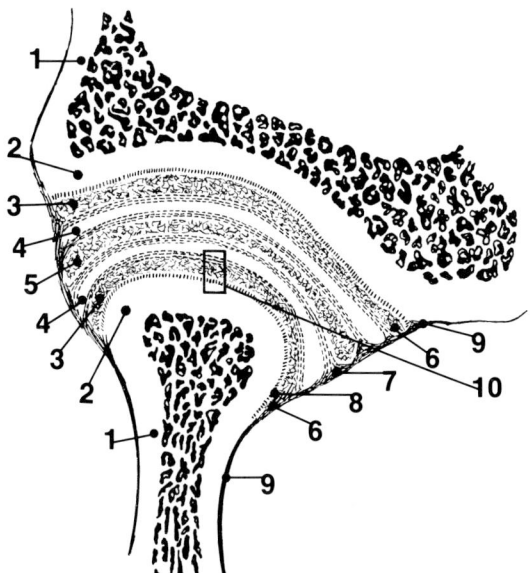

Figure 4–1. Frontal section through the temporomandibular joint. The cortical (1) and subchondral (2) bone of the mandible and temporal bones are covered by articular cartilage (3) encased in a fibrous capsule (7) and separated by an articular disk (5). The joint space (4) separates the articular cartilages from the articular disk. At its deepest portion the articular cartilage is anchored to bone by the calcified zone (8) and at its periphery (6) to the periosteum (9) and capsule (7). For details of articular cartilage (10) see Figure 4–2.

consist of a richly vascularized, loose connective tissue matrix containing fibrocytes, lipocytes, macrophages, mast cells, and nerve fibers.[8] The proximity of blood vessels to the joint cavity provides ready access of nutrients to the synovial fluid and to the cells and solid matrices that this fluid bathes. Normal synovial membrane consists of two types of cells:[7, 9] Type A, which constitutes the majority, and Type B. Type A cells contain a large Golgi apparatus and many smooth-walled vacuoles, which are thought to be involved in the synthesis and export of hyaluronan, or hyaluronic acid (HA), the major component of synovial fluid.[10] These cells are also phagocytes; thus, their activity is particularly increased in arthritic states.[8]

Type B cells have an extensive, rough-surfaced endoplasmic reticulum and appear to be involved principally in the synthesis and export of proteins. Although most of the protein in synovial fluid is derived as a dialysate from blood plasma, approximately 2% is tightly bound to the HA molecule and may be derived from Type B cells.[11, 12] In certain

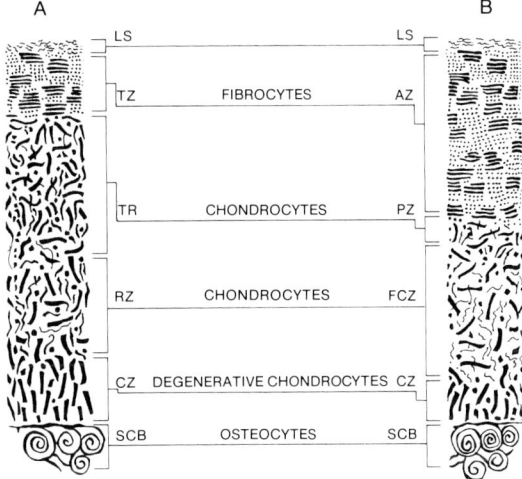

Figure 4–2. Diagrammatic representation of the collagen fibril architecture of normal human articular cartilage from (A) diarthrodial joints and (B) the temporomandibular joint. The surfaces are covered by a condensation of hyaluronan molecules, the lamina splendens (LS), several microns thick. The outer covering of articular cartilage—tangential zone (TZ) of A and articular zone (AZ) of B—consists of tightly woven bundles of collagen fibrils arranged parallel to the articular surface and at right angles to each other, with little intervening ground substance except for hyaluronan molecules. The cells of this zone are fibrocytes. This covering of the articular cartilage is approximately 5 to 10% of the thickness of diarthrodial cartilage and 50% of the thickness of the temporomandibular articular cartilage at its summit. It is thinnest at the summit and thickest at the periphery of the joint, where it is anchored to the capsule and periosteum. This "skin" covers two zones of hyalin articular cartilage—the transitional (TR) and radial (RZ) zones in A and the proliferated (PZ) and fibrocartilaginous (FCZ) zones in B. The cells of these zones are chondrocytes and the matrix consists of larger, randomly arranged collagen fibrils embedded in a glycosaminoglycan ground substance. In its depths the articular cartilage is anchored to the subchondral bony end plate (SCB) by the calcified zone (CZ), which consists of calcified collagen fibrils of larger diameter and degenerating chondrocytes.

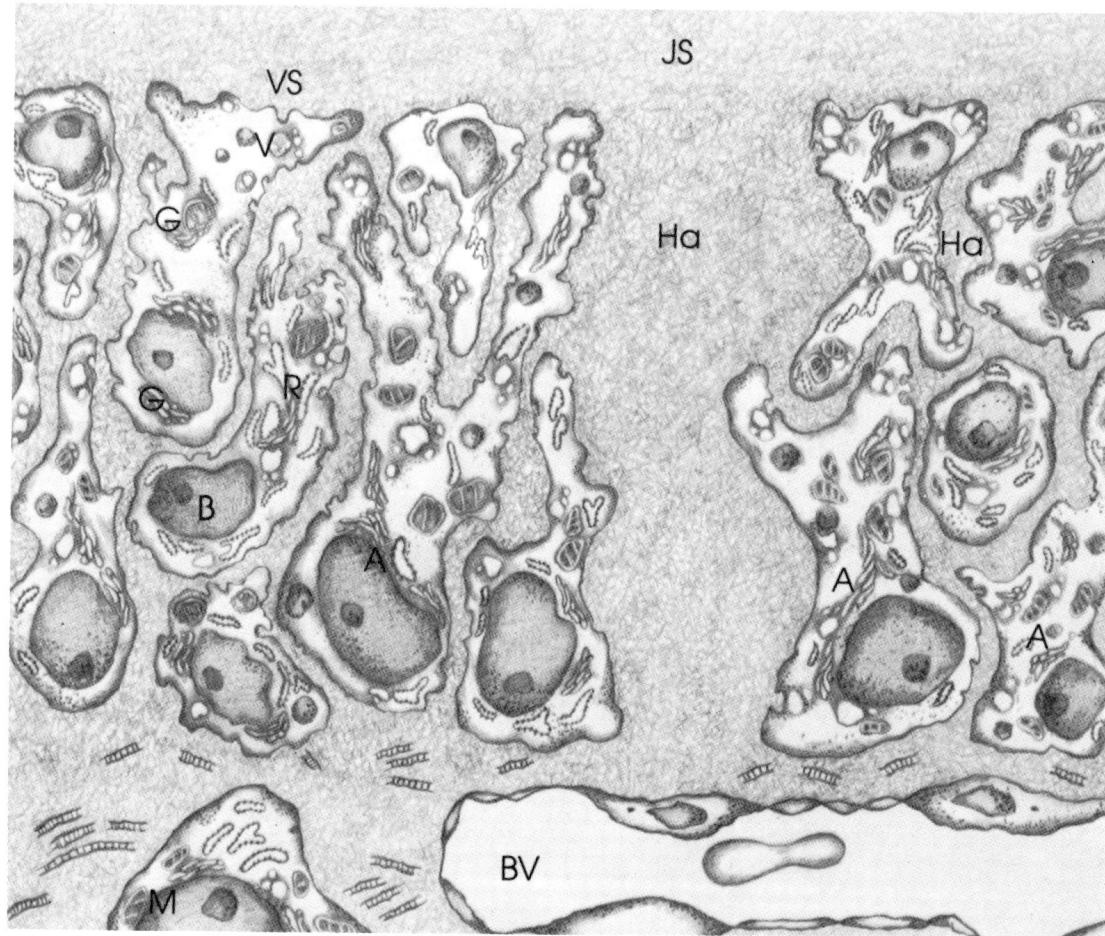

Figure 4–3. Schematic representation of normal synovial membrane. Type A and type B cells lie suspended in a network of hyaluronic acid molecules (Ha). Blood vessels (BV) lie in close proximity to the joint space (JS). Loose bundles of collagen fibers as well as lymphocytes, fibrocysts, and macrophages (M) underlie the surface cells. Type A cells have prominent Golgi apparatuses (G), micropinocytosis vesicles (VS), and many vacuoles (V). Type B cells have extensive rough endoplasmic reticulum (R). (Reprinted with permission from Weiss C: The basic structure of diarthrodial joints. In Parisien JS (ed): Arthroscopic Surgery. New York: McGraw-Hill, 1988.)

acid and N-acetylglucosamine) (Fig. 4–4), synthesized by the synovial A cells, and small amounts of protein, synthesized by the synovial B cells. The concentration of HA in normal synovial fluid is approximately 3.3 mg/ml. Because of the extraordinarily large volume of fluid occupied by each of these polyanionic molecules (spheroidal domain of 0.3 μm), this concentration is approximately ten times that required to entirely fill its volume of solvent (see Fig. 4–4). Synovial fluid therefore may be viewed as an extremely concentrated overlapping network of HA molecules in which water and various ions are trapped.[1] The size, shape, and volume of the HA molecules and their interaction with water and dissolved ions are expressed as the limiting viscosity number of HA. Change in this number is not correlated with a patient's age, but it is significantly diminished in patients with arthritis.[1, 17]

HA is not evenly distributed within the joint. The lowest concentration fills the joint space, whereas the highest concentrations occur on the surfaces of articular cartilage and the articular disc, forming a highly concentrated layer several micra in thickness and penetrating into the depths of these tissues to a distance of 50 to 100 μm.[1, 18, 19] This highly concentrated layer serves three distinct yet interrelated functions. First, it permits the free diffusion of small nutrients,

A. Synovium ■ 23

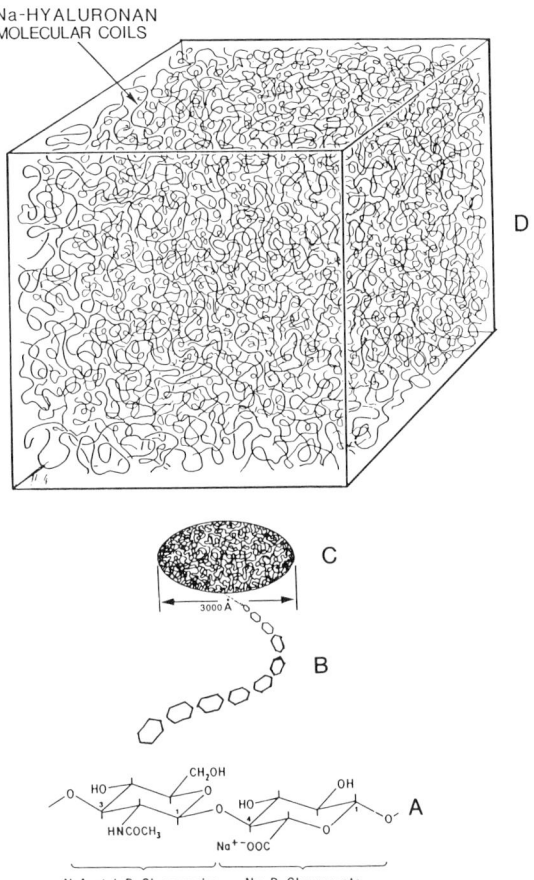

Figure 4–4. Diagrammatic representation of hyaluronan, a glycosaminoglycan containing N-acetyl-D-glucosamine and Na-D-glucuronate, with each molecule occupying a spheroidal domain of 3000 Å and existing in synovial fluid in a concentration of 3.3 mg/ml or ten times the amount required to fill its entire volume of solvent.

ions, and water into and out of articular cartilage, menisci, articular discs, and other tissues to provide cellular nutrition and the exodus of waste products from cellular metabolism in these avascular structures. Second, it forms an impenetrable barrier to the leakage of large molecules, such as proteoglycans, from the depths of articular cartilage; thus, it preserves the mechanical integrity of these tissues and provides a constant macro- and micromolecular extracellular environment. Finally, it serves as a lubricant.

BIOLOGIC LUBRICATION

Lubrication in biologic terms differs somewhat from the mechanical concept of "slipperiness"; it is concerned with the protection of cells and surfaces from compressive loads, shear stress, surface contact, and the dissipation of energy. HA exhibits both viscous and elastic properties, depending on the strain frequencies applied to the molecule (Fig. 4–5). At low strain frequencies, normal synovial fluids behave predominantly as viscous fluids, whereas at high strain frequencies they behave as elastic solids.[1, 14, 17, 20, 21] At low frequencies such as occur during joint movement without excessive pressure, the HA molecular chains are able to adjust their shape and slip easily one by the next, thus resulting in viscous flow. The movement between articulating surfaces takes place at the level of these flowing HA molecules; therefore the collagen fibers on the surface of the articular cartilage and the articular disc do not abrade one another, since there is no direct contact. Under higher strain frequencies, the molecules are unable to adjust configurationally; they become entangled and deform sinusoidally, thereby forming elastic solids,[2] which store the mechanical energy in their interstices. Once stress is released, the elastic solid gradually unwinds, a viscous flow is established, and the energy is gradually dissipated as heat. Therefore, under high strain frequencies, collagen surfaces are separated by the elastic solid formed by the HA molecule, which absorbs the mechanical energy and prevents collagen deterioration. These rheologic changes from viscous fluid to elastic solid occur without degradation of HA.

In traumatic, degenerative, or inflammatory arthritis, the HA molecule is decreased in size. In this state of reduced viscosity, it behaves primarily as a viscous fluid[1, 14] and is unable to provide collagen surface protection under high strain frequency (high impact loading), thus starting a cycle of increased surface damage, increased joint inflammation, and decreased HA viscosity, leading to progressive joint deterioration. The restoration of normal synovial fluid viscosity, therefore, is essential to the preservation of normal TMJ surface protection.

ARTICULAR DISC

The articular disc appears during the eighth intrauterine week as a condensation of mesenchymal cells attached to the capsule.

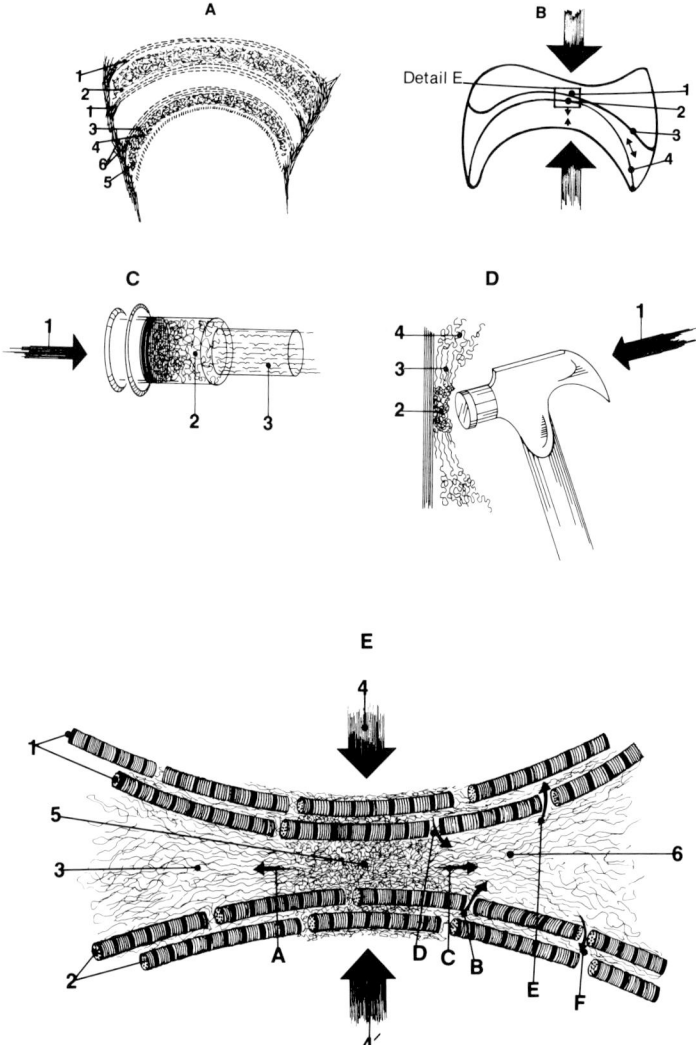

Figure 4–5. Biologic lubrication. *A*, Normal temporomandibular joint frontal section through the articular disc (1 and 2) and articular cartilage (3 and 4). The articular zone (3) is anchored to the periosteum at the joint margin (5) and to the joint capsule (6). The superficial zone of the articular disc (1) is anchored to the capsule. The outward pressure of the fibrocartilaginous zone (4) is constrained by the articular zone (3). *B*, Under compression (*large arrows*) the primary joint contours change; the area under compression flattens (1 and 2) and the peripheral portion of the joint surfaces bulges (3 and 4). The random arrangement of collagen fibers and high concentration of proteoglycans in the fibrocartilaginous zone of the articular cartilage resists compression ($\updownarrow$) and the thick tangential zone (articular zone) bulges and is subjected to tensile forces ($\leftrightarrow$). *C*, At the molecular level, hyaluronan molecules randomly arranged (2) and subjected to low strain frequencies (1) configurationally adjust and act as viscous fluids (3). *D*, When subjected to high strain frequencies (1) the molecules become entangled (2), forming an elastic, solid storing energy within the molecules. At a distance from the point of highest strain frequency, the molecules establish a viscous flow (3), slowly releasing energy and finally establishing their normal random arrangement (4). *E*, High-magnification molecular view of two surfaces (1 and 2) composed of collagen fibrils with an intervening layer of hyaluronan molecules (3) subjected to compressive forces (4 and 4′). At the point of highest strain frequency, hyaluronan forms an elastic solid (5) separating the collagen fibrils from direct contact. Water leaves the domain of the collagen surfaces and hyaluronan (arrows A–D). At a distance from the point of greatest compression the hyaluronan establishes a viscous flow (6) and water returns to the collagen surface (arrows E and F).

This disc-shaped, highly collagenous, and relatively acellular structure consists of bundles of collagen fibers of variable diameter[22] arranged at varying angles to one another, parallel in an anteroposterior direction to the articulating surfaces of the disc in its superficial portions and more randomly arranged in the interior of the disc (see Fig. 4–1).[23] The collagen fiber arrangement of the articular disc suggests that the superficial layers resist shear forces and tension in the anteroposterior direction and that the deeper zones resist compression in the cephalocaudad direction.[23, 24]

The chondrocytes and fibrocytes of the disc receive their nutrition by diffusion of nutrients from the joint cavity through the dense hyaluronan covering its surfaces.[23] This surface covering is identical to the fine fibers and filamentous fibrils that compose the lamina splendens covering the articular cartilage.[1, 3, 4, 6, 10, 25–29] The articular disc serves to assist efficient lubrication of the TMJ by increasing the cross-sectional area covered by synovial fluid and the number of lubricated surfaces that transmit compressive loads and shear forces between the articulating ends of the mandible and maxilla that compose the TMJ.[8, 23]

The peripheral few millimeters of the articular disc attached to the capsule is its only vascularized area and the only area having significant potential for healing.[25, 30–34] Experimental animal models of meniscal healing suggest that tears in avascular areas can heal, provided they receive nutrition from a vascularized synovial flap. The scar that forms this healing is derived by metaplasia of synovial cells.[25] The long-term clinical application of this technique is yet to be studied in the temporomandibular articular disc.

ROLE OF SYNOVIAL ENZYMES IN OSTEOARTHRITIS

Osteoarthritis is characterized chemically by the progressive loss of proteoglycan and collagen, which parallels roughly the severity of the disease.[35, 36] In the past decade, enzymes (metalloproteases) have been found in the chondrocytes of articular cartilage and in the cells of the synovial membrane which are capable of breaking down protein polysaccharides and collagen at neutral pH.[37–41] These enzymes, however, require an activation factor.[42, 43] The levels of these enzymes are increased three- to fourfold in osteoarthritic cartilage, paralleling the extent of the disease.[44] It is only in the end stage, when the cartilage has been depleted of its proteoglycan content, that the enzymatic levels diminish.[43] The initial cellular response to matrix loss is an accelerated synthesis of collagen and proteoglycan by the remaining cells of articular cartilage,[45–47] stimulated by the release of transforming growth factor B (TGF-B) from synovial cells.[48, 49] However, this increased synthetic capacity is insufficient to counteract the progressive loss of matrix components resulting from enzymatic degradation.[50, 51]

Ehrlich and colleagues have found a non–lysosomal-dependent collagenase present in inactive form in normal cartilage, which increases in an amount paralleling the level of the disease in osteoarthritic cartilage.[42, 52, 53] This, like the metalloglycan-proteinases, is also calcium-dependent.[52] Although the enzymes responsible for the breakdown of proteoglycan and collagen of articular cartilage in osteoarthritic lesions are derived from local chondrocytes within the lesional area, the activity of these enzymes is markedly increased by the presence of synovium, owing to a low molecular weight protein called cytokine (activation factor) that is synthesized by the synovium.[43] This activation factor is similar to interleukin-1, has a molecular weight of 15,000, and stimulates the proliferation of activated T cells as well as chondrocytes to produce collagenase and a neutral metalloprotease.[40, 54–56] The increase in activity of these enzymes in synovial-conditioned media of arthritic articular cartilage suggests that the enzymes responsible for the breakdown of cartilage are derived from chondrocytes and triggered by the release of these activation proteins from the synovium.[48, 49, 55, 57]

Articular degradation appears common to all types of articular cartilage (see Fig. 5–9). Physical, chemical, or metabolic stress sufficient to injure the articular zone of cartilage results in the loss of HA from the surface of the joint and the leakage of proteoglycans into the synovial fluid. This, in turn, stimulates already injured synovial lining cells to increase the rate of phagocytosis, produce a shorter-chain HA molecule, release enzymes (which increase capillary leakage, further dilute the concentration HA in synovial fluid, and stimulate pain fibers in the joint capsule), and release cytokine, a small molecular weight protein (activation factor), similar to interleukin-1, which diffuses into articular cartilage.

Chondrocytes stimulated by the trauma synthesize and release enzymes (neutral metalloproteases and collagenases), which when activated degrade cartilage matrix. The loss of cartilage matrix stimulates both reparative and degenerative responses by chondrocytes, resulting in (along with the release of synovial TGF-B) chondrocyte proliferation, increased matrix synthesis, and increased chondrocyte death and the release of additional degradative enzymes. The net result of these activities is that the repair response is insufficient to compensate for the loss of proteoglycan and of collagen matrix components, thereby resulting in further mechanical deterioration of the articular matrix and further stress to the articular cartilage, thus a closed circle or cascade of degenerative changes is instituted.

There are many points at which this closed circle of progressive degenerative changes may be disrupted and even reversed. Factors that may affect this closed circle include increased joint surface protection by enhancing the body's own lubrication capacity; chemical, enzyme, and enzyme activator inhibitors; and enhancement of the innate reparative response of the chondrocytes. These represent encouraging avenues for the protection and maintenance of joint homeostasis and disruption of the arthritic cascade.

References

1. Balazs EA: The physical properties of synovial fluid and the special role of hyaluronic acid. In Helfet AJ (ed): Disorders of the knee, Vol 4. Philadelphia: Lippincott, 1982, p 61.
2. Weiss C: The Basic Structure of Diarthrodial Joints. Arthroscopic Surgery. Parisien JS (ed): New York: McGraw-Hill, 1988, pp 3–18.
3. Weiss C: Microstructure and biochemistry of joints, In Helfet AJ (ed): Disorders of the Knee, Vol 3. Philadelphia: Lippincott, 1982, p 37.
4. Weiss C: Light and electron microscopic studies of normal articular cartilage. In Simon WH (ed): The Human Joint in Health and Disease. Philadelphia: University of Pennsylvania Press, 1978, pp 9–21.
5. Weiss C: Normal and osteoarthritic articular cartilage. Orthop Clin North Am 10:175, 1979.
6. Weiss C, Rosenberg L, Helfet AJ: An ultrastructural study of normal young adult human articular cartilage. J Bone Joint Surg 50A:663, 1968.
7. Novikoff AB, Hamerman D: Electron microscopy of the human synovial membrane. J Cell Biol 14:207, 1962.
8. Ghadially FN, Roy S: Ultrasound of Synovial Joints in Health and Disease. New York: Appleton-Century-Crofts, 1969.
9. Ghadially FN, Crane WAJ: Synovial membrane in traumatic effusion. Ultrastructure and autoradiography with tritiated leucine. Ann Rheum Dis 25:259, 1966.
10. Hamerman D, Rosenberg LC, Schubert M: Diarthrodial Joints Revised. J Bone Joint Surg 52A:725, 1970.
11. Sandson J, Hamerman D: Isolation of hyaluronate-protein from human synovial fluid. J Clin Invest 41:1817, 1962.
12. Schubert M, Hamerman D: A Primer on Connective Tissue Biochemistry. Philadelphia: Lea & Febiger, 1968.
13. Hammerman D, Sandson J: Unusual Properties of Hyaluronate-Protein Isolated From Pathological Synovial Fluids. J. Clin Invest 42:1882, 1963.
14. Balazs EA, Watson D, Duff IF, et al: Hyaluronic acid in synovial fluid: I. Molecular parameters of hyaluronic acid in normal and arthritic human fluids. Arthritis Rheum 10:357, 1967.
15. Deck B, McKenzie BF, McGuckin WF: Zone electrophoretic studies of proteins and glycoproteins of bovine serum and synovial fluid. Proc Soc Exp Biol Med 102:616, 1959.
16. Schmidt K, MacNair MB: Characterization of the proteins of certain post-mortem human synovial fluids. J Clin Invest 37:708, 1958.
17. Balazs EA: Some aspects of the aging and radiation sensitivity of the intercellular matrix with special regard to hyaluronic acid in synovial fluid and vitreous, In Engel A, Loarsson T (eds): Thule International Symposium: Aging of Connective and Skeletal Tissue. Stockholm: Nordiska Bokhandelns Forlag, 1969.
18. Balazs EA: Structure and metabolism of connective tissue under physiological and pathological conditions. In Ruttner J, et al (eds): Arthritis and Osteoarthritis. Wein: Verlag Hans Huber, 1971.
19. Balazs EA, Bloom GD, Swann DA: Fine structure and glycosaminoglycan content of the surface layer of articular cartilage. Fed Proc 25:1813, 1966.
20. Balazs EA: Viscoelastic properties of hyaluronic acid and biological lubrication. Univ Mich Ctr J [Special Issue]: 255, December, 1968.
21. Balazs EA, Gibbs DA: The rheological properties and biological function of hyaluronic acid. In Balazs EA (ed): Chemistry and Molecular Biology of the Intercellular Matrix. London: Academic Press, 1970, pp 1241–1254.
22. Zambrano NZ, Montes GS, Shigihara KM, et al: Collagen arrangement in cartilages. Acta Anat 113:26–38, 1982.
23. de Bont LGM, Liem RSB, Havinga P, Boering G: Fibrous component of the temporomandibular joint disc. J Craniomandib Pract 3 (4):368–373, 1985.
24. Minns RJ, Steven FS: The collagen fibril organization in human articular cartilage. J Anat 123:437–457, 1979.
25. Arnoczky SP, Stone RG, Hungerford DH, and other panel members: American Association of Orthopaedic Surgeons. Course on Advanced Arthroscopy—Complications and Problems. Philadelphia, July, 1982.

26. de Bont LGM, Boering G, Havinga P, Liem RSB: Spatial arrangement of collagen fibrils in the articular cartilage of the mandibular condyle: A light microscopic and scanning electron microscopic study. J Oral Maxillofac Surg 42:306–313, 1984.
27. Meachim G, Stockwell RA: The matrix. In Freeman MAR (ed): Adult Articular Cartilage, 2nd Ed. London: Pitman Medical, 1979, p 1.
28. Meachim G, Roy S: Surface ultrastructure of mature adult human articular cartilage. Ann Rheum Dis 27:544–558, 1968.
29. Weiss C: An ultrastructural study of aging human articular cartilage. [Abstract] J Bone Joint Surg 53A:803, 1971.
30. Arnoczky SP, Warren RF: Microvasculature of the human meniscus. Am J Sports Med 10(2):90, 1982.
31. Schneider DA: Peripheral detachment of the meniscus—arthroscopic and clinical correlations. Orthop Rev 6:55, 1977.
32. Seedhorn BB, Dowson D, Wright V: Function of the menisci: A preliminary study. [Abstract] Ann Rheum Dis 33:111, 1965.
33. Smillie IS: Injuries of the Knee Joint, 4th Ed. Edinburgh: Churchill Livingston, 1970.
34. Stone RG: Peripheral detachment of the menisci of the knee: A preliminary report. Ortho Clin North Am 10(3):643, 1979.
35. Mankin HJ, Dorfman H, Lippiello L, et al: Biochemical and metabolic abnormalities in articular cartilage from osteoarthritic human hips. II. Correlation of morphology with biochemical and metabolic data. J Bone Joint Surg 53A:523, 1971.
36. Mankin HJ, Lippiello L: Biochemical and metabolic abnormalities in articular cartilage from osteoarthritic human hips. J Bone Joint Surg 52A:424, 1970.
37. Ehrlich MG, Mankin HJ, Vigliani G, et al: Pattern of proteoglycan subunit breakdown by human degradative enzymes at neutral pH. Trans Orthop Res Soc 2:7, 19.
38. Harris ED Jr, Parker HG, Radin EL, Krane SM: Effects of Proteolytic Enzymes On Structure and Mechanical Properties of Cartilage. Arthritis Rheum 15:497, 1972.
39. Martel-Pelletier J, Pelletier JP, Cloutier JM, et al: Neutral proteases capable of proteoglycan digesting activity in osteoarthritic and normal human cartilage. Arthritis Rheum 27:305, 1984.
40. Ridge SC, Oronsky AL, Kerwar SS: Induction of the synthesis of latent collagenase and latent neutral protease on chondrocytes by a factor synthesized by activated macrophages. Arthritis Rheum 23:448, 1980.
41. Sapolsky AI, Keiser H, Howell DS, Woesnner JF Jr: Metalloproteases of human articular cartilage that digest cartilage proteoglycans at neutral and acid pH. J Clin Invest 58:1030, 1976.
42. Ehrlich MG: Degradative enzyme systems in osteoarthritis cartilage. J. Orthop Res 3:170, 1985.
43. Ehrlich MG, Armstrong A, Treadwell BV, Mankin HJ: Degradative enzyme systems in cartilage. J Orthop Res 3:170, 1985.
44. Lahey PJ, Ehrlich MG, Mankin HJ: Neutral protease activity vs. severity of osteoarthritis. Trans Orthop Res Soc 4:46, 1979.
45. Calandruccio RA, Gilmer WS: Proliferation, regeneration, and repair of articular cartilage of immature animals. J Bone Joint Surg 44A(3):431, 1962.
46. Mankin HJ: Current concepts review: The reaction of articular cartilage to mechanical injury. J Bone Joint Surg 64A:460, 1982.
47. Weiss C, Mankin HJ, Zarins A: Autoradiographic studies of matrix synthesis in articular cartilage. Surg Forum 19:485, 1973.
48. Bandara G, Lin CW, Georgescu HI, Evans CH: The synovial synthesis of TGF-B and its consequences for chondrocyte activation. Trans Orthop Res Soc 15:313, 1990.
49. Recklies, White C: Differential effects of transforming growth factor-B on matrix synthesis in cartilage explants and isolated chondrocytes. Trans Ortho Res Soc 15:316, 1990.
50. Mankin HJ: The reaction of articular cartilage to injury and osteoarthritis (second of two parts). N Engl J Med 291: pp 1335, 1974.
51. Mankin HJ, Boyle CJ: The acute effects of lacerative injury on DNA and protein synthesis in articular cartilage. In Bassett CAL (ed): Cartilage Degradation and Repair. Washington: NAS–NRC, 1967.
52. Ehrlich MG, Houle PA, Vigliani G, Mankin HJ: Correlation between articular cartilage collagenase activity and osteoarthritis. Arthritis Rheum 21:761, 1978.
53. Ehrlich MG, Mankin HJ, Jones H, et al: Collagenase and collagenase inhibitors in osteoarthritis and normal human cartilage. J Clin Invest 59:6, 1977.
54. de Bont LGM, Liem RSB, Havinga P, Boering G, van der Korst JK: Collagen network of human femoral head cartilage; A light microscopic and scanning electron microscopic study. Acta Anat 1985.
55. Dinarello CA: Interleukin-1 and the pathogenesis of the acute-phase response. N Engl J Med 311:1413, 1984.
56. Gowen M, Wood DP, Ihrie EJ, et al: Stimulation by human interleukin-1 of cartilage breakdown and production of collagenase and proteoglycanase by human chondrocytes but not by human osteoblasts in vitro. Biochem Biophys Acta 797:186, 1984.
57. Chandrasekhar AK Sr, Harvey PS, Hrubey AR. Intra-articular administration of IL-1 causes prolonged suppression of cartilage proteoglycan synthesis. Trans Orthop Res Soc 15:321, 1990.
58. Hukins DWL: Biomechanical properties of collagen. In Weiss JB, et al (eds): Collagen in Health and Disease. Edinburgh: Churchill Livingstone, 1982.
59. Walker PS, et al: Mode of aggregation of hyaluronic acid protein complex in the surface of articular cartilage. Ann Rheum Dis 29:591, 1970.

☐ B. Articular Cartilage

*LAMBERT G.M. DE BONT, D.D.S., PH.D.,
BOUDEWIJN STEGENGA, D.D.S., and
GEERT BOERING, D.D.S., PH.D.*

Temporomandibular joint (TMJ) disorders usually are accompanied by a complex of signs and symptoms in which clicking, limitation of movement, and pain occur most frequently.[1] TMJ studies commonly deal with TMJ dysfunction, internal derangement, or osteoarthrosis and accompanying signs and symptoms.

The number of publications about the TMJ dealing with microscopy of the articular cartilage is restricted. Few ultrastructural studies on TMJ articular cartilage are available. Degenerative changes in synovial joints, described in the literature as osteoarthrosis, osteoarthritis, degenerative arthritis, degenerative joint disease, and arthrosis deformans, arise in the articular cartilage and subchondral bone.[2] The degenerative process can be characterized as disintegration of the collagen network and loss of ground substance, which consists of proteoglycans.[3, 4]

Knowledge about the structure of the TMJ articular cartilage from the mandibular condyle, the disc, and the articular eminence (Fig. 4–6) has been poorly developed.[5, 6] Fortunately, when comparing the articular cartilage of the TMJ with that of other synovial joints (i.e., the knee or hip joint), several morphologic similarities are detectable on a light and electron microscopic level. The aim of this chapter is to survey the recent literature on articular cartilage structure and normal physiology of synovial joints in general and that of the TMJ in particular.

STRUCTURE AND FUNCTION OF ARTICULAR CARTILAGE

The cartilage of synovial joints is predominantly composed of chondrocytes, collagen fibrils, proteoglycans, and water. Collagen fibrils and proteoglycans form the articular cartilage matrix. Glycoproteins and small fractions of lipids and inorganic material are also present in this matrix. The collagen

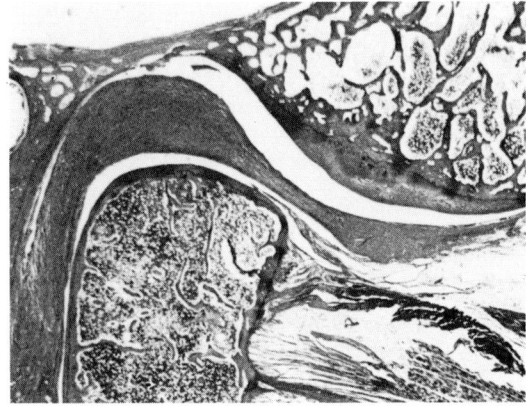

Figure 4–6. Midsagittal survey section of the temporomandibular joint. The articular cartilage covering of the mandibular condyle and the articular eminence as well as the cartilage of the articular disc are clearly observable. (Magnification × 5). (Reprinted with permission from de Bont LGM, de Haan P, Boering G: Struktuur en bouw van het kraakbeen van het Kaakgewricht. Ned Tijdschr Tandheelkd 92:184–189, 1985.)

fibrils create a three-dimensional network. Proteoglycans are entangled in this network not only mechanically but probably also chemically. The supposed biochemical interactions between proteoglycans and some parts of the collagen fibrils are not yet clearly specified. Because of the hydrophilic character of proteoglycans, the articular cartilage ground substance contains a large proportion of water. The ground substance resembles a hydrophilic gel that swells by infusion of water from the synovial fluid via osmosis. Expansion of the gel is counteracted by the tension of the collagen fibrils in the network. By this mechanism, collagen fibrils are under continuous tension stress, even when the joint is unloaded. In this way, the presence of internal hydrostatic pressure in the articular cartilage can be explained.[4] When the articular surfaces become loaded, the internal pressure of the articular cartilage and the tension in the collagen fibrils simultaneously increase. Thus, the function of the collagen fibrils in cartilage is to resist the internal pressure, just as the walls of a tire withstand air pressure. If the internal pressure, as the result of heavy loading, exceeds the osmotic pressure of the matrix, water and waste products squeeze out of the cartilage matrix, which contributes to the lubrication of the joint surfaces.[7] This mechanism has been called "weeping" lubrication. When the loading is reduced and the osmotic pressure exceeds the hydrostatic pressure, water and nutrients penetrate back into the cartilage matrix.[8]

Because of the mechanisms outlined in the preceding paragraph, articular cartilage has the following properties:[9]

1. It accepts high loads and distributes these to the underlying bone.
2. It accepts long-lasting loads, applied locally to the joint surface. These loads are transformed into tension stresses in the collagen fibrils, dispersed, and therefore reduced.
3. It enhances movement with little friction.
4. It absorbs shocks.

During loading, and even in an unloaded state, the equilibration mechanisms between the different components of the matrix are complex. These mechanisms involve the mechanical entanglement of collagen and proteoglycans, the tensile resistance of collagen fibrils, the swelling pressure and compression resistance of proteoglycans, and the diffusion resistance generated as interstitial fluid flows through the matrix.[8, 10]

Articular cartilage is an avascular, alymphatic, and aneural tissue. The articular surface is not covered by a perichondrium but by synovial fluid, the presence of which is essential for sufficient joint lubrication. Nutrition of the articular cartilage cells occurs by diffusion of molecules from the synovial fluid. This diffusion is stimulated by alternate loading. Immobilization of a joint severely deteriorates it, causing either atrophy or pressure-induced necrosis of the articular cartilage. Joints need appropriate motion and functional stress to maintain their health.[11] The thickness of the articular cartilage covering of large joints, such as the hip and the knee joint, varies from 2 to 4 mm.[12] The mandibular condyle is covered by a cartilage layer approximately 0.5 mm thick.[13]

Articular cartilage varies considerably in terms of cellular content, fiber density, and chemical composition. The temporomandibular and sternoclavicular joint surfaces are covered with fibrocartilage, in contrast to other synovial joints, which are covered with hyaline cartilage. The main differences between fibrocartilage and hyaline cartilage are reported to be a higher fiber content and Type I collagen in the fibrocartilage compared with Type II collagen in hyaline cartilage.[12] The nonfibrous components of the fibrocartilage matrix also differ from hyaline cartilage, containing a lower percentage of water and proteoglycans.[12, 14] Different zones are distinguishable by light microscopy (LM) in the fibrocartilage of the mandibular condyle and in the hyaline cartilage of other synovial joints.[14–17]

Cells

Only about 0.01 to 0.1% of the volume of articular cartilage consists of cartilage cells. These cells produce the articular cartilage matrix components collagen and proteoglycans.[9]

In the articular zone of the articular cartilage of the mandibular condyle, both chondrocytes and fibrocytes are found. Chondrocytes and fibrocytes can be found as undifferentiated and as differentiated cells with signs of aging and degeneration.[18] The proliferative zone contains undifferentiated mesenchymal cells. Cell division is observed occasionally.[15, 19]

Collagen

The collagen content of articular cartilage is generally more than 50% of its dry weight. The collagen fibrils are organized in bundles, layers, or lamellar structures that form a network.[9] The smallest, threadlike collagen structure detectable by transmission electron microscopy (TEM) is called filament. If the characteristic banding, with periodicity ranging from 52 to 64 nm, is detectable by TEM, it becomes a fibril (Fig. 4–7.). The diameter of a collagen fibril varies from 30 to 110 nm. Collagen fibrils form bundles or rope-like structures called fibers. As mentioned previously, collagen layers or sheets and lamellae may also be formed. Thus a collagen fiber is composed of collagen fibrils,

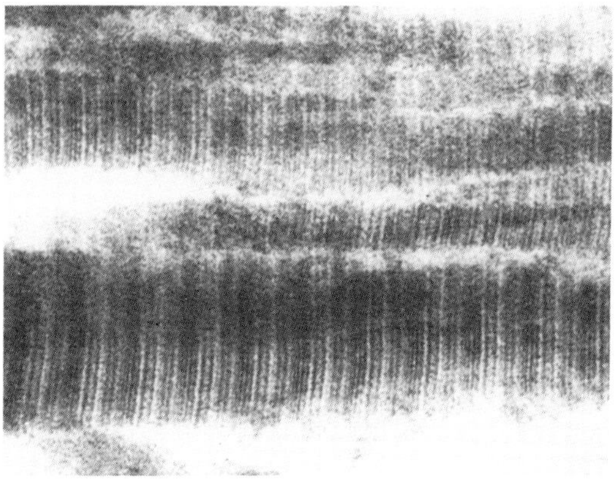

4 Normal Physiology of Synovial Joints

Figure 4–7. Transmission electron microscopic image of collagen fibrils showing alternating dark and light bands and fine cross-striations. (Magnification × 133,000.) (Reprinted with permission from de Bont LGM, de Haan P, Boering G: Structuur en bouw van het kraakbeen van het Kaakgewricht. Ned Tijdschr Tandheelkd 92:184–189, 1985.)

and these fibers can be arranged in bundles (Fig. 4–8) that are clearly distinguishable by LM.[9]

Collagen consists of tropocollagen molecules. Chondrocytes and fibrocytes produce these molecules in the same manner, in accordance with the general rules for protein synthesis. Each tropocollagen molecule consists of three helical polypeptide α-chains that wind round each other, creating a triple helix 280 nm in length (Fig. 4–9). The tropocollagen molecules are arranged in chains and side by side in an approximately quarter staggered arrangement,[20] with polar and apolar areas alternating. Heavy metal ions lead and uranyl from lead citrate and uranyl acetate staining solutions, fix the polar areas, and in this way they produce the alternating dark and light bands of the collagen fibrils in TEM ultra-thin sections (Figs. 4–7 and 4–9).

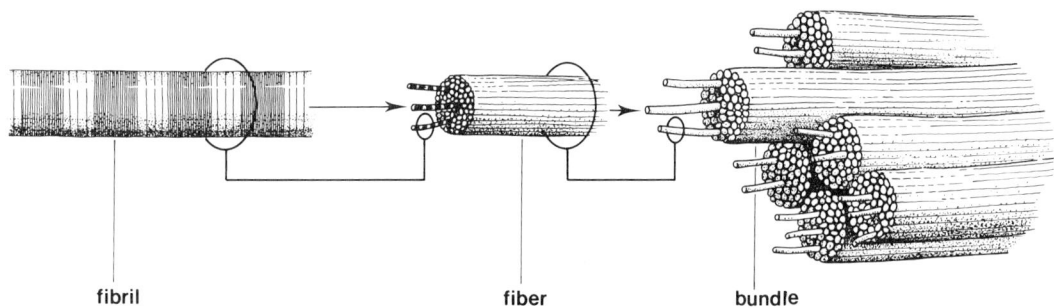

Figure 4–8. Diagram showing the organization of collagen from fibril to fiber and fiber bundle. (Reprinted with permission from de Bont LGM, de Haan P, Boering G: Structuur en bouw van het kraakbeen van het Kaakgewricht. Ned Tijdschr Tandheelkd 92:184–189, 1985.)

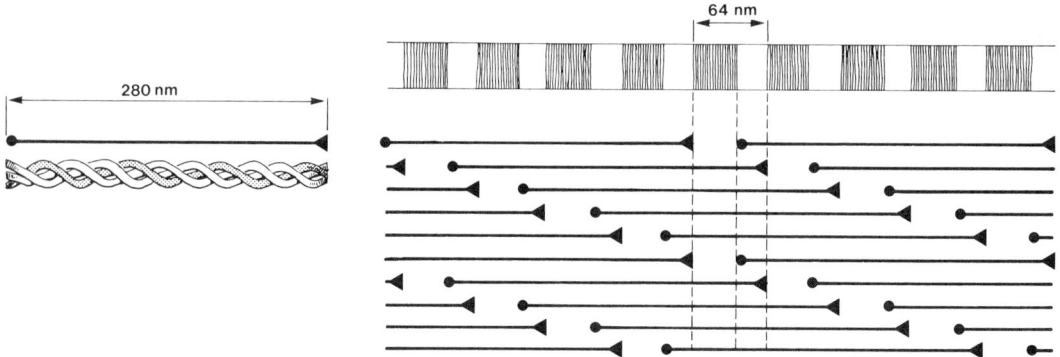

Figure 4–9. Diagram of the arrangement of tropocollagen molecules, which consist of three helical polypeptide α-chains, and the collagen fibril periodicity. (Reprinted with permission from de Bont LGM, de Haan P, Boering G: Structuur en bouw van het kraakbeen van het Kaakgewricht. Ned Tijdschr Tandheelkd 92:184–189, 1985.)

Between the individual tropocollagen molecules, covalent bindings (so-called intermolecular cross-links) exist. In this way, collagen fibrils get their strength. The process that determines fibril length and width is unknown.

There are different types of collagen, based on variations in amino acid composition and sequence and on the extent of glycosylation of the hydroxylysine residues in the α-chains. The tropocollagen molecules of Type I collagen are composed of two identical $\alpha_1(I)$-chains and one $\alpha_2(I)$-chain. Type II collagen consists of three identical $\alpha_1(II)$-chains.[12, 21, 22]

Proteoglycans

The ground substance of the articular cartilage matrix consists predominantly of proteoglycans associated with hyaluronic acid, creating large complexes of hydrophilic molecules (Fig. 4–10).[23] Proteoglycan synthesis occurs in the chondrocytes. A proteoglycan is a complex molecule composed of a protein core and glycosaminoglycan chains. These chains, consisting of chondroitin sulfate and keratan sulfate, are the extensions positioned away from the protein core that are responsible for the bottle-brush appearance of proteoglycans. Hyaluronic acid and proteoglycans form molecule complexes that are situated between the collagen fibrils of the articular cartilage, occupying all the interstitial spaces in the matrix, and are intertwined throughout the collagen network (Fig. 4–11).[24] Binding between proteoglycans and collagen has been suggested but not yet been proved biochemically. The exact nature of these interactions is still unknown.[25] The mechanical relationship between proteoglyans and collagen fibrils has been demonstrated in a model in which ping-pong balls are entrapped by threads and ropes that form a network.[26]

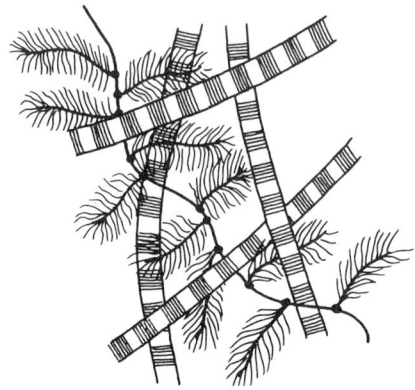

Figure 4–11. Diagram showing intertwinement of proteoglycans and collagen fibrils. (Reprinted with permission from de Bont LGM, de Haan P, Boering G: Structuur en bouw van het kraakbeen van het Kaakgewricht. Ned Tijdschr Tandheelkd 92:184–189, 1985.)

Fibrous Architecture of Hyaline Cartilage and Fibrocartilage

Fibrocartilage and hyaline cartilage cells are surrounded by a dense intercellular matrix of collagen fibrils and ground substance. The collagen fibrils of hyaline cartilage (Type II) are completely, randomly arranged throughout the tissue, creating a dense network without a clear zonal or bundle-like orientation.[17] The collagen fibrils of fibrocartilage (Type I), in comparison, are arranged in several distinct zones (Figs. 4–12 and 4–13). In the articular zone of mandibular condylar cartilage, the collagen fibrils are arranged in sheets running nearly parallel to

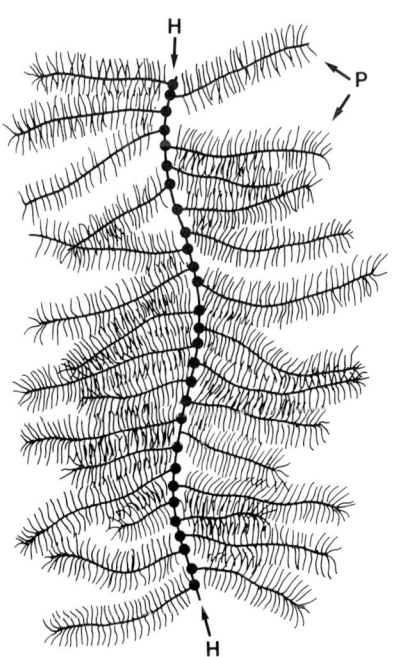

Figure 4–10. Diagram showing proteoglycans (P) associated with hyaluronic acid (H). (Reprinted with permission from de Bont LGM, de Haan P, Boering G: Structuur en bouw van het kraakbeen van het Kaakgewricht. Ned Tijdschr Tandheelkd 92:184–189, 1985.)

4 Normal Physiology of Synovial Joints

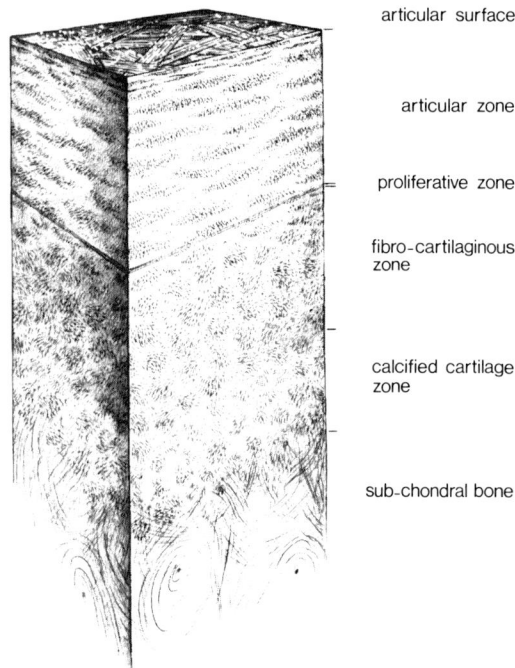

Figure 4–12. Diagram of the spatial arrangement of collagen fibrils in the articular cartilage of the mandibular condyle. (Reprinted with permission from de Bont LGM, Boering G, Havinga P, Liem RSB: Spatial arrangement of collagen fibrils in the articular cartilage of the mandibular condyle: An LM and SEM study. J Oral Maxillofac Surg 42:306–313, 1984).

the articular surface. A layer of undifferentiated mesenchymal cells (the proliferative zone) marks the border between the collagen network of the articular and fibrocartilaginous zones. The collagen fibrils in the latter zone are organized in bundles with a random orientation. A similar organization can be found in the calcified cartilage zone.[16] The collagen fibrils of the articular disc are also organized in bundles. In the surface layer, an anteroposterior orientation is present.[27] The bundles spread out in various directions into the anterior and posterior bands and toward the attachments.

In both hyaline cartilage and fibrocartilage, the collagen fibrils create a three-dimensional network in which the proteoglycan aggregates are entangled (Figs. 4–14 and 4–15).[16, 17] This similarity suggests that both types of cartilage have comparable mechanical properties. Therefore, it seems likely that the mechanisms on which these properties are based also occur in the fibrocartilage of the TMJ, including the articular disc.

DISCUSSION

One of the early degenerative changes due to osteoarthrosis in synovial joints is an increase of water content in the articular cartilage.[4] Proteoglycans are able to swell only by imbibing water when not counteracted by the collagen fibrils. Thus, changes in collagen fibril organization probably permits proteoglycans to bind more water and subsequently to swell. Therefore, as postulated by Freeman and Meachim,[3] collagen network disintegration most likely is the starting point of osteoarthrosis. From this point of view, knowledge about the structure and biochemistry of the fibrous component of the articular cartilage is important for the understanding of both the normal physiology and the initial pathologic alterations of synovial joints, particularly of the articular cartilage.

The arrangement of collagen fibrils in articular hyaline cartilage according to a system of arcades has been described by Benninghoff.[28] According to this investigator,

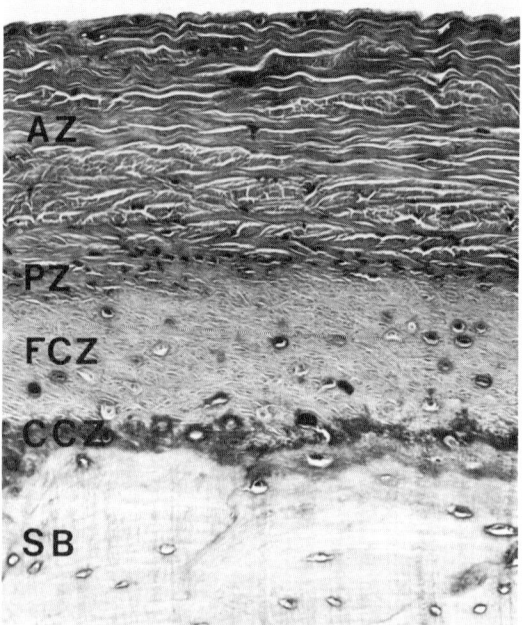

Figure 4–13. Detail of normal articular cartilage of the mandibular condyle showing the different zones. AZ = Articular zone; PZ = proliferative zone; FCZ = fibrocartilaginous zone; CCZ = calcified cartilage zone; SB = subchondral bone. (Transmitted light, hematoxylin and eosin, magnification × 200.) (Reprinted with permission from de Bont LGM, de Haan P, Boering G: Structuur en bouw van het kraakbeen van het Kaakgewricht. Ned Tijdschr Tandheelkd 92:184–189, 1985.)

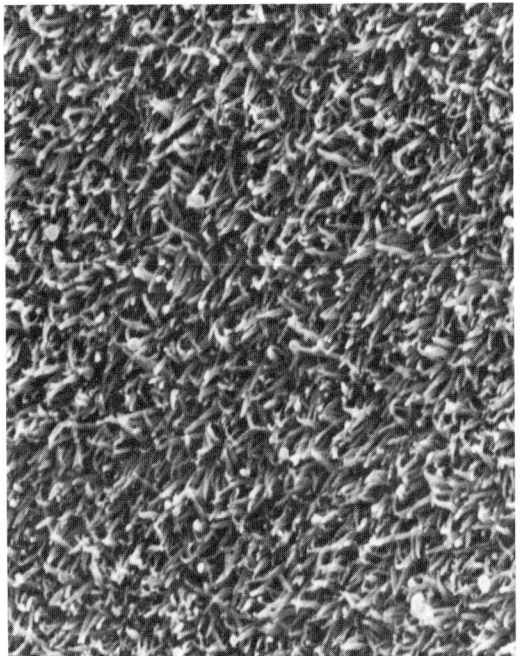

Figure 4–14. Scanning electron microscopic image of femoral articular cartilage (hyaline cartilage) at a saw-cut surface showing the individual collagen fibrils in a dense homogeneous network, without a zonal or bundle-like orientation. (Magnification × 6440.)

the collagen fibrils are anchored in the subchondral bone, radiating toward the surface, where they form an arc, and running back to the subchondral bone. The same features, concerning the arrangement of collagen fibrils in the articular fibrocartilage of the mandibular condyle, have been described by Steinhardt.[29] However, Benninghoff's and Steinhardt's results were based on observations by polarized LM, a method with several limitations. The individual collagen fibril, which should normally have a width of less than 110 nm, is not observable by LM. Therefore, for investigations of the arrangement of collagen fibrils, a more sophisticated imaging technique such as electron microscopy is needed (see Figs. 4–14 and 4–15). Electron microscopic studies show that the collagen fibrils in hyaline cartilage are organized in a three-dimensional network of randomly oriented fibrils and that the collagen fibrils in fibrocartilage are organized in a network with different arrangements of the fibrils in the different zones of the articular cartilage.[16, 17]

Collagen fibril arrangement is more complicated than can be concluded from studies using LM. Due to the interdependence of form and function, the organization and arrangement of collagen fibrils, like the organization of bone trabeculae in cancellous bone, is likely to be related to the pattern of forces working on the articular cartilage.[30] Therefore, it is to be expected that the organization of the fibrils in the different zones of the articular cartilage of the TMJ is in accordance with the function of each zone (see Figs. 4–12 and 4–13).

Remodeling, which is functional adaptability in response to mechanical loading, takes place in articular cartilage and subchondral bone.[31] The TMJ obeys the same biologic laws as all other synovial joints and their associated musculoskeletal components.[32] Nevertheless, when comparing articular cartilage of the TMJ with that of other synovial joints, there are differences, such as the presence of undifferentiated mesenchymal cells in the proliferative zone of the cartilage covering of the mandibular condyle. These cells probably give the TMJ a great re-

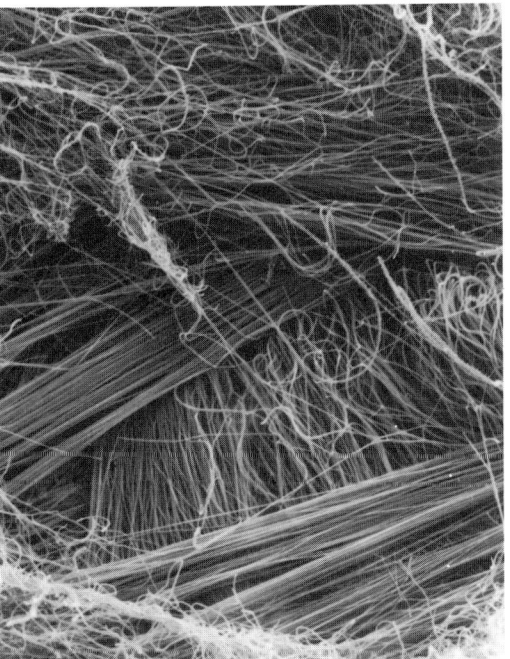

Figure 4–15. Scanning electron microscopic image of the articular surface of the mandibular condyle (fibrocartilage), showing the individual fibrils in the interwoven collagen fiber bundles. (Magnification × 1400.) (Reprinted with permission from de Bont LGM, de Haan P, Boering G: Structuur en bouw van het kraakbeen van het Kaakgewricht. Ned Tijdschr Tandheelkd 92:184–189, 1985.)

modeling potential and repair capacity.[33-36]

The role of synovial fluid as a lubricant in the normal TMJ is underestimated. Articular cartilage receives its nutrition from the synovial fluid that is produced by the synovial membrane. Therefore, the synovial membrane seems to play a key role in the normal physiology of synovial joints.

ACKNOWLEDGMENT

Illustrations and several parts of this chapter are reprinted from the Dutch Dental Journal *(Nederlands Tijdschrift voor Tandheelkunde)*[6] *with permission of the publisher.*

References

1. Boering G: Temporomandibular joint arthrosis: An analysis of 400 cases. Leiden: Stafleu & Tholen, 1966.
2. Sokoloff L: The pathology of osteoarthrosis and the role of ageing. In Nuki G (ed): The Aetiopathogenesis of Osteoarthrosis. London: Pitman Medical, 1980, pp 1–15.
3. Freeman MAR, Meachim G: Ageing and degeneration. In Freeman MAR (ed): Adult Articular Cartilage, 2nd Ed. London: Pitman Medical, 1979, pp 487–540.
4. Maroudas A. Physiochemical properties of articular cartilage. In Freeman MAR (ed): Adult Articular Cartilage, 2nd Ed. London: Pitman Medical, 1979, pp 215–290.
5. Boering G: Anatomical and physiological considerations regarding the temporomandibular joint. Int Dent J 29:245–251, 1979.
6. de Bont LGM, de Haan P, Boering G: Structuur en bouw van het kraakbeen van het Kaakgewricht. Ned Tijdschr Tandheeld, 92:184–189, 1985.
7. Myers ER, Mow VC: Biomechanics of cartilage and its response to biomechanical stimuli. In Hall BK (ed): Cartilage, Vol 1. New York: Academic Press, 1983, pp 313–341.
8. Hukins DWL: Biomechanical properties of collagen. In Weiss JB, et al (eds): Collagen in Health and Disease. Edinburgh: Churchill Livingstone, 1982, pp 49–72.
9. Ghadially FN: Fine structure of synovial joints. A Text and Atlas of the Ultrastructure of Normal and Pathological Articular Tissues. London: Butterworths, 1983.
10. Mow VC, Holmes MH, Lai WM: Fluid transport and mechanical properties of articular cartilage: A review. J Biomech 17:377–394, 1984
11. Helminen HJ, Jurvelin J, Kivirante I, et al: Joint loading effects on articular cartilage: A historical review. In Helminen HJ, et al (eds): Joint Loading. Biology and Health of Articular Structures. Bristol: Wright, 1987, pp 1–46.
12. Meachim G, Stockwell RA: The matrix. In Freeman MAR (ed): Adult Articular Cartilage, 2nd Ed. London: Pitman Medical, 1979, pp 1–67.
13. Hansson T, Öberg T, Carlsson GE, Kopp S: Thickness of the soft tissue layers and the articular disk in the temporomandibular joint. Acta Odontol Scand 35:77–83, 1977.
14. Stockwell RA: Biology of Cartilage Cells. Cambridge: Cambridge University Press, 1979.
15. Blackwood HJJ: The temporomandibular joint: Development, structure and function. In Cohen B, et al (eds): Scientific Foundations of Dentistry. London: Heinemann, 1976, pp. 590–595.
16. de Bont LGM, Boering G, Havinga P, Liem RSB: Spatial arrangement of collagen fibrils in the articular cartilage of the mandibular condyle: An LM and SEM study. J Oral Maxillofac Surg 42:306–313, 1984.
17. de Bont LGM, Liem RSB, Havinga P, et al: Collagenous network in cartilage of human femoral condyles. A light microscopic and scanning electron microscopic study. Acta Anat 126:41–47, 1986.
18. de Bont LGM, Liem RSB, Boering G: Ultrastructure of the articular cartilage of the mandibular condyle: Ageing and degeneration. Oral Surg Oral Med Oral Pathol 60:631–641, 1985.
19. Toller PA: Ultrastructure of the condylar articular surface in severe mandibular pain-dysfunction syndrome. Int J Oral Surg 6:297–312, 1977.
20. Junqueira LC, Carneiro J: Functionele Histologie. 2e dr. (Vert. James J, et al.) Utrecht: Bunge, 1982.
21. Weiss JB, Ayad S: An introduction to collagen. In Weiss JB, et al (eds): Collagen in Health and Disease. Edinburgh: Churchill Livingstone, 1982, pp 1–17.
22. Mayen R, Von der Mark K: Collagens of cartilage. In Hall BK, (ed): Cartilage, Vol 1. New York: Academic Press, 1983, pp 181–214.
23. Muir IHM: The chemistry of the ground substance of joint cartilage. In Sokoloff L (ed): The Joints and Synovial Fluid, Vol 2. New York: Academic Press, 1980, pp 28–94.
24. Hascall VC, Hascall GH: Proteoglycans. In Hay ED (ed): Cell Biology of Extracellular Matrix. New York: Plenum, 1981, pp 39–63.
25. Lash JW, Vasan NS: Glycosaminoglycans of cartilage. In: Hall BK (ed): Cartilage, Vol 1. New York: Academic Press, 1983, pp 215–251.
26. Broom ND, Marra DL: New structural concept of articular cartilage demonstrated with a physical model. Connect Tissue Res 14:1–8, 1985.
27. de Bont LGM, Liem RSB, Boering G: Fibrous component of the temporomandibular joint disc. J Craniomandib Pract 3:368–373, 1985.
28. Benninghoff A: Form und Bau der Gelenkknorpel in ihren Beziehungen zur Function. II. Der Aufbau des Gelenkknorpels in seinen Beziehungen zur Funktion. Z Zellforsch Mikrosk Anat 2:783–862, 1925.
29. Steinhardt G: Funktion und strukturelle Veränderungen der Kiefergelenke. In Schön F, et al (eds): Eruopäische Prothetik heute. Berlin: Quintessenz, 1978, pp 515–525.
30. Bollough P, Goodfellow J: The significance of the fine structure of articular cartilage. J Bone Joint Surg (Br) 50:852–857, 1968.
31. Sokoloff L: Loading and motion in reaction to ageing and degeneration of joints: Implications for prevention and treatment of osteoarthritis. In Helminen HJ, et al (eds): Joint Loading. Biology and Health of Articular Structures. Bristol: Wright, 1987, pp 412–424.
32. Moffett BC: Classification and diagnosis of temporomandibular joint disturbances. In Solberg WK, et al

(eds): Temporomandibular Joint Problems. Biologic Diagnosis and Treatment. Chicago: Quintessence 1980, pp 21–31.
33. Blackwood HJJ: Cellular remodeling in articular tissue. J Dent Res 45:480–489, 1966.
34. Hansson T, Nordström B: Thickness of the soft tissue layers and articular disk in temporomandibular joints with deviations in form. Acta Odontol Scand 35:281–288, 1977.
35. Durkin JF, Heeley JD, Irving JT: Cartilage of the mandibular condyle. *In* Zarb GA, et al (eds): Temporomandibular Joint Function and Dysfunction. St. Louis: Mosby, 1979, pp 43–100.
36. Öberg T, Carlsson GE: Macroscopic and microscopic anatomy of the temporomandibular joint. *In* Zarb GA, et al (eds): Temporomandibular Joint Function and Dysfunction. St. Louis: Mosby, 1979, pp 101–118.

Chapter 5

PATHOPHYSIOLOGY OF TEMPOROMANDIBULAR JOINT DISORDERS

ROBERT D. SCHWARTZ, D.M.D.

By definition, pathophysiology is the study of how normal physiologic processes are altered by disease.[1] To understand the various temporomandibular joint (TMJ) disorders and physiologic processes that are affected, an appreciation of the basic joint and supporting structures is a prerequisite. This includes the relationships between muscles, tendons, ligaments, cartilage, capsule, bone, and synovial fluid and how those structures interact to distribute biomechanical forces or stresses.

The basic structures of synovial joints consist of articular cartilage, disc, synovium, capsule, and subchondral bone.[2] The articular structures require a thin layer of healthy synovial fluid for an optimal functional relationship, allowing for low-friction load-bearing.[3] Effective joint lubrication is accomplished through a complex biomechanical mechanism and, although not fully understood, is imperative for normal function.[4-6]

The functional demands placed on synovial joints elicit biochemical, biomechanical, and biosynthetic adaptive mechanisms (remodeling and reparative processes) from these structures. Connective tissue cells in both condensed and loose tissues are embedded in an abundant extracellular matrix composed of collagen, proteoglycans, elastin, fibronectin, and other proteins. The majority of connective tissues have a great regenerative capacity, displaying remarkable cellular proliferation and biosynthetic activity, particularly in response to injury. Under normal conditions a relatively active turnover exists, with continuous degradation and replacement of macromolecular components.[7]

When the physiologic limits of adaptive capacity (repair and remodeling) of the joint structures are exceeded, a degradation process prevails. This process consists of complex interactions between biomechanical, biochemical, inflammatory, immunologic, and metabolic reactions that can lead to dysfunctional and disease states. In diffuse connective tissue diseases, critical events take place not only in the synovium but also in the interstitial tissue throughout the body. The interaction between the primary cellular and macromolecular components of the connective tissue (fibroblasts and their relatives, extracellular proteins, and ground substance) and inflammatory cells (monocytes, lymphocytes, mast cells, and polymorphonuclear leukocytes) and their products is probably crucial to the pathogenesis and outcome of many rheumatic diseases.[7, 8] Degradative enzymes located in the chondrocytes of articular cartilage and in the cells of the synovial membrane are capable of breaking down proteoglycans. An activation factor that is synthesized by synovium stimulates the proliferation of activated T cells as well as the chondrocytes to produce collagenase and a neutral metalloprotease.[9-12]

These degradative mechanisms can alter and affect the integrity of the articular cartilage (chondromalacia), the cellular response of the synovium (nutritional and lubrication deficiency, inflammation, activation of degradative enzymes, and fibrosis), the disc (position, mobility, morphology, and histopathology), the capsule (fibrosis and contracture), and the subchondral bone (microfracture, osteophyte formation, subchondral cysts, and eburnation), as seen in osteoarthritis.[2]

The articular cartilage is composed of two basic elements. The first is the cellular component, which is composed of chondrocytes and fibrocytes that sustain the cartilage. The second element is the matrix, which surrounds these cells and gives the cartilage its compressibility, tensile strength, and shock-absorbing mechanism. The matrix is mainly composed of collagen fibrils and hydrophilic proteoglycans; glycoproteins, small fractions of lipids, and inorganic material are also present. The mechanical function of the collagen fibers is to resist tensile loads. Any change in the integrity or orientation of the fibers may alter the tensile strength of the cartilage as a whole. The ground substance is that part of the matrix that does not possess collagen. The ground substance of the articular cartilage contains a significant amount of water due to the hydrophilic nature of the proteoglycans.[2, 13, 14] The osmotic pressure of the ground substance causes the water from the synovial fluid to infuse into the articular cartilage. The collagen fibrils resist the expansion of the ground substance, which places them under tension when the joint is unloaded. When the joint is loaded, hydrostatic pressure exceeds the osmotic pressure of the matrix, and water is compressed out of the matrix and into the joint space.[13] Depletion of ground substance causes water loss, reduced turgor, and softening of the articular cartilage.[15]

Several physiologic processes contribute to the normal dynamics of the TMJ. When these processes are interfaced with systemic disease or localized pathology and dysfunction, pathophysiologic processes become involved, including nutritional deprivation of articular cartilage and the disc, impairment of joint lubrication, inflammation, proliferation of fibrous connective tissue (adhesions), and the activation and synthesis of degradative enzymes.

NUTRITIONAL IMPAIRMENT OF ARTICULAR CARTILAGE

The avascular, alymphatic, and aneural tissue of the articulating cartilage derives its nutrition from the synovial fluid through diffusion gradients. Mechanical activities (intermittent loading) act as a pump to aid in this diffusion process.[15]

In the synovium, essential nutrients are present in the blood stream perfusing the local tissue. Synovial microvessels contain fenestrations that appear to be sites of diffusion exchange between plasma and the surrounding interstitium (Fig. 5-1). Free diffusion provides equilibration of small solutes between plasma and the immediate interstitial space. Further diffusion extends this equilibration process to include all other intracapsular spaces including the synovial fluid and the interstitial fluid of cartilage. The narrow pathway between synovial cells

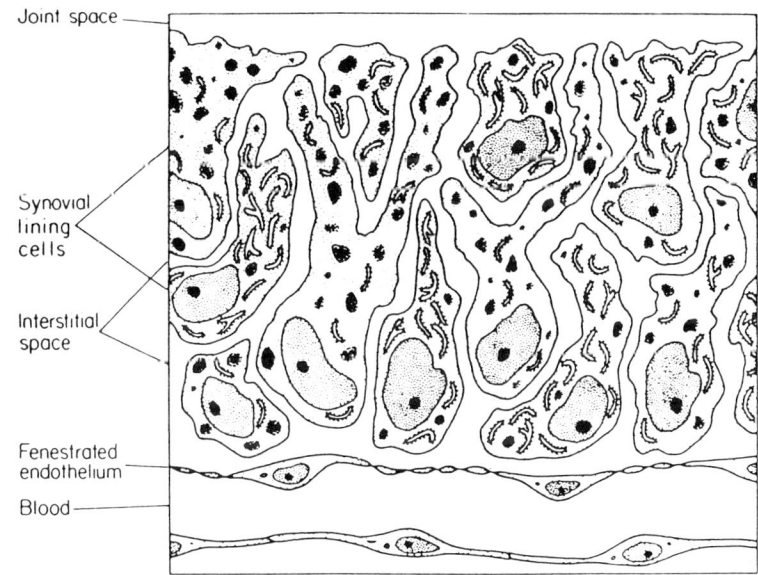

Figure 5-1. Diffusion exchange between blood plasma and synovial tissue is determined by molecular size. The narrow pathways of the interstitial spaces are filled with large hyaluronate molecules. Those molecules, as well as the endothelial fenestrations, serve to limit the overall exhange of nutrients. (Reprinted with permission from Simkin PA: Synovial physiology. *In* McCarty DJ (ed): Arthritis and Allied Conditions. Philadelphia: Lea & Febiger, 1989.)

appears to be the principal barrier limiting the overall exchange between plasma and synovial fluid of nutrients and of metabolic waste products in the opposite direction. This unidirectional transport system of plasma proteins enhances the delivery of glucose across this barrier. No other specific transport systems have yet been identified.[16-18]

Local evidence of intrasynovial circulatory metabolic imbalance provides a second instance when the delivery and removal of small solutes become clinically relevant. In normal TMJs, as well as in most pathologic effusions, essentially full equilibrium exists between plasma and synovial fluid. The gradients that drive the net exchange of nutrients (glucose and oxygen) and removal of wastes (lactate and carbon dioxide) are too small to be detectable. In some cases, however, the synovial microvascular supply is unable to meet the local metabolic demand, and significant gradients develop. In these joints, the synovial fluid develops low oxygen pressure (PO_2), low glucose, low pH, high lactate, and high carbon dioxide pressure (PCO_2). Such fluids are found in septic arthritis, often in rheumatoid disease, and infrequently in other kinds of synovitis.[17]

Plasma proteins also can enter synovial fluid by passive diffusion. The microvasculature is the major barrier limiting the escape of plasma proteins into the synovial interstitium. The protein path across the endothelium is not yet clear. Conflicting experimental evidence tends to indicate that fenestrae, intercellular junctions, and cytoplasmic vesicles are predominant sites of plasma protein escape. What is clear is that the process follows diffusion kinetics regardless of the exact pathway. This means that smaller proteins, which have faster diffusion coefficients, will enter the joint space at rates proportionately faster than large proteins with relatively slow diffusion coefficients. Large proteins such as IgM and α_2-macroglobulin are under-represented, whereas smaller proteins are present in relatively higher concentrations.[16, 19] Some evidence, although limited, suggests that ion charge may also be important. However, size appears to be the principal determinant of relative synovial permeability among different plasma proteins.[20]

In contrast, proteins leave synovial fluid by bulk flow through lymphatic vessels. This process does not seem to be size-selective or even constant between joints or between individuals. In particular, joints of patients affected by rheumatoid arthritis experience significantly more rapid removal of proteins than do those of patients with osteoarthritis.[21] Thus, in all joints, there is a continuing passive transport of plasma proteins involving the synovial microvasculature, diffusion across the epithelium, and ultimate return to the venous plasma through lymphatic vessels.[16, 19]

The intrasynovial concentration of any protein represents the net contributions of plasma concentration, synovial blood flow, microvascular permeability, and lymphatic removal. In addition, specific proteins may be produced or consumed within the joint space. For instance, lubricin normally is synthesized within synovial cells and released into synovial fluid, where it facilitates boundary layer lubrication of the cartilage-on-cartilage bearing. In disease, additional proteins may be synthesized, such as IgG rheumatoid factor in rheumatoid arthritis, or released by inflammatory cells, such as lysosomal enzymes. Similarly, intra-articular proteins may be depleted by local consumption, as are complement components in rheumatoid disease. Examining and quantifying the contributions of these various factors in determining the intrasynovial concentrations of any protein are now possible. Drawing conclusions about any one factor unless the other contributing mechanisms have also been examined could be dangerously simplistic.[19]

Clinicians have often used the concentration of protein to determine whether a given effusion represents a transudate or an exudate in cavities other than joints. By implication, the former is thought to represent a fluid collection driven by changes in the balance of microvascular hydrodynamics, whereas the latter is attributed to inflammation-induced changes in the microvascular permeability of proteins. In synovial fluid, however, protein concentrations vary little between highly inflamed rheumatoid joints and modestly involved osteoarthritic articulations. Microvascular permeability to protein is, in fact, more than twice as great in rheumatoid arthritis than it is in osteoarthritis. This marked difference to permeability, however, leads to only a minimal increase in protein concentration, because the resultant enhanced ingress of proteins is largely offset by a comparable rise in lymphatic egress. These findings illustrate the fact that synovial microvascular permeability cannot be evaluated from protein concentrations unless the kinetics of delivery or removal are concurrently assessed.[16, 19] Any change in the quality of synovial fluid or the pump action jeopardizes nutrition of the articular cartilage, leading to chondromalacia. Diseases involving the synovial membrane that change the viscosity or alter the elements of the synovial fluid, such as rheumatoid disease, sepsis, or any metabolic disorder such as gout or pseudogout, can lead to depletion of the ground substance and eventually to degeneration of the joint surface.

Nutrient qualities can be impaired by a decrease in the production and quality of the synovial fluid, hemorrhage (hemarthrosis), and granulation tissue or fibrin deposits within the synovium.[22] Certain specific clinical situations can also lead to nutritional impairment. Recurrent hemorrhage into a joint can lead to chondromalacia. Unfavorable loads (i.e., chronic bruxism) may cause excessive sustained loads to the articular cartilage, interfere with nutrition of the articular cartilage, and result in loss of chondrocytes and ground substance. Inactivity, such as prolonged immobilization of the joint, slows down the diffusion of nutrients to articular cartilage, also leading to chondromalacia. Repetitive intra-articular injection of cortical steroid results in depletion of ground substance, in turn causing articular cartilage to become soft and fibrillated.[15]

IMPAIRMENT OF JOINT LUBRICATION

In normal human synovial joints, a thin layer of synovial fluid covers the surfaces of the synovium, disc, and cartilage within the joint space. The synovial fluid penetrates the surface layer of the articular cartilage, thereby separating synovial cells, chondrocytes, and fibrocytes from the collagen fibrils and preventing direct contact between them.[2] The mechanics of joint lubrication have been the focus of productive investigations. Although all questions have not been resolved, certain principles are generally accepted. One of these rests on the fact that articular cartilage is elastic, fluid-filled, and supported by a relatively impervious layer of calcified cartilage and bone. This means that compression of a loaded area will force underlying fluid to flow laterally and to then be expressed through the surface of adjacent, unloaded cartilage. As that area in turn slides under the load, its surface is partially protected by the newly expressed fluid. This is a special form of hydrodynamic lubrication, so-named because the dynamic motion of the surface-bearing areas continually produces an aqueous layer that serves to separate and protect the bearing surface. This has also been termed "weeping" lubrication.[16, 23, 24]

Boundary layer lubrication is the second major mechanism considered important in achieving the low-friction load-bearing characteristic of normal joints. Here, a layer of water is physically bound to the cartilaginous surface. The binding agent is a small glycoprotein called lubricin. A number of independent lines of investigation all support the critical role of this synovium-derived molecule. Its lubricating properties are highly specific and are dependent on its ability to bind to articular cartilage and retain water molecules at the site of this interaction. Lubricin is not an effective lubricant in artificial systems and therefore cannot be used to lubricate artificial joints.[16, 25]

Thus, boundary lubrication properties and hydrodynamic lubrication properties are occurring simultaneously. The combination of these two properties has been termed elastohydrodynamic lubrication.[2]

A number of lubricating mechanisms have been proposed, some of which remain under active investigation. It is interesting, however, that hyaluronic acid, the molecule that makes synovial fluid viscous, has been largely excluded as a significant contributor to lubrication of the cartilage-on-cartilage bearing surfaces. Instead, hyaluronate is now thought to lubricate quite different sites of surface contact, those of synovium on cartilage and synovium on synovium.[26] Surrounding the load-bearing areas of articular cartilage are even larger surface areas of synovial lining. This well-vascularized, well-innervated tissue must alternately fold upon itself and then expand to cover nonloaded cartilage surfaces as each joint moves through its normal range of motion.

The coefficient of friction between the surfaces of synovial joints is approximately 1.002, where a friction-free coefficient would be 1.[27, 28] Synovial fluid viscosity is due to the presence of sodium hyaluronate, which is a sulfate-free glycosaminoglycan. Synovial fluid exhibits viscous properties owing to the number, size, configuration, and interaction of sodium hyaluronic acid molecules. Normal synovial fluid behaves as a viscous fluid at low-strain frequencies (slow-moving joint), exhibiting thixotropic flow properties.[2, 29] The more slowly it flows, the more viscous it becomes. Synovial fluid viscosity is determined by hyaluronate concentration and provides lubrication peripherally between the synovial lining surfaces and both the articular surface and other synovial lining surfaces.

Pathologic fluids found in arthritis and other joint traumas (e.g., infection, inflammation, hemorrhage, and arthroscopy) exhibit diminished viscosity due to decreased hyaluronate concentrations.[2] Under those conditions, the functional integrity of the synovial surfaces is vulnerable to increased frictional wear and abrasion as those surfaces slide by each other. Thus, a reduction in synovial fluid viscosity leads to irritation of the synovial lining (Fig. 5–2).

Balazs has described another property of synovial fluid that involves transformation from a viscous fluid to an elastic body.[30, 31] This phenomenon occurs in response to high-strain frequencies (rapidly moving loaded joint) and serves to function as a shock absorbing mechanism to protect articular cartilage from damage. With aging and in osteoarthritic joints, synovial fluid loses its capacity to form elastic bodies, owing to an alteration in quality and quantity of synovial fluid. Thus, under conditions of high loading, the articular surfaces become abraded, resulting in chondromalacia and degenerative changes. Leakage of proteoglycans into the joint space produces irritants that perpetuate the inflammatory response of the synovium. A decrease in viscosity of the synovial fluid also leaves the articular cartilage vulnerable to the inflow of enzyme activators (catabolins), which are derived from the synovium. The catabolins (mononuclear cell factor, interleukin-1), which are low molecular weight proteins, stimulate the proliferation of activated T cells and stimulate the cells of the articular cartilage to produce degradative enzymes (neutral metalloproteinases, collagenases, and proteoglycanase). These enzymes are capable of degrading the protein core of proteoglycans and the collagen fibrils of the articular cartilage. This process leads to chondromalacia and degenerative joint disease.[9–12]

Summary

The effects of impairment of lubrication and nutrition of the articular surfaces as a result of the pathophysiologic processes described may be summarized as follows:

1. Deterioration of collagen fibrils.
2. Depletion of ground substance causing water loss, reduced turgor, and softening, which leads to fissuring of the articular cartilage.

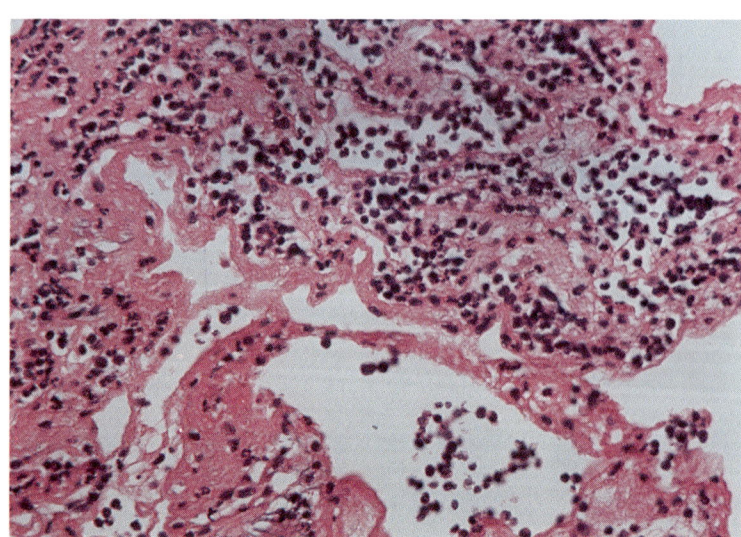

Figure 5–2. Acute synovitis with an intense inflammatory infiltrate and capillary proliferation.

3. Adherence of discal tissues and their attachments to articulating surfaces secondary to a decrease in viscosity of synovial fluid, inflammation and its by-products, and the proliferation of fibrous connective tissue adhesions.

INFLAMMATION

By definition, inflammation is the response of living tissues to injury. The vascular response is an essential component of inflammation, serving to deliver molecular components important to inflammation, as well as most mononuclear cellular elements, neutrophils, and mononuclear leukocytes, to sites of inflammation in the extracellular connective tissues. Under normal conditions, only small molecules are capable of being mobilized into the interstitial connective tissue.[33] If inflammation is present, larger molecules such as immunoglobulins, immune complexes, and complement components are able to migrate into the tissue. Inflammatory and immunologic events can influence both the synthesis and degradation of connective tissue in a number of circumstances in vitro. Inflammatory joint disease presents a histologic picture of an advancing edge of proliferating synovium and antibody-producing cells creeping along a cartilage surface and destroying it locally.[8]

The inflammatory process is necessary for protecting the host from sequelae resulting from various forms of injury. These include bacterial, viral, and parasitic infections, and thermal and mechanical wounds.

An integral component of inflammatory reactions is repair. In certain types of tissue injury, repair is the major beneficial result of inflammation, as in clean lacerations. In others, such as acute bacterial infections, the pathogens are eliminated and inflammation is resolved with a small amount of destruction. The same process initiated by the host to destroy foreign organisms and to repair injuries may be injurious to the host. This is readily observed in the tissue destruction associated with acute abscess formation or in chronic inflammatory diseases such as rheumatoid arthritis.[34]

Inflammation may be considered in two forms: acute and chronic. Both of these are often present simultaneously. Acute inflammation is usually the initial response, involving vascular responses with neutrophils or mast cells playing dominant roles. Chronic inflammation usually occurs later or is of longer duration, and is characterized by the presence of mononuclear cells, macrophages, lymphocytes, and plasma cells and by the proliferation of connective tissue fibroblasts (Fig. 5–3).[36, 37]

Local signs of inflammation include heat, redness, swelling, and pain. The first three of these largely result from the response of the vasculature to injury. A transient period of vasoconstriction occurs, followed by vasodilation of the microvasculature, resulting in arteriolar dilation. This may result in transudation of fluid with low protein content into the extracellular space.[33, 34] Subsequently, increased permeability of microvasculature through gaps in junctions between endothelial cells develops, resulting in exudation of fluid containing all plasma components into the extravascular spaces.[17, 19] The loss of plasma results in stasis of erythrocytes in the microvasculature from increased blood viscosity. Leukocytes will then adhere to the vascular endothelium, a process called margination, and will subsequently migrate through widened gap junctions between endothelial cells, and ultimately through the basement membrane into the extravascular spaces.[33, 34]

Bacteria, cell debris, foreign particles, or crystals, which precipitate the inflammatory process, are engulfed at the sites of inflammation by neutrophils and monocytes.[36, 37] Phagocytosis often results in elimination of injurious particles but, in the process, may lead to the release of degradative materials and cause further injury to normal tissue. Phagocytosis consists of a series of events that are preceded by recognition of foreign particles.[33] Most microorganisms are not recognized by phagocytes unless they are coated by serum constituents called opsonins. Opsonins include IgG antibodies to antigens on the surface of the microorganisms or the C3b fragment of the complement component, C3. Opsonins are recognized by specific receptors on the surfaces of neutrophils and macrophages, and binding of the opsonins initiates the process of phagocytosis.[39]

Synovial Type A cells found at the surface of the synovial membrane frequently have filopodia and micropinocytotic vesicles, and appear to act as phagocytes, keeping the joint free of debris. This activity is particularly

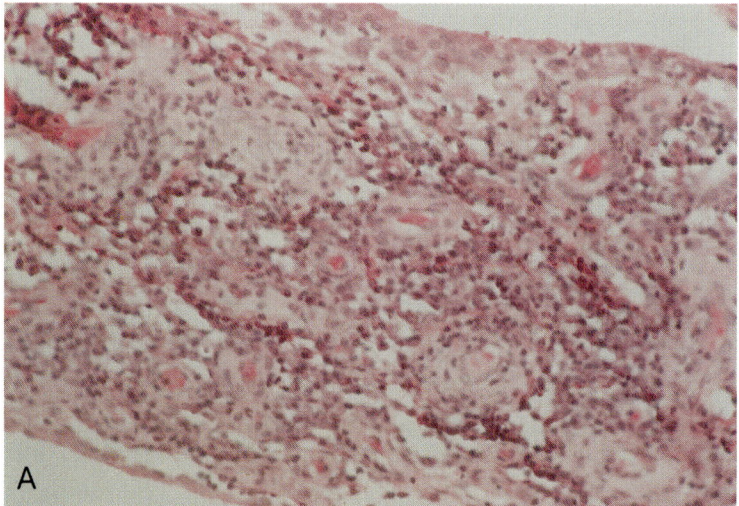
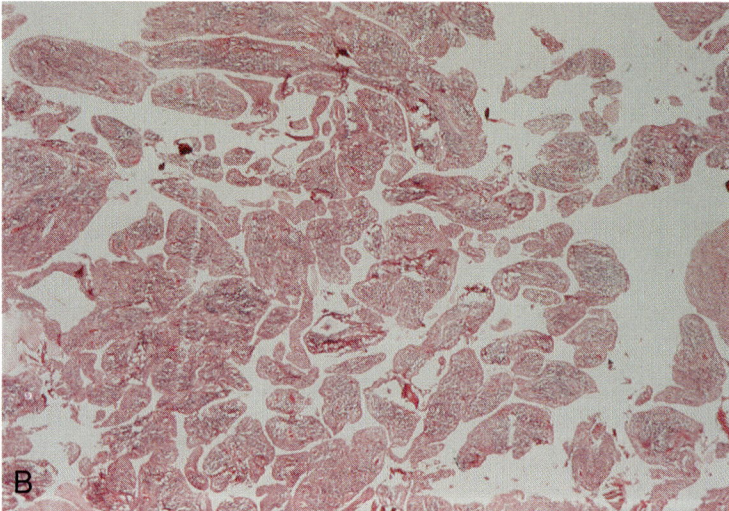

Figure 5–3. *A,* Synovial hyperplasia (low power). Villous hypertrophy with focal nodular inflammatory infiltrates. *B,* Hyperplastic lining of synovial cells with capillary proliferation and an intense plasmacytic infiltrate (high power).

noticeable in arthritic states, and these cells appear similar to subsynovial macrophages in this function.[2]

Phagocytosis begins when phagocytes surround particles with pseudopods or extensions of cytoplasmic membranes that are eventually used to enclose particles in phagocytic vacuoles that, in turn, fuse with membranes of lysosomes. Discharge of the contents of the lysosome into the phagolysosome exposes the engulfed particle to a variety of enzymes and oxygen free radicals potentially capable of degrading the particle. Some of these agents are lost into the extracellular environment, which may cause degradation of normal tissue and perpetuate the inflammatory process.[34] In rheumatoid arthritis, the antigens and antibodies interact in synovial tissues, fluid, and cartilage and give rise to an extravascular immune complex disease (Fig. 5–4). These complexes activate the complement cascade and generate a number of biologically active materials from the complement proteins.[35]

Mediators of Inflammation

The vascular and cellular events described previously, as well as destruction of microorganisms and other injurious agents, are brought about by a large number of chemicals and enzymes (mediators of inflammation). Many chemicals and enzymes have been described as having the capacity to elicit the responses of inflammation, and several of

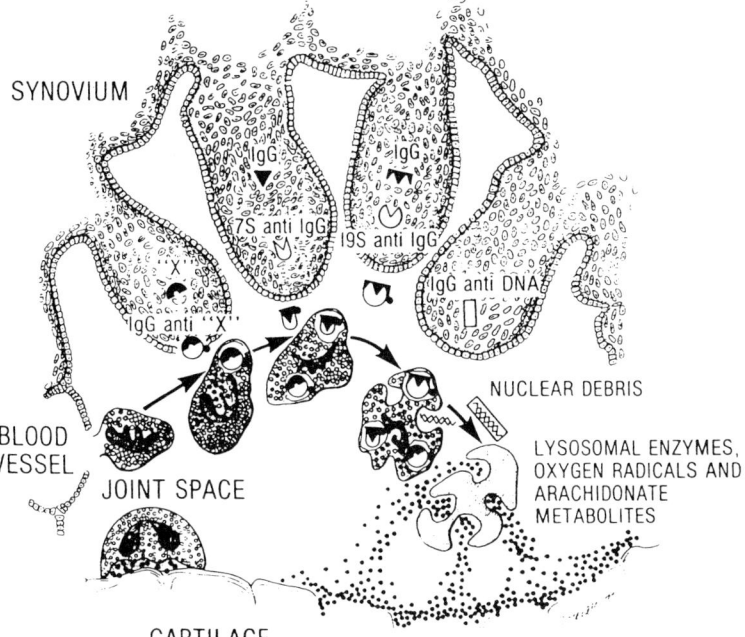

Figure 5-4. Schematic illustration of immune complex interaction in structures involved by rheumatoid arthritis. (Reprinted with permission from Zvaifler NJ: Etiology and pathogenesis of rheumatoid arthritis. *In* McCarty DJ (ed): Arthritis and Allied Conditions. Philadelphia: Lea & Febiger, 1989.)

these agents have similar activities. It is likely that two or more mediators acting synergistically can produce inflammatory effects that neither mediator is capable of producing alone. The inflammatory reactions resulting from various stimuli also may be dictated by different mediators.[34, 40]

Several classes of mediators have important roles in inflammation. These include the vasoactive amines, the complement system, the kinin system, the clotting system, prostaglandins (lipid-like agents), and a series of peptides known as chemotactic agents.[33, 40] Characteristics of these mediators (except the chemotactic agents) include the ability to increase vascular permeability (edema formation) and, in some types (e.g., bradykinin), to produce pain. All can change the blood flow to the inflammatory site by their ability to alter the bore of arterioles, since they can relax or constrict the smooth muscle of these vessels. The prostaglandins are particularly noteworthy because they not only have the properties mentioned above but also amplify the inflammatory properties of kinins and histamine.[34, 40]

Prostaglandins

One of the significant groups of chemical mediators are the prostaglandins. Prostaglandins are lipid-like molecules that are synthesized in almost all tissues from arachidonic acid. The synthesis is carried out by a number of enzymes present in the tissue that are generally termed prostaglandin synthetase. The synthesis is rapid, as is the release. There is no cell storage of prostaglandins. The many different prostaglandins are named by letter (D, E, F, I, etc.), based on their chemical structure.[41] A major property of the prostaglandins is their ability to amplify the pharmacologic properties of bradykinin and histamine, thus enhancing the action of these mediators by increasing vascular permeability (edema), as well as pain.[33, 34, 40] In addition, various prostaglandins have other properties of inflammation. They are synthesized and released in response to mechanical as well as chemical stimuli. Mechanical stimuli are involved during stretching and tugging of tissues. Chemical stimuli are agents such as kinins or histamine. Once kinins are released, they not only set up an inflammatory response but also may induce the synthesis and release of prostaglandins that amplify their actions.[39]

More specifically, a large number of biologically active metabolites are derived from reactions of oxygen with arachidonic acid to form prostaglandins, thromboxane, and leukotrienes (Fig. 5-5).[41] Arachidonic acid is an

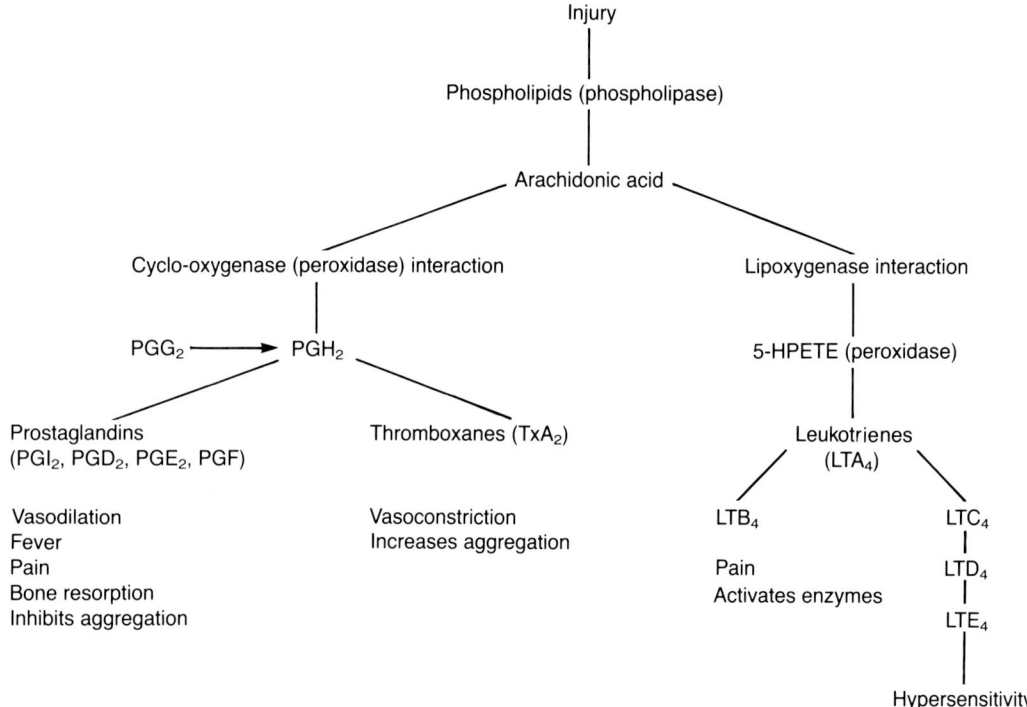

Figure 5–5. Arachidonic acid metabolites. Arachidonic acid is released from tissue phospholipids by phospholipase. Arachidonic acid interacts with oxygen through two processes. The cyclo-oxygenase process forms prostaglandin G_2 (PGG_2) and ultimately is catalyzed into various types of prostaglandins and thromboxanes. The lipoxygenase processes produce various leukotrienenes.

abundant fatty acid in the phospholipids of most tissues. Before conversion of arachidonic acid into mediators can occur, this fatty acid must be released by phospholipase. Cyclo-oxygenases are specialized lipoxygenases that catalyze the addition of molecular oxygen to arachidonic acid to form the endoperoxide intermediate compound prostaglandin G_2 (PGG_2). Peroxidase catalyzes the reduction of PGG_2 to form PGH_2. PGH_2 then may react with one of a number of enzymes called isomerases to become one of the prostaglandins (PGI_2, PGD_2, PGE_2, PGF_2) or thromboxanes. These compounds differ markedly in their biologic effects in spite of their similarities in structure.[41] Thromboxane A_2 is a powerful vasoconstrictor and causes platelet aggregation, whereas prostacyclin (PGI_2) causes vasodilation and opposes platelet aggregation.[42] Two prostaglandins, PGE_2 and PGI_2, are mediators of the vascular phase of inflammation. Both are potent vasodilators and act synergistically with certain other vasoactive mediators, such as histamine and kinins, to increase microvasculature permeability.[34, 41] Prostaglandins E_2 and I_2 also stimulate osteoclastic bone resorption, suggesting that bone erosion in chronic inflammatory diseases may be mediated, at least in part, by prostaglandins produced in inflamed tissues.[34, 41]

Although prostaglandins generally are incapable of causing tissue injury, it has been demonstrated that PGE_2 stimulates bone resorption in vitro and in vivo.[42–44] PGE_2 produced by rheumatoid synovia promotes resorption of bone in the absence of other major products of the rheumatoid tissue. In addition, rheumatoid synovial tissue in culture produces approximately 10 times more PGE_2 than does normal synovial tissue. It appears likely, therefore, that prostaglandins (particularly PGE_2) produced by hypertrophic and hyperplastic synovial tissue contribute to the destruction of the juxta-articular bone in rheumatoid arthritis. Since PGE compounds also inhibit collagen biosynthesis in vitro, enhanced production of prostaglandins by rheumatoid synovium may lead to additional detrimental effects in adjacent connective tissue.[34, 41]

Lipoxygenases catalyze the addition of oxygen in specific double bonds to polyunsaturated fatty acids, leading to a large number of hydroperoxy and hydroxy derivatives.[42, 45] The most important lipoxygenase pathway is the 5-lipoxygenase, which leads to several important derivatives. The distribution of 5-lipoxygenase products is more restricted than that of cyclo-oxygenase products. Leukocytes, including neutrophils, monocyte-macrophages, mast cells, and eosinophils, are the major sources of leukotrienes. The 5-lipoxygenase reaction involves the addition of molecular oxygen to the double bond in the 5 position of arachidonic acid to form 5-HPETE. The next step is a peroxidase reaction producing leukotriene A_4 (LTA_4). The LTA_4 intermediate is hydrolyzed to the stereospecific product leukotriene B_4 (LTB_4) by LTA_4 epoxide hydrolase. Alternatively, LTA_4 may react with glutathione, a glutathione-S-transferase catalyzed reaction, to form LTC_4. The three compounds LTC_4, LTD_4, and LTE_4 are called sulfidopeptide leukotrienes, and collectively they are responsible for the activity of the slow-reacting substance in anaphylaxis, an important mediator of immediate hypersensitivity reactions.[34, 41]

Products of the 5-lipoxygenase pathway are potentially important mediators of inflammation. Leukotriene B_4 is a chemoattractant for leukocytes, promotes the adherence of leukocytes to endothelial cells, and activates the secretion of active oxygen species and degradative enzymes from neutrophils. LTC_4, LTD_4, and LTE_4 contract smooth muscle in vascular, respiratory, and intestinal tissues.[34]

Quinn found significant concentrations of PGE_2 and LTB_4, via biochemical assay, in the synovial fluid of nineteen inflamed TMJs.[46] This clinical study corroborates the hypothesis that arachidonic acid metabolites play a role as a chemical mediator of inflammation in the TMJ. This information supports the hypothesis that arachidonic acid metabolites that lead to pain, dysfunction, and disease states in other synovial joints also afflict the TMJ.[47, 48]

Summary

The effects of the inflammatory process on synovial joints as a result of the pathophysiologic processes described may be summarized by the following:

1. Alteration of synovial fluid viscosity leading to impairment of lubrication and nutrition to the articular cartilage and disc.
2. Activation of degradative enzymes that have deleterious effects on synovium and articular cartilage.
3. Fibrosis of the synovial membrane in the form of adhesions.
4. Reactive and proliferative forms of synovitis.

CONNECTIVE TISSUE ADHESIONS

The arthroscopic observation of connective tissue adhesions in the TMJ has had a major impact on understanding the pathophysiology of TMJ disorders, particularly the dysfunctional aspects of disc-condylar mechanics.[49-51] Developing an appreciation of their development and their effects on joint mobility is an important step in understanding their role in the pathophysiology of TMJ disorders.

Adhesions are the result of an inflammatory process. If the process is severe, localized areas of synovial necrosis are produced and fibrin deposition occurs on the synovial surfaces. The fibrin and the areas of synovial necrosis form a scaffold on which permanent adhesions may be established (Fig. 5-6). The extent to which the synovial membrane is involved directly determines the loss of mo-

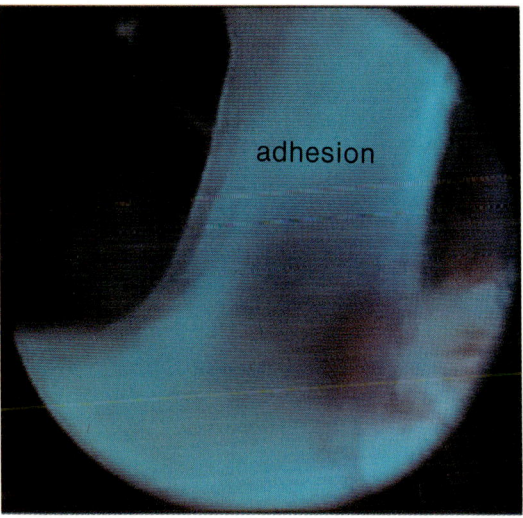

Figure 5-6. Fibrous adhesion in the anterior recess of the upper joint space of the right temporomandibular joint.

tion that results from this process.[51,52] It may be that in the majority of internal derangements the location of the disc may not be as important as its mobility, the elimination of the inflammatory process, and the identification and elimination of its etiology. This concept may be valid when the role of mesenchymal cells in repair and adaptive mechanisms is better understood. Mesenchymal cells have the potential to differentiate into synovial cells, fibrocytes, and chondrocytes, which contribute to the reparative and adaptive processes of synovium and articular cartilage in dysfunctional and diseased synovial joints.[53,54]

GROWTH FACTORS AND INFLAMMATION

A variety of growth factors, or cytokines, may contribute to the inflammatory process as well as affecting the cellular and matrix components of articular cartilage. Recent work has focused attention on both tumor necrosis factor (TNF), also called cachectin, and interleukin-1 (IL-1).[2,9,55]

TNF appears to have a broad range of activities on mesenchymal cells, including the chondrocyte-mediated breakdown of matrix proteoglycans in vitro. TNF, like IL-1, also can promote the release of collagenase and prostaglandin E_2 (PGE_2) by chondrocytes and synovial cells.[56]

IL-1 was originally identified as a factor activating lymphocytes but is now known to affect a variety of connective tissue cells as well. It appears to have binding sites on synovial cells and similar metabolic effects on mesenchymal target cells, such as synovial cells and chondrocytes.[57] Recent studies have also shown that IL-1 can affect collagen metabolism in explant cultures of cartilage by limiting the formation of Type II collagen in the chondrocyte.[58] In osteoarthritic cartilage, IL-1 may activate neutral, metal-dependent enzymes that degrade proteoglycans and produce proteoglycan species with a limited capacity to aggregate with hyaluronic acid. The intimate relationship between the synovial membrane and cartilage is relevant to the potential role of IL-1 in osteoarthritis.[12,59,60] IL-1 has been isolated from cells of the synovial lining[61] and is present in the synovial fluids from osteoarthritic joints.[62] As a consequence of the multiple factors contributing to cartilage damage, components of the matrix (e.g., proteoglycans and collagen) enter the joint fluid and are taken up by the cells in the synovial lining and induce the release of IL-1 and other cytokines. These in turn gain access to the cartilage, where they promote a metabolic function in the chondrocyte that is deleterious to the matrix and perpetuates a vicious cycle.[63]

BIOMECHANICAL STRESS DISTRIBUTION

The role of biomechanical loading (stress distribution) in the development of TMJ disorders depends on the integrity of a number of factors that contribute to the overall stability of a synovial joint.

In general, the load that is generated to the actively mobile joint is accompanied by kinetic energy. This energy is dissipated and distributed to the supporting articular components of the joint.[16] Synovial joints constantly adapt to functional demands by means of remodeling and repair.[64] When the load to the joint exceeds its adaptive capacity, the equilibrium between form and function may become disturbed, and degradation processes may commence.[65]

The loading phenomenon has been described in terms of either absolute or relative overloading, both of which have the potential to disturb the equilibrium between form and function and give rise to degradation of articular structures as seen in osteoarthritis.[66] Absolute overloading exists when abnormal and repetitive mechanical stresses exceed the functional capacity of normal articular tissues. Freeman and Meachim hypothesized that fatigue failure due to repetitive overloading results in a decreased collagen network stiffness, which leads to increased hydration of the proteoglycan-water gel.[63] Radin and colleagues hypothesized that cartilage breakdown is induced by a reduction in the resilience of subchondral bone due to microfractures as a result of excessive loading.[67,68]

Relative overloading occurs when normal loads are applied to a joint in which the functional capacity is intrinsically reduced. This may be seen when the quality or quantity of synovial fluid is impaired where the effects of frictional wear of articular cartilage and nutrient deprivation lead to the impairment of joint function. Biochemical, biomechanical, and inflammatory processes may contribute to the cycle that reduces the intrinsic capacity of the joint to adapt and repair.[66]

Normal joints distribute loading energy throughout their component parts. The greatest load of energy is taken up within the muscles and tendons supporting each joint. Effective reflexes normally ensure that impact forces are delivered to flexed joints. This means that the stress of loading is primarily opposed by involuntary contraction of striated muscles.[69]

Loading stress that is not absorbed by surrounding muscles, tendons, and ligaments impacts directly on the opposing cartilage surfaces and their underlying trabecular bone.[24] Despite the viscoelastic properties of articular cartilage, most loading energy is transmitted to the subchondral bone, as the cartilage is quite thin. Immediately beneath the cartilage is a continuous plate of subchondral bone supported by a complex meshwork of underlying trabeculae.[70]

The condylar heads of TMJs have trabecular patterns, which indicates that functional loading does occur in this joint.[71] The trabecular bone patterns of the condylar heads exhibit characteristic loading patterns in different types of maxillomandibular skeletal relationships. Loading of the condylar head influences trabecular size, number, alignment, and structural organization. Force vector analysis of compression loading indicates that trabecular alignment is parallel to the load force. Structural reinforcement is arranged so as to offer strength in parallel alignment to the forces applied.[72]

In a Class I skeletal relationship, condylar trabecular patterns exhibit loading in a posterior/inferior direction from the anterior aspect of the articular surface. The force vector is perpendicular to the plane of the eminence. Skeletal Class II open bites have a trabecular pattern that is sparse, with no distinct orientation. The lack of trabecular organization indicates that the condyle functions primarily in rotation without much translatory loading. Skeletal Class III relationships exhibit a trabecular and functional pattern similar to that of a Class II open bite. Skeletal Class II deep bites have a more dense trabecular pattern than any other skeletal relationship.[73]

These loading patterns correlate with known information regarding muscular function during mastication. Skeletal Class II open bites exhibit impaired muscular function. There is diminished electromyographic activity, decreased bite force, and decreased mechanical advantage. Skeletal Class II deep bites, however, exhibit significantly increased values in all these parameters.[74]

The nature of biomechanical load and its distribution to the subchondral bone appear to play a role in the degenerative changes of articular cartilage. Since osteoarthritic hyaline cartilage and fibrocartilage show a striking ultrastructural similarity, it is reasonable to believe that osteoarthritis in both types of cartilages develops with similar mechanisms where stress loading may be an important factor in the pathogenesis of osteoarthritis of the TMJ.[75]

DEGRADATIVE ENZYMES AND TISSUE INJURY

The proteinases are among the most important mediators of tissue injury and degradation.[33, 74, 77] Some are stored within lysosomes of leukocytes, whereas others are synthesized and secreted in response to inflammatory stimuli. They can be divided into two classes: those active in acid pH and those active in neutral pH. The former probably function to degrade bacteria and cell debris at low pH within phagolysosomes. At neutral pH, the extracellular activity of these enzymes does not appear to be significant. In the latter, several neutral proteinases (those active in neutral pH) degrade extracellular proteins in connective tissues. Both types of proteinases are derived from neutrophils, monocyte macrophages, fibroblasts, and other cells.[34]

Neutral proteinases can be divided into two groups: the metalloenzymes, which require metal ions such as zinc or calcium as a cofactor, and the serine proteinases, which have a serine hydroxyl group in their catalytically active sites. Collagenase initiates the degradation of extracellular or interstitial collagens. It is highly specific and cleaves both Type I (fibrocartilage) and Type II (hyaline cartilage) collagen, the major form of collagen in articular cartilage. Collagen must be in its native, triple-helical form to be cleaved by collagenase. One form of collagenase is produced by fibroblasts, macrophages, synovial cells, and endothelial cells whereas a different form of collagenase is produced by neutrophils.[78, 79]

Proteoglycanase is an enzyme that is capable of degrading proteoglycans by cleaving the proteoglycan core protein. It has been found in articular cartilage and may also be produced by rheumatoid synovial tissue (Fig. 5–7).[79]

Serine proteinases are located in the serum and represent a number of proteolytic enzymes that arise from the activation of compounds of several systems of proteins. Proteolytic enzyme activity is closely regulated in order to avoid uncontrolled degradation of tissue. Some metalloproteinases are stored in granules or lysosomes of neutrophils.[37] Release of stored enzymes can be stimulated by substances that activate neutrophils such as C5a and leukotriene B_4. Other proteolytic enzymes are synthesized in response to various stimuli. IL-1 markedly activates the synthesis of collagenase and their secretion by synovial cells, chondrocytes, and macrophages.[34, 79]

Metalloproteinases often are secreted as inactive precursors or proenzymes, which are activated by other proteolytic enzymes and certain chemical agents. Inhibitors of proteolytic enzymes normally are abundant in plasma and tissues and are essential in preventing undesired tissue degradation. Both metalloproteinases and serine proteinases are inhibited by α_2-microglobulin, a 720-kilodalton protein abundant in plasma. Another important inhibitor is called tissue inhibitor of metalloproteinases (TIMP), a 28-kilodalton molecular weight protein that inhibits proteases by complexing with them.[34]

It is apparent that the degradative enzymes play a major role in the progressive destruction of collagen and proteoglycans in articular cartilage in certain disease states. The effects of their activity can also perpetuate the inflammatory processes, leading to a vicious degradative cycle.[63] Until this cycle is interrupted by reducing the inflammatory process and creating an environment for repair, healing will remain impaired.

REPAIR, REMODELING, AND ADAPTATION

As previously described, synovial joints constantly adapt to the functional demands placed on the articular cartilage, disc, synovial membranes, and subchondral bone. TMJ articular cartilage demonstrates shifting equilibria in changes in form and function by tissue remodelings, as is seen in all synovial joints.[80]

Increased loading, either absolute or relative, may stimulate the biosynthesis of collagen fibrils and proteoglycans. The proliferative zone of the articular cartilage appears to play an important role in the remodeling process and repair capacity.[64] The repair process is limited by the ability of cartilage cells to proliferate and by the rate of cartilage matrix formation by these cells.[15] Undifferentiated mesenchymal cells located in the proliferative zone appear to play a role in repair

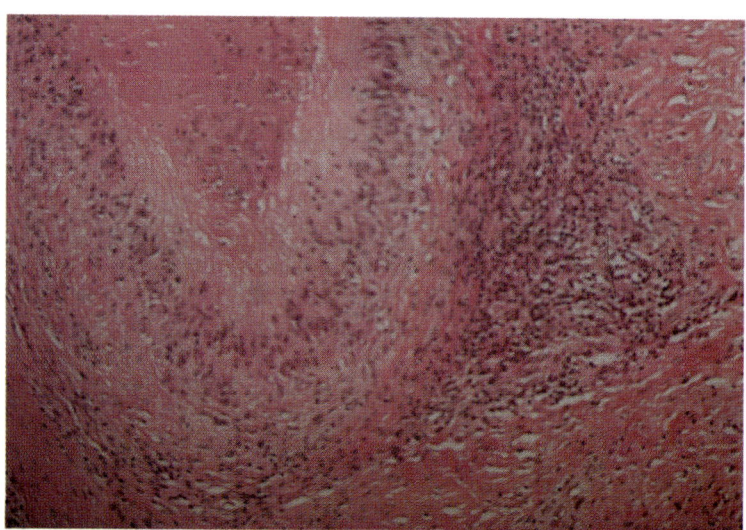

Figure 5–7. Histopathologic representation of a rheumatoid nodule. Note peripheral palisading histiocytes and central fibrinoid necrosis associated with a lymphocytic infiltrate.

by having the potential to differentiate into synovial cells, fibrocytes, and chondrocytes.[53, 54]

In osteoarthrosis, there is a gradual enlargement of the area of bone exposure secondary to abrasive wear. This leads to flattening and loss of bone. In the remodeling process, new bone and fibrous tissue may form in the periphery of the region of tissue destruction (peripheral remodeling), which can be visualized radiographically as osteophyte lipping (Fig. 5–8).[81, 82]

Even though it has been shown that articular surface irregularities are more often associated with deformed discs, and more severe changes are seen in completely anteriorly displaced discs, caution should be used before serial radiographic changes are inter-

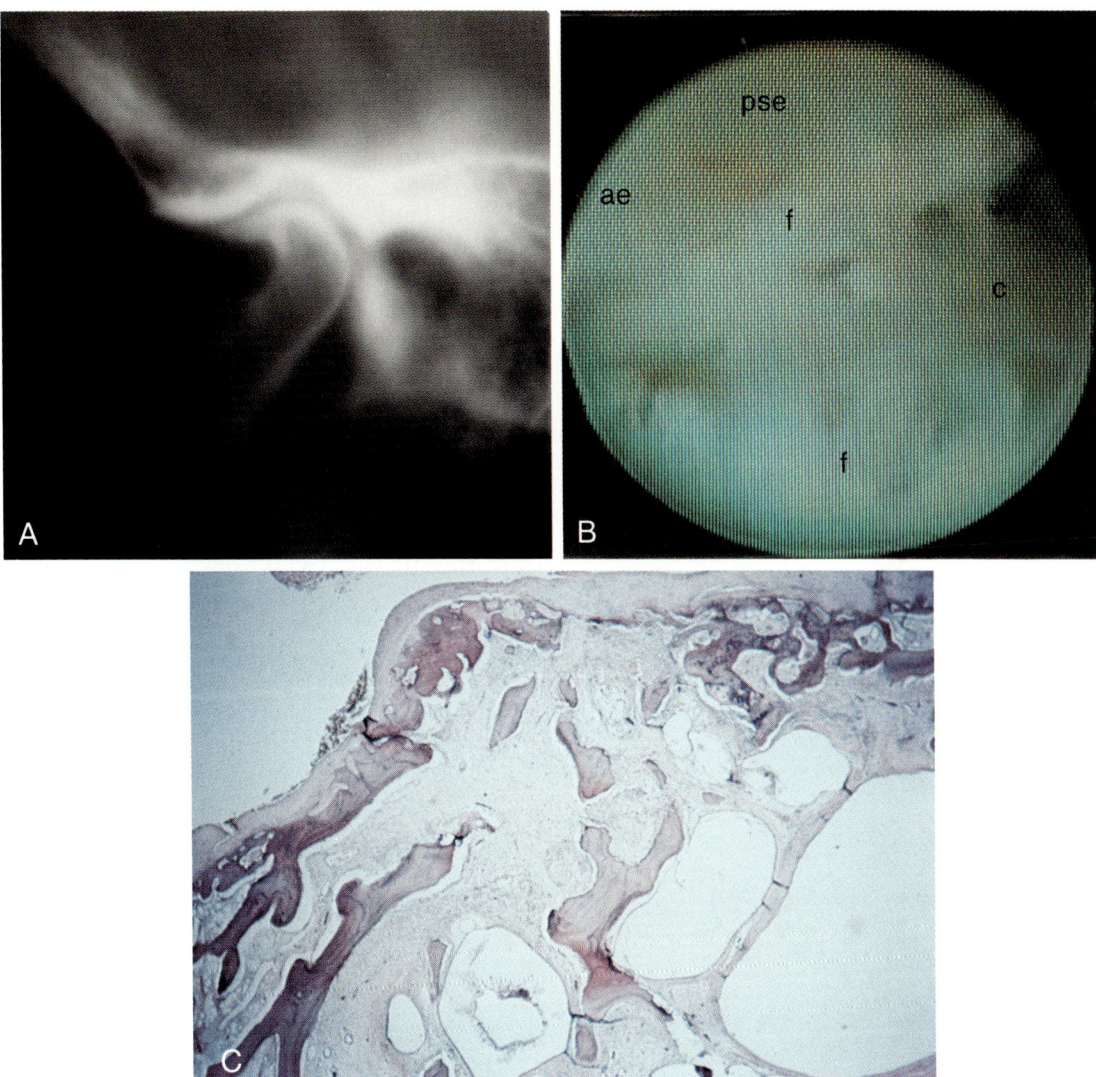

Figure 5–8. *A*, Radiograph of osteoarthrosis of the temporomandibular joint (TMJ) exhibiting flattening of anterior surface of condyle with peripheral remodeling. *B*, Arthroscopic view of osteoarthrosis demonstrating a central area of bone exposure on the condylar head of the left TMJ as well as the posterior slope of the eminence. Note the decrease of joint space, absence of the disc and its attachments, and fibrillation at the periphery. (ae = articular eminence; pse = posterior slope of articular eminence; f = fibrillations). *C*, Histopathology of osteoarthrosis. Note cartilage cover is markedly thinned with focal areas of complete disintegration. The subchondral bone is permeated by pink intertrabecular fibrocollagenous tissue. The fibrous component has undergone cystic changes. Subchondral cysts occur in both osteoarthritic and rheumatoid disease; cysts in rheumatoid bone characteristically are filled with granulation tissue (pannus) or dense fibrous scar; the cysts in osteoarthritic bone characteristically are filled with synovial fluid, gelatinous coagulum, or dense fibrous scar.

preted as degenerative when they might be described more accurately as adaptive remodeling.[83]

Inflammatory and immunologic events can influence both the synthesis and the degradation of connective tissue. Increased stress on articular cartilage, whether biomechanical, biochemical, or metabolic, can stimulate several of the pathophysiologic mechanisms previously discussed that contribute to the degradation of articular cartilage. At the same time, the reparative process of cartilage is stimulated in an effort to interrupt the degradation cycle and its effects (Fig. 5–9).

In order to enhance the reparative process, therapeutic goals should be aimed at providing the proper environment for repair. These goals include reducing the inflammatory process, control of excessive loading, and reducing hyperactivity of masticatory and cervical spine musculature. This necessitates the elimination of the cause of the above factors as well as their effects.

Internal derangement of the TMJ has been described as an abnormal relationship between the disc, condyle, and fossa in a closed jaw position where there is a mechanical displacement of the disc permitted by elongation of its attachments with possible perforation.[84]

Even though osteoarthrosis can develop without disc displacement, in several autopsy studies internal derangement appears to be correlated with TMJ osteoarthrosis.[75, 85] It has been suggested that internal derangement of the TMJ is a primary cause of osteoarthrosis. Others believe that disc displacement in the TMJ should in many cases be regarded as an accompanying sign of osteoarthritis rather than its cause.[66] Factors such as direct trauma, prolonged extended opening, and constitutional joint laxity may also be responsible for elongation of disc attachments and subsequent disc displacement, which may lead to cartilage breakdown and osteoarthrosis.

Until recently, little regard has been given to the role of joint lubrication and its importance in normal disc-condylar mechanics, as well as the role of the synovial inflammatory response and its effects on viscosity of synovial fluid. The effects of arthrosis on articular surfaces and the alterations of synovial fluid viscosity increase the coefficient of friction, leading to adhesive wear and loss of disc mobility.[66] This process initially can be observed as disc hesitation,[86] progressing to a reducible disc displacement, and ultimately to a permanent displacement (closed lock) resulting in impairment of condylar transla-

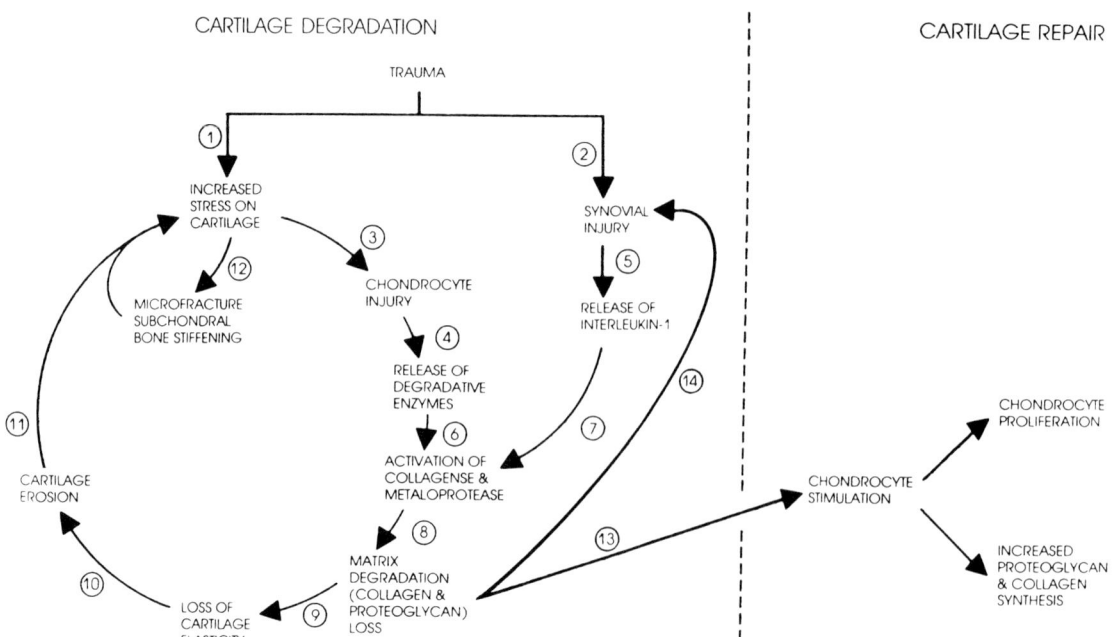

Figure 5–9. Schematic representation of the cycle of degradation and repair in osteoarthritis.

tion in the upper joint space.[66]

The author has observed arthroscopically several patients with permanent disc displacement associated with impaired translation and has found the anterior recess of the upper joint space completely obliterated with fibrous connective tissue that was confluent with the anterior lateral capsular wall. An explanation of this phenomenon may be that, as the disc becomes permanently displaced, the condyle meets resistance from the disc that is fixed in a forward and medial position along with the anterior lateral wall of the capsule. The synovial membrane of the capsule may be caught between the anterior slope of the eminence and the displaced disc. The chronic insult to the synovial membrane ultimately may lead to the proliferation of the fibrous connective tissue (capsular fibrosis) (Fig. 5–10), resulting in the loss of volume of the anterior recess (see Chapter 13A).

Several questions remain unanswered. Do all disc displacements represent pathology or are most functional adaptations? Do the posterior attachment tissues have the capability to adapt to "disclike" tissue? Can a TMJ function without pain or dysfunction if the disc is not located in a normal anatomic position? The answer to the first question can be derived from epidemiology studies that demonstrate that most TMJ clicking does not progress to locking or even problem clicking.[87–89] These findings clearly indicate that the patient with asymptomatic clicking (anterior displacement with reduction) is not

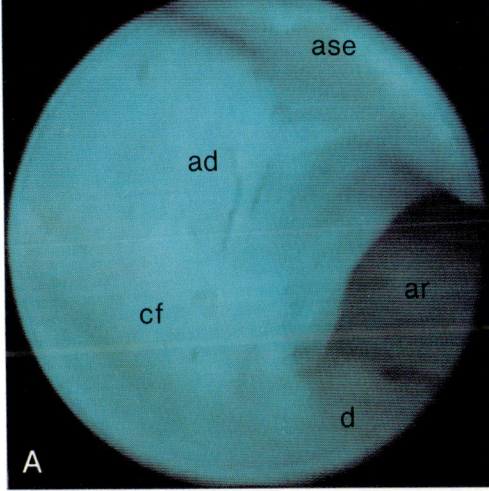

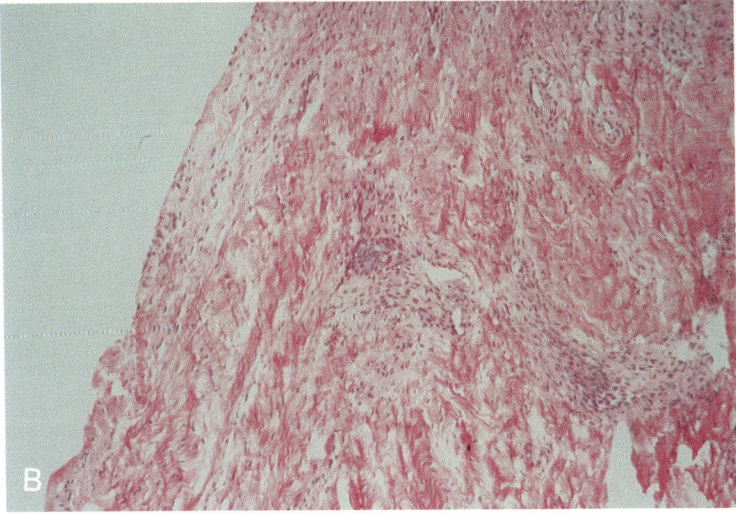

Figure 5–10. *A*, Capsular fibrosis, anterior lateral capsular wall of upper joint space of left temporomandibular joint seen on arthroscopic examination of anterior recess. cf = capsular fibrosis; d = disc; ar = anterior recess; ase = anterior slope of articular eminence; ad = adhesion. *B*, Histopathologic photomicrograph demonstrating fibrous thickening of capsule consistent with capsular fibrosis.

necessarily destined for a permanent displacement and degenerative joint disease. Another study showed anterior disc displacement by magnetic resonance imaging in 32% of the asymptomatic joints studied.[90] This finding suggests that some anteriorly displaced discs may reflect a functional adaptation rather than pathology.

The question of whether the posterior attachment has the ability to adapt to disclike tissue has been discussed. The specific adaptive changes in the bilaminar zone consist of a decrease in vascularity and elastin content, the presence of cartilage cells, and fibrosis of the anterior part of the bilaminar zone (Fig. 5–11).[91–93]

Finally, the question of whether the TMJ can function without pain or dysfunction if the disc is not located in a normal anatomic position can best be answered from clinical studies and observations.[94, 95] These studies were conducted on patients with a clinical diagnosis of internal derangement. All patients underwent arthroscopic surgery (lysis and lavage) of the upper joint compartment and also underwent pre- and postoperative magnetic resonance imaging to assess the effects of lysis and lavage on discal position.

One study consisted of 92 patients (152 TMJs) with anteriorly displaced discs.[94] Of the joints operated, 92% had no change in disc position, 80% of the patients had marked improvement of disc mobility, and 92% of the total patient sample had a significant reduction in pain and restoration of normal mandibular function. The follow-up period ranged between 1 and 32 months, with an average of 19 months.

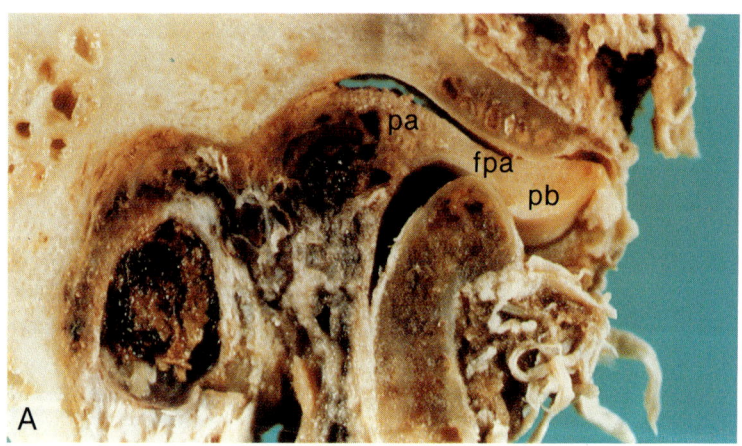

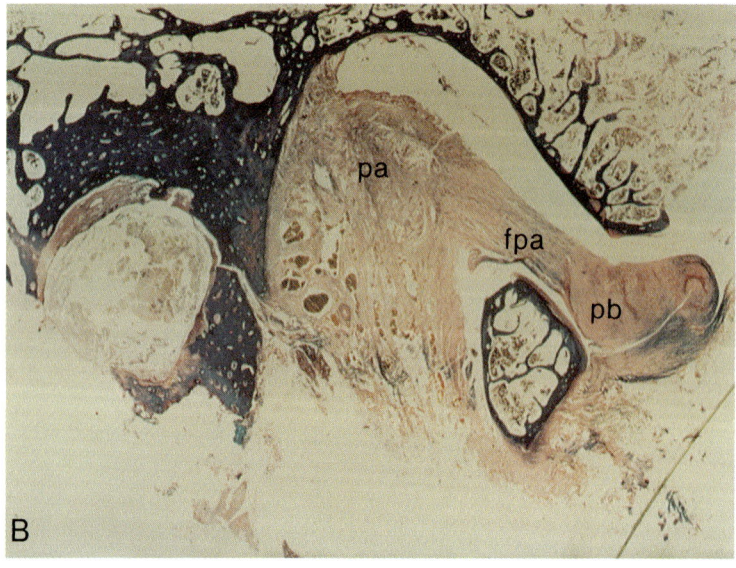

Figure 5–11. A, Adaptation of posterior attachment (fpa) of cadaveric specimen with internal derangement of right temporomandibular joint. Note that the posterior band (pb) has undergone morphologic deformation and is located anterior to the condyle. pa = posterior attachment; fpa = fibrosed posterior attachment; pb = posterior band. B, Histologic section of A demonstrating fibrosis of posterior attachment (fpa), illustrating adaptation potential of posterior attachment. (A and B courtesy of Dr. M. Franklin Dolwick.)

These data suggest that the clinical success of arthroscopic surgery (lysis and lavage) does not rest on disc relocation, and that other factors such as disc mobility, the removal of the resistance of condylar translation, and the elimination of etiologic and perpetuating factors may have a more significant influence.

SUMMARY

This chapter has been written in the belief that the TMJ, a synovial joint, obeys the same biologic laws as do all synovial articulations and their associated musculoskeletal components, despite the differences between the TMJ and most other synovial joints. On that basis, several of the pathophysiologic processes that afflict synovial joints have been discussed, in order to provide a better understanding of the pathophysiology of TMJ disorders.

ACKNOWLEDGMENT

My sincere gratitude to Mr. Dennis Bewyer for his endless time and guidance in the production of this manuscript.

References

1. Thomas L: Tabor's Cyclopedic Medical Dictionary. Philadelphia: FA Davis, 1989.
2. Weiss C: Basic structures of diarthrodial joints. In Parisien JS (ed): Arthroscopic Surgery. New York: McGraw-Hill, 1988.
3. Ghadially FN, Roy S: Ultrastructure of Synovial Joints in Health and Disease. New York: Appleton-Century-Crofts, 1969.
4. Radin EL, Swann DA, Weisser P: Separation of a hyaluronate free lubricating fraction from synovial fluid. Nature 288:377–378, 1970.
5. Swann DA, Radin EL, Nazmiec M, et al: Role of hyaluronic acid in joint lubrication. Ann Rheum Dis 33:318–326, 1974.
6. Swann DA, Radin EL: The molecular basis of articular lubrication. I. Purification and properties of a lubricating fraction from bovine synovial fluid. J Biol Chem 274:8069–8073, 1972.
7. Jimenez SA: The connective tissue: Structure, function, and metabolism. In Schumacher HR (ed): Primer on the Rheumatic Diseases, 9th Ed. Atlanta: Arthritis Foundation, 1988, pp 6–14.
8. Howell DS, Manicourt DH: Complex polysaccharides. In Schumacher HR (ed): Primer on the Rheumatic Diseases, 9th Ed. Atlanta: Arthritis Foundation, 1988.
9. Dinarello CA: Interleukin-1 and the pathogenesis of the acute-phase response. N Engl J Med 311:1413, 1984.
10. Deshmuke-Phadke K, Nanda S, Lee K: Macrophage factor that induces neutral protease secretion by normal rabbit chondrocytes. Eur J Biochem 104:175, 1980.
11. Gowen M, Wood DP, Ihrie EJ, et al: Stimulation by human interleukin-1 of cartilage breakdown and production of collagenase and proteoglycanase by human chondrocytes but not by human osteoblasts in vitro. Biochim Biophys Acta 797:186, 1984.
12. Martel-Pelletier J, Pelletier JP, Malemud CJ: Activation of neutral metalloprotease in human osteoarthritic knee cartilage: Evidence for degradation in the core protein of sulfated proteoglycan. Ann Rheum Dis 47:801–808, 1988.
13. de Bont LGM, de Haan P, Boering G: Cartilage of the temporomandibular joint. In Temporomandibular Joint, Articular Cartilage Structure and Function. [Thesis] Groningen, The Netherlands: University of Groningen, 1985, pp 3–7.
14. Ghadially SN: Structure and function of articular cartilage. Clin Rheum Dis 7:3, 1981.
15. Shahriaree H: Chondromalacia. Contemp Orthop 27:27–39, 1985.
16. Simkin PA: Joints: Structure and function. In Schumacher HR (ed): Primer on the Rheumatic Diseases, 9th Ed. Atlanta: Arthritis Foundation, 1988.
17. Simkin PA, Pizzorno JR: Transsynovial exchange of small molecules in normal human subjects. J Appl Physiol 36:581–587, 1974
18. Levick JR: Blood flow and mass transport in synovial joints. Handb Physiol 4(2):917–947, 1984.
19. Simkin PA: Synovial physiology. In McCarty DJ (ed): Arthritis and Allied Conditions, 11th Ed. Philadelphia: Lea & Febiger, 1989, pp 207–239.
20. Levick JR: Permeability of rheumatoid and normal human synovium to specific plasma protein. Arthritis Rheum 24:1550–1560, 1981.
21. Wallis WJ, Simkin PA, Nelp WB: Protein traffic in human synovial effusions. Arthritis Rheum 30:57–63, 1987.
22. O'Connor RL, Salisbury RB, Shahriaree H: Synovial disease. In Shahriaree H (ed): O'Connor's Textbook of Arthroscopic Surgery. Philadelphia: Lippincott, 1984, pp 277–288.
23. Maroudas A. Physiochemical properties of articular cartilage. In Freeman MAR (ed): Adult Articular Cartilage, 2nd Ed. Kent, England: Pitman, 1979, pp 215–290.
24. Mow VC, Roth V, Armstrong CG: Biomechanics of joint cartilage. In Frankel VH, Nordin M (eds): Basic Biomechanics of the Skeletal System. Philadelphia: Lea & Febiger, 1980, pp 61–86.
25. Swann DA, Silver FH, Slayter HS, et al: The molecular structure and lubricating activity of lubricin isolated from bovine and human synovial fluids. Biochem J 225:195–201, 1985.
26. Linn FC, Sokoloff L: Movement and composition of interstitial fluid of cartilage. Arthritis Rheum 8:481–493, 1965.
27. Toller PA: The synovial apparatus and the temporomandibular joint function. Br Dent J 111:355, 1961.
28. Bewyer DC: Biomechanical and physiologic processes leading to internal derangement with adhesion. J Craniomandib Disord 3:44–49, 1989.

29. Maukin HJ, Radin E: Structure and function of joints. *In* McCarty DJ (ed): Arthritis and Allied Conditions, 11th Ed. Philadelphia: Lea & Febiger, 1989, pp 189–206.
30. Balazs EA: The physical properties of synovial fluid and the special role of hyaluronic acid. *In* Helfet AJ (ed): Disorders of the Knee, Vol 4. Philadelphia: Lippincott, 1982, p 61.
31. Balazs EA: Viscoelastic properties of hyaluronic acid biological lubrication. Univ Mich Med Ctr J (Special Issue): 225, December, 1968.
32. Balazs EA, Watson D, Duff IF, et al: Hyaluronic acid in synovial fluid: Arthritis Rheum 10:357, 1967.
33. Robbins SL, Cotran RS, Kumar V (eds): Robbins' Pathologic Basis of Disease, 3rd Ed. Philadelphia: Saunders, 1984, pp 40–84.
34. Robinson DR: Mediators of inflammation. *In* Schumacher HR (ed): Primer on the Rheumatoid Diseases, 9th Ed. Atlanta: Arthritis Foundation, 1988, pp 24–30.
35. Zvaifler NJ: Etiology and pathogenesis of rheumatoid arthritis. *In* McCarty DJ (ed): Arthritis and Allied Conditions, 11th Ed. Philadelphia: Lea & Febiger, 1989.
36. Cronstein BN, Weismann G: Neutrophil structure and function. *In* McCarty DJ (ed): Arthritis and Allied Conditions, 11th Ed. Philadelphia: Lea & Febiger, 1989, pp 346–365.
37. Snyderman R, Pike MC: Structure and function of monocytes and macrophages. *In* McCarty DJ (ed): Arthritis and Allied Conditions, 11th Ed. Philadelphia: Lea & Febiger, 1989, pp 306–335.
38. Stobo JD: Lymphocytes: Structures and function. *In* McCarty DJ (ed): Arthritis and Allied Conditions, 11th Ed. Philadelphia: Lea & Febiger, 1989, pp 336–345.
39. Fearon DT: Complement mediators of inflammation. *In* McCarty DJ (ed): Arthritis and Allied Conditions, 11th Ed. Philadelphia: Lea & Febiger, 1989, pp 399–408.
40. Greenbaum LM: Inflammation and the role of endogenous pain producing substances. Dent Clin North Am 22(1): 47–50, 1978.
41. Goetzl EJ, Goldstein IM: Arachidonic acid metabolites. *In* McCarty DJ (ed): Arthritis and Allied Conditions, 11th Ed. Philadelphia: Lea & Febiger, 1989, pp 409–425.
42. Needleman P, Turk J, Jakschik BA, et al: Arachidonic acid metabolism. Ann Rev Biochem 55:69–102, 1986.
43. Klein DC, Raisz LG: Stimulation of bone resorption in tissue culture. Endocrinology 86:1436–1440, 1970.
44. Seybert HW: Prostaglandins as mediators of hypercalcemia associated with certain types of cancer. N Engl J Med 193:1273–1283, 1975.
45. Samuelsson B, Dahlen SC, Lindgren JA, et al: Leukotrienes and lipoxins: structures, biosynthesis, and biological effects. Science 237:1171–1176, 1987.
46. Quinn JH: Pathogenesis of TMJ chondromalacia and arthralgia. Oral Maxillofac Surg Clin North Am 2(1):47–57, 1989.
47. Egg A: Concentrations of prostaglandin D_2, E_2, F_2a, 6-keto Fla and thromboxane B_2 in synovial fluids from patients with inflammatory disorders in osteoarthritis. Z Rheumatol 43:89, 1984.
48. Henderson C, Higgs GA: Synthesis of arachidonate oxidation products by synovial joint tissue during the development of chronic erosive arthritis. Arthritis Rheum 30:1149, 1987.
49. Sanders B: Arthroscopic surgery of the temporomandibular joint: Treatment of internal derangement with persistent closed lock. Oral Surg Oral Med Oral Pathol 62(4):361, 1986.
50. Sanders B, Buoncristiani R: Diagnostic and surgical arthroscopy of the temporomandibular joint: Clinical experience with 137 procedures during a two year period. J Craniomandib Disord 1(3):202, 1989.
51. Kaminishi RM, Davis CL: Temporomandibular joint arthroscopic observations of superior space adhesions. Oral Maxillofac Surg Clin North Am 1(1):103–109, 1989.
52. O'Connor RL: Intra-articular adhesions and fibrous ankylosis of the knee. *In* Shahriaree H (ed): O'Connor's Textbook of Arthroscopic Surgery. Philadelphia: Lippincott, 1984, pp 289–298.
53. Carlsson GE, Oberg T, Bergman F, et al: Morphological changes in the mandibular joint disc in temporomandibular joint pain dysfunction syndrome. Acta Odontol Scand 25:163, 1967.
54. Helmy ES, Bays RA, Sharwy MM: Histopathological study of human TMJ perforated discs with emphasis on synovial membrane response. J Oral Maxillofac Surg 47:1048–1052, 1989.
55. Beutler B, Cerami A: Cachectin: more than a tumor necrosis factor. N Engl J Med 316:379–385, 1987.
56. Hammerman D: The biology of osteoarthritis. N Engl J Med 320:1322–1330, 1989.
57. Krane SM, Goldring MB, Goldring SR: Cytokines. *In* Evered D, Harnett S (eds): Cell and Molecular Biology of Vertebrate Hard Tissues. New York: John Wiley & Sons, 1988, pp 239–256.
58. Tyler JA, Benton HP: Synthesis of type II collagen is decreased in cartilage cultured with interleukin-1 while the rate of intracellular degradation remains unchanged. Coll Relat Res 8:393-406, 1988
59. Dingle JT, Tyler JA: Role of intercellular messengers in the control of cartilage matrix dynamics. *In* Kuettner R, Schleyerbach R, Hascall VC (eds): Articular Cartilage Biochemistry. New York: Raven Press, 1986, pp 181–191.
60. Caputo CB, Sygowski LA, Patton SP, et al: Degradation of rat chondrosarcoma proteoglycans by a neutral metalloprotease from rabbit chondrocytes. Connect Tissue Res 18:191–203, 1988.
61. Wood DD, Ihrie EJ, Hamerman D: Release of interleukin-1 from human synovial tissue in vitro. Arthritis Rheum 28:858–862, 1985.
62. Wood DD, Ihrie EJ, Dinarello CA, Cohen PL: Isolation of an interleukin 1–like factor from human joint effusions. Arthritis Rheum 26:975–983, 1983.
63. Hamerman D, Klagsbrun M: Osteoarthritis: Emerging evidence for cell interactions in the breakdown and remodeling of cartilage. Am J Med 78:495–499, 1985.
64. Meikle MC: Remodeling. *In* Sarnat BG, Laskin DM (eds): The Temporomandibular Joint: Biologic Diagnosis and Treatment, 3rd Ed. Springfield, IL: Thomas, 1979, pp 205–226.
65. Freeman MAR, Meachim G: Aging and Degeneration. *In* Freeman MAR (ed): Adult Articular Cartilage, 2nd Ed. London: Pitman, 1979, pp 316–406.
66. Stegenga B, de Bont LGM, Boering G: Osteoarthrosis as the cause of craniomandibular pain and dysfunction: A unifying concept. J Oral Maxillofac Surg 47:249–256, 1989.

67. Radin EL, Paul IC, Rose M: Osteoarthritis as a final common pathway. *In* Nuki G (ed): The Aetiopathogenesis of Osteoarthritis. London: Pitman, 1980, p 88.
68. Radin EL: Biomechanical considerations. *In* Moskowitz RW, Howell DS, Goldborg VM, Mankin HJ (eds): Osteoarthritis: Diagnosis, and Management. Philadelphia: Saunders, 1984, p 104.
69. Nordin M, Frankel VH: Biomechanics of the knee. *In* Frankel VH, Nordin M (eds): Basic Biomechanics of the Skeletal System. Philadelphia: Lea & Febiger, 1980, pp 113–148.
70. Radin EL: Mechanics of joint degeneration. *In* Radin EL, Simon SR, Rose RM, Paul IL (eds): Practical Biomechanics for the Orthopaedic Surgeon. New York: John Wiley & Sons, 1979.
71. Hinton RJ: Form and function in the temporomandibular joint. Craniofacial Biology, Ann Arbor: University of Michigan, 1981, pp 37–60.
72. Curry JD: The adaptation of bones to stress. J Theor Biol 20:91–106, 1968.
73. O'Ryan F, Epker B: Temporomandibular joint function and morphology: Observation of the spectra of normalcy. Oral Surg Oral Med Oral Pathol 58:272–279, 1984.
74. Gonyea WS, Throckmorton GS, Finn RA, et al: Masticatory muscles and dentofacial deformities. *In* Bell WH, Profitt WR, White RP (eds): Surgical Correction of Dentofacial Deformities. Philadelphia: Saunders, 1985, pp 227–258.
75. de Bont LGM, Boering F, Liem RSB, et al: Osteoarthritis of the temporomandibular joint. A light microscopic and scanning electron microscopic study of the articular cartilage of the mandibular condyle. J Oral Maxillofac Surg 43:481, 1985.
76. Barrett AJ, Saklatvala J: Proteinases in joint disease. *In* Kelley WN, Harris ED Jr, Ruddy S, Sledge CB (eds): Textbook of Rheumatology. Philadelphia: Saunders, 1985, pp 1–182.
77. Mainardi CL: Biochemical mechanics of articular destruction. Rheum Dis Clin North Am 13:215, 1987.
78. Krane SM: Mechanics of tissue destruction in rheumatoid arthritis. *In* McCarty DJ (ed): Arthritis and Allied Conditions, 11th Ed. Philadelphia: Lea & Febiger, 1989, pp 698–714.
79. Howell DS: Etiopathogenesis of osteoarthritis. *In* McCarty DJ (ed): Arthritis and Allied Conditions, 11th Ed. Philadelphia: Lea & Febiger, 1989, pp 1595–1604.
80. Moffett BC: Classification and diagnosis of temporomandibular disturbances. *In* Solberg WK, Clark GT (eds): Temporomandibular Joint Problems. Chicago: Quintessence, 1980, p 23.
81. Meachim G, Brooke G: The pathology of osteoarthritis. *In* Moskowitz RW, Howell DS, Goldberg VM, Mankin HJ (eds): Osteoarthritis, Diagnosis and Management. Philadelphia: Saunders, 1984, pp 29–42.
82. Boering G: Temporomandibular Joint Arthrosis: An Analysis of 400 Cases. Leiden: Stafler & Tholen, 1966.
83. Pullinger AG: Natural history and pathologic progression of internal derangements with persistent closed locks. *In* Sanders B, Murakami K, Clark GT (eds): Diagnostic and Surgical Arthroscopy of the Temporomandibular Joint. Philadelphia: Saunders, 1989, pp 159–189.
84. Dolwick MF, Katzberg RW, Helms CA: Internal derangements of the temporomandibular joint: Fact or fiction? J Prosthet Dent 49:415–418, 1983.
85. Westesson P-L, Rohlin M: Internal derangement related to osteoarthrosis in temporomandibular autopsy specimens. Oral Surg Oral Med Oral Pathol 57:17, 1984.
86. Ogus H: The mandibular joint: Internal derangement. Br J Oral Maxillofac Surg 25:218 1987.
87. Pullinger AG, Monterio AA: Functional impairment in TMJ patients and non-patient groups according to a disability index and symptom profile. J Craniomand Pract 6:156–164, 1988.
88. Solberg WK, Woo MW, Houston JB: Prevalence of mandibular dysfunction in young adults. J Am Dent Assoc 98:25–34, 1979.
89. Lundh H, Westesson P-L, Kopp S: A three year follow-up of patients with reciprocal temporomandibular joint clicking. Oral Surg Oral Med Oral Pathol 63:530–533, 1987.
90. Kircos LT, Ortendahl DA, Mark AS, Arakawa M: Magnetic resonance imaging of the TMJ disc in asymptomatic volunteers. J Oral Maxillofac Surg 45:852–854, 1987.
91. Hall MB, Brown RW, Baughanan RA: Histological appearance of the bilaminar zone in internal derangement of the temporomandibular joint. Oral Surg Oral Med Oral Pathol 58:375–381, 1987.
92. Scapino RP: Histopathology associated with malposition of human temporomandibular disc. Oral Surg Med Oral Pathol 59:382–397, 1983.
93. Isberg A, Isacsson G: Hyperplastic soft tissue formation in the temporomandibular joint associated with internal derangement: A radiographic and histologic study. Oral Surg Oral Med Oral Pathol 61:32–38, 1986.
94. Moses JJ, Sartoris D, Glass R, et al: The effect of arthroscopic surgical lysis and lavage of the superior joint space on TMJ disc position and mobility. J Oral Maxillofac Surg 47:674–678, 1989.
95. Gabler MJ, Greene C, Palacios E, Perry HT: Effect of arthroscopic temporomandibular joint surgery on articular disc position. J Craniomandib Disord 3:191–202, 1989.

Chapter 6

FUNCTIONAL ANATOMY OF THE TEMPOROMANDIBULAR JOINT

SIDNEY L. BRONSTEIN, D.D.S., M.Sc.D., F.A.C.D.

DISTINCTIVE FEATURES

Surely the temporomandibular joints (TMJs) must be the most complex, least understood, and unique synovial joints of the body, sharing, as they do, one bone with bilateral opposing articulations. Each side has been described as being just one-half of a larger joint, the craniomandibular articulation, and they have been described as being separate articular facets of a larger joint.[1] However, these facets are far apart (not in close proximity) as seen on the first vertebra and the femoral-tibial articulation.[2] The action of one side greatly influences that of the other, and their normal functioning requires a highly developed synchrony. The craniomandibular articulation is a bilateral configuration acting as one functional unit, composed of paired joints, muscles, and ligaments with both command and reflex movements. "Thus . . . the craniomandibular articulation is a peculiar, roving fulcrum around which moments of force turn in a complex jaw-lever system."[3]

Synovial joints have no perfectly flat surfaces, and even surface curvatures vary. No opposing surfaces are completely congruous; they fit together imperfectly. Pressures are not concentrated in one spot for long. However, in certain positions of articulation, broad areas of the two surfaces are matched exactly. This is the "close-packed" position, and it is at this time that the joint transmits pressures most effectively.[3]

The TMJ, as we know it, is a joint found only in mammals and develops late in embryonic life.[1] It is associated with Meckel's cartilage, which is derived from the first branchial arch. This is seen the seventh week in utero, extending from the symphysis to the base of the skull on each side (Fig. 6–1). This embryologic structure remains in this form, functioning as a support against which the mandible develops. The proximal segment of Meckel's cartilage continues posterosuperiorly through the petrotympanic fissure into the tympanic cavity and is the progenitor of the head and body of the malleus. It also gives rise to the anterior ligament of the malleus in the tympanic cavity and to the sphenomandibular ligament in the infratemporal fossa (Fig. 6–2). The stapes develops from the second branchial arch, as does the stylomandibular ligament (Fig. 6–3).[4]

Within the primordial joint regions, the articular disc develops first, from the first branchial arch, and seems to be related also to the muscular derivatives of this arch. There is evidence that the lateral pterygoid attachment inserts on Meckel's cartilage and contributes to the formation of the medial part of the disc.[4] The fetal disc is vascularized prior to being compressed between the developing condyle and the temporal bone; it later becomes avascular, first in its central portion and subsequently posteriorly and anteriorly. The articular eminence is the last structure of the joint to form and assumes its adult morphology gradually during growth

6 Functional Anatomy of the Temporomandibular Joint ■ 57

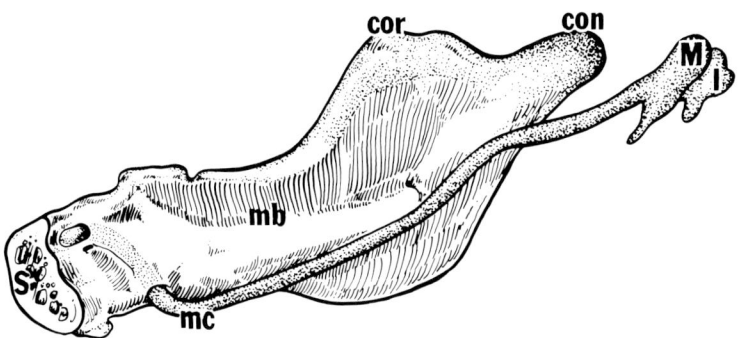

Figure 6–1. Ossification and growth of the human mandible. Relationship of Meckel's cartilage. Medial view. mc = Meckel's cartilage; mb = membranous bone; cor = coronoid process; con = condyle; M = malleus; I = incus; S = symphysis. (Redrawn with permission from Arey LB: Developmental Anatomy. Philadelphia: WB Saunders, 1947.)

and development.[1] Figure 6–4 depicts the development of the tympanic portion of the temporal bone.

Healthy temporomandibular joint function is related closely to the presence of the teeth, acting as both guides and stops, and to their positions in the dental arches. Jaw interrelationships can acutely affect joint response and function and can predispose to dysfunction. These joints mature and function during the eruption of two sets of teeth and the loss of at least one set, calling for tremendous adaptive ability.[2] Seemingly small dental and/or occlusal changes can produce, over time, when certain predisposing joint-destabilizing factors are present, severe painful and dysfunctional symptoms. Although there is little scientific evidence that loss of teeth, malocclusion, "high" fillings, jaw malrelationships, and so forth actually produce TMJ arthropathy in and of themselves, many patients presenting with painful dysfunctional joint display advanced dentofacial abnormalities and significant dental or occlusal discrepancies.

This articulation is characterized by two types and four directions of joint movement. An initial hinge, or rotational, movement and a continuing gliding, or translatory, component are seen. By cooperative and synchronous control opening, lateral and protrusive excursions are produced. Pure rotational and translational movements probably do not occur in normal TMJ function. Rotational movement starts at the beginning of opening up to mid-opening, when the anterior capsule tightens. Translation then begins and continues until it is limited by the collateral ligaments.[5] During masticatory function both sides sustain pressure, but the load varies from side to side as jaw position changes. Some studies suggest that this contralateral articulation—the balancing side—may bear the greater pressure when hard biting forces are applied.[3]

Another significant feature of this joint is

Figure 6–2. Fate map of Meckel's cartilage. Mandibular segment undergoes resorption. mc = Meckel's cartilage; sm = sphenomandibular ligament; S = spine of sphenoid; alm = anterior ligament of malleus; apm = anterior process of malleus; I = incus. Arrows indicate petrotympanic fissure. (Redrawn with permission from Coleman RD: Temporomandibular joint: Relation of the retrodiscal zone to Meckel's cartilage and lateral pterygoid muscle. J Dent Res 49(3):626–630, 1970.)

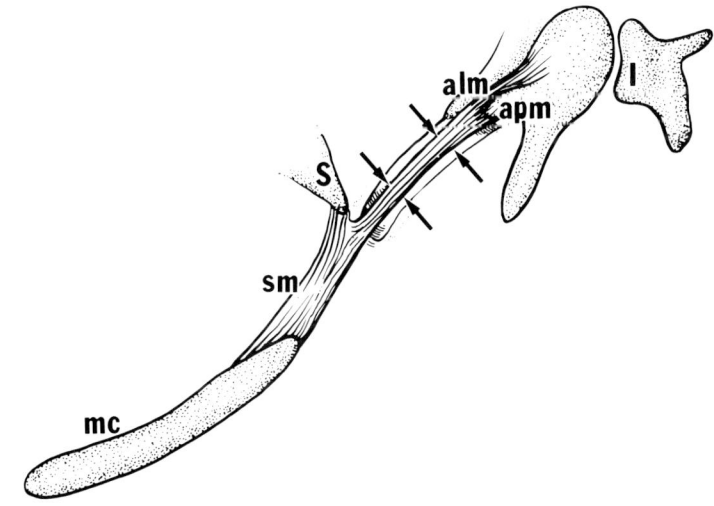

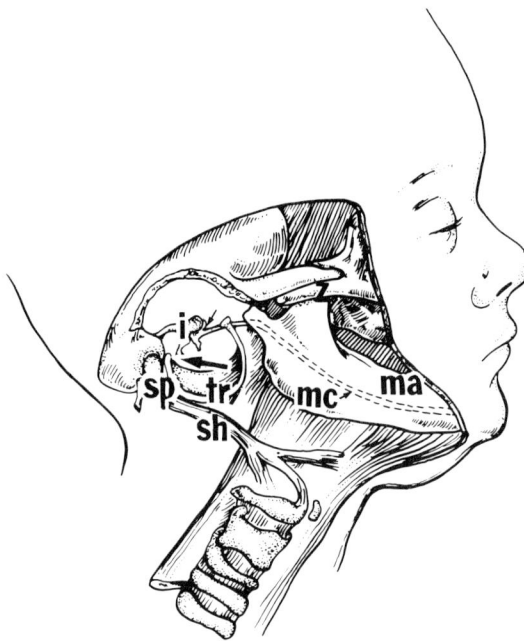

Figure 6–3. Derivatives of the human branchial arches (I and II). i = Incus [I]; sp = styloid process; tr = tympanic ring; sh = stylohyoid ligament [II]; mc with arrow = Meckel's cartilage [I]; ma = mandible; z = zygoma. Small arrow at right of i indicates malleus [I]; large arrow indicates stapes; bracketed inclusions indicate branchial arch of origin. (Redrawn with permission from Arey LB: Developmental Anatomy. Philadelphia: WB Saunders, 1947.)

its proximity to the middle ear. Certain studies have shown that the remnants of the fetal discomalleolar ligament, which extended from the disc to Meckel's cartilage and the malleus, are continuous in the adult retrodiscal tissue with the origin of the anterior ligament of the malleus and are attached within the walls of the petrotympanic fissure (Fig. 6–5).[6]

JOINT COMPONENTS AND THEIR FUNCTIONAL SIGNIFICANCE

The TMJ is composed of the head of the condylar process of the mandible articulating through a disc with the temporal bone. On the temporal bone the posterior slope of the articular eminence is the point of function, whereas its zygomatic arch attaches the capsule, the movable bony portion of the joint, of course, being the condylar head (Fig. 6–6). The glenoid fossa merely provides space for the disc to occupy during rest.[7] The condylar head has been described as being convex both sagittally and frontally and is made up of spongy bone with a thin cortical border. Its trabeculae are stress-oriented, according to Wolff's law, and are directed primarily upward and forward perpendicular to the surface.[7]

During growth, the condylar head is divided histologically into four zones. The articular zone (1) has a dense covering of fibrous tissue, covering the condyle, in which the collagen fibers are arranged parallel to the surface. The proliferative zone (2) contains many small closely packed cells; their mitotic division into eventual chondrocytes provides the main growth center of the hypertrophic zone (3). Here the cells secrete cartilage matrix, hypertrophy, and become the zone of enchondral ossification (4) where the cartilage mineralizes, then resorbs, and is finally replaced by enchondral bone.[7] The hyaline cartilage growth center, after cessation of mandibular maturation, remains to allow remodeling to occur.[8]

Modification occurs in the developmental zones of the adult condylar head. Only a thin articular covering with merely a few cartilage cells is seen. Below this covering is a very narrow proliferative zone which enters into the repair and remodeling of the articular zone in younger adults. Next is the fibrocartilaginous zone, thicker and more cellular in young adults than in older individuals. A calcified cartilage zone is then identified over the zone of subarticular bone[7] (see Figs. 4–13 and 4–14, Chapter 4).

The articular eminence corresponds to a pulley in its formation: convex in the sagittal plane and concave frontally.[1] These contours can be modified during life by articular remodeling secondary to mechanical stimuli, a method by which form and function can remain in equilibrium.[1] The eminence surface consists of fibrocartilage over a thin cortical layer covering spongy bone.[7]

Articular surface coverings of the TMJ, unlike other synovial joints, are composed of fibrocartilage. This difference may be traced to the embryologic development of the joint from discontinuous condensations of mesenchyme;[8] however, the fibrocartilage responds to injury much like hyalin cartilage. In studies by Hansson and co-workers,[9] the articular surfaces of the condyle and eminence were measured (Fig. 6–7). Histologic studies showed the articular surface layers to be

Figure 6-4. Development of tympanic ring and tympanic portion of temporal bone from the newborn stage to adolescence. The arms of the tympanic ring grow toward each other and finally fuse, dividing the space they enclosed into the external auditory meatus and foramen of Huschke. (Reprinted with permission from Anson BJ, Donaldson, JA: Surgical Anatomy of the Temporal Bone, 3rd Ed. Philadelphia: WB Saunders, 1981, p 122.)

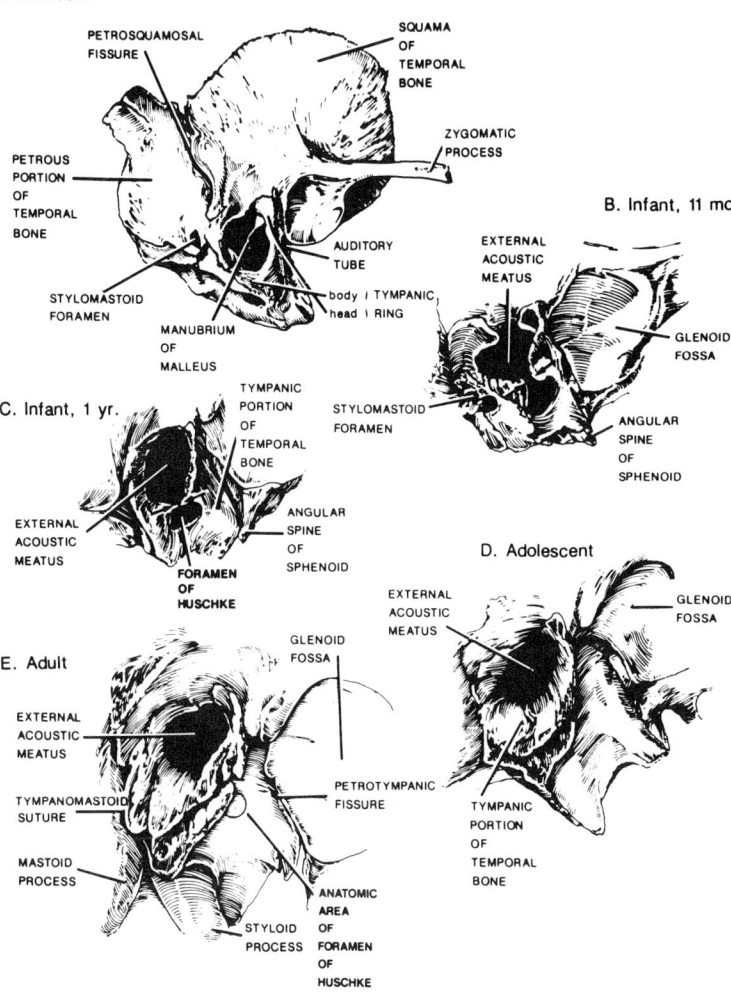

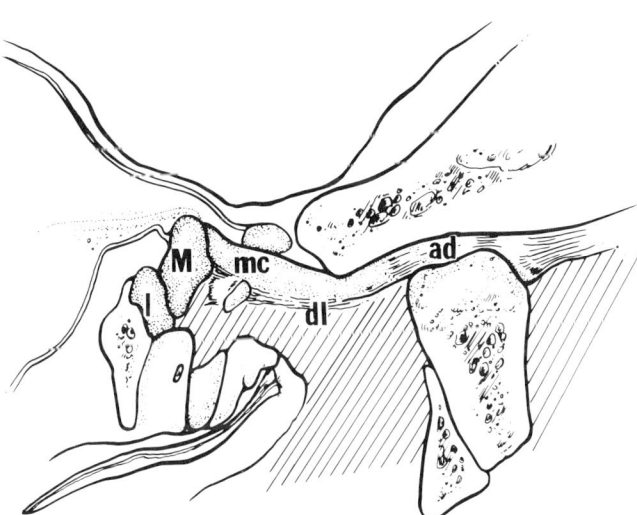

Figure 6-5. Sagittal section of right fetal temporomandibular joint and tympanic cavity. ad = Articular disc; dl = discomalleolar ligament; I = incus; M = malleus; mc = Meckel's cartilage. (Redrawn with permission from Coleman RD: Temporomandibular joint: Relation of the retrodiscal zone to Meckel's cartilage and lateral pterygoid muscle. J Dent Res 49(3):626–630, 1970.)

60 ■ 6 Functional Anatomy of the Temporomandibular Joint

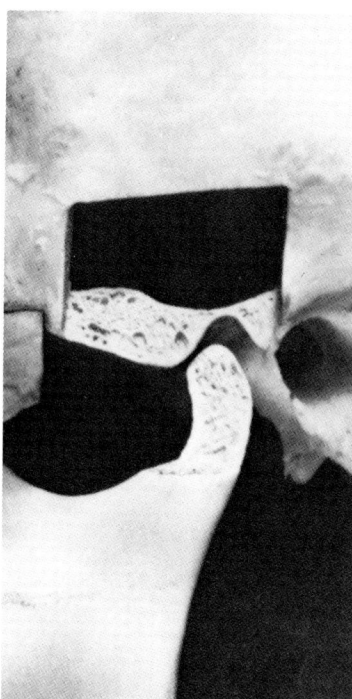

Figure 6–6. Sagittal section with teeth in occlusion. Note (1) forwardly bent condyle facing posterior slope of articular eminence, (2) closest match of opposing articular surfaces (close packed position), and (3) bulkiness of articular eminence versus thinness of bone in depth of fossa. (Reprinted with permission from DuBrul EL: The craniomandibular articulation. *In* Sicher and Dubrul's Oral Anatomy, 8th Ed. St. Louis: CV Mosby, 1988.)

attempt to decrease force per unit area by spreading the forces over a surface of increased area.[12]

Soft tissue components of the joint consist of the dense fibrous articular disc, the highly neurovascular retrodiscal pad or tissues (posterior attachment, bilaminar zone),[13] and the capsule. The TMJ disc often is incorrectly referred to as a meniscus. The meniscus is a lunate-shaped structure open on one side in relation to its position in the joint. As can be

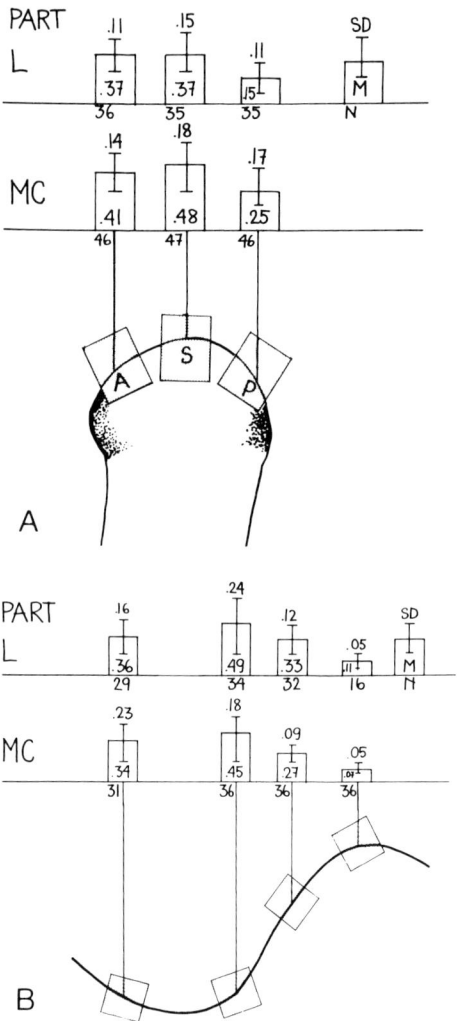

Figure 6–7. Total thickness in millimeters of the soft tissue layers of the condyle (*A*) and temporal component (*B*). M = Mean, N = number of joints examined, SD = standard deviation; L = lateral; MC = mediocentral; A = anterior; S = superior; P = posterior. (Reprinted with permission From Hansson T, Oberg T, Carlsson GE, Kopp S: Thickness of the soft tissue layers and the articular disc in the temporomandibular joint. Acta Odont Scand 35:77–83, 1977.)

thickest on the condyle anterosuperiorly (0.4–0.5 mm) and on the posteroinferior slope of the eminence (0.5 mm). A composite drawing depicts this relationship in Figure 6–8. These are the areas most heavily loaded during function; the thickness of these tissues depends heavily on an increase in cartilage from the undifferentiated mesenchyme situated in these locations.[9] It is interesting to note that in patients receiving Silastic HP temporary disc substitutes, the wear facets were almost invariably located at the upper medial part of the posterior slope of the eminence (Fig. 6–9).[10] DuBrul[3] describes this point of contact as the entoglenoid process (Fig. 6–10).

These bony components undergo both progressive and regressive remodeling, influenced by mechanical stresses. If the articular tissue breaks down, then the process evolves into osteoarthritis.[11] Flattening of articular surfaces of osseous joint components secondary to mechanical loads is thought to be an

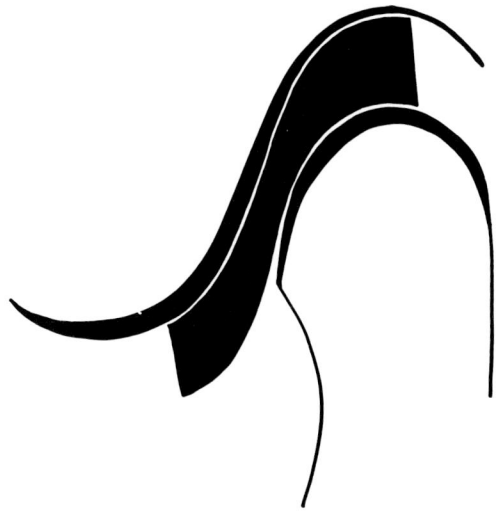

Figure 6–8. Drawing depicting total thicknesses of covering soft tissue layers in the temporomandibular joint components. (Reprinted with permission from Hansson T, Oberg T, Carlsson GE, Kopp S: Thickness of the soft tissue layers and the articular disc in the temporomandibular joint. Acta Odont Scand 35:77–83, 1977.)

seen in the knee, the menisci only partially cover the articulating joint surfaces and thus are actually three-sided; the TMJ disc, when intact, is complete on all four sides, covering the entire joint surface.

This disc functions as a protective and cushioning shock absorber, a stabilizing force in conjunction with the lateral pterygoid muscle, and a partitioning structure that divides the joint into two compartments, "smoothing" the abrupt translatory curvatures of its articular path as it travels its arcical S-shaped course forward and backward during function. It has also been described as the structure by which the superior head of the lateral pterygoid muscle controls the condyle, by stabilizing it and the disc against the eminence during function.[13] Rees's landmark investigations in 1954[13] established the disc as having four zones: a narrow anterior band, a thin intermediate zone, and a thick posterior band (all of which consist of dense white fibrous tissue with flat fibrocytes and occasional chondroid cells), and a bilaminar zone with a loose fibroelastic superior lamina and a fibrous inferior stratum (Fig. 6–11).[13] The thin central portion appears to carry most of the functional forces. Hansson's histologic measurements of the disc revealed its thickest portion to be the posterior band (2.9 mm). This is normally situated against a fossa roof about 0.1 mm thick (Fig. 6–12).[8]

The capsule functions to enclose the joint and, by specialized changes laterally, offers additional ligamentous stability with a thick-

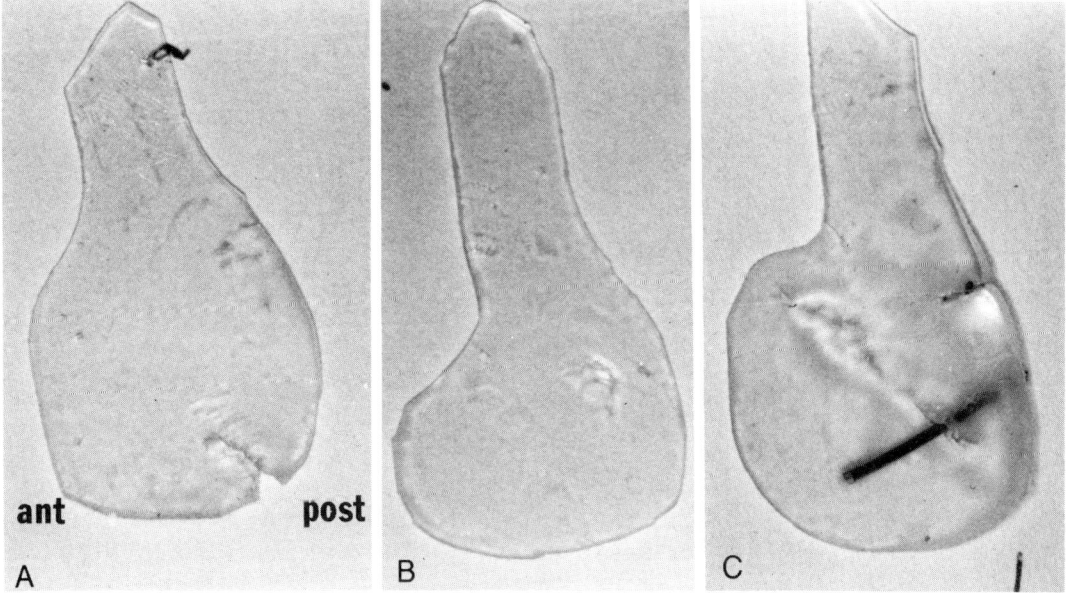

Figure 6–9. Clinical photographs of silicon elastomer temporary implants removed after 1 to 3 months. All were from left temporomandibular joints. Anterior (Ant) is to the reader's left. *A*, Splitting of the implant at the point of maximum articulation; *B*, wear facet at point of maximum contact; *C*, splitting, wear facet, and perforation at contact areas.

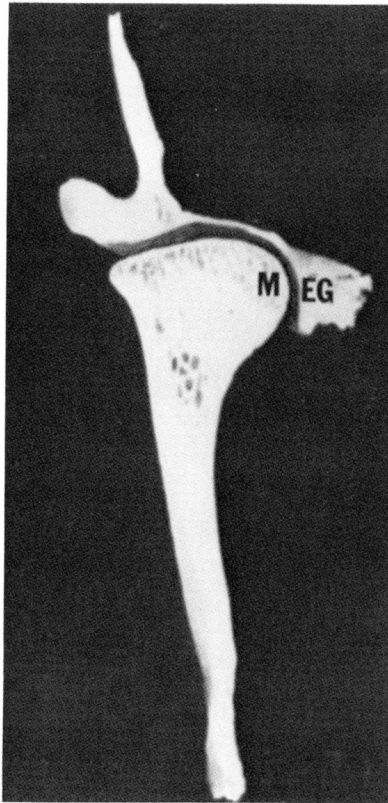

Figure 6–10. Coronal section with teeth in full occlusion. Note the increased curvature at the medial pole (M) of condyle, opposing entoglenoid process (EG), and thinness of bone between glenoid and middle cranial fossae. (Reprinted with permission from DuBrul EL: The craniomandibular articulation. *In* Sicher and Dubrul's Oral Anatomy, 8th Ed. St. Louis: CV Mosby, 1988.)

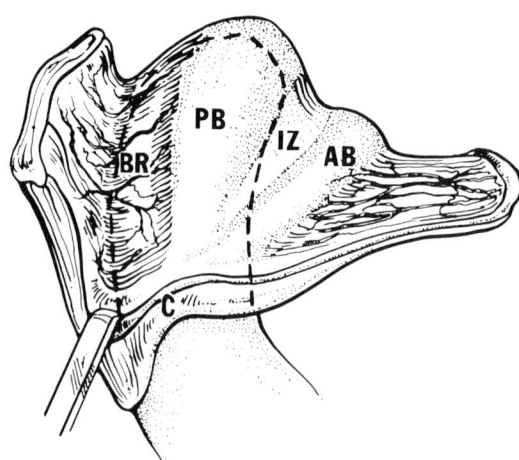

Figure 6–11. Relationships of parts of the articular disc to the condyle. BR = Bilaminar region; PB = posterior band; IZ = intermediate zone; AB = anterior band; C = capsule. Condyle is outlined. (Redrawn with permission from Rees LA: The structure and function of the mandibular joint. Br Dent J 96(6):125–133, 1954.)

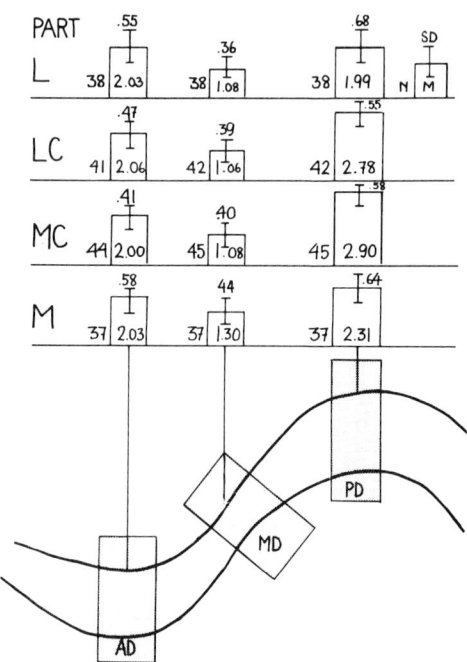

Figure 6–12. Thicknesses in millimeters of various areas of the articular portion of the disc. M (in small type, at right) = Mean; N = number of joints examined; SD = standard deviation; L = lateral; LC = laterocentral; MC = mediocentral; M (in large type) = medial; AD = anterior dense part; MD = middle dense part; PD = posterior dense part. The end points of vertical bar correspond to M ± SD. (Reprinted with permission from Hansson T, Oberg T, Carlsson GE, Kopp S: Thickness of the soft tissue layers and the articular disc in the temporomandibular joint. Acta Odont Scand 35:77–83, 1977.)

ened portion coursing from the articular tubercle on the lateral surface of the eminence to the condylar neck (Fig. 6–13).[3] The right and left temporomandibular "ligaments" allow all normal joint movements without being stretched and form a unit to keep the joint surfaces close together during function; they resist lateral movements.[7] Clinically, it seems that the main disruptive event promoting acute internal joint derangement, with anterior and often also medial disc displacement, is traumatically produced release of the lateral capsular and condylar attachments.[10]

The capsule attaches on each side of the skull, to the disc medially and laterally at the condylar poles, to the lateral pterygoid muscle, to the deep fibers of the deep belly of the masseter muscle, to the most posterior fibers of the temporalis muscle, and to the bilaminar zone above and below (Fig. 6–14).[13] Its mandibular connection is farther inferiorly

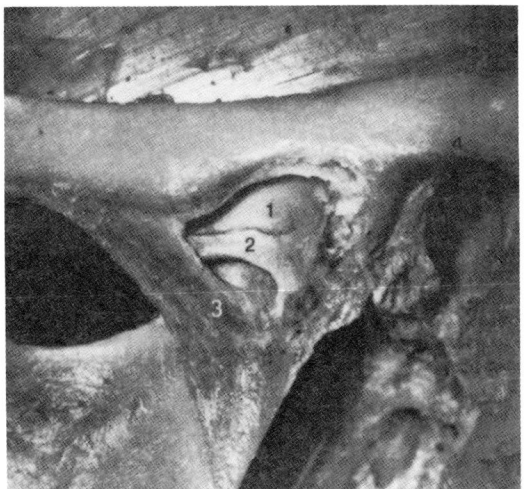

Figure 6–13. Lateral view of temporomandibular ligament complex. 1 = Articular disc; 2 = inner horizontal ligament; 3 = outer oblique ligament; 4 = roof of acoustic meatus. (Reprinted with permission from Dubrul EL: The craniomandibular articulation. In Sicher and Dubrul's Oral Anatomy, 8th Ed. St. Louis: CV Mosby, 1988.)

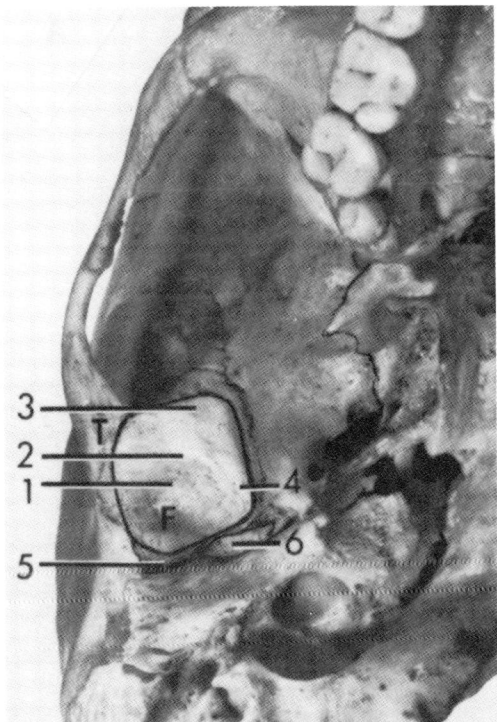

Figure 6–14. Articulating surface of mandible with line of attachment of capsule. 1 = Slope of articular eminence; 2 = crest of eminence; 3 = preglenoid plane; 4 = entoglenoid process with medialglenoid plane; 5 = postglenoid process; 6 = tegmen tympani; F = mandibular fossa, T = articular tubercle. (Reprinted with permission from DuBrul EL: The craniomandibular articulation. In Sicher and Dubrul's Oral Anatomy, 8th Ed. St. Louis: CV Mosby, 1988.)

on the condylar neck and is independent of the lateral and medial margins of the disc.

Muscles and ligaments commonly associated with the TMJ are the lateral pterygoid, probably the major muscle of concern; the medial pterygoid and masseter, primary closing muscles; the temporalis, an active closer and retractor of the mandible; the suprahyoid muscles, accessory opening muscles; and the sphenomandibular and stylomandibular ligaments, accessory ligaments of the joint. The sphenomandibular ligament travels from the spinous process of the sphenoid bone to the lingula of the mandibular foramen. It gives off fibers which travel posteriorly through the medial portion of the petrotympanic fissure to attach there and to become continuous within the fissure with the anterior ligament of the malleus.[6] Its possible effect in this area has already been mentioned.

The lateral pterygoid muscle is composed of two heads, inferior and superior, enveloped individually in fascia, with a fat pad between (Fig. 6–15).[14] This muscle is considered to stabilize the disc by its superior head and to translate the condyle forward in opening and lateral movements by its inferior head.

The detailed anatomy of the lateral pterygoid muscle and study of its function have come under intense scrutiny. Honee[14] stressed that this muscle has two separate portions: a lower part inserted into the anterior face of the condyle and an upper head inserted into the joint capsule and to the disc along the medial two-thirds of its anterior border.

The superior head arises from the infratemporal surface of the greater wing of the sphenoid bone, well above the joint. Its fibers are directed down and back to the anterior portion of the capsule and then move horizontally to attach to the neck of the mandible and the anteromedial corner of the disc through the capsule. At rest, these fibers can move the disc and jaw forward; in function, however, the direction of pull of the upper head becomes more and more vertical, pulling the condyle up against the disc and the articular eminence. This will insure stability of the "joint fulcrum" (Fig. 6–16).[3]

A cadaver study has described and histologically confirmed insertion of the inferior head to the medial ligamentous portion of the joint capsule as well as to the anterior aspect of the condyle.[15] This suggests that

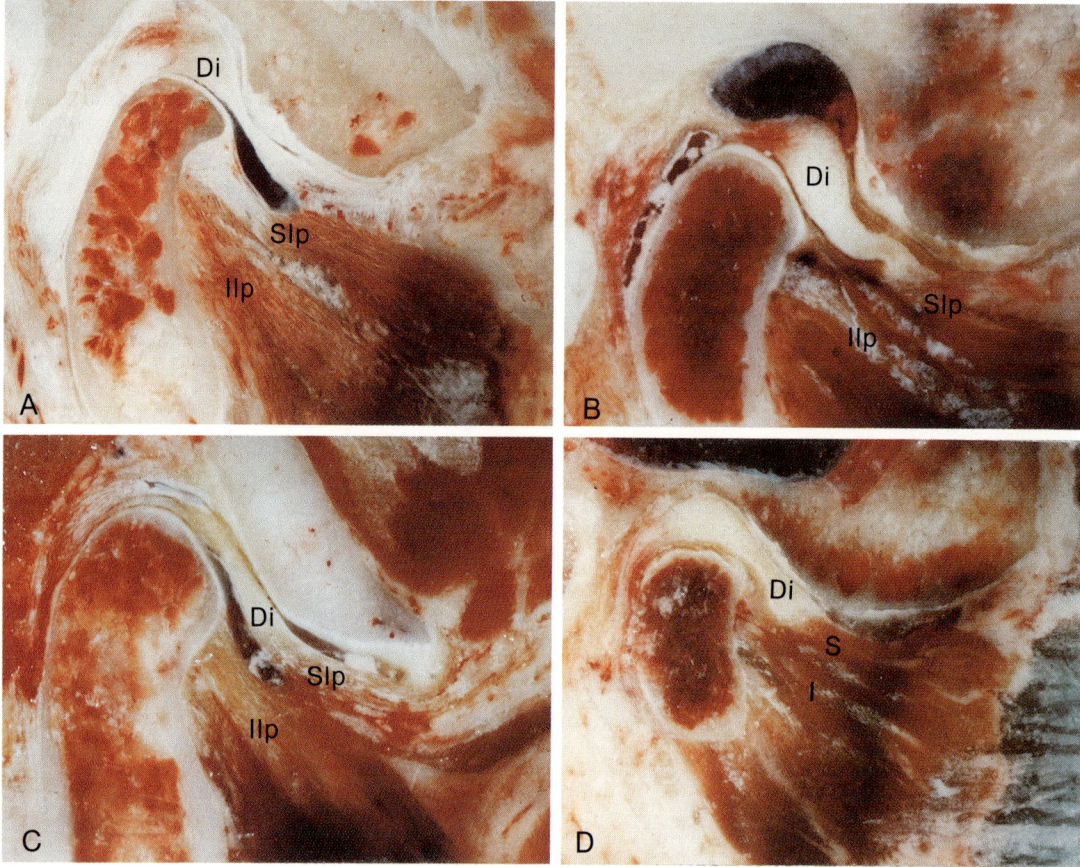

Figure 6–15. Cryosections of human cadaver joints showing attachments of the superior and inferior heads of the lateral pterygoid muscle. *A*, Essentially no attachment to the disc; *B*, slight disc attachment; *C* and *D*, more anatomic continuity between muscle and disc. Di = disc; Slp and S = superior head; Ilp and I = inferior head.

the inferior head may thus also affect medially directed disc displacements.

Occasionally the lingual and possibly the inferior alveolar nerves will vary from their normal courses and travel through the substance of the lateral pterygoid muscle. Continuous contraction or spasm of this muscle, such as might occur during joint disorders, may then produce a dysesthesia or paresthesia of these nerves (Fig. 6–17).[16] Consideration of such an unusual anatomic situation on the medial side of the joint may clarify an otherwise difficult diagnosis.

Other important soft tissue components contribute to the normal function of this joint: the synovium and the articular coverings. The synovium, or synovial membrane (Fig. 6–18), is located on the nonbearing surfaces of both joint compartments and, aided by its specialized villi formation, provides lubricity, nutrition, phagocytosis, and repair,

as theorized in studies with experimentally produced disc perforations.[17]

The retrodiscal tissue, along with the condyle, has a close positional relationship with the external auditory canal and middle ear (Fig. 6–19). Pathologic changes in this bilaminar zone may contribute to the etiology of certain ear- or auditory-related signs and symptoms accompanying TMJ arthropathy, although no direct anatomic confirmatory evidence exists at this time. On the other hand, the psychological effects of coincident tinnitus and baroacousia (stuffiness), can exaggerate patients' responses to their articular symptoms.

In one study, adult retrodiscal tissue was reported as showing a continuous ligamentous connection between a "tiny ligament" from the disc, capsule, and sphenomandibular ligament to the malleus.[18] This has not been confirmed by other investigators, but

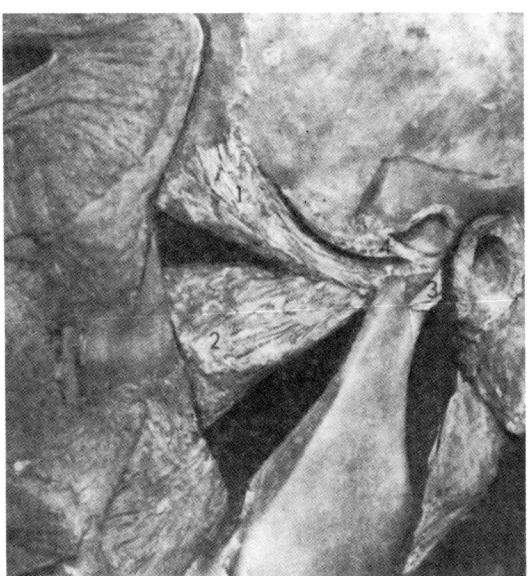

Figure 6-16. Dissection of lateral pterygoid muscle. Zygomatic arch and coronoid process have been removed. The muscle travels down and back to the lip of the root of the zygoma, where it turns to continue horizontally to the neck of the mandible. As the jaw translates, the vertical direction of the muscle increases, pulling the condyle up to firm contact against the apex of the eminence. 1 = upper head; 2 = lower head; 3 = reflected segment of oblique band of ligament. (Reprinted with permission from DuBrul EL: The craniomandibular articulation. *In* Sicher and Dubrul's Oral Anatomy, 8th Ed. St. Louis: CV Mosby, 1988.)

condylar heads.[8] The sliding motion contributes to wide opening and to right and left lateral and protrusive excursions. Hinge motion results in the initial opening movement and, in fact, probably suffices for most jaw functions not requiring extremely wide opening. Some people can probably open to 35 or 40 mm with only hinge opening. The disc is thicker medially than laterally, and this appears mainly to be due to the fact that the tendons of the superior head of the lateral pterygoid muscle are incorporated into its structure at this point.[20] The superior head also may be inserted partly into the condylar head (see Fig. 6–14).[21] Grant[22] demonstrated through measurement of moments of force that the two heads differ mechanically, the inferior head functioning more on opening and the superior head more on closing. McNamara[21] also demonstrated this in monkeys, and Juniper[23] confirmed this in adult humans.

The joint is innervated principally by fibers from the retrodiscal tissue do insert into the petrotympanic fissure along with the anterior ligament of the malleus; they probably do not induce mobility of the malleus.[6] However, a recent study on cadavers has shown that tension applied on the sphenomandibular ligament, whose fibers were continuous with the anterior ligament of the malleus, resulted in movement of the malleus in some cases, whereas tension on the discomalleolar ligament did not.[19] This investigation indicated that middle ear damage might result from undue tension on the sphenomandibular ligament.

Functionally the TMJ is a bicompartmental synovial joint. The superior compartment functions as a sliding or translatory joint between the disc, eminence, and condyle. The condyle and disc slide forward together, but the condyle travels the greater distance to its end position.[13] The inferior joint compartment functions as a hinge joint between the condyle and the disc on an axis through both

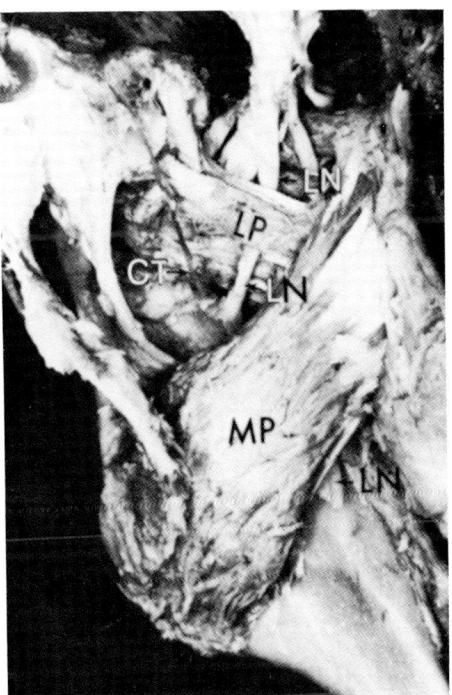

Figure 6-17. Medial view of lingual nerve entrapment. LN = Lingual nerve; CT = chorda tympani; LP = lateral pterygoid muscles; MP = medial pterygoid muscle; A = angle of mandible. (Reprinted with permission from Isberg AM, Isacsson G, Williams WN, Loughner BA: Lingual numbness and speech articulation deviation associated with temporomandibular joint disc displacement. Oral Surg 64(1):9–14, 1987.)

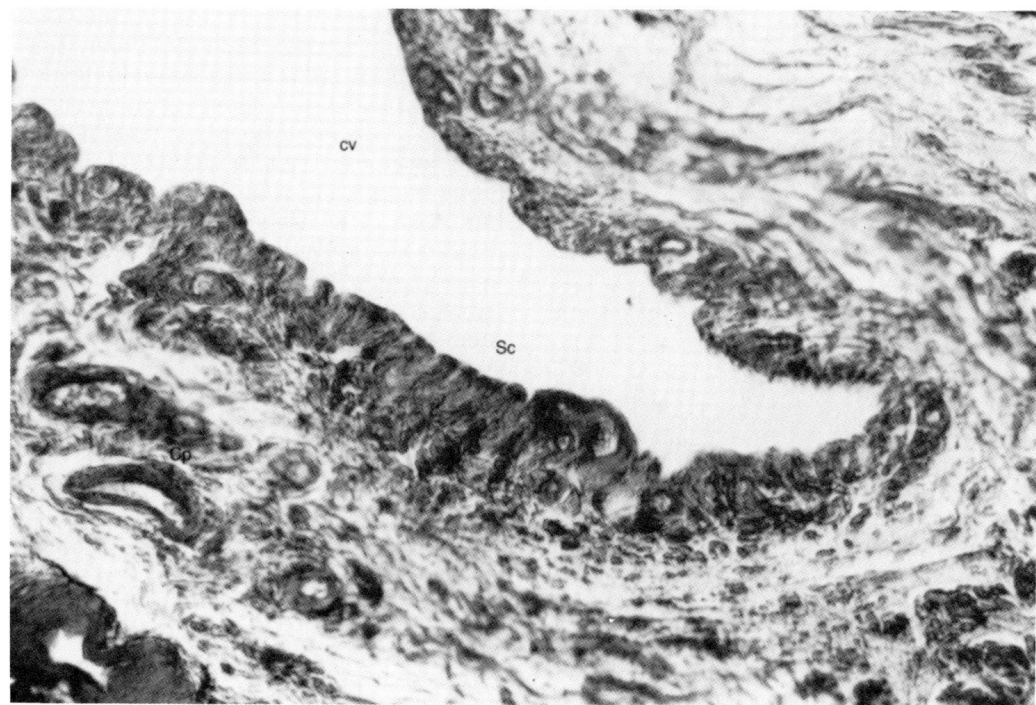

Figure 6–18. Photomicrograph of sagittal section of the left upper posterior synovial pouch, depicting synovial membrane. Cv = Upper joint cavity; Sc = synovial cell layer; Cp = capillaries. (Reprinted with permission from Murakami K-I: Arthroscopic anatomy. *In* Sanders B, Murakami K-I, Clark G (eds): Diagnostic and Surgical Arthroscopy of the Temporomandibular Joint. Philadelphia: WB Saunders, 1989.)

branches of the auriculotemporal nerve, and also by branches of the posterior deep temporal and masseteric nerves.[24] Because the auriculotemporal nerve sends branches to the external auditory canal and tympanic membrane as well as to the temporal area, joint pain may be referred to the ear and temporal areas in just under 50% of patients.[6] Additional innervation comes from the auricular branch of the vagus nerve for the external auditory canal and from the tympanic branch of the glossopharyngeal for the tympanic

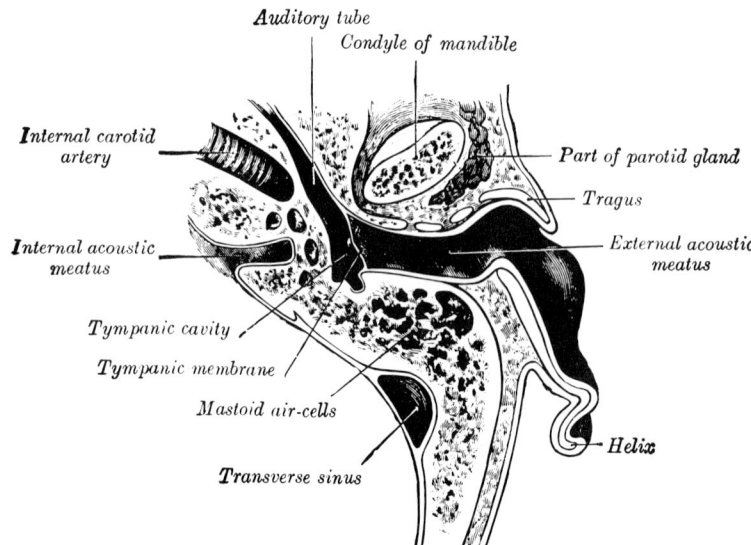

Figure 6–19. Coronal section through the left ear. (Redrawn with permission from Goss CM (ed): Gray's Anatomy of the Human Body, 25th Ed. Philadelphia: Lea & Febiger. 1948.)

membrane. Perhaps the symptoms of vertigo, tinnitus, and stuffiness result from the proximity of these branches to arthropathy in the joints. Certain nerve fibers in the TMJ may also contribute to the production of pain mediators during disease states. Substance P–like immunoreactive nerve fibers have been identified in monkey TMJ soft tissues and are thought to influence inflammation and contribute to painful joint symptoms. These fibers have been demonstrated in human tibial bone but not yet in the TMJ. Since the nerve supply of monkey and human TMJs is similar, this may explain the genesis of at least a portion of joint pain.[25]

The vascular supply of the TMJ is from the superficial temporal and maxillary arteries posteriorly, the maxillary artery anteriorly, and the facial veins.[3] These vascular channels form extensive plexuses around the joint (Fig. 6–20). During function, blood variously enters the joint area during opening and exits during closure, to accommodate changes in hydrostatic needs. Griffin[20] has identified a mechanism within the TMJ—a glomus body—which can regulate the blood supply to the TMJ. He also cites a study in which a pressure transducer connected to a needle placed within the bilaminar zone was able to measure intra-articular pressures during function. Opening, protrusive, and contralateral movements produced a negative pressure, whereas closing, retrusive, and ipsilateral movements caused a positive pressure.[20]

Receptors within the joint and associated muscles exert some regulation over joint responses. Deep proprioceptors and stretch receptors in the masticatory muscles will affect opening and closing movements. Many free nerve endings and specialized nerve end-organs have been identified in parts of the lateral capsule and temporomandibular ligament. It is believed that these are involved in proprioceptive control of the joint.[7] Mechanoreceptors in the TMJ itself affect control of the compression and functional forces produced on the joint through arthrokinetic reflexes on the mandibular musculature.[7]

ROLE OF TEMPOROMANDIBULAR JOINT FUNCTION IN THE QUALITY OF LIFE

Although patients may tolerate less than optimum service from some joints, smooth, noiseless, painless function of the craniomandibular articulation is sorely missed. Normal jaw function serves nutritional needs by providing a method of food mastication and by supporting deglutition; both are most necessary and desirable. Normal TMJ function also contributes to one's demands in speech and expression. While the TMJ is not normally a direct provider of facial form, a patient's desire for a more pleasing appearance can involve the TMJ inappropriately in a damaging quest for facial harmony.

The first-mentioned functions above require little embellishment. It is obvious that the TMJ must function well to fully serve the requirements of food mastication and subsequent painless tooth contact during swallowing. Isotonic muscle contraction requires little effort, as in speaking or merely moving food around the mouth, but when the molars are almost in contact and food is being chewed and ground vigorously the muscles act in an isometric manner. Muscle forces and, consequently, joint stresses, are greatly increased.[2] Although everyday speech and expression generally may not require significant joint movement, it is difficult to prevent significant painful jaw dysfunction from affecting facial expression and verbal communication.

Voluntary forward posturing of the mandible by persons exhibiting retrognathia or micrognathia is well known. This anterior posturing of the condylar head may result, in some cases, in the formation of a new and irreversible articulating junction forward on the eminence. As time goes on, the disc may become nonexistent, having suffered degeneration at the point of articulation. Early radiographs can show an intact articulation farther forward than normal, and arthrography may confirm such a condition. When the disease or disorder is in a late stage, the anatomy becomes abnormal and radiographic demonstration of its status becomes difficult.

The importance of the TMJ in certain vocations, professions, and occupations can be observed in singers, announcers, auctioneers, divers, musicians, and so forth. Some of these individuals not only predispose themselves to an arthropathy, but, should a painful joint dysfunction occur (as from acute trauma, for example), it will seriously interfere with the everyday involvement in their occupation or profession.

Daily social and business interaction very often produce adverse effects indirectly on

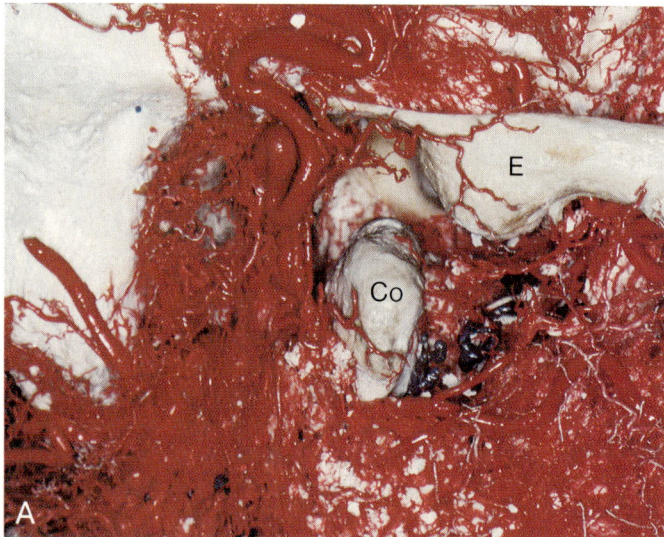
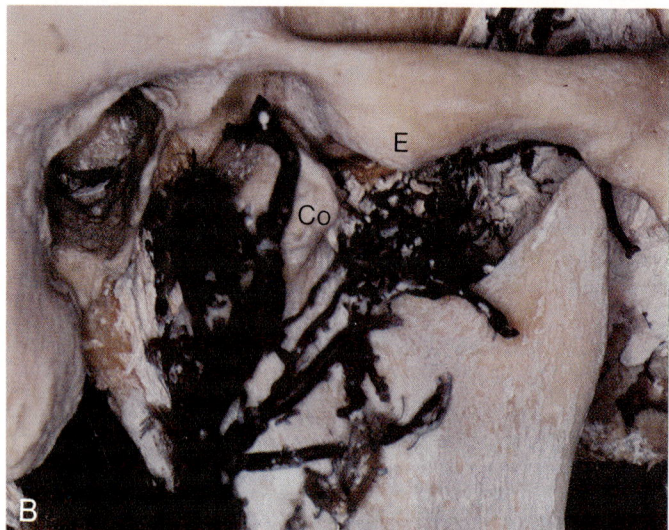
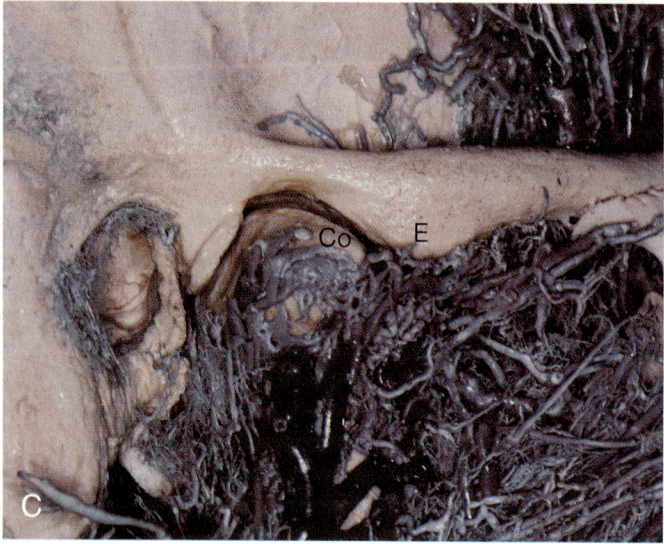

Figure 6–20. Anatomic corrosion specimens depicting vascular supply of the temporomandibular joints. *A*, Arterial supply; *B* and *C*, deep and superficial venous drainage. Co = Condyle; E = eminence. (Courtesy of Dr. O. V. Batson, University of Pennsylvania.)

the TMJ apparatus. Stress, anger, pressures, tensions—all can be manifest in the parafunctional habits of bruxism, both diurnal and nocturnal. This constant, complete rhythmic contraction of the major jaw closing muscles can produce severe damage to the major TMJ components and associated muscles.

Stresses on the TMJ appear to be concentrated on the condylar neck and less within the condylar head, due to its elliptical shape. Directions of stress within the condylar head vary with varying mandibular positions. This supports the concept that the condyle is designed to withstand light, varied forces rather than concentrated, heavy unidirectional forces.[26]

Diligent study and close scrutiny of the components of the TMJ and their anatomic relationships in normal and abnormal function assist in the diagnosis and treatment of TMJ disorders. It is of extreme importance to consider these articulations as an interplay of form and function governed by biologic and physiologic principles.

References

1. Moffett B: Anatomy and physiology of the temporomandibular joint. Distributed material. Continuing Education Symposium. University of Colorado School of Dentistry, 1983.
2. Batson OV: The anatomist looks at the temporomandibular joint. Trans Am Acad Opthalmol Otol May–June:413–418, 1956.
3. DuBrul EL: The craniomandibular articulation. In DuBrul EL (ed): Sicher's Oral Anatomy, 7th Ed. St. Louis: CV Mosby, 1980.
4. Arey LB: Developmental Anatomy. Philadelphia: WB Saunders, 1947, pp 384–385.
5. Bewyer DC: Biomechanical and physiologic processes leading to internal derangement with adhesion. J Craniomandib Disord Facial Oral Pain 3:44–49, 1989.
6. Coleman RD: Temporomandibular joint: Relation of the retrodiscal zone to Meckel's cartilage and lateral pterygoid muscle. J Dent Res 49(3):626–630, 1970.
7. Boering G: Anatomical and physiological considerations regarding the temporomandibular joint. Int Dent J 29(4):245–251, 1979.
8. Manzione JV, Katzberg RW, Manzione TJ: Internal derangements of the temporomandibular joint I. Normal anatomy, physiology and pathophysiology. Int J Periodont Rest Dent 4:9–15, 1984.
9. Hansson T, Oberg T, Carlsson GE, Kopp S: Thickness of the soft tissue layers and the articular disc in the temporomandibular joint. Acta Odont Scand 35:77–83, 1977.
10. Bronstein SL: Personal experience.
11. Moffett BC, Johnson LC, McCabe JB, Askew HC: Articular remodeling in the adult human temporomandibular joint. Am J Anat 115:119–142, 1962.
12. Hatcher DC, Blom RJ, Baker CG: Temporomandibular joint spatial relationships: Osseous and soft tissues. J Prosthet Dent 56(3):344–353, 1986.
13. Rees LA: The structure and function of the mandibular joint. Br Dent J 96(6):125–133, 1954.
14. Honee GLJM: The anatomy of the lateral pterygoid muscle. Acta Morphol Neerl Scand 10:331–340, 1972.
15. Helmy E, Bays R, Sharawy M: A new observation on clinical significance on the insertion of the inferior head of the lateral pterygoid muscle in humans. [Abstract] American Association of Dental Research, 1986.
16. Isberg AM, Isacsson G, Williams WN, Loughner BA: Lingual numbness and speech articulation deviation associated with temporomandibular joint disc displacement. Oral Surg 64(1):9–14, 1987.
17. Stewart HM, Hann JR, DeTomasi DC, et al: Histologic fate of dermal grafts following implantation for temporomandibular joint meniscal perforation: A preliminary study. Oral Surg 62:481–485, 1986.
18. Pinto OF: A new structure related to the temporomandibular joint and middle ear. J Prosthet Dent 12(1):95–132, 1962.
19. Loughner BA, Larkin LH, Mahan PE: Discomalleolar and anterior malleolar ligaments: Possible causes of middle ear damage during temporomandibular joint surgery. Oral Surg 68:14–22, 1988.
20. Griffin CJ, Hawthorn R, Harris R: Anatomy and histology of the human temporomandibular joint. Monogr Oral Sci 4:1–26, 1975.
21. McNamara JA Jr: The independent functions of the two heads of the lateral pterygoid muscle. Am J Anat 138:197–206, 1973.
22. Grant PG: Lateral pterygoid: Two muscles? Am J Anat 138:1–10, 1973.
23. Juniper RP: The superior pterygoid muscle. Br J Oral Surg 19:121–128, 1981.
24. Thilander B: Innervation of the temporomandibular joint capsule in man. Transactions Royal Schools, Stockholm, Umea, Vol. 71, 1961.
25. Johansson A-S, Isacsson G, Isberg A, Granholm A-C: Distribution of substance P–like immunoreactive nerve fibers in temporomandibular joint soft tissues of monkey. Scand J Dent Res 94:225–230, 1986.
26. Standlee JP, Caputo AA, Ralph JP: The condyle as a stress-distributing component of the temporomandibular joint. J Oral Rehab 8:391–400, 1981.

Chapter 7

NATURAL HISTORY OF INTERNAL DERANGEMENT OF THE TEMPOROMANDIBULAR JOINT

ANDREW S. KAPLAN, D.M.D., F.A.C.D., F.I.C.D.

Researchers and clinicians have long recognized a natural progression of temporomandibular joint (TMJ) disorders. In 1951, Ireland[1] observed progression of disease in his patients that started with clicking, progressed to intermittent limitation of mandibular movement and then to permanent limited movement, and ended with crepitation. He postulated that the progression was due to a displaced disc.

In the late 1960s Laskin,[2] in his paper describing myofascial pain dysfunction syndrome, outlined a disease progression that started with dental problems and/or stress, progressed to muscular parafunction, and often manifested with joint symptoms.

Farrar[3] proposed that anterior displacement of the disc was the cause of the TMJ clicking. He believed that clicking was a result of the condyle traversing over the thick posterior band of the disc, which was displaced in a forward position. He also thought that the stretching of the "joint ligaments" over a period of time resulted in further disc displacement and limited opening.

In clinical follow-up studies, Rasmussen[4,5] identified six phases of TMJ arthropathy: (1) clicking, (2) periodic locking, (3) TMJ pain at rest, (4) TMJ pain on function, (5) residual symptoms other than pain, and (6) absence of symptoms. He paired these phases, creating three clinical stages: initial, intermediate, and terminal. He reported that 80% of his patients passed through at least two of these stages.

Dolwick and co-workers[6] discussed the progression of internal derangement in a manner similar to that proposed by Farrar, describing four stages: (1) clicking, (2) clicking with intermittent locking, (3) disappearance of clicking (limited opening), and (4) crepitus (perforation of the disc).

The idea of a natural progression of internal derangement of the TMJ has been supported in many scientific papers and textbooks. The existence of these stages is documented by anatomic, histologic, and clinical research. The exact sequence of disease progression for a given patient and the percentage of patients who will pass through these stages still remains open to discussion.

Fricton and colleagues[7] divided the natural history of internal derangement into five clinical stages. (Most of the articles discussed reflect similar stages.) Fricton's progression is adapted here to more fully describe the clinical presentation of each stage (Fig. 7–1 A through D).

Stage I: Reciprocal Clicking (Internal Derangement Secondary to Anterior Disc Displacement with Reduction). The patient complains of clicking in both opening and closing movements. Generally the clicks do not occur at the same time in jaw movement; the opening click occurs when there is a greater interincisal distance than during the closing click, reflecting "play" in movement of the disc. It is generally believed that the later the opening click, the more advanced the disc displacement. Clicking occurring at the same time, particularly late opening and early closing, likely represents a

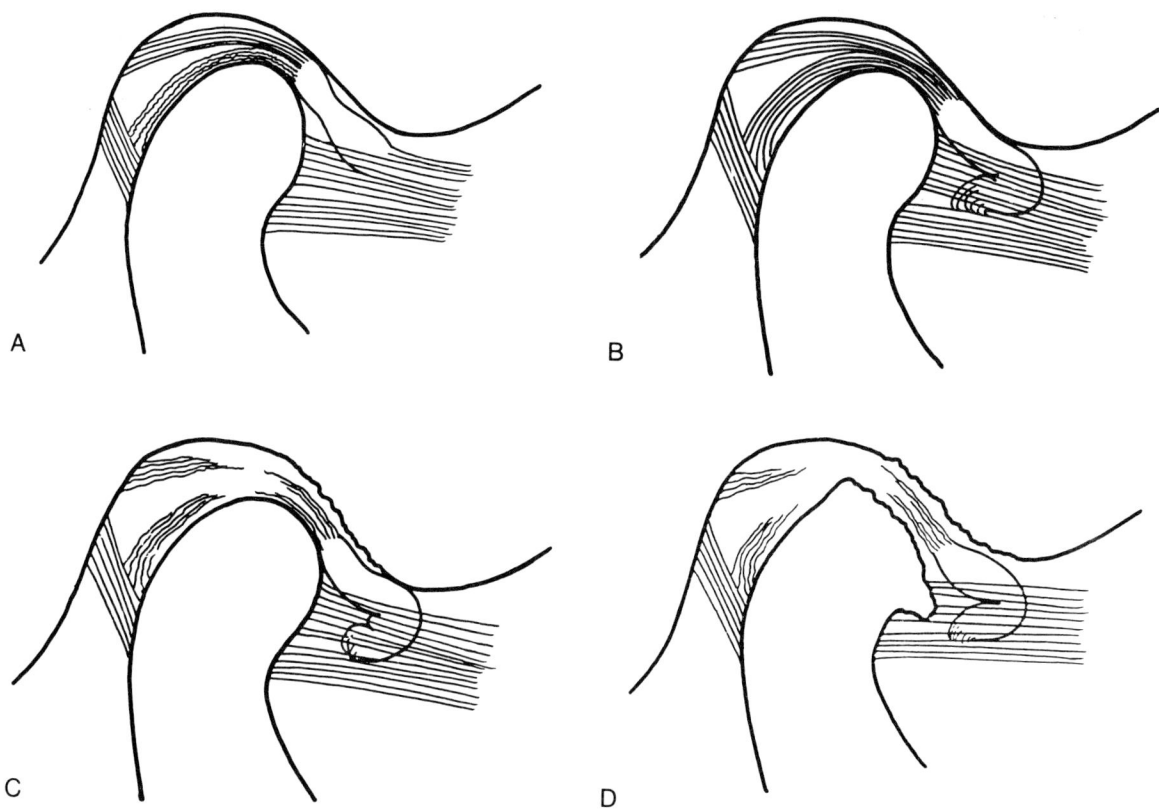

Figure 7-1. Stages in the "classic" progression of internal derangement of the temporomandibular joint. *A*, Internal joint derangement secondary to anterior disc displacement with reduction (intermittent locking may occur); *B*, anterior disc displacement without reduction; *C*, perforation of the bilaminar zone; *D*, osteoarthrosis.

hypermobile condyle traversing the articular eminence.

The presence of a loud click probably indicates disc displacement without significant change in shape. A disc with the normal biconcave shape is thought to exhibit louder joint noise than a disc that is convex or flattened and elongated.[8] Eriksson and co-workers[9] have shown in an arthrographic study that anterior disc displacement with reduction can exist without joint noises. Conversely, a clicking joint does not always indicate disc displacement with reduction. Significant regressive remodeling of the condylar head, seen in advanced cases of osteoarthrosis, can also cause clicking.[10]

Joint and related muscular pain may or may not be present with an internal derangement. Both maximal interincisal opening and lateral excursive movements should be within normal range. Lateral deviation may be evident in opening or closing. If a unilateral anterior disc displacement with reduction is present, the opening deviation will be to the affected side before returning to midline. Bilateral internal derangement with reduction will produce more complex mandibular deviations.

Disc displacement is visible on arthrograms and magnetic resonance images (Fig. 7-2). The film will reveal anterior disc displacement in the maximal intercuspal position, but the disc will appear normal in the open position. Regressive osseous changes are unlikely at this stage.

Stage II: Internal Derangement Secondary to Anterior Disc Displacement with Reduction and Intermittent Locking. In this stage all the characteristics of Stage I are evident, except that the patient begins to complain of periodic limitation of movement. This limitation is often described by the patient as "hitting an obstruction" when opening is attempted. The limitation may last from a few minutes to a number of days. During the locking episode, no joint noise is evident.

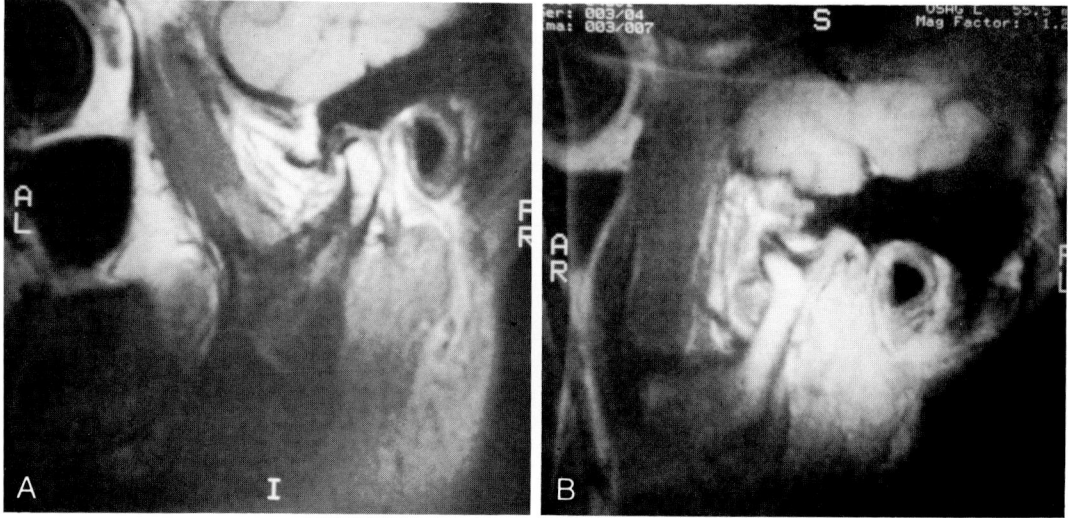

Figure 7–2. Stage I: Internal derangement with reduction as seen on a magnetic resonance image. *A*, View demonstrating anterior displacement of the disc in the closed position; *B*, open-mouth view demonstrating normal positioning of the disc.

Some patients report that the limited movement spontaneously disappears; others report that they are able to manipulate the mandible beyond the "obstruction." A few patients can demonstrate how they are able to manually manipulate the mandible to allow it to open fully. When the patient overcomes the intermittent lock, reciprocal clicking usually will begin again. Radiographic presentation is similar to that described for Stage I. Disc position relative to the condyle will be dependent on joint dynamics as the study is done.

Pain is a more common finding at this stage and is localized over the TMJ. Masticatory muscle pain may be present, particularly if the patient has related parafunction.

Stage III: Acute Closed Lock (Internal Derangement Without Disc Reduction). The patient now complains of chronic limited opening, usually less than 30 mm. Clicking and other joint noise are absent. Pain localized to the TMJ is a common finding; masticatory muscle pain also is often present, because of the associated parafunction and/or muscle splinting.

The mandible deviates to the affected side on opening and with protrusive movements. Maximal lateral excursive movement is normal toward the affected side and limited toward the contralateral side. If the condition is bilateral, lateral movement will be limited in both directions. Pain may accompany border movements. The mandible can sometimes be unlocked at this stage by manipulation with or without anesthesia. If this is done, splint therapy should be initiated immediately.

Arthrographic and magnetic resonance imaging will show anterior disc displacement in both maximal intercuspal and maximal open positions (Fig. 7–3). Limited condylar translation will also be revealed.

Stage IV: Internal Derangement Without Disc Reduction (Chronic Phase). With function, the retrodiscal tissue gradually stretches, and the patient begins to regain some of the lost range of motion. As the retrodiscal tissue continues to be stretched, it becomes subject to thinning and perforation. Pain may continue at this stage or diminish, owing to fibrous changes that may occur in the retrodiscal tissue.[11] No joint noise is grossly evident, but occasionally fine crepitus may be detected, using a stethoscope.

The radiographic appearance will reflect changes similar to those described for Stage III. A greater amount of condylar translation will usually be evident (Fig. 7–4). Lower joint space arthrography may reveal contrast material entering the upper joint space, indicating perforation.

Stage V: Hard Tissue Remodeling (Osteoarthrosis). Gradually, the hard tissue of the temporal and condylar components remodels. In truth, remodeling probably takes place

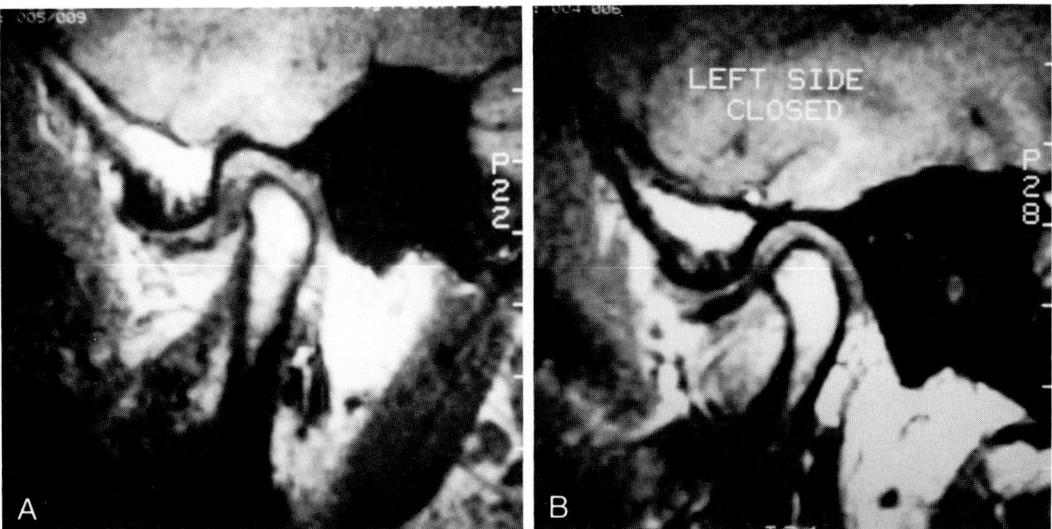

Figure 7–3. Stage III: Internal derangement without reduction, acute stage, as seen on a magnetic resonance image. *A,* Closed position (note anterior displacement); *B,* open position (note anterior disc displacement and limited condylar translation).

throughout all stages, but regressive changes become particularly evident in Stage V. Osteoarthrosis first appears on the temporal component but may be difficult to detect radiographically. Flattening, eburnation, and roughened articular surfaces will be noted on transcranial radiographs or tomograms (Fig. 7–5) but constitute late findings. Perforation may be evident on arthrography, and irregular articular surfaces along with disc displacement will be evident on magnetic resonance imaging.

In the early stages of osteoarthrosis, the patient may exhibit tenderness over the TMJ and complain of pain with function. The maximal interincisal opening will be normal unless there is significant pain restriction due to muscle splinting or unless the disc

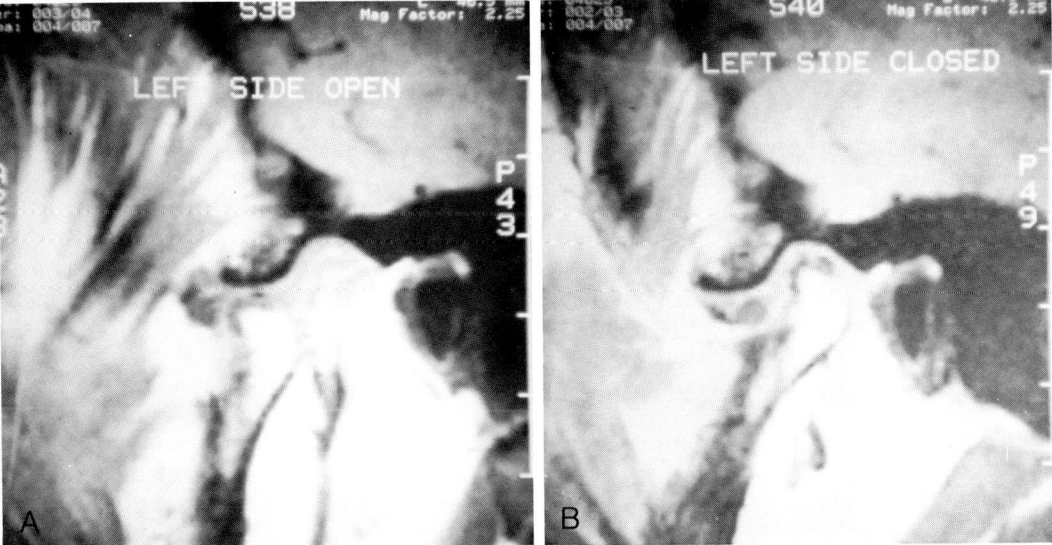

Figure 7–4. Stage IV: Internal derangement without reduction, chronic stage, as seen on a magnetic resonance image. *A,* Closed position (note anterior displacement); *B,* open position (note anterior disc displacement, disc deformity, and normal condylar translation).

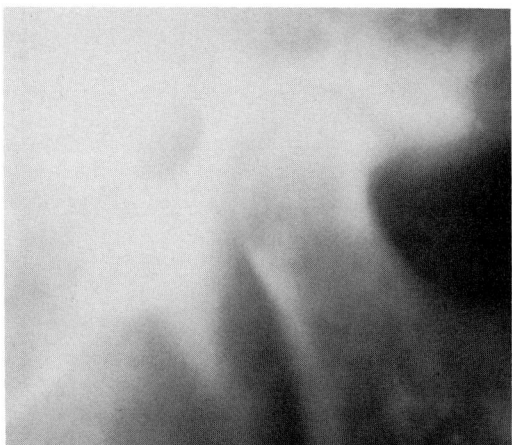

Figure 7-5. Stage V: Tomograms in the closed position demonstrating the regressive remodeling seen in osteoarthrosis.

continues to osbstruct condylar translation. The chronic stage (Stage IV) is characterized by coarse crepitus in a surprisingly pain-free patient. As is the case with clicking, one cannot assume that all crepitus is associated with osteoarthrosis.[10]

Although unquestionably many cases "fit" into the stages of progression described above, it is evident that many patients develop osteoarthrosis without passing through these stages. Osteoarthrosis, as pointed out by Solberg,[12] is the end stage of many possible disease processes. Toller,[13] in a microscopic study of osteoarthrotic condyles, stated that the specimens he studied had intact discs, and he believed that the presence of an intact disc aided in the natural process of repair.

Pullinger and Seligman,[14] in a study of 122 patients with TMJ disorders, identified five groups of patients, based on history, age, sex, and previous trauma.

Group 1: Disc Displacement with Reduction and No Sign of Osteoarthrotic Change. This group of 45 patients had reciprocal clicking only. The subjects on the average were older than those in Group 2 described subsequently (34.6 years vs. 28.8 years). Theoretically, if all patients passed through the classic disease progression, then those in the locking group would expected to be older; this was not the case.

Group 2: Locking Without Signs of Arthrosis but with a History of Clicking. The mean age of this group of 14 patients was 28.8 years, compared with the mean age of the group with osteoarthrosis who had progressed through all the stages (34.7 years). At least some of these patients would be likely candidates to progress to locking.

Group 3: Locking Without Arthrosis and Without a History of Clicking. This was the smallest group, consisting of only two patients. In these patients the locking was of sudden onset. The patients were both women in their 20s.

Group 4: Osteoarthrosis with a History of Locking. This group consisted of 29 patients who progressed through the classic stages as outlined. The average age of this group was 34.7 years.

Group 5: Osteoarthrosis Without a Prior History of Locking. This group of 32 patients was generally older than the classic progression group, with a mean age of 46.3 years. The authors noted that men with osteoarthrosis tend to be included in this group. Men rarely exhibit a history of internal derangement. The authors theorized that the TMJs of these patients had undergone a process similar to that which takes place in other joints throughout the body as a result of the aging process.

Trauma was more commonly a factor in patients with disc displacement with or without locking than in patients with osteoarthrosis (71% and 50%, respectively). The frequency of trauma associated with all groups, however, was quite high (53% in Groups 1 and 2; 38% in Groups 3 and 4).

ANATOMIC STUDIES OF INTERNAL DERANGEMENT

Scapino's classic study[11] described the gross appearance and histopathology of disc displacement. By sectioning human TMJ cadaver specimens and also looking at discs removed at the time of surgery, he was able to observe and describe changes associated with anterior and anteromedial disc displacement.

Grossly the discs appeared misshapen. Deviations from the normal biconcave appearance included biplanar and biconvex configurations, thickened posterior bands, and loss in distinction of the posterior, middle, and anterior bands. Abnormal flexure and changes in the normal orientation of the collagen fibers were also noted.

In some of the specimens, the normal architecture of the retrodiscal tissue was disrupted. Elongation in cases of advanced disc displacement was observed. The junction of the posterior band and retrodiscal tissue appeared fibrosed. This fibrosis, which may partly account for asymptomatic patients with clicking joints, demonstrates the capacity of the retrodiscal tissue to remodel in the face of changes in functional demand.

Akerman and colleagues[15] studied histopathologic specimens of 21 elderly individuals. Discs anteriorly positioned were found to be biplanar or biconvex. Perforation was correlated with regressive remodeling.

Rohlin et al and co-workers[16] studied joint sounds in dissected cadaveric specimens and found a high correlation of clicking with anterior displacement. The discs in this study also had biplanar or biconvex appearance. Crepitus was correlated with arthrosis and perforation. In most specimens the disc and temporal and condylar components exhibited regressive changes. Interestingly, one-third of the TMJs that did not exhibit any joint noise had anterior disc displacement. Remodeling of the articular surfaces (deviations in form) was evident in all but four of the 32 TMJs studied.

The correlation of joint sounds with anterior disc displacement has been studied using high-speed cinematographic techniques and arthrography. Isberg-Holm and Westesson[17] exposed the lateral aspect of the TMJ in five specimens and observed rapid movements of the disc and condyle in association with clicking. Joint sounds were correlated with the slipping of the condyle over the anteriorly displaced disc.

Findings at the time of open TMJ surgery[18] also have supported the existence of the theoretical stages of clicking (anterior disc displacement with reduction), locking (anterior disc displacement without reduction), and osteoarthrosis. Radiographic studies using single- and double-contrast arthrography and, more recently, magnetic resonance imaging support the existence of these clinical stages.[19,20]

Diagnostic arthroscopy has demonstrated pathologic changes in the synovium, retrodiscal tissue, condyle, and temporal component that are associated with disc displacement without reduction or osteoarthrosis.[21-23]

Patients presenting with limited movement and disc displacement without reduction show stretching of the retrodiscal tissue, fibrous changes in the junction between the retrodiscal tissue and the disc, and disc deformity. Anteromedial displacement and hyperemia of the retrodiscal tissue and the synovium are commonly reported findings. Fibrillation of the temporal component also has been associated with internal derangement.

Sanders[24] described the occurrence of "surface stickiness" on the posterior slope of the articular eminence and superior surface of the disc, which may limit movement and contribute in some patients to the findings of crepitation. He called this a "suction-cup effect" and described the formation of fibrous adhesions between the disc and the temporal component, preventing free movement of the disc.

Acute traumatic arthritis, as described by Murakami,[25] showed evidence of acute hyperemia, microbleeding, and congestion. The author also described the proliferation of a capillary network into the disc. The chronic stage showed a swollen hyperemic synovium with areas of fibrotic change and occasional extensive fibrillation. Denuded bone with an eburnated appearance also was described. No doubt, as more studies are done utilizing arthroscopy, and as that technology advances, our knowledge of the changes occurring in various pathologic states will increase.

REMODELING

Joints throughout the body are in a constant state of adaptation. The TMJ is no exception and undergoes progressive or regressive remodeling as its functional demands change.

Oberg,[26] in an autopsy study, reported a higher frequency of deviation in form (progressive remodeling) in the condylar head than in the temporal component; conversely, he found a higher frequency of osteoarthrosis in the temporal component (regressive remodeling). These changes are seen most often on the lateral and central aspects and rarely on the medial aspect of the TMJ.

Solberg and colleagues,[27] in a study of 51 young adult autopsy specimens, also found a higher frequency of deviation in form of the condyle, whereas osteoarthrotic changes were more evident in the temporal component. It seems as if the disc adapts passively to changes in the temporal and condylar articulating surfaces. If the adaptive capacity of the articular surfaces is surpassed, regressive changes take place. The changes begin with deviations in form and progress to disc displacement, as previously described. The final stage is osteoarthrosis.

LONGITUDINAL STUDIES

The often quoted studies of Rasmussen[4,5] describing the six clinical phases of internal derangement have been criticized on the grounds that his subjects comprised a group of patients who had enough pain or discomfort to seek care. Observations on true progression were confounded because his patients had been treated with nonsurgical techniques.

Observations made of a nonrandom group of subjects are valid only for that particular group. Rasmussen's results are valid for a group of patients who have undergone nonsurgical or no therapy. The data have little validity for non-patients with asymptomatic clicking. Since only about 5% of individuals with one or more symptoms of TMJ disorders seek treatment,[28] it is dangerous to assume progression of disease for all.

Unfortunately, there have been few longitudinal studies of large groups of subjects. Existing research has focused on disease progression in groups of children and young adults. These studies provide *limited* insight as to the natural history of signs and symptoms in non-patient populations; they do not provide a definitive answer to the question of what percentage of clicking TMJs go on to locking and ultimately to osteoarthrosis.

Magnusson and co-workers[29] followed a group of 135 children over a 5-year period. Histories and examinations were done at ages 15 and 20. The authors noted that signs and symptoms were common at both time periods (70%) but were mostly mild and occasional. During the 5 years between follow-ups there was an increase in the frequency of clicking, bruxing and/or clenching, and headaches. The maximal interincisal distance was correlated with the severity of the subjective symptoms.

Three of the 135 children had severe signs and symptoms initially but had little or no symptoms on 5-year follow-up. At the initial examination only one patient exhibited locking; at the follow-up, another patient exhibited locking. The authors reported that half the patients who exhibited clicking at age 15 no longer did so at age 20, and about half of those who did not exhibit clicking at age 15 developed clicking. In other words, the probability that TMJ clicking will disappear in a symptomatic individual is about the same as the probability that clicking will occur in an asymptomatic subject.

In a 4-year longitudinal study of schoolchildren between the ages of 7 and 11 and 11 and 15, Magnusson and colleagues[30] observed similar results. The most interesting difference was that subjective symptoms did not increase between the ages of 11 and 15 but the clinical signs did. The authors attributed this to a possible developmental "calm" period for the subjective symptoms studied.

De Boever and van den Berghe[31] also conducted a 5-year longitudinal study of 75 Flemish children. Their results showed a dramatic increase in the frequency of signs and symptoms of "mandibular dysfunction." This included pain on palpation, deviation in opening, clicking, and restricted lateral movement. These authors stressed that the signs and symptoms were, for the most part, mild to moderate, and that very few subjects were judged to need treatment. In a cross-sectional study, Pullinger and colleagues[32] demonstrated that, in a non-patient sample, signs and symptoms occurred with much higher frequency than did actual impairment in function.

Wanaman and Agerberg[33] looked at signs and symptoms in 285 adolescents, first at age 17 and again at age 19. The frequency of clicking increased over the 2-year period for females; recurrent headache was reported more frequently as well. The prevalence of clinical signs was greater in the 19-year-old subjects but tended to fluctuate longitudinally. Clinical symptoms also fluctuated, and improvement and exacerbation of symptoms occurred equally often.

Longitudinal studies of clinic patients with TMJ disorders may give insight into disease progression, as long as the limitations of the data are recognized. Greene and Laskin[34] conducted a telephone follow-up of patients who had been treated nonsurgically for "myofascial pain dysfunction syndrome" and who had complained of clicking. At the follow-up, which was done after a minimum of 5 years, 73% of patients reported that clicking had stopped; 26% had continued clicking; one patient reported that the condition was worse. As for overall condition, 67% of patients were fully or partially recovered, and 15% thought that they had recovered despite continued clicking. Because techniques such as arthrography, magnetic resonance imaging, and computed tomography were not used in these studies, it is not possible to know whether the TMJ disorders in patients with a decrease in frequency or cessation in clicking had progressed to locking with or without pain.

Brooke and co-workers[35] followed a group of 93 patients who had TMJ clicking; 55 presented with or developed intermittent locking during the observation period. All were treated with jaw-opening exercises, and 31 patients were given "non-repositioning" splints worn for 10 days, and then for 3 weeks but only at night. The patients were followed from 1 to 10 years. The authors' data showed that 70% of patients eventually developed pain, with onset occurring in about 6% each year. This study supports the notion of disease progression; however, the observations were confined to the group of patients who generally presented clinically with intermittent locking and were symptomatic enough to seek care.

Rothwell[36] examined disease progression in 400 patients with TMJ disorders. The most common pattern, which constituted 21.8% of his sample, was joint noise progressing to pain and limitation with no joint noise. This pattern was more common in females than males. Pain/noise/limitation without progression and pain/noise without progression were the next two most common patterns.

Although it appears that the signs and symptoms of TMJ disorders increase in frequency longitudinally, the studies that have been done form only the tip of the iceberg. Before definitive statements can be made about the natural history of internal derangement, research must be conducted on different non-patient populations with different socioeconomic and ethnic backgrounds and in different age groups and over a longer period of time.

TREATMENT IMPLICATIONS

If one assumes that disease progression can take place in patients with internal derangement, it is important to understand the effects of treatment on progression. The literature contains many follow-up studies of the clinical effectiveness of various treatment modalities.

The clinician should attempt to evaluate the stage of disc displacement during clinical work-up. A determination should be made of the degree of displacement as well as of the degree of distortion from the normal biconcave structure. This can be done by evaluating range of motion and the nature of joint sounds and by careful examination of arthrograms or magnetic resonance images in both sagittal and coronal views.

The following variables affecting treatment outcome have been studied and give insight about factors that may or may not affect the prognosis in a given patient.

Age. Agerberg and Carlsson,[37] in a long-term follow-up study of nonsurgical therapy, noted that many of their treatment failures tended to occur in elderly patients. However, a more recent study by Gerke and colleagues,[38] demonstrated that age had no effect on treatment outcome. Other well-controlled studies have supported these workers' results.

Sex. Other than the well-known high percentage of females seeking care for TMJ disorders and the unusual occurrence in males of TMJ disorders that undergo the classic progression,[14] no significant correlation with sex has been identified with regard to outcome.

Sociocultural Background and Sociomedical Orientation. Lipton and Marbach,[39] in a study of 170 patients with TMJ disorders, identified variables useful in predicting treatment outcome. Among these variables were the patient's ethnic background, degree of emotionality and expressiveness to pain, skepticism regarding medical care, and the number of different types of physicians consulted. These authors found these variables to be more predictive than history and findings on clinical examination.

Signs and Symptoms. Wedel and Carlsson[40, 41] reported that patients with pain of less than 6 months' duration are more likely to have successful outcomes. In addition, the length of treatment and the number of visits have been shown to have a positive correlation with the severity of the symptoms. No relationship between the initial severity of the TMJ disorder and treatment outcome has been shown, but the duration of the initial symptom correlates negatively with the treatment results. Carraro and colleagues[42] studied the time elapsed between the date of onset of the first symptom, the date of first examination, and the initial response to treatment. They were unable to find any correlation.

Radiographic Diagnosis. Changes on plain and tomographic radiographs have failed to be useful predictors of treatment outcomes.[43] Prognostic studies using arthrography and magnetic resonance imaging have yet to be done.

Psychological Factors. Significant differences in treatment outcome have been shown with psychological variables. Schwartz and co-workers,[44] in a study of successfully and unsuccessfully treated patients with TMJ disorders, found that the Minnesota Multiphasic Personality Inventories (MMPIs) did not differ in profile but did differ in significantly higher scores in unsuccessfully treated patients. This indicated a greater degree of emotional distress. However, Millstein-Prentky and Olson[45] were unable to develop a scaled-down version of the MMPI to predict treatment outcome. They believed that a single scale to predict treatment outcome was unrealistic because of the absence of consistent personality characteristics among patients with the myofascial pain–dysfunction syndrome.

Gerke and Goss[46] reported that patients with TMJ disorders had higher scores for disease conviction, affective disturbance discriminative function, disease affirmation, affective state, and lower values for psychological versus somatic focusing.

Occlusal Factors. Loss of molar support and the presence of a lateral slide between retruded contact position and intercuspal position were correlated with the presence of a TMJ disorder,[46] but no variable of occlusion has been shown to correlate with success or failure of nonsurgical therapy.

IMPLICATIONS OF ARTHROSCOPIC SURGERY

Because arthroscopy is a relatively new technique in the management of internal derangements, only short-term follow-up data (from a few months to 2 years), are available regarding its use. The published literature has reported almost exclusively on upper joint space arthroscopy with lysis and lavage.[24, 47-49] Most patients studied have had preoperative diagnoses of internal derangements without reduction or osteoarthrosis. Some studies have included patients with internal derangement with reduction[48] and patients with previously placed TMJ implants.[47] Follow-up care included orthotic and physical therapy for the majority of patients. Most studies have included patients who have undergone appropriate nonsurgical therapy with poor results. Therefore, comparing the results of nonsurgical therapy to arthroscopic surgery may have little statistical meaning.

Short-term longitudinal studies have shown improvement in 60 to 100% of patients treated.[24, 47-49] Kaminishi and colleagues,[50] using data collected from 13 different centers with a total of 1344 patients, reported an overall success rate of 84%. Israel and Roser[48] looked at the change in levels of pain, joint noise, and mandibular movement and reported that the greatest improvement in the symptoms of pain and joint sounds was seen at about 1 month. The improvement was generally stable over a longer follow-up period, with a mean of 7.5 months' duration. Interestingly, with regard to postoperative interincisal opening, these clinicians found a mean increase of 5.9 mm. In patients with preoperative opening of 30 mm or less, the mean improvement jumped to 11.4 mm. This result is similar to that of Clark and co-workers,[51] who reported a mean improvement of 14 mm in a 6-month follow-up study of six patients with closed lock.

Initial reports of arthroscopy treatment compelled clinicians to believe that the release of adhesions was sufficient to improve the position of nonreducing anteriorly displaced discs. Sanders[24] noted that the shorter the period that the disc was displaced, the better the chance for successful arthroscopic treatment. In a study of 122 patients, Moses and colleagues,[52] using pre- and postsurgical arthrography and/or magnetic resonance imaging, found that there was a "recapture" of the disc in only 13% of the TMJs studied. In comparison, 67% showed improved disc mobility compared with presurgical imaging. In addition, range of motion improved in 86% of the treated patients, and 92% had symptomatic relief and painless mandibular function. These workers also reported that perforations of the bilaminar zone and the presence of osteoarthrosis did not affect prognosis, whereas patients with perforations under the meniscus, myofascial pain, and condylar osteophytes had poorer prognoses. The concept of an "anatomically normal joint" for successful treatment of internal derangement needs to be re-evaluated; the key may be the normalization of joint mobility. It may be more useful to direct treatment at improving pain levels and function than to strive for an anatomically correct disc/condyle/fossa relationship.

References

1. Ireland V: The problem of "the clicking jaw." Proc R Soc Med 44:191, 1951.
2. Laskin D: Etiology of the pain-dysfunction syndrome. J Am Dent Assoc 89:147–153, 1969.
3. Farrar W: Diagnosis and treatment of anterior dislocation of the articular disc. NY Dent J 51:191, 1971.
4. Rasmussen O: Clinical findings during the course of temporomandibular arthropathy. Scand J Dent Res 89:283–288, 1981.
5. Rasmussen O: Description of population and progress of symptoms in a longitudinal study of temporomandibular arthropathy. Scand J Dent Res 89:196–203, 1981.
6. Dolwick F, Katzberg R, Helms C: Internal derangements of the temporomandibular joint: Fact or fiction? J Prosthet Dent 49:(3)415–418, 1983.
7. Fricton J, et al: Joint Disorders: Derangement and Degeneration. *In* Fricton J, Kroening R, Hathaway K (eds): St. Louis: Ishiyaku EuroAmerica, 1988, pp 87–89.
8. Moffett B: Histological aspects of TMJ derangements. In Moffett B (ed): Diagnosis of Internal Derangements of the TMJ, Vol 1. Seattle: Univ of Wash Contin Ed, 1984, pp 47–49.
9. Eriksson L, Rohlin M, Westesson P-L: Temporomandibular joint sounds correlated to morphology in autopsy specimens. J Oral Maxillofac Surg 1984.
10. Westesson P-L: A diagnostic analysis of TMJ sounds. *In* Moffett B (ed): Diagnosis of Internal Derangements of the TMJ, Vol. 1. Seattle: Univ of Wash Contin Ed, 1984, pp 43–45.
11. Scapino R: Histopathology associated with malposition of the human temporomandibular joint disc. Oral Surg 55(4):382–397, 1983.
12. Solberg W: Temporomandibular disorders: Clinical significance of TMJ changes. Br Dent J 160:232–236, 1986.
13. Toller P: Temporomandibular arthropathy. Proc R Soc Med 67:153–159, 1974.
14. Pullinger A, Seligman AD: TMJ osteoarthrosis: A differentiation of diagnostic subgroups by symptom history and demographics. J Craniomandib Dis Facial Oral Pain 1(4):251–256, 1987.
15. Akerman S, Kopp S, Rohlin M: Histological changes in temporomandibular joints from elderly individuals: An autopsy study. Acta Odontol Scand 44:231–239, 1986.
16. Rohlin M, Westesson P-L, Eriksson L: The correlation of TMJ sounds with joint morphology in fifty-five autopsy specimens. J Oral Maxillofac Surg 43:194–200, 1985.
17. Isberg-Holm A, Westesson P-L: Movement of the disc and condyle in TMJs with and without clicking: A high-speed cinematographic study on autopsy specimens. Acta Odontol Scand 40:167–179, 1982.
18. Bronstein SL, Tomasetti B, Ryan D: Internal derangements of the TMJ: Correlation with surgical findings. Oral Surg 39:572–584, 1981.
19. Ross J: Diagnostic criteria and nomenclature for TMJ arthrography in sagittal section: Part I. Derangements. J Cranio 1:(3)185–201, 1987.
20. Helms C, et al: Staging of internal derangements of the TMJ with magnetic resonance imaging: preliminary observations. J Craniomand Dis 3(2):93, 1989.
21. Westesson P-L, Bronstein SL, Liedberg J: Correlation between single contrast videoarthrography and post mortem morphology. Radiology 160(3):767–771, 1986.
22. Murakami K-I, et al: Diagnostic arthroscopy of the TMJ: Differential diagnoses in patients with limited jaw opening. J Cranio Pract 4:(2)117–126, 1986.
23. Murakami K-I: Diagnostic arthroscopy. In Sanders B, Murakami K-I, Clark G (eds): Diagnostic and Surgical Arthroscopy of the TMJ. Philadelphia: WB Saunders, 1989.
24. Sanders B: Arthroscopic surgery of the TMJ: Treatment of internal derangement with persistent closed lock. Oral Surg 62:361–372, 1986.
25. Murakami K-I: Diagnostic arthroscopy. In Sanders B, Murakami K-I, Clark GT (eds): Diagnostic and Surgical Arthroscopy of the TMJ. Philadelphia: WB Saunders, 1989.
26. Oberg T, Carlsson G, Fajers C: The TMJ: A morphologic study on human autopsy material. Acta Odontol Scand 29:349–384, 1971.
27. Solberg W, Hansson T, Nordstrom B: The TMJ in young adults at autopsy: A morphological classification and evaluation. J Oral Rehab 12:303–321, 1985.
28. Solberg W, Woo M, Houston J: Prevalence of mandibular dysfunction in young adults. J Am Dent Assoc 98:25–34, 1979.
29. Magnusson T, Egermark-Eriksson I, Carlsson G: Five year longitudinal study of signs and symptoms of mandibular dysfunction in adolescents. J Cranio Pract 4(4)339–344, 1986.
30. Magnusson T, Egermark-Eriksson I, Carlsson G: Four year longitudinal study of mandibular dysfunction in children. Community Dent Oral Epidemiol 13:117–120, 1985.
31. de Boever J, van den Berghe L: Longitudinal study of functional condition of the masticatory system in Flemish children. Community Dent Oral Epidemiol 15:100, 1987.
32. Pullinger A, Monteiro A: Functional impairment in TMJ patient and non-patient groups according to a disability index and symptoms profile. J Craniomandib Dis 6:(2)156–164, 1988.
33. Wanaman A, Agerberg G: Two year longitudinal study of symptoms of mandibular dysfunction in adolescents. Acta Odontol Scand 44:321, 1986.
34. Greene C, Laskin D: Long-term status of clicking in patients with myofascial pain and dysfunction. J Am Dent Assoc 17:461–465, 1988.
35. Brooke R, Leeds L, Grainger R: Long term prognosis for the clicking jaw. Oral Surg 65:668, 1988.
36. Rothwell P: Symptoms of temporomandibular pain dysfunction in 400 patients: Time to revise the classical profile? J Dent 15:6, 1987.

37. Agerberg G, Carlsson G: Late results of treatment of functional disorders of the masticatory system. J Oral Rehab 1:309–316, 1974.
38. Gerke D, Goss A, Pilowsky I: The relation of age to temporomandibular joint dysfunction. Clin J Pain 4:17–26, 1988.
39. Lipton J, Marbach J: Predictors of treatment outcome in patients with myofascial pain-dysfunction syndrome and organic TMJ disorders. J Prosthet Dent 51:(3)387–393, 1984.
40. Wedel A, Carlsson G: Factors influencing the outcome of treatment in patients referred to a TMJ clinic. J Prosthet Dent 54:420–426, 1985.
41. Wedel A, Carlsson G: A four year follow up by means of a questionnaire of patients with functional disturbances of the masticatory system. J Oral Rehab 12:105–113, 1986.
42. Carraro J, Caffesse R, Albano E: TMJ syndrome: Influence of the first symptom on the initial therapeutic response. J Prosthet Dent 30:(1)87–90, 1973.
43. Hansson L, Petersson A, Vallon-Christersson D: Clinical and radiologic six year follow up study of patients with crepitation of the TMJ. Swed Dent J 8:277–287, 1984.
44. Schwartz R, Greene C, Laskin D: Personality characteristics of patients with myofascial pain-dysfunction syndrome unresponsive to conventional therapy. J Dent Res 58:(4)1435–1439, 1979.
45. Millstein-Prentky S, Olson R: Predictability of treatment outcome in patients with myofascial pain-dysfunction syndrome. J Dent Res 58(4):1341–1346, 1979.
46. Gerke A, Goss A: Factors affecting the outcome of treatment for TMJ dysfunction. J Cranio Pract 6:(2)165–171, 1988.
47. Tarro A: Arthroscopic diagnosis and surgery of the temporomandibular joint. J Oral Maxillofac Surg 46:282–289, 1988.
48. Israel H, Roser S: Patient response to TMJ arthroscopy. J Oral Maxillofac Surg 47:570–573, 1989.
49. Sanders B: Surgical arthroscopy. *In* Sanders B, Murakami K-I, Clark GT (eds): Diagnostic and Surgical Arthroscopy for the Temporomandibular Joint. Philadelphia: WB Saunders, 1989, p 95.
50. Kaminishi R, Davis C, Moses J: A multicenter study and evaluation of the efficacy of arthroscopic surgical procedures of the TMJ. *In* Course Manual for a Diagnostic and Therapeutic Approach for TMJ Disorders. San Diego: University of California San Diego Medical Center, 1988.
51. Clark GT, Moody D, Sanders B: Analysis of arthrographically treated TMJ derangement and locking. *In* Sanders B, Murakami K-I, Clark GT (eds): Diagnostic and Surgical Arthroscopy of the Temporomandibular Joint. Philadelphia: WB Saunders 1989, p 95.
52. Moses J, Sartor D, Glass R, et al: Correlation studies of effects of TMJ arthroscopic surgical lysis of superior joint compartment adhesions and lavage on disc position and mobility. *In* Course Manual for a Diagnostic and Therapeutic Approach for TMJ Disorders. San Diego: University of California San Diego Medical Center, 1988.

Chapter 8

CLINICAL DIAGNOSIS OF TEMPOROMANDIBULAR JOINT ARTHROPATHY

MOHAN THOMAS, D.D.S., F.A.C.D.,
RICHARD H. HAUG, D.D.S.

In order to treat any surgical problem effectively, a satisfactory diagnosis must first be made. Following this, an appropriate modality of therapy may then be administered. When dealing with temporomandibular joint (TMJ) afflictions, a plethora of diagnoses have been placed in the category of TMJ syndrome (Table 8–1). Although approximately two thirds of these afflictions are of the myofascial pain dysfunction subgrouping, the remaining third are disorders of organic origin. It is necessary to establish an accurate diagnosis so that arthroscopic surgical therapy may be carried out. The particular subclassifications of TMJ arthropathy that are most amenable to arthroscopic surgery are as follows:
1. Hypomobility secondary to anteriorly displaced discs with or without reduction
2. Hypermobility
3. Degenerative joint disease (osteoarthritis).

Diagnosis is made by correlating the history, clinical examination, and imaging results to rule out or support clinical impressions. The history surrounding the patient's affliction will provide the guidelines for a good clinical examination. The diagnostic information provided by the clinical examination will ultimately provide a diagnosis that can be supported by imaging modalities. The following discussion reviews appropriate history taking and clinical examination, with emphasis on diagnosing those subclassifications of TMJ disorders most amenable to arthroscopic surgery.

HISTORY

The history of the particular TMJ symptomatology as reported by the patient will direct the clinical examination and indicate appropriate imaging studies. The ability of the patient to relate the history, and the patient's reliability, must be considered in recording the data.

Pain is the most common symptom that the patient with TMJ arthropathy relates to the clinician. The patient should be asked to describe the location of the pain. If the patient points to the preauricular region, the problem is most likely due to an affliction of the joint. If the patient puts his or her hand on the side of the face or head, the pain is more likely myofascial in origin. A history of headaches is indicative of a vascular or muscular etiology rather than joint problems primarily. If the patient describes a constant dull ache, a joint problem may be suspected; intermittent pain with varying intensity may identify muscular problems. Pain on awakening may identify nighttime bruxism, whereas acute pain when chewing or talking or with other jaw functions can be indicative of joint dysfunction. Pain that radiates to other portions of the head and neck is less likely to be of articular origin. The onset of pain following a deceleration injury, assault, or other jaw trauma must be noted.

Another symptom that the patient with TMJ arthropathy may describe is joint noise. Noises may be categorized by the patient as popping, clicking, snapping, grinding, or grating. The time of occurrence and any

Table 8–1. CLASSIFICATION OF TEMPOROMANDIBULAR JOINT DISORDERS*

I. Craniomandibular disorders of organic origin
   A. Articular disturbances
      1. Disc derangements
         a. Disc dysfunction
         b. Disc displacement
         c. Disc dyscrasias
      2. Condylar displacement
      3. Inflammatory conditions
         a. Synovitis
         b. Discitis
         c. Capsulitis
         d. Contusion
         e. Rupture
      4. Arthritides
         a. Osteoarthritis (arthrosis)
         b. Rheumatoid arthritis
         c. Polyarthritis (gout, lupus, Reiter's syndrome)
         d. Rheumatoid variants (psoriatic, juvenile)
         e. Infectious arthritis
      5. Ankylosis
         a. Fibrous
         b. Osseous
      6. Fractures
      7. Neoplasias
         a. Chondroma
         b. Osteoma
      8. Developmental abnormalities
         a. Hyperplasia
         b. Hypoplasia
         c. Agenesis
   B. Nonarticular disturbances
      1. Neuromuscular conditions
         a. Myofascitis (muscle tenderness)
         b. Contracture (mechanical shortening)
         c. Trismus/spasm (reflex splinting)
         d. Dyskinesia (weakness and incoordination)
      2. Dental occlusal conditions
         a. Unstable occlusion (structural imbalance)
         b. Premature posterior tooth contacts (posterior fulcruming)
         c. Lack of posterior occlusal support
         d. Distal thrust to mandible
      3. Disturbances involving referral of secondary symptoms
         a. Latent myofascial tenderness
         b. Active myofascial trigger points
II. Craniomandibular disorders of nonorganic (functional) origin
   A. Myofascial pain dysfunction syndrome
   B. Phantom pains
   C. Positive occlusal sense
   D. Conversion hysteria
III. Craniomandibular disorders of nonorganic origin combined with secondary organic tissue changes
   A. Articular
   B. Nonarticular
      1. Neuromuscular
      2. Oral
         a. Teeth
         b. Periodontium
         c. Soft tissues

*Classification agreed upon by the recently formed Regional Workshop Committees of the American Academy of Craniomandibular Disorders.

Reprinted with permission from McNeill C, Danzig WM, Farrar W, et al: Craniomandibular (TMJ) disorders—the state of the art. J Prosthet Dent 44:434–437, 1980.

event that triggers these noises should be recorded. Popping and snapping generally are caused by reducing discs and give a better prognosis, whereas grinding and grating noises may be indicative of disc perforations and provide a more guarded prognosis. Noises and pain should be correlated. Also, any identifiable incident that causes the noise should be elicited.

The range of motion of the jaw may in itself be diagnostic. The unafflicted patient should be able to open to 45 mm interincisally without deviation, to protrude 5 to 10 mm anteriorly without deviation, and to demonstrate 5 to 10 mm lateral excursions. Inability to open beyond 20 to 25 mm is commonly indicative of an anterior disc displacement; deviation will be to the affected side. Loss of lateral excursions is indicative of more severely displaced discs on the contralateral side, often medially. The patient who is able to open fully after a click and the patient who can manipulate the jaw into a position that allows full opening will have a better prognosis.

Other medical illnesses and psychogenic factors should be elicited in the history. Altered interpersonal relations, domestic disputes, problems at work, and psychological disturbances must be considered in making diagnoses. Mastoiditis, middle ear infection, and odontogenic infections must be identified. Other orthopedic or musculoskeletal disorders should be investigated, including rheumatoid arthritis and cervical spine degeneration.

CLINICAL EXAMINATION

The clinical examination should begin when the patient first enters the office. Observation of the patient's demeanor and habitus may identify psychosocial problems. An unusual gait may provide information regarding arthritides or other musculoskeletal problems. Dyskinetic movements, parafunctional habits, and muscle twitching should be noted. A gross examination should identify facial asymmetry, obvious edema, erythema, or fluctuance of any facial tissues.

An intraoral examination should identify gross caries, pericoronitis, periodontitis, and serviceability of dentition. Balancing or working side occlusal contacts should be recorded, and retrognathic or prognathic dental and skeletal relationships should be identified.

Next, bimanual palpation should be performed. Masses, swellings, and asymmetries need to be identified in the osseous structures and musculature of the jaws. The condyle should be palpated laterally and with a finger tip in the external auditory meatus (Fig. 8–1A). As the mouth opens, the movement of the condyles will be felt. Deviation, fremitus, and popping should be recorded. The temporalis muscles are palpated externally to elicit tenderness (Fig. 8–1B). The thumb and forefinger should be used to examine the masseter muscles. The forefinger should identify the coronoid, palatoglossal fauces, and lateral pterygoid muscle, from an intraoral approach. A tender coronoid process is usually indicative of pain of myofascial origin (Fig. 8–1C). The forefinger may then be run along the medial ramus to test the superior constrictor and medial pterygoid muscles for tenderness (Fig. 8–1D). The forefinger of the dominant hand is placed intraorally along the floor of the mouth to palpate the suprahyoid musculature, while the opposite hand provides counterpressure (Fig. 8–1E). The sternocleidomastoid and trapezius muscles may then be examined.

During the examination, interincisal opening protrusion and lateral excursions are measured. The position of both deviation and realignment should be recorded (Figs. 8–2A and 8–2B). At this time, an auscultatory examination with a stethoscope can be performed (Fig. 8–3); any noises, their positions, and their time of occurrence should be recorded.

At the completion of the history and physical examination, additional diagnostic mo-

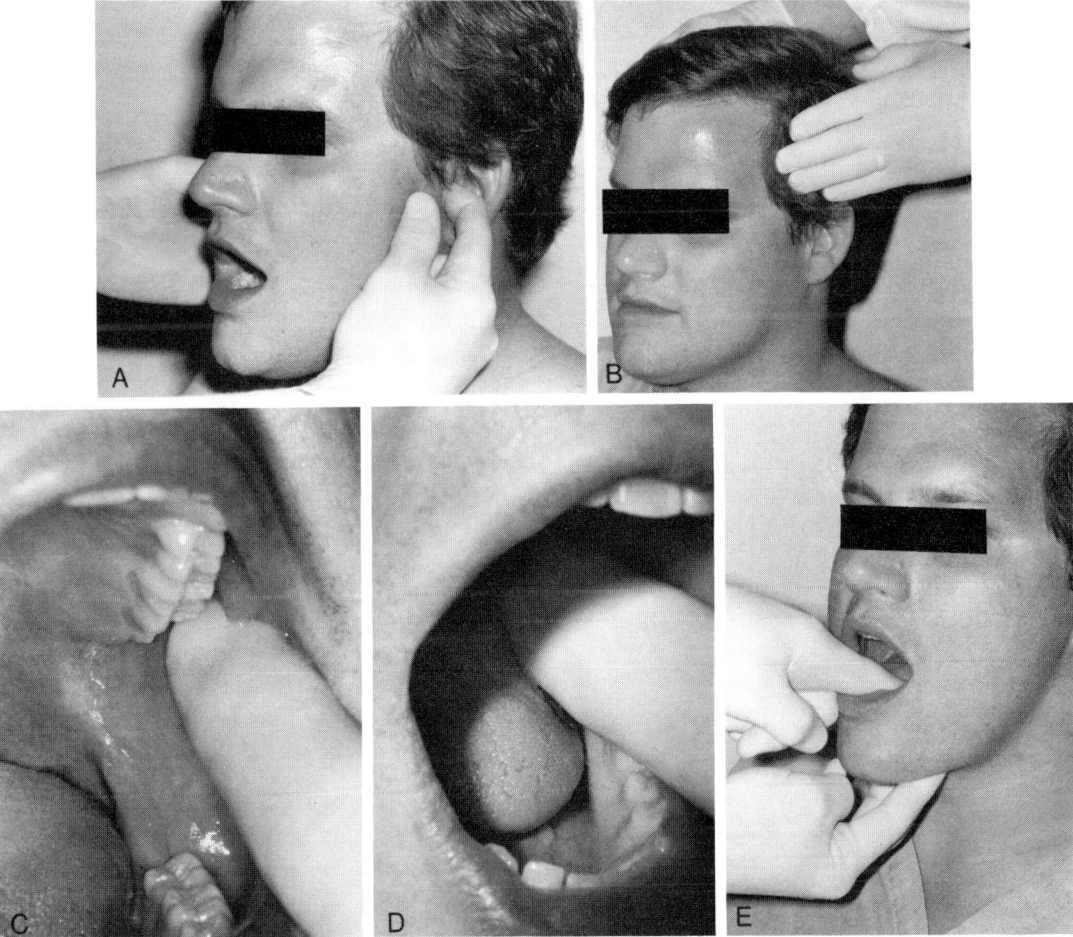

Figure 8–1. A, Manual palpation of condylar head; B, manual palpation of temporalis muscle; C, manual palpation of coronoid; D, manual palpation of lateral pterygoid muscle; E, bimanual palpation of floor of mouth.

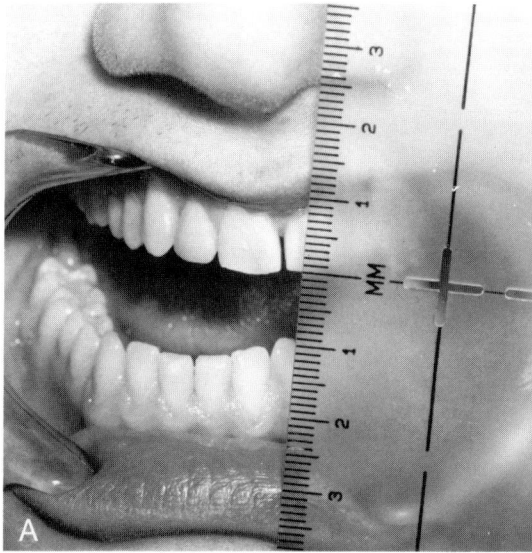
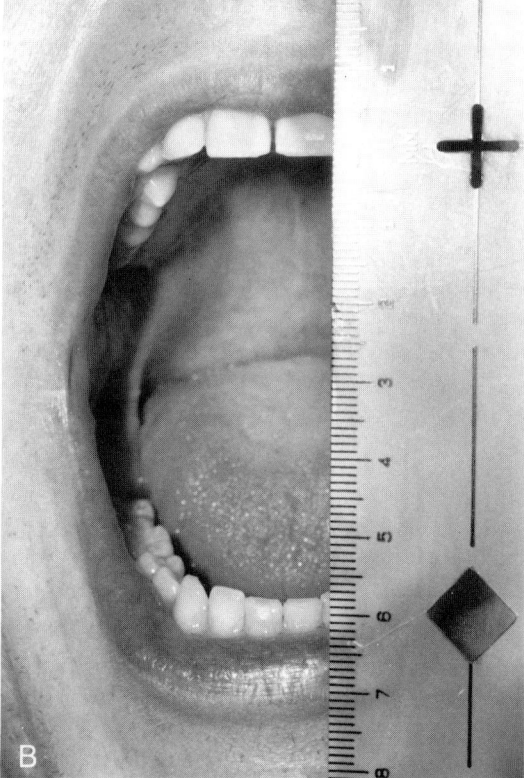

Figure 8–2. *A*, Anterior view of opening with deviation and lock; *B*, anterior view of click and return to midline.

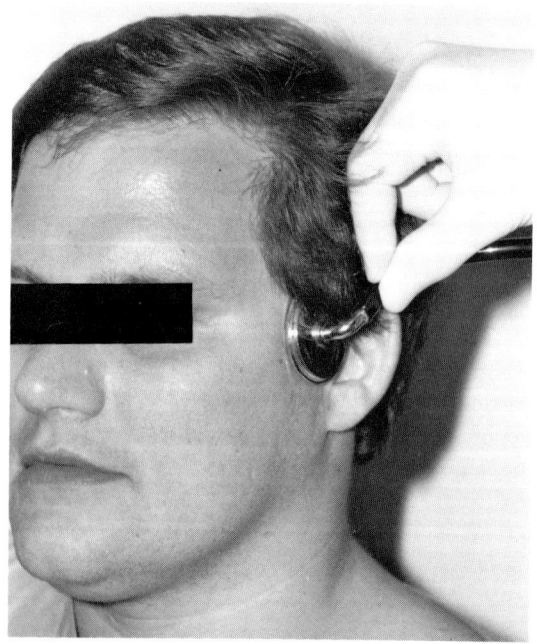

Figure 8–3. Stethoscope placed over the TMJ.

dalities may be considered. A diagnostic block may be indicated. Imaging and laboratory data will help confirm clinical impressions.

Diagnostic Block. The diagnostic block is actually a misnomer and is best performed as a sterile diagnostic infiltration. Various local anesthetics may be used, depending on the practitioner's preference. For a short-acting anesthetic, mepivacaine (Carbocaine) 3% or lidocaine 2% may be used. For a longer-lasting anesthetic, lidocaine 2% with 1:100,000 epinephrine may be utilized. If prolonged effects are desired, bupivacaine (Marcaine) 0.5% or Marcaine 0.5% with 1:100,000 epinephrine may be used.

The patient is approached from the posterior and lateral sides, and the head of the condyle is identified by palpation with the forefinger. A 27-gauge 1½-inch needle should be introduced through the skin at the 11 o'clock position to touch the head of the condyle (Fig. 8–4*A*). With needle contact on the head

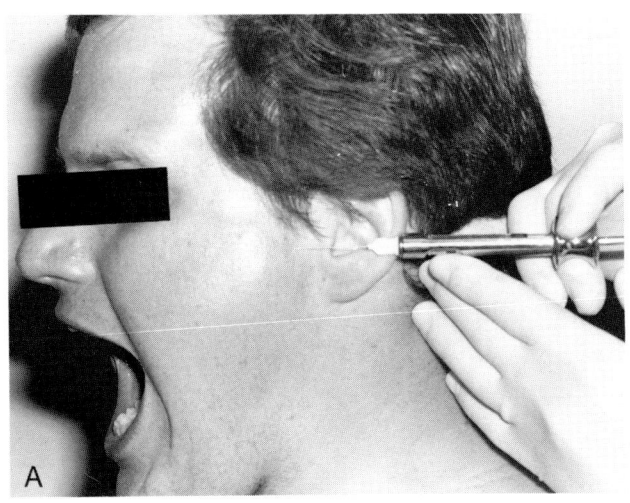
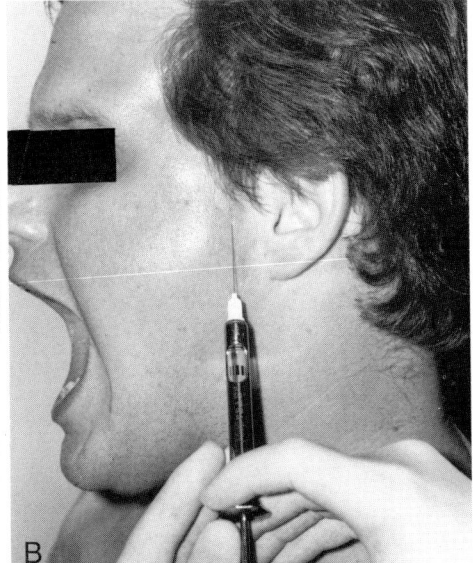

Figure 8-4. Diagnostic block. *A*, Inferior space; *B*, superior space.

of the condyle, the patient is asked to slowly open the mouth. The needle will then slide into the lower joint space. Less than 1.0 ml should be deposited. The needle is then retracted and redirected superiorly until the glenoid fossa is touched (Fig. 8–4B). The needle will now be in the superior joint space. Less than 1.5 ml should be deposited.

Relief of pain will occur within 5 minutes if the etiology is organic and within the joint. If there is no pain relief, pain of muscular or vascular origin should be considered.

DIFFERENTIAL DIAGNOSIS

Hypomobility Secondary to Anterior Disc Displacement with Reduction

The history and symptoms associated with the anteriorly displaced disc with reduction are unique and allow ready evaluation. The patient frequently will exhibit joint noise at various positions in the movement of the mandible. There will be a history of intermittent preaurical pain. The hallmark of this entity, however, is the inability of the patient to open the mouth normally until a pop or click occurs; the patient will then be able to open fully. Associated findings include deviation of the mandible to the affected side, with occasional pain at the time of the click.

Patients may be able to induce disc reduction with manual palpation over the condylar head.

The clinical examination will be significant for preauricular pain on the affected side. When the patient opens the mouth, a deviation in the condylar path toward the displaced disc will be noted and can be palpated with the forefinger in the external auditory meatus. Upon reaching the obstruction by the disc, the patient will experience pain and limitation. After the disc is reduced, the examiner will hear a click and may also feel the disc reduction with his fingers. The amount of opening that the patient has at the time of the click should be recorded. At this time, the deviation will be eliminated, and the patient will be able to open fully. The measurement at full opening also should be recorded. As the patient begins to close, an additional, reciprocal closing click will be heard and felt, and the amount of closing should be recorded in this position as well.

To support these impressions, magnetic resonance images or arthrograms displaying the anteriorly displaced disc in the closed and partially open position, and the recaptured disc in the open position, are obtained. Plain radiographs are unreliable for this diagnosis (Table 8–2).

Table 8–2. SIGNS AND SYMPTOMS OF HYPOMOBILITY SECONDARY TO ANTERIORLY DISPLACED DISC WITH REDUCTION

History	Joint noise
	Intermittent preauricular pain
	Intermittent inability to open mouth until a pop occurs; then ability to open fully
Clinical Examination	Preauricular pain
	Deviation in condylar path
	Opening click
	Reciprocal click (closing)
Imaging	Magnetic resonance image—reveals an anteriorly displaced disc in closed and partially open positions
	Arthrogram—reveals anteriorly displaced disc in closed and partially open positions
	Plain radiograph or tomogram—may reveal an increased anterior joint space

Table 8–3. SIGNS AND SYMPTOMS OF HYPOMOBILITY SECONDARY TO ANTERIOR DISC DISPLACEMENT WITHOUT REDUCTION

History	Intermittent joint pain
	Limited opening
	History of prior click or trauma
Clinical Examination	Preauricular pain
	Deviation on opening to affected side
	Obstruction restricting opening of less than 25 mm
Imaging	Arthrogram and magnetic resonance image—reveal disc displacement without reduction
	Plain radiographs—not diagnostic

Hypomobility Secondary to Anterior Disc Displacement Without Reduction

The history related by the patient with anterior disc displacement without reduction resembles that for anterior disc displacement with reduction, but without the "pop" and the subsequent ability to open further. There will be associated joint pain. The patient will have had a prior click or trauma with deviation that previously resulted in full opening after the pop or click. The patient will now have completely limited opening and may feel pressure or the presence of something obstructing full opening.

Examination will reveal preauricular pain and deviation upon opening to the affected side. Obstruction restricting opening to less than 25 mm interincisally will be noted, despite movements of the jaw and despite manual palpation. The nonreducing disc will not allow any further opening.

Radiographs are not particularly diagnostic in this situation. The arthrograms and magnetic resonance images show anteriorly displaced discs in the closed, semi-open, and fully open positions (Table 8–3).

Hypermobility

Patients with temporomandibular joint hypermobility will have mandibular condyles that translate anterior to the articular eminence. If the condyle remains trapped anteriorly, it is termed a dislocation, whereas a condyle that self-reduces is termed a subluxation. The hypermobility may be bilateral or unilateral.

The patient presents with a history of dislocation or subluxation caused by yawning, shouting, eating, or long dental procedures. Acute problems tend to be painful. Patients with chronic subluxation tend to exhibit less pain and can "pop" the mandibular condyle anterior and posterior to the articulating eminence.

The clinical examination will be dramatic. Opening beyond 40 to 45 mm will cause a "bump" or "jump" with the head of the condyle translating anterior to the articulating eminence on the affected side or sides. Open-mouth plain radiographs, tomograms, and magnetic resonance images will confirm this (Table 8–4).

Arthritis

The history related by the patient with arthritis will include significant pain, swelling, redness, stiffness, and warmth and progressively worsening symptoms in the affected joint. The patient with a history of trauma and associated traumatic capsulitis may present with similar hallmarks of inflammation.

Clinical examination will reveal preauricular pain, especially when in function. Edema and erythema may also be present. Occasionally, crepitus with grinding noises and

Table 8-4. SIGNS AND SYMPTOMS OF HYPERMOBILITY

History	Pain associated with anterior displacement of jaw
	Subluxation with or without entrapment and open lock of jaws in position
Clinical Examination	Preauricular pain with protrusive movement
	Subluxation with or without entrapment of head of condyle in protrusive position
Imaging	Plain radiograph, tomogram, and magnetic resonance image—reveal condylar head at lowest portion or anterior to articular eminence

Table 8-5. SIGNS AND SYMPTOMS OF ARTHRITIS

History	Significant pain, swelling, redness, stiffness, warmth; progressive involvement in all affected joints if rheumatoid or osteoarthritis
	History of trauma if traumatic arthritis
Clinical Examination	Preauricular pain, especially in function
	Occasional swelling, edema, crepitus
	Fever if infectious arthritis
	Ecchymosis if traumatic arthritis
Imaging	Radiograph—may reveal irregularities of bony density and loss of lamina dura
Laboratory Data	Antinuclear antibody—elevated if rheumatoid arthritis
	Rheumatoid factor—elevated if rheumatoid arthritis
	Erythrocyte sedimentation rate—elevated if rheumatoid arthritis or chronic infection
	White blood cell count—elevated if infectious arthritis
	Normochromic anemia in rheumatoid arthritis

fremitus will be noticed. If the arthritis is infectious in nature, an elevated temperature may be present. If the arthritis is traumatic in nature, ecchymosis may be noted.

Radiographic characteristics are specific. Degenerative and rheumatoid arthritis show irregular densities in the bone with a loss of lamina dura. Traumatic arthritis with a posterior capsulitis may show an increased joint space. Infectious arthritis, if acute, shows no radiographic changes.

The clinical examination must be supplemented with a laboratory examination to further establish a diagnosis. In the case of rheumatoid arthritis, an elevated antinuclear antibody, erythrocyte sedimentation rate, and rheumatoid factor will be present. Normochromic anemia will be identified in the vast majority of arthritic patients (Table 8-5). If the arthritis is infectious in nature, an elevated white blood cell count and temperature will be noted.

SUMMARY

Clinical examination of the patient with a TMJ disorder should follow the same sequence and methods as physical examination of all patients. The history of the presenting complaint is particularly important in the investigation of the problem. Physical evaluation will provide further diagnostic material to establish a differential diagnosis. This, followed by imaging and laboratory data, will usually allow the practitioner to make a positve diagnosis and direct patient therapy. An accurate diagnosis is especially important in order to direct arthroscopic surgical therapy successfully.

Suggested Reading

Dawson PE: Differential diagnosis of temporomandibular joint disorders. *In* Dawson PE: Evaluation, Diagnosis, and Treatment of Occlusal Problems. St. Louis: CV Mosby, 1989.

Dawson PE: Understanding and diagnosing intra-articular problems. *In* Dawson PE: Evaluation, Diagnosis, and Treatment of Occlusal Problems. St. Louis: CV Mosby, 1989.

Dolwick MF: Clinical diagnosis of temporomandibular joint internal derangement and myofascial pain and dysfunction. Oral Maxillofac Surg Clin North Am 1:1-6, 1989.

Dolwick MF: Diagnosis and etiology. *In* Internal Derangements of the Temporomandibular Joint. San Francisco: Radiology Research and Education Foundation, 1983.

Gelb H: Patient evaluation. *In* Gelb H (ed): Clinical Management of Head, Neck, and TMJ Pain and Dysfunction. Philadelphia: WB Saunders, 1977.

Johnson WB: New method for reduction of acute dislocations of the temporomandibular articulations. J Oral Surg 16:501–504, 1958.

McNeill C, et al: Craniomandibular (TMJ) disorders—the state of the art. J Prosthet Dent 44:434, 1980.

Ross JB, Sanders B, Murakami K-I: Treatment planning. *In* Sanders B, Murakami K-I, Clark GT (eds): Diagnostic and Surgical Arthroscopy of the Temporomandibular Joint. Philadelphia; WB Saunders, 1989.

Ware W: Clinical presentation. *In* Helms CA, Katzberg RW, Dolwick MF (eds): Internal Derangements of the Temporomandibular Joint. San Francisco: Radiology Research and Education Foundation, 1983.

Chapter 9

NONSURGICAL MANAGEMENT OF TEMPOROMANDIBULAR JOINT DISORDERS

A. Occlusal Diagnosis and Splint Therapy

TERRY T. TANAKA, D.D.S.

Successful management of temporomandibular joint disorders depends upon many factors and must include a clear understanding of the following: the etiology of the disorder; the chronicity, which determines the degree of pathology and dysfunction; and the host resistance, which includes physical as well as psychological responses to the disorder.

This chapter is designed to increase the clinician's understanding of how muscle hypertonicity, occlusal disorders, and inflammation can affect joint arthrokinematics and result in internal joint derangement. Special emphasis is placed on several clinically successful treatment modalities, including occlusal adjustments, splint therapy, physical therapy, and the use of anti-inflammatory medications.

The clinical decision of how and what to treat is obviously of great importance, but more often the essential question is when and when not to treat. The solution to this dilemma should be based on the development of a careful diagnosis reached by a thorough case history, patient interview, and physical examination.

CASE HISTORY

Almost all physicians agree that the case history, if properly taken, will furnish over 80% of the information required to make a diagnosis.[1] There are no shortcuts to taking a history.

The simplest way to take a history is to request all the pertinent information from patients before they are seen in the office. Once this information is obtained and reviewed, the patient interview and physical examination can proceed swiftly and efficiently.

PATIENT INTERVIEW

While each patient is unique and requires an individualized approach to questioning, several cardinal rules must be observed. The most important ones are to *observe the patient carefully and to listen effectively.*[2] If the clinician observes the patient carefully, he or she will be able to note physical signs of disease and dysfunction that may be visible on the skin of the face, hands, knuckles, wrists, fingernails, eyes, and feet. If one listens effectively, one may notice that the patient will describe the origin of his or her disorder by the adjectives used to describe the dysfunction or pain.

Certain information, of course, has to be obtained by direct questioning. The clinician must be prepared to guide the questioning, being careful not to interject any of his or her own biases and feelings. Also, the clinician should not expect that the patient has everything nicely outlined and sorted out. These skills must be developed through diligent practice. Regardless of the ultimate diagnosis, particular attention should be paid to the particular concerns of the patient, even though they may eventually turn out to be inconsequential.

If a thorough history and interview have been reviewed, the clinician will have a good idea of what the diagnosis is and what treatment should be proposed. The physical examination is done to obtain additional significant information and to confirm or refute this preliminary diagnosis.

ETIOLOGY

The etiology and current status of the patient's disorder can be determined by asking a series of questions that will provide the following information.

Chief Complaint. What is your problem or problems? Several complaints may be described by the patient; therefore, the patient should be asked to list them in order of importance.

Onset and Progression of the Problem. When did the pain or disorder begin and how has it progressed? Did it begin gradually, or did it occur suddenly, as the result of an accident?

Description of the Pain or Problem. Generally, this will identify the source of the patient's discomfort: for example, *vascular pain* will be described as throbbing, pounding, beating, and constant; *neurogenic pain* will be described as sharp, stabbing, numbing, and tingling; and *muscle contraction pain* will be described as a dull, achy, sore, or tight feeling.[3]

Muscle Contraction Pain (Myalgia)

This is the most frequent cause of head and face pain and can be precipitated by a variety of factors, including increased masticatory function. This can occur in stressful states, in which the patient continues to brace or contract the muscles, or as the result of trauma to the face or mandible.

Muscle hyperactivity can also occur as a result of oral habits, such as parafunctional clenching and bruxing, and can result in an increased level of muscle tonus.

Functional and parafunctional activities are quite different clinical entities. The former are very controlled muscle activities that allow the masticatory system to perform necessary functions with minimal damage to any structure. Protective reflexes are constantly present that guard against undesirable tooth contacts, such as interfering tooth contacts during function, which have inhibitory effects on functional muscle activity.[4] Functional activities, therefore, are directly influenced by the occlusal condition.

Parafunctional activities are controlled by an entirely different mechanism. Some authors have suggested that parafunctional activities, instead of being inhibited by tooth contacts, are actually provoked by certain tooth contacts.[5,6] Current electromyographic research in this field by Rugh and Orbach[5] and others should provide valuable information for clinicians.

Occlusion

The definition of an *ideal occlusion* serves realistically only as a basis with which to compare other physiologic types of occlusion. Ideal occlusions rarely occur in humans, and occlusal discrepancies or slides exist as the norm, in addition to skeletal abnormalities. In most instances, the adult patient has adapted to a physiologic occlusion, and no significant pathologic manifestations or dysfunctional problems are experienced in the teeth, periodontium or temporomandibular joint (TMJ). New muscle engrams are programmed to avoid these occlusal discrepancies while still providing efficient function.

Obviously, the patient and his or her functional needs have adapted and continue to adapt to the occlusal variation. In instances when the patient remains asymptomatic, occlusal treatment is generally not indicated.[7]

In symptomatic patients with occlusal discrepancies or skeletal open bites, when a definite cause-and-effect relationship can be made, appropriate treatment must be recommended to alleviate pain and dysfunction. The treatments recommended will depend on the etiology and acuteness of the dysfunction and will usually consist of some type of splint therapy and, when the patient is comfortable, possible occlusal correction by selective grinding.

The initial examination, therefore, should include an analysis of the dental occlusion to determine if pathologic parafunction is present.

Parafunction

Clenching and bruxism are the most frequently encountered oral habits that produce destructive or pathologic forces on the teeth and joint structures. Every attempt should be made to control these habits before any type of irreversible occlusal treatment is initiated.[5] In addition, occlusal correction by selective grinding should not be attempted in the presence of any muscle dysfunction or inflammation of the TMJ. As a general rule, these causes usually can be addressed successfully with proper physical, behavioral, and splint therapy and anti-inflammatory medications.

It is highly recommended that any occlusal correction beyond the removal of a few interfering cusps or ridges in working and balancing movements be preceded by a similar exercise on study models of the patient's dentition mounted on an articulator.

Inflammatory Disorders

Although it is well documented that arthrosis of the TMJ affects most adults by the age of 50, only a small percentage of these adults have pain severe enough to seek medical or dental care. Inflammatory disorders, however, are usually secondary, where synovitis is the result. In patients with synovitis, pain usually occurs during functional movements of the mandible or during any movement that involves joint loading. Most often a combination of muscle splinting, inflammation, and proliferative tissue in the joint causes distraction of the joint parts and an acute malocclusion. Therefore, one must have a clear understanding of arthrosis and arthritis and how they affect the dental occlusion.

Primary Osteoarthrosis

Primary osteoarthrosis may involve remodeling of the articular surfaces of the eminence and the anterior superior surface of the condyle. Osteophytes may be present on the condyle and a decreased joint space may be evident on TMJ radiographs. Generally, however, pain, inflammation, and mandibular dysfunction are not seen. When arthrosis is encountered in this stage, usually no treatment is recommended. If parafunction is present, an orthosis may be prescribed to stabilize the occlusion and to prevent further wear on the dentition.

Secondary Osteoarthrosis (Osteoarthritis)

Osteoarthritis usually results in remodeling of the eminence and condylar surfaces as a result of secondary inflammation of the tissues of the TMJ.[8-10]

In osteoarthritis, hydroxyapatite crystals are shed into the joint and attract macrophages. These macrophages cause an increase in the production of collagenase enzymes in the joint. Collagenase produces active inflammation with degradation of the cartilage matrix and eventually of the surface of the condyle.

The principal treatment for osteoarthritis is anti-inflammatory medication. It should be remembered, however, that in the treatment of osteoarthritis or rheumatic diseases, we are not altering the course of the disease; we are only treating the symptoms of the disease.

The current model for the treatment of osteoarthritis (OA) and rheumatoid arthritis (RA) is based on the following assumptions:

1. OA and RA are treatable diseases.
2. OA and RA are chronic diseases, mandating that the patient participate in his/her care.
3. All medications have side effects; therefore risk/benefit ratios are specifically important.

Those patients with a better prognosis are men less than 40 years of age with acute onset of disease occurring less than 1 year before therapy. Patients with a poor prognosis are those with continuous disease activi-

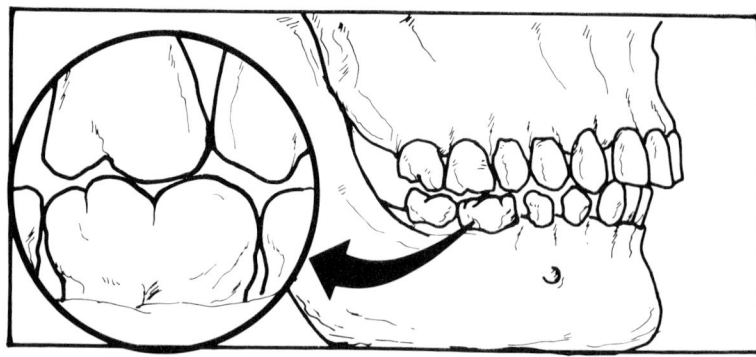

Figure 9–1. Drawing of the dental arches, with enlarged inset, depicting the removal of centric interferences from the mesial inclines of the maxillary teeth and the distal inclines of the mandibular teeth.

ty, bony erosions, extra-articular manifestations (nodules), and a positive rheumatoid factor.[11]

TREATMENT
Indications for Occlusal Adjustment

Occlusal adjustment is recommended (1) in treatment of occlusal trauma (particularly primary occlusal traumatism associated with periodontal disease), (2) in treatment of major occlusal interferences affecting jaw closure (extruded third molars and tilted or rotated teeth), (3) post-orthodontically where indicated, and (4) often before and/or after prosthetic or restorative procedures. Occlusal correction by selective grinding should follow a step-by-step outline in order to produce a finished result that is both stable in centric relation as well as functional in all of the lateral and protrusive excursions (Figs. 9–1 and 9–2).

Splint Therapy

Splint therapy is currently one of the dental profession's most popular and most misused treatment modalities. The existence of so many theories about and techniques for the use of splint therapy points out the lack of a rational understanding of the biomechanics, anatomy, and physiology of the TMJ. Few people understand how and why splints work and for this reason splints are often misused, causing increased suffering for the patient and aggravation and frustration for the dentist.

This section addresses the rational indications and uses of splint therapy for muscle contraction pain of the head and neck and for internal derangement of the TMJ. These are the two most frequently encountered disorders for which splint therapy is effective.

Splints are effective because of their ability to (1) alter muscle proprioception, (2) stabilize the occlusion and condyle-fossa relationship, and (3) alter adverse loading forces in the TMJ.[12, 13]

Types of Appliances

Three basic types of orthoses (splints) are recommended. They are classified here as Types A, B, and C.

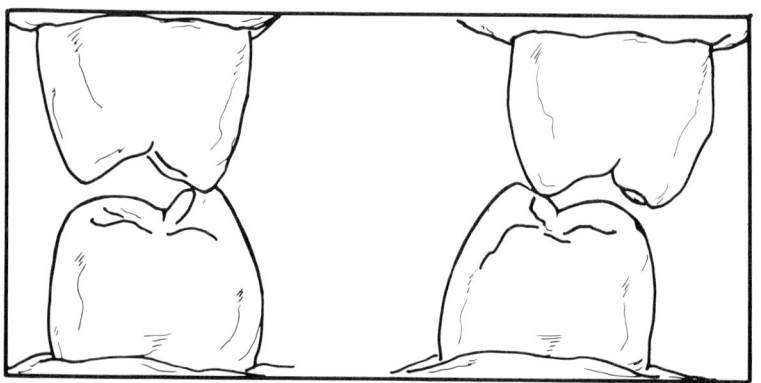

Figure 9–2. In lateral working excursions, interferences should be removed from the buccal cusps of the maxillary teeth and the lingual cusps of the mandibular teeth.

Type A

This orthosis is a *rotational*, full occlusal contact appliance with anterior guidance that contacts all of the opposing teeth in centric occlusion (maximal intercuspation) (Fig. 9–3). It is made of hard acrylic with a minimal vertical thickness posteriorly (1.0–1.5 mm) between the molars. It is intended for patients with parafunctional habits, such as bruxism and clenching, and malocclusion and occlusal interferences. The orthosis can be placed on either maxillary or mandibular teeth, depending on the condition of the existing supporting dentition, missing teeth, and type of occlusion or malocclusion.

This orthosis should be placed on the maxilla when possible. The patient is instructed to wear the appliance at night while sleeping if he or she is a nocturnal bruxer. If the patient is a nocturnal clencher-bruxer, the appliance should be adjusted or equilibrated against the opposing teeth while the patient is reclined in the dental chair (reclined postural centric).

If there is parafunction during the day, the appliance should be placed on the maxilla and should be equilibrated initially in centric occlusion, with the patient seated in an upright position. If the parafunction occurs during both day and night, the appliance must be equilibrated in both positions, with the patient seated and lying down. This type of appliance is useful for minor derangement

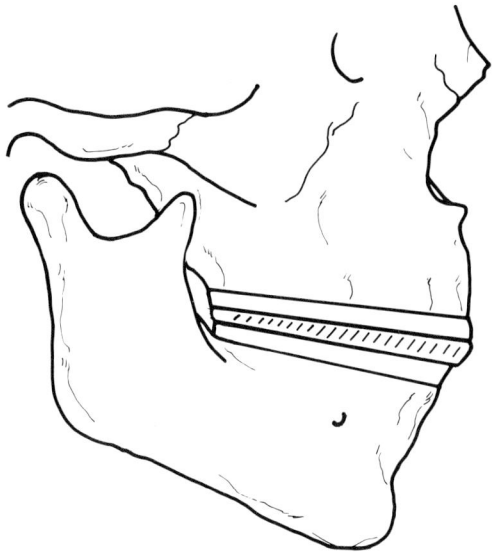

Figure 9–4. Type B (rotational) splint. This appliance is designed to be used for Class II, Division II malocclusions or severely abraded dentition with decreased vertical dimension.

of the TMJ and for relief of minor pain and dysfunction from adverse loading due to muscle contraction pain.

As the muscle and joint dysfunction are resolved, the splint can be adjusted to a centric relation position and the natural dentition adjusted to the centric relation position. Eventually, the splint can be worn only at night and as needed during the day. At this time the splint surface can be relined with acrylic to stabilize the centric position. Approximately 80% of splints will be of this type.

Type B

Like Type A, this orthosis is a *rotational*, full occlusal contact appliance with anterior guidance that usually contacts all of the opposing teeth in centric occlusion at maximal intercuspation. The purpose of this appliance is to restore the lost vertical dimension from tooth wear, to physically affect the loading and splinting muscles through their mechanoreceptors, and to restore a more normal resting length to the muscles. Therefore, it must be thicker (1.5–2.0 mm) in the posterior occlusal areas but should not interfere with the freeway space. Type B appliances are used most frequently in Class II—Div. II deep bite cases (Fig. 9–4).

Neither the Type A or Type B splint will

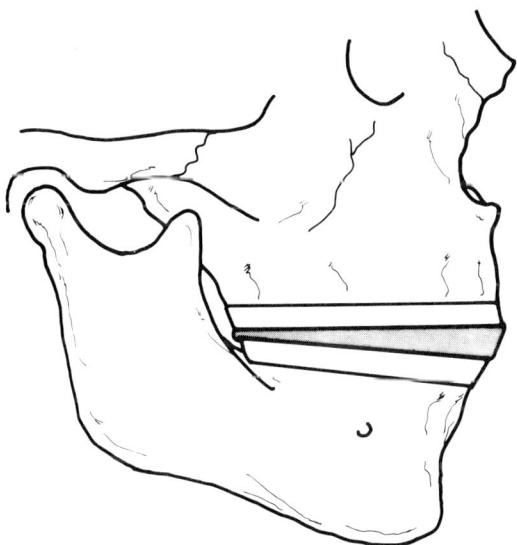

Figure 9–3. Type A (rotational) splint, constructed with 1.5 mm thickness between the posterior teeth.

alter the position of the condyle in the fossa, because both are made at different thicknesses along the same arc of closure and around the same center of rotation.

Even though the early clicking and popping sounds diminish and may eventually disappear, the Type B appliance height must be maintained. At this time the patient can be instructed to wear the Type B orthosis only at night. When the patient begins to feel better, however, he or she must continue to wear the appliance 24 hours a day, until the vertical dimension is restored permanently by orthodontic therapy or by fixed or removable prosthodontic appliances. Patients with deep bites (Class II—Division II) should continue use night and day for at least 6 to 9 months before final treatment is started with orthodontics or rehabilitation.

Type A and Type B appliances should be worn day and night during therapy. The complete arch, full occlusal contact appliances rarely intrude the dentition when used properly. If the clinician is in doubt as to whether the appliance is too thick, he can ask the patient to repeat the letters "M, M, M" or "N, N, N" or the sound, "hummmm, hummmm." If the splint is too thick and encroaches upon the freeway space, the patient's teeth will contact the appliance. The appliance can be reduced in height slightly to clear the interference. Both Type A and Type B appliances are fabricated in centric occlusion initially and then may be adjusted to an ideal condyle fossa position as the symptoms diminish.

Type C

This orthosis is a condyle *repositioning* appliance that occludes throughout the arch. The condyles are repositioned, using the corrected TMJ tomograms as a guide, as follows:

Step 1: Mount study models on an articulator with a face-bow (Fig. 9–5).

Step 2: The incisal pin is opened at least 2 mm before repositioning the condyle in the fossa. This is done to prevent breaking the teeth on the models when repositioning the mandible (Fig. 9–6).

Step 3: The condyles are then repositioned either to increase the joint space or to locate the condyle more centrally in the fossa in order to decrease adverse loading of the joint structures (Fig. 9–7).

Step 4: The patient should be able to bite immediately into the new splint position

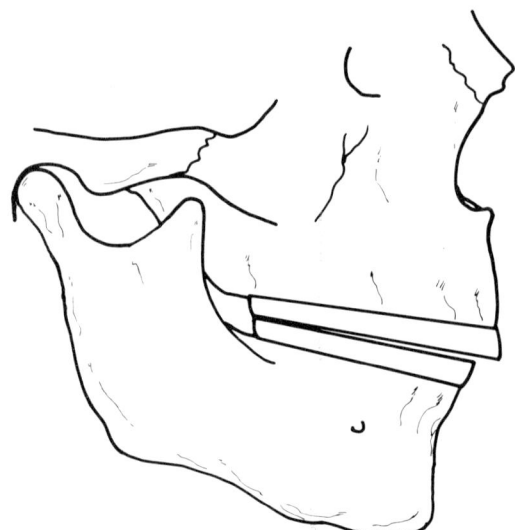

Figure 9–5. Type C repositioning splint (step 1). Severe posterior condylar displacement is depicted in this schematic drawing. This relationship would be transferred onto an articulator.

without difficulty. All repositioning splints should be made at a minimal thickness and should not encroach on the freeway space (Fig. 9–8).

In cases of acute displacement, as the painful symptoms diminish and the disc returns to a more normal anatomic position interposed between the articular eminence and the condyle, the appliance can be adjusted

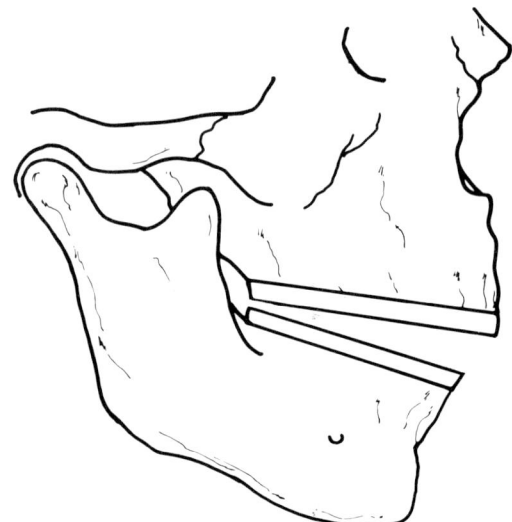

Figure 9–6. In step 2, the incisal pin is opened approximately 2 mm before repositioning the condyles on the articulator.

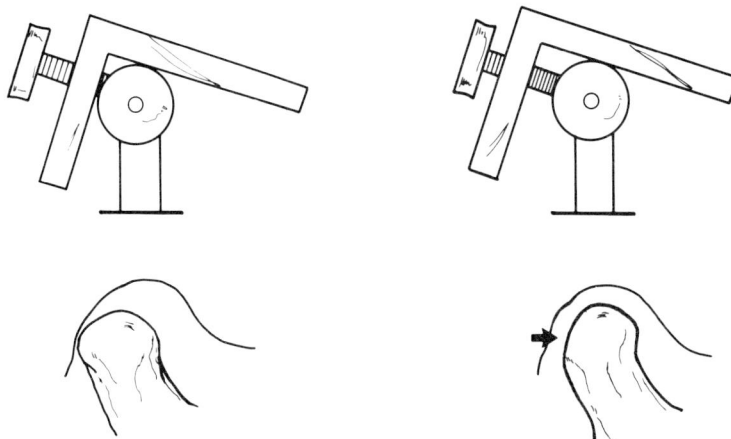

Figure 9–7. In step 3, the condyles are repositioned on the articulator into more central positions in the fossae. Radiographic assistance can be used.

back to the physiologic centric position. This same procedure can be followed in cases in which the disc does not reduce but the painful symptoms have remitted and restoration of function has been re-established.

In cases of severe condylar displacement, once the condyles have been repositioned, they are left in that position. At this time, the patient should be sent to the radiology laboratory to have a tomogram taken of each TMJ with the splint in place. A middle sagittal view with the teeth closed in the splint will reveal whether the condyle has been repositioned in the fossa in the same position as it was on the articulator.

The use of this type of appliance allows proper repositioning of the displaced disc within 1 to 5 days if the displacement was of recent onset. In cases in which the displacement occurred 4 to 6 months prior to splint therapy, the Type C appliance may provide symptomatic relief, but disc repositioning is doubtful.

If the disc cannot be repositioned within the first 3 to 4 weeks with the Type C splint and physical therapy, further conservative therapy will probably be unsuccessful.

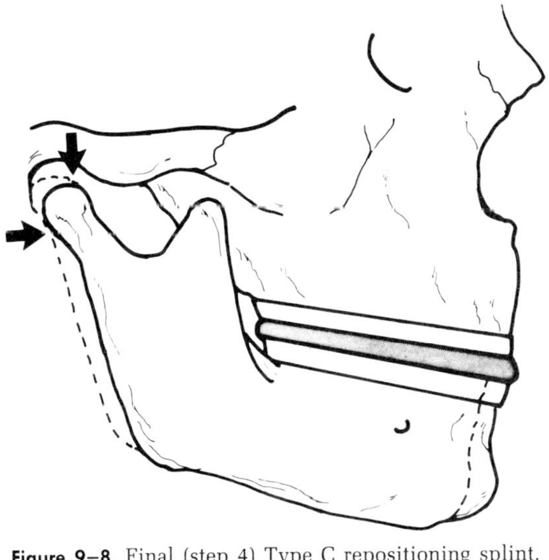

Physical Therapy

Physical therapy should be utilized concurrently with splint therapy in all cases of internal derangement when splints are used. The physical therapy treatment modalities are especially effective for muscular disorders, for discs that are displaced, and for painful capsulitis.

Once the disc has been repositioned and the patient's signs and symptoms have diminished, the patient must continue to wear this appliance for at least 1 month in this position before attempting to lower or thin down the appliance. It is during this period that remodeling of the retrodiscal tissues takes place.

Figure 9–8. Final (step 4) Type C repositioning splint. The patient should be able to close immediately into the new repositioning splint. The new position can be verified by tomograms.

Orthodontic therapy is usually the preferable treatment following disc repositioning appliance therapy, because long, involved reconstruction procedures with protracted mouth opening maintain the joint structures in a hyperextended position and can cause trauma to the healing joint structures and possible recurrence of the initial disorder.

SUMMARY

The rational use of occlusal adjustments, anti-inflammatory medications, physical therapy, and splint therapy must be based on a thorough understanding of TMJ anatomy and associated musculature and how these structures function. With this knowledge, dysfunctions can be diagnosed readily and accurately and proper treatments rendered, resulting in prompt resolution for the benefit of the patient.

References

1. Assessment. *In* Potter D O, et al (eds): Nursing 84 Books, Springhouse, PA: Springhouse, 1984, pp 15–51.
2. Part I: Medicine as a Learned Profession. Wyngaarden J B, Smith L H (eds): Cecil Textbook of Medicine. Philadelphia: W B Saunders, 1985, pp 1–15.
3. Bell W E: Orofacial Pains, 4th Ed. Chicago, Year Book 1989, pp 77–92.
4. Sessle B J: *In* Roth G I, Calmes R (eds): Oral Biology. St Louis: CV Mosby, 1989, p 61.
5. Rugh J D, Orbach R: Occlusal parafunction. *In* Mohl N, et al (eds): Textbook of Occlusion. Lombard, IL, Quintessence, 1988, pp 249–261.
6. Okeson J P: Management of Temporomandibular Disorders, 2nd Ed. St Louis: CV Mosby, 1989, pp 152–172.
7. Majersjo C, Carlsson G E: Analysis of factors influencing the long-term effect of treatment of TMJ dysfunction. J Oral Rehab, 11:289–297, 1984.
8. Carlsson G E: Mandibular dysfunction and pathosis. J Prosthet Dent 43:658, 1980.
9. Carlsson G E, Kopp S, Oberg T: Arthritis and allied diseases of the TMJ. *In* Zarb G A, Carlsson G E (eds): Temporomandibular Joint Function and Dysfunction, Copenhagen: Ejnor Munkegaard Forlag, 1979, pp 269–320.
10. Castelli W A, et al: Histologic findings in temporomandibular joints of aged individuals. J Prosthet Dent 53:415, 1985.
11. Weisman M: Rheumatology for dentists. *In* Tanaka T T (ed): A Diagnostic and Therapeutic Approach for Head, Neck and TMJ Disorders for Restorative Dentists, 3rd Ed. San Diego: Clinical Research Foundation, 1988, pp N1–6.
12. Okeson J P: Management of TM Disorders and Occlusions, 2nd Ed., St Louis: CV Mosby, 1989, pp 297–425.
13. Tanaka T T: (ed): A Diagnostic and Therapeutic Approach for Head, Neck and TMJ Disorders for Restorative Dentists, 4th Ed. Chula Vista: Clinical Research Foundation, 1989, pp 11–21.

☐ B. Splint Treatment of Patients with Disc Displacement with Reduction: A Research Perspective

HÅKAN LUNDH, D.D.S., PH.D.,
PER-LENNART WESTESSON, D.D.S., PH.D.

HISTORICAL BACKGROUND

Identification and Definition of Disc Displacement

Disc displacement of the temporomandibular joint (TMJ) (Fig. 9–9) was mentioned as early as 1823 by Sir Astley Cooper,[1] and the first description of treatment of this disorder was by Annandale in 1887,[2] who described two patients in whom "the interar-

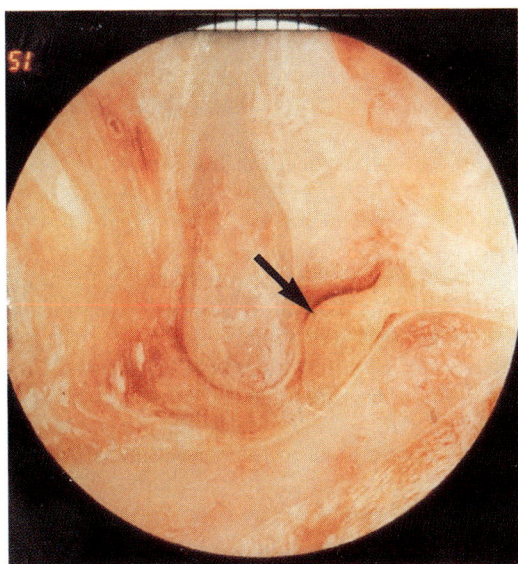

Figure 9–9. Cryosection of a temporomandibular joint with disc displacement. Arrow indicates the location of the posterior band of the disc.

ticular cartilage was seized, drawn into position, and secured to the periostium." Treatment of disc displacement later on was mentioned in the literature on several occasions,[3-8] but the mechanism of TMJ clicking and its association with disc displacement remained obscure to most clinicians until the late 1970s, when arthrographic documentation of disc displacement became available.[9, 10] However, based on clinical observations, Ireland[11] accurately described the mechanism of TMJ clicking in 1951; he reported that "during the final few millimeters of the closing movement, the thickened upper part of the disc rotates forward to lie between the condyle and the posterior-inferior surface of the eminence. This movement of the disc causes the faint click heard during this movement." Ireland was not, however, able to support his observation with radiographic or other documentation and his description of the mechanism of clicking was not adopted by many clinicians until almost 30 years later.

In 1978, Wilkes[9, 10] combined clinical, arthrographic, and surgical observations of a group of patients who presented with pain, clicking, and TMJ dysfunction and stated that displacement of the disc is a frequent source of these symptoms. A dual-space, double-contrast arthrogram of a patient with anterior disc displacement is shown in Figure 9–10. Wilkes' observations confirmed earlier studies[12, 13] and were later verified by several investigators.[14-18]

Reduction of a displaced disc implies that the relationship between the condyle and the disc is normal during mouth opening. In 1979, this terminology was adopted from the Sixth Annual TMJ Research Seminar, in Chicago.[14] Accordingly, disc displacement without reduction implies that the disc remains in the displaced position relative to the condyle during all mandibular movement (Fig. 9–11).

Development of Treatment Modalities

Immediately following the demonstration that disc displacement is frequent in patients with TMJ disorder,[9, 10] there was much interest in the treatment of this condition. The interest was initially concentrated on surgical correction of disc displacement,[15, 19-22] but there were also publications about the nonsurgical treatment of this condition.[12, 13, 20, 21, 23] Thus, Farrar[12, 13] suggested that a displaced disc could be repositioned by positioning the mandible anteriorly, using a so-called protrusive splint (Fig. 9–12). This type of treatment was adopted with enthusiasm by many clinicians, and several reports on the initial results of treatment with protrusive splints were published.[24-30]

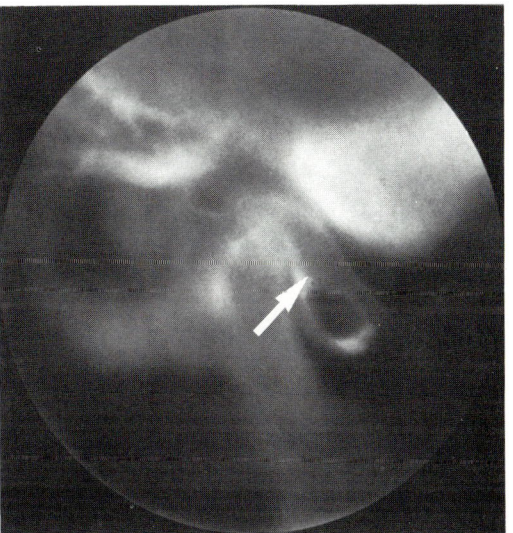

Figure 9–10. Double-contrast arthrogram of a patient with anterior disc displacement. Contrast medium and air have been injected into the upper and lower joint spaces. Arrow indicates the location of the posterior band of the disc.

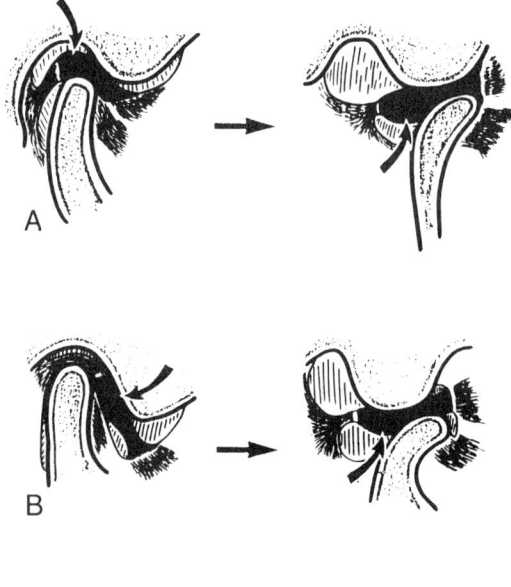

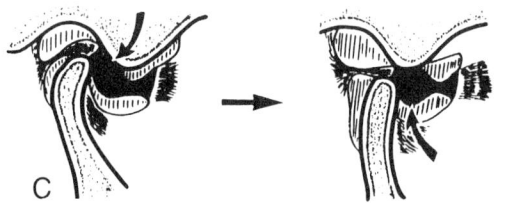

Figure 9–11. Schematic drawings of the temporomandibular joint illustrating normal disc position *(A)* and anterior disc displacement with *(B)* and without *(C)* reduction.

The treatment, however, was questioned because of the risk of induced malocclusion,[31, 32] failure to relieve pain,[31] and the need for difficult and time-consuming follow-up treatment with rather low success rates.[33]

Traditionally TMJ disorders have been treated using a flat occlusal splint (Fig. 9–13), either alone or combined with other methods such as occlusal adjustment or physical therapy.[34–50] A high success rate has been reported for these methods in patients with nonspecific TMJ pain and dysfunction.[34–50] Therefore, some authors have suggested that these methods should also be used for patients with disc displacement, and a few studies have indicated that the same methods are successful for this group of patients.[51–53] These recommendations, based on studies without control groups, however, contradict findings in another study[28] that systematically compared the results of treatment with a flat occlusal splint to those with a protrusive splint in patients with disc displacement with reduction (Table 9–1). This study found that treatment with the flat occlusal splint resulted in no significant change in either anamnestic or clinical dysfunction indexes in patients with a clinical diagnosis of disc displacement with reduction.[28]

In the light of these contradictory findings we initiated a series of studies to evaluate treatment with a protrusive splint[12, 13] in patients with disc displacement with reduction and compared findings to those with nontreated controls and with patients treated with a flat occlusal splint.[54–57] The following results are based on these studies[54–57] and on other information in the literature.

DISC REPOSITIONING SPLINT

Study Design

In our first study,[54] 70 patients with a clinical diagnosis of disc displacement with re-

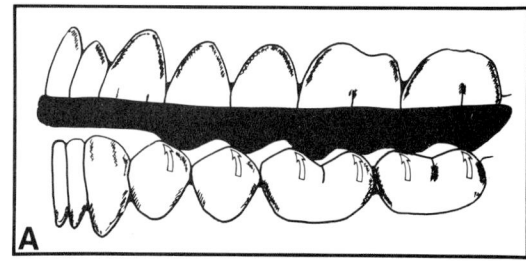

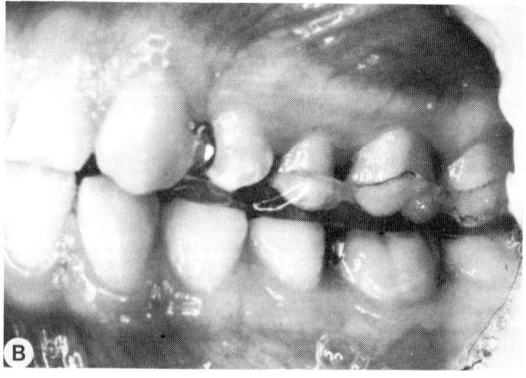

Figure 9–12. *A*, Schematic drawing of an anterior repositioning splint showing how the mandible is guided to close in an anterior position (splint designed according to Farrar[12]). *B*, Anterior repositioning splint in vivo. The splint maintains the mandible in the therapeutic position.

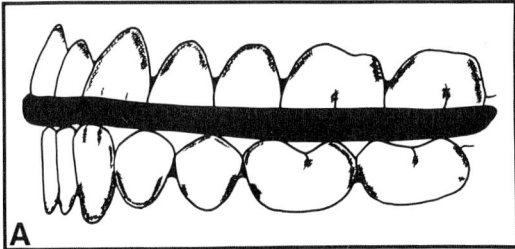

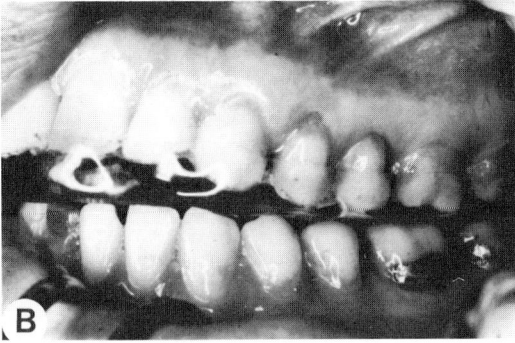

Figure 9–13. *A,* Schematic drawing of a flat occlusal splint (splint designed according to Posselt[35]). *B,* Flat occlusal splint in vivo showing even occlusal contacts without interferences.

duction manifested as reciprocal clicking were randomly assigned to be treated with (a) an anterior repositioning splint, (b) a flat occlusal splint, or (c) to serve as an untreated control group. Two thirds of the patients were females and one third were males. The median age was 30 years, with a range of 15 to 62 years. Patients were selected on the basis of having reciprocal clicking that could be eliminated with a protrusive splint (see Fig. 9–12). No consideration was given to the intensity of the pain (some patients had severe pain, whereas others had only mild pain).

The anterior repositioning splint was designed to keep the mandible in an anterior, non-clicking, position such that the disc was not displaced.[12, 13, 20] The anterior position of the mandible was maintained through inclines on the occlusal surface of the splint, which forced the mandible to occlude only when the splint was in the anterior position (Fig. 9–12A). If the patient attempted to move the mandible posteriorly, this immediately increased the vertical dimension through these inclines. By this method the disc was kept in the reduced position. The anterior repositioning splint was used for 24 hours a day for 6 weeks; its use was gradually reduced during the following 2 weeks.

The flat occlusal maxillary splint (see Fig. 9–13) was designed according to Posselt.[34] It was adjusted to maximal occlusal contacts in the centric relation and in centric occlusion. There was no intention, by using this splint, to actually recapture the disc although it may happen in some cases. The splint was used nightly,[50, 58] which is the traditional way of using this type of splint. The splint was used for 6 weeks; its use was gradually reduced during the following 2 weeks.

Patients in the untreated control group were not given any active occlusal treatment, although they received pain medication as needed. They were reassured that this was a benign condition that would gradually improve over time.

Results of Treatment (Table 9–2)

At follow-up after 6 weeks, the patients treated with an anterior repositioning splint showed less pain at rest, during chewing, and during protrusion, compared with the

Table 9–1. COMPARISON (NUMBER OF PATIENTS) OF FLAT OCCLUSAL SPLINT AND ORTHOPEDIC MANDIBULAR REPOSITIONING SPLINT (20 PATIENTS)

	Flat Occlusal Splint	Orthopedic Mandibular Repositioning Splint
Anamnestic Index		
Improved	0	6
Unchanged	10	4
Clinical Dysfunction Index		
Improved	1	7
Unchanged or Exacerbated	9	3

Reprinted with permission from Anderson GC, Schulte JK, Goodkind RJ: Comparative study of two treatment methods for internal derangement of the temporomandibular joint. J Prosthet Dent 53:392–397, 1985.

Table 9–2. DISTRIBUTION (NUMBER OF PATIENTS) OF CLINICAL FINDINGS BEFORE TREATMENT AND AT FOLLOW-UP AFTER 6 AND 17 WEEKS IN THREE TREATMENT GROUPS (70 PATIENTS)

Clinical Findings	Treatment Groups		
	Anterior Repositioning Splint (24 Patients)	*Flat Splint (23 Patients)*	*Control Group (23 Patients)*
Reciprocal clickings			
Before treatment	24	23	23
After 6 weeks	2	23	21
After 17 weeks	19*	21	23*
Tenderness laterally over the joint			
Before treatment	9	9	9
After 6 weeks	2	2	11
After 17 weeks	7	5	8
Tenderness laterally of pterygoid muscle			
Before treatment	17	14	20
After 6 weeks	8	13	19
After 17 weeks	13	14	18
Tenderness of insertion of temporal muscle			
Before treatment	19	15	19
After 6 weeks	7	12	21
After 17 weeks	12	12	17
Tenderness of superficial masseter muscle			
Before treatment	9	8	8
After 6 weeks	4	5	16
After 17 weeks	8	8	12

*One of these patients demonstrated limitation of opening and deviation to the affected side.

initial status before treatment. Tenderness of the TMJ and the masticatory muscle also was less frequent than before treatment.

After removal of the anterior repositioning splint, the favorable effect of the treatment disappeared and the symptoms returned in most patients, as noted at the 17-week follow-up. In patients treated with a flat occlusal splint, a decreased frequency of tenderness over the joint was observed, but there were no other changes compared with the initial recordings. In the untreated control patients, increased tenderness in the superficial masseter muscle was noted, but there were no other changes compared with the initial recordings.

A comparison between the three treatment groups is shown in Table 9–3. The greatest difference was noted between patients with the anterior repositioning splint and the control group. However, there were also differences between patients with the flat occlusal splint and the control group. It was not possible to demonstrate any statistically significant differences between the groups receiving the anterior repositioning splint and the flat occlusal splint, except for the disappearance of reciprocal clicking in the former.

DISC REPOSITIONING ONLAYS

The observation in the previous study that the symptoms returned when the use of the splint was terminated led us to believe that a longer treatment period is necessary to maintain the favorable results of the disc repositioning treatment. Therefore, in this study,[55] we used cemented disc repositioning onlays (Fig. 9–14). These onlays were cemented on the lower, unprepared premolars and molars and were used for 6 months.

The principal function of these onlays was the same as that of the anterior repositioning splint, but these were more convenient to use. Also, the onlays were guaranteed to stay

Table 9-3. LEVEL OF STATISTICAL SIGNIFICANCE (FISHER'S EXACT TEST) FOR COMPARISON OF CLINICAL FINDINGS IN THREE TREATMENT GROUPS (70 PATIENTS) AFTER 6 WEEKS OF TREATMENT

Clinical Observation	Level of Statistical Significance		
	Anterior Repositioning Splint Compared with Control Group	*Flat Occlusal Splint Compared with Control Group*	*Anterior Repositioning Splint Compared with Flat Occlusal Splint*
Reciprocal clicking	<0.001	n.s.*	<0.001
Palpatory tenderness laterally over joint	<0.006	<0.007	n.s.
Palpatory tenderness of lateral pterygoid muscle	<0.001	n.s.	n.s.
Palpatory tenderness of insertion of temporal muscle	<0.001	<0.007	n.s.
Palpatory tenderness of superficial masseter muscle	<0.001	<0.003	n.s.

*n.s. = not significant (p>0.05).

in place during the entire treatment period, which may not always be true with anterior repositioning splints, since patients could remove these.

Study Design

In this study, there were 63 patients, 54 females and 9 males, whose ages ranged from 13 to 74 years, with a median age of 24 years. All patients had had an arthrographic diagnosis of anterior disc displacement with re-

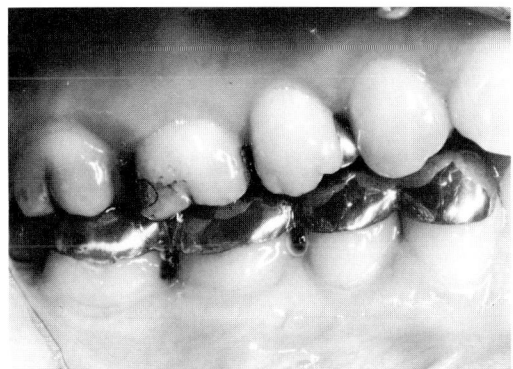

Figure 9-14. Disc repositioning onlays cemented on the unprepared lower molars and premolars. The onlays are cast in silver.

duction, and the mandibular positions for disc repositioning onlays were determined during arthrography as previously described (Fig. 9-15).[27, 59, 60] Double-contrast arthrograms in the closed mouth position are shown in Figure 9-16, with the disc being anteriorly displaced (Fig. 9-16A) and immediately after disc repositioning (Fig. 9-16B). The patients also were selected with respect to the intensity of pain; those with no pain or only mild pain (less than 5 on a scale of 0 to 10) were excluded in order to be able to better differentiate between the treatment results in the different groups. One third of the patients were treated with disc repositioning onlays, one third were treated with a flat occlusal splint in the same way as in the previous study, and the last third did not receive any active treatment and served as untreated controls. The patients were randomly assigned to the different treatment groups.

Results of Treatment

Follow-up after 6 months of treatment showed that the intensity of subjective complaints, pain during protrusion, and degree of disturbed joint function were significantly lower in patients treated with disc repositioning onlays, compared with the untreated

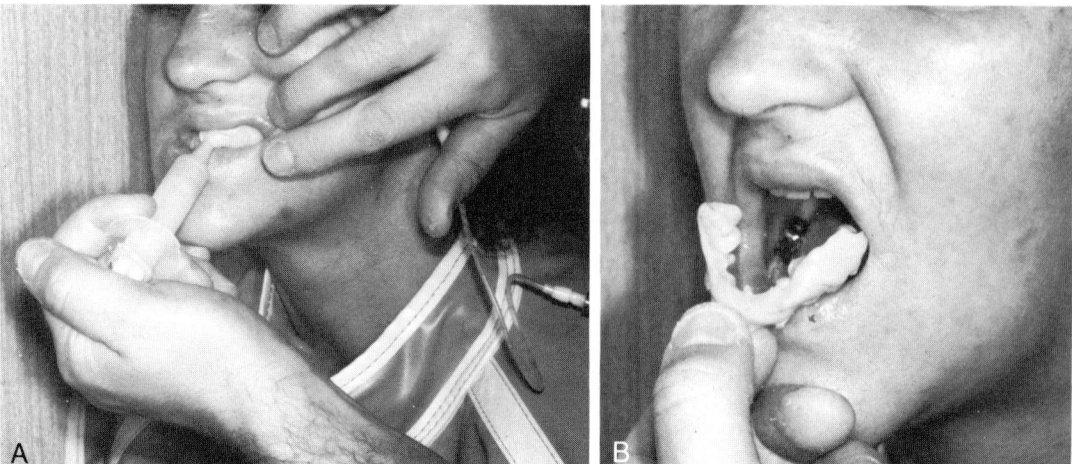

Figure 9–15. *A*, Therapeutic position for disc repositioning established in association with arthrography and documented with fast-setting material. *B*, Bite registration index of the therapeutic position is removed.

controls (Tables 9–4 through 9–7). The intensity of subjective complaints was also lower in the onlay group compared with the flat occlusal splint group. The group treated with the flat occlusal splint did not show any statistically significant improvement compared with the untreated control group, and the untreated control group did not show improvement during the 6-month observation period.

After 6 months the treatments were discontinued. Reciprocal clicking or locking returned in all but one patient within 6 weeks (median = 1 week). TMJ and masticatory muscle pain returned with clicking and locking.

Post-treatment Arthrography

Arthrography was performed before removal of the onlays in 18 of the 20 patients so treated.[55, 56] Arthrography at follow-up after 6 months of treatment showed that the disc

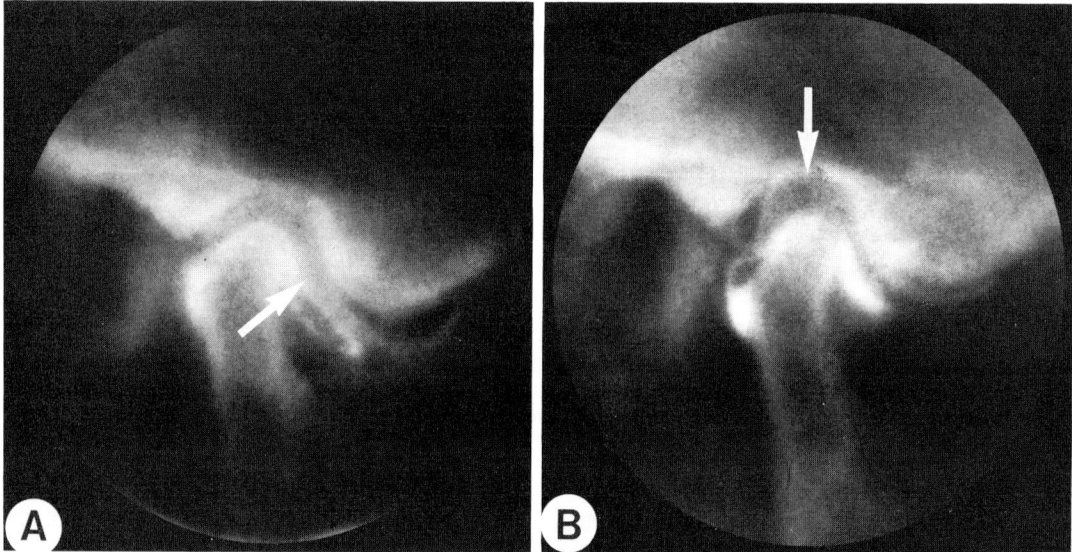

Figure 9–16. *A*, Double-contrast arthrogram showing disc displacement at the closed mouth position. Arrow indicates the location of the posterior band of the disc. *B*, The same temporomandibular joint after the disc has been recaptured. The posterior band (arrow) of the disc is now on top of the condyle.

Table 9-4. MEDIAN OF SUBJECTIVE SYMPTOMS AS EVALUATED BY 63 PATIENTS*

Subjective Symptoms	Treatment Groups		
	Disc Repositioning Onlays (20 Patients)	Flat Occlusal Splint (21 Patients)	Control Group (22 Patients)
Intensity of chief complaint			
Before treatment	6	5	6
After 6 months	0	2	4.5
Pain during chewing			
Before treatment	2.5	3	3.5
After 6 months	0	1	2.5
Pain during protrusion			
Before treatment	1	1	3.5
After 6 months	0	2	1.5
Disturbed joint function			
Before treatment	4.5	5	6
After 6 months	0	3	3

*Using visual analog scales with 0 and 10 as end points.

Table 9-5. DISTRIBUTION (NUMBER OF PATIENTS) OF CLINICAL FINDINGS BEFORE TREATMENT AND AT FOLLOW-UP AFTER 6 MONTHS IN THREE TREATMENT GROUPS (63 PATIENTS)

Clinical Findings	Treatment Groups		
	Disc Repositioning Onlays (20 Patients)	Flat Occlusal Splint (21 Patients)	Control Group (22 Patients)
Reciprocal clicking			
Before treatment	20	21	22
After 6 months	1	16	17
Palpatory tenderness laterally over the joint			
Before treatment	12	17	19
After 6 months	3	10	14
Palpatory tenderness of lateral pterygoid muscle			
Before treatment	14	18	14
After 6 months	4	14	19
Palpatory tenderness of insertion of temporal muscle			
Before treatment	11	17	16
After 6 months	3	17	18
Palpatory tenderness of anterior portion of temporal muscle			
Before treatment	6	6	6
After 6 months	2	8	10
Palpatory tenderness of superficial masseter muscle			
Before treatment	8	10	12
After 6 months	4	14	13

Table 9-6. LEVEL OF STATISTICAL SIGNIFICANCE (WILCOXON'S RANK SUM TEST) FOR COMPARISON OF TREATMENT GROUPS CONCERNING THE REDUCTION OF SUBJECTIVE SYMPTOMS AFTER 6 MONTHS (63 PATIENTS)

Subjective Symptoms	Treatment Groups		
	Disc Repositioning Onlays Compared with Control Group	Disc Repositioning Onlays Compared with Flat Occlusal Splint	Flat Occlusal Splint Compared with Control Group
Intensity of chief complaint	++	++	n.s.
Pain during chewing	n.s.	n.s.	n.s.
Pain during protrusion	+	n.s.	n.s.
Disturbed joint function	+	n.s.	n.s.

Abbrev.: n.s. = not significant (p>0.05); + = p≤0.05; ++ = p≤0.01.

remained in the superior position in 12 patients but was displaced again in six patients. Thus, in one third of the patients treated with disc repositioning onlays, the discs were displaced during treatment, and symptoms returned in these patients.

A retrospective analysis of the pretreatment arthrogram suggested that there could have been a medial component to the disc displacement in four of the six patients in whom the disc became displaced during treatment. Medial disc displacements were not seen in patients with a successful treatment outcome. This suggests that medial disc displacement is more difficult to treat with disc repositioning than is straight anterior disc displacement.

Table 9-7. LEVEL OF STATISTICAL SIGNIFICANCE (FISHER'S EXACT TEST) FOR COMPARISON OF CLINICAL FINDINGS BETWEEN TREATMENT GROUPS AFTER 6 MONTHS (63 PATIENTS)

Clinical Findings	Treatment Groups		
	Disc Repositioning Onlays Compared with Control Groups	Disc Repositioning Onlays Compared with Flat Occlusal Splint	Flat Occlusal Splint Compared with Control Group
Reciprocal clicking	+++	+++	n.s.
Palpatory tenderness laterally over joint	++	n.s.	n.s.
Palpatory tenderness of lateral pterygoid muscle	+++	++	n.s.
Palpatory tenderness of insertion of temporal muscle	+++	+++	n.s.
Palpatory tenderness of anterior portion of temporal muscle	+	n.s.	n.s.
Palpatory tenderness of superficial masseter muscle	+	++	n.s.

Abbrev.: n.s. = not significant (p>0.05); + = p≤0.05; ++ = p≤0.01; +++ = p≤0.001.

LONG-TERM RESULTS OF DISC REPOSITIONING

Review of the Literature

Results of long-term follow-up after disc repositioning therapy have been presented by several authors. Clark[25] in 1984 published the result of a 1- to 3-year follow-up of 14 patients who were found on clinical examination to have internal derangement of the TMJ and who had been treated with disc repositioning appliances. The results were evaluated using a patient questionnaire in which they were asked to judge frequency of jaw clicking, amount of functional limitation caused by their jaw problem, and percentage of improvement of the subjective symptoms. A marked decrease in the frequency of clicking and some improvement in joint function were reported by 12 of the 14 patients.

Another long-term study of the results of treatment of TMJ reciprocal clicking was presented by Le Bell and Kirveskari in 1985.[30] They followed 18 patients with reciprocal clicking and symptoms of mandibular dysfunction who had been treated with repositioning splints in combination with occlusal adjustment. The results were assessed clinically after 2½ years. They reported that clicking disappeared in about one half of the patients and that all the patients were free of symptoms at the final evaluation. In 1986, Moloney and Howard[33] reported an overall success rate of 36% with anterior repositioning therapy in 241 patients from whom the records were reviewed after a period of about 3 years.

Thus, different studies have reported substantially different long-term results of disc repositioning therapy. No long-term studies have been published comparing the results of treatment with disc repositioning, treatment with surgical disc repositioning, and no treatment (untreated control group).

Long-term Follow-up Study of Our Patients

Our long-term follow-up study was based on 15 patients (13 females and 2 males) with ages ranging from 17 to 64 years and a median age of 38 years.[57] This was a consecutive series of patients treated by one of us (HL). All but one of the patients in this study had been treated unsuccessfully, before disc repositioning treatment was initiated, using conventional methods; these included counseling, occlusal adjustment, medication, flat occlusal splint, and physical therapy. All patients had a clinical diagnosis of disc displacement that was confirmed with arthrography in six patients. The median follow-up period was 41 months, with a range of 15–86 months.

Initially, the patients were treated with anterior repositioning devices such as acrylic onlays (Fig. 9–17), removable metallic onlays (Fig. 9–18), and metallic onlays with acrylic veneering (Fig. 9–19). In one patient, light-cured composite material was used to maintain the mandible in such a position that the disc was not displaced. The temporary repositioning devices were used for 24 hours a day for 6 to 32 months (average, 10 months) before permanent reconstruction of the occlusion to the therapeutic position was performed.

Permanent Change of Occlusion to the Therapeutic Position

Provided that the patient was free of clicking, intermittent locking, pain, and other symptoms during the observation period with a temporary device, a permanent change of the occlusion was performed. The occlusion was permanently changed to the therapeutic position by prosthodontic methods in 11 patients (Figs. 9–8 and 9–20) and by orthodontic methods in 4 patients (Fig. 9–21). The extent of the orthodontic treatment or the prosthodontic reconstruction was individually determined based on the need to stabilize the occlusion in the therapeutic position. The treatment was first performed on one side; on completion, the onlays were removed and the other side was completed. In this way, one side always served as an accurate indicator to transfer the temporary therapeutic position to the permanent reconstruction.

The orthodontic technique to permanently change occlusion to the therapeutic position aimed specifically at closing the bilateral posterior open bites that occurred when the onlays or the anterior repositioning splints were removed. This was done by modifying the maxillary anterior repositioning splint to function like a Sved bite plate.[61, 62] Thus the appliance covered the upper second molars, incisors, and cuspids, and the teeth in be-

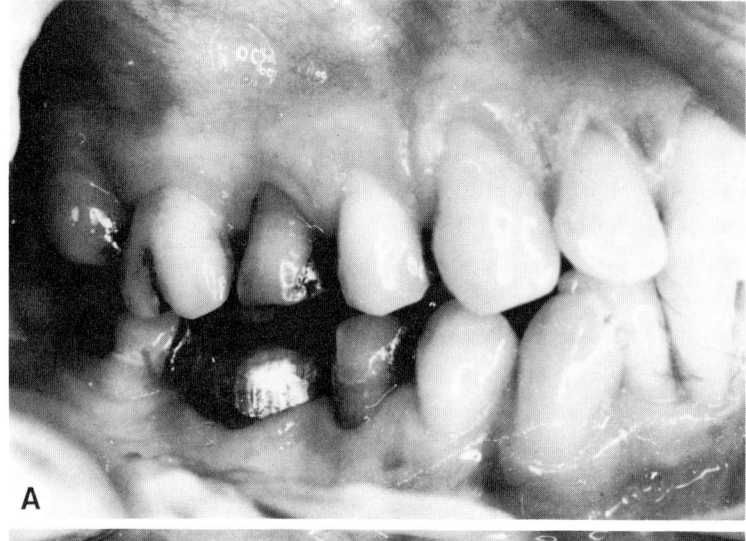
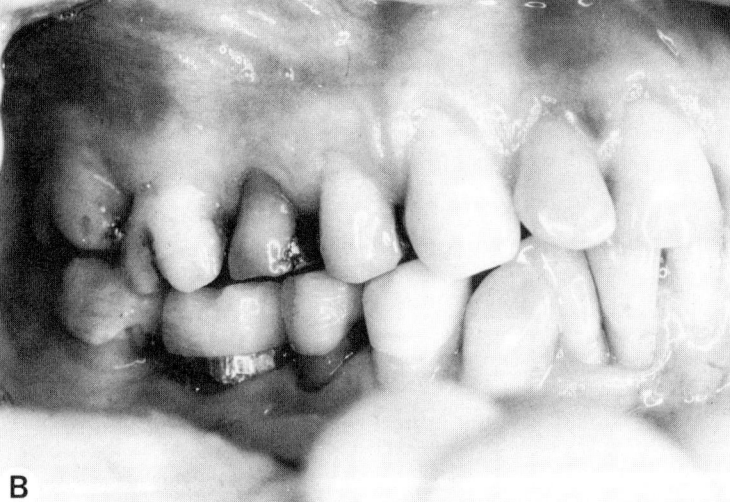

Figure 9–17. *A*, Lateral open bite in the premolar and molar region when the mandible is in the therapeutic position. *B*, Acrylic onlays on the lower molars and premolars eliminate the open bite and maintain the mandible in the therapeutic position.

tween were allowed to erupt. When stable occlusal contacts were established on these teeth, the bite plate was removed, and the second molars erupted to occlusal contacts. Finally, minor occlusal adjustments were performed to create a stable occlusion. In two patients, the closure of the posterior open bite was accelerated by the use of interocclusal elastics as previously described (see Fig. 9–21).[61, 62] The median time for the orthodontic treatment was 4 months, with a range of 2 to 12 months.

Long-term Results

Follow-up examination about 3 years after initiation of treatment showed that joint function was improved, intensity of pain was reduced, and joint and muscle tenderness occurred less frequently than before treatment (Tables 9–8 and 9–9). Furthermore, intermittent locking, use of analgesics, sleep disturbances, and absence from work because of TMJ symptoms were also less frequent (Table 9–10).

Radiographic examination, including arthrography, was performed in 11 of the 15 patients at follow-up. Tomography performed in 11 patients revealed inferior, anterior condylar position in five patients, central position in four, and posterior condylar position in two patients. There were only minor hard-tissue changes (Fig. 9–22). Arthrography showed the disc to be in a correct

9B Splint Treatment of Patients with Disc Displacement with Reduction ■ 107

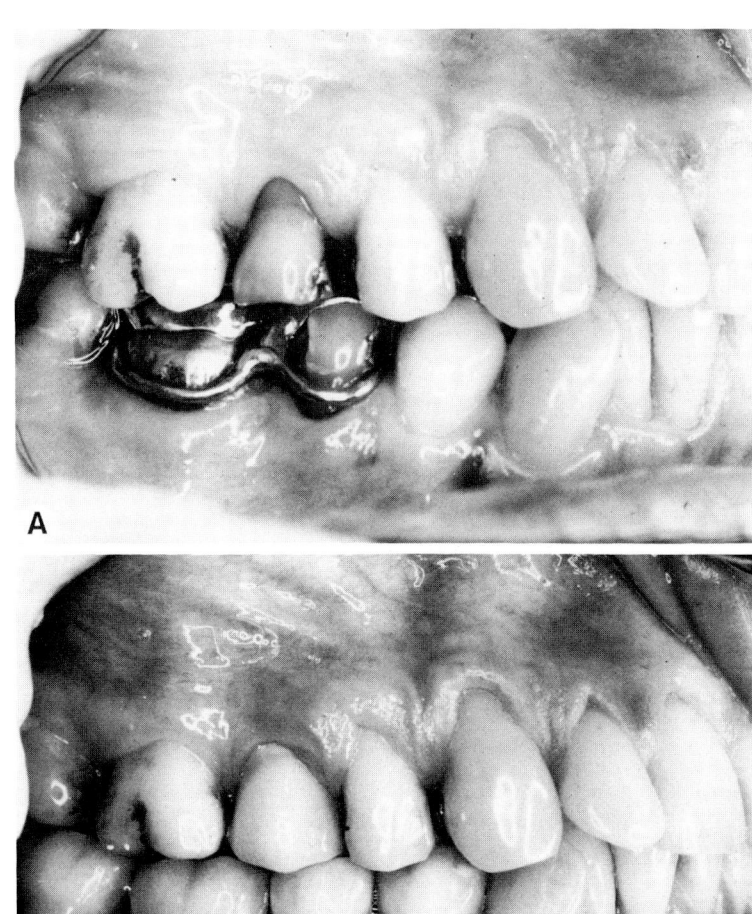

Figure 9–18. *A*, Removable metal onlays for maintaining the therapeutic position. The onlays were cast in Vitallium. *B*, The same patient shown in Figures 9–17 and 19–18*A* after prosthodontic treatment.

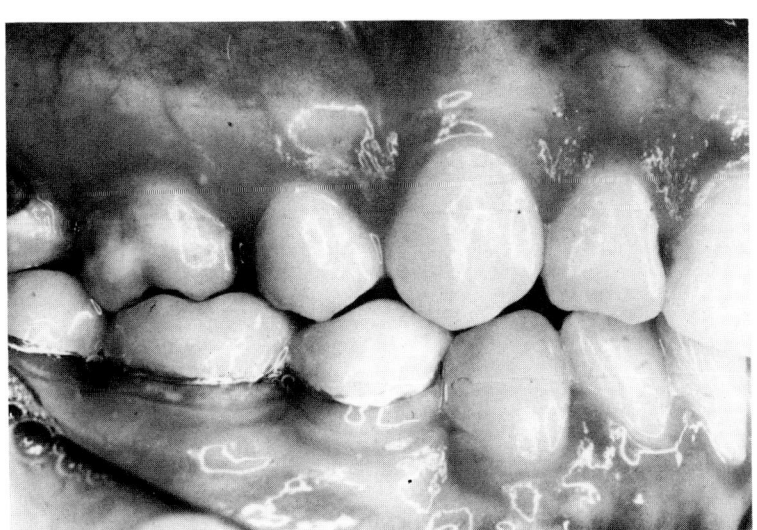

Figure 9–19. Metal onlays with acrylic veneering to maintain the therapeutic position.

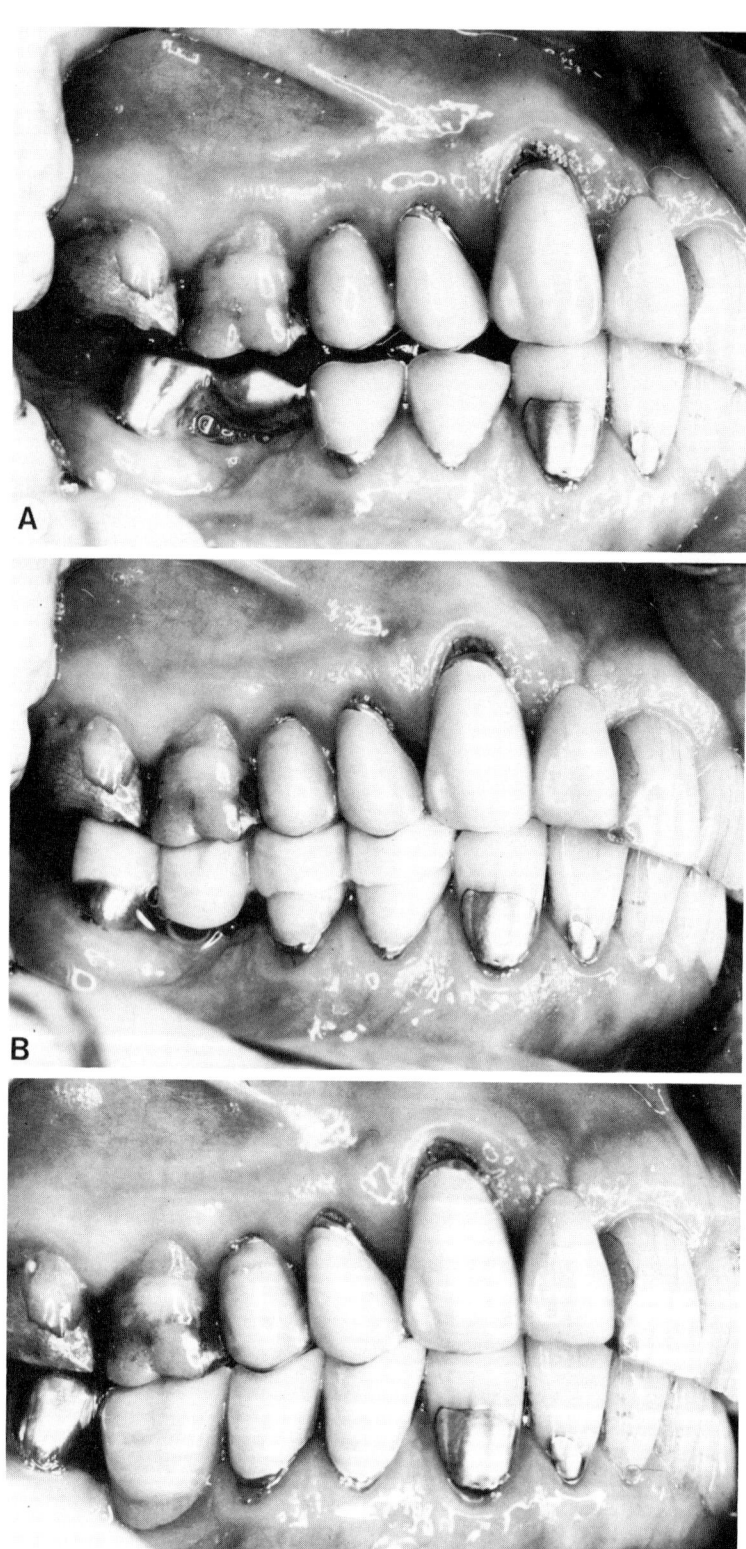

Figure 9-20. *A,* Lateral open bite in the therapeutic position. *B,* Acrylic occlusal onlays cemented on the unprepared premolars and molars. *C,* The same patient shown in *A* and *B* after prosthodontic treatment.

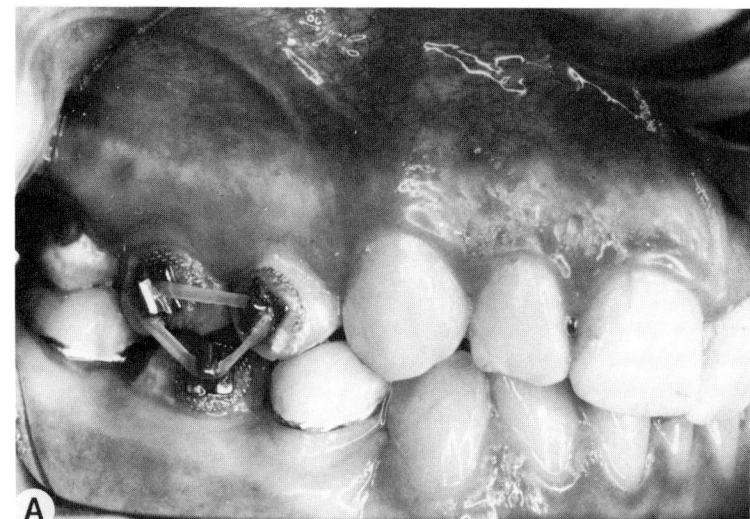
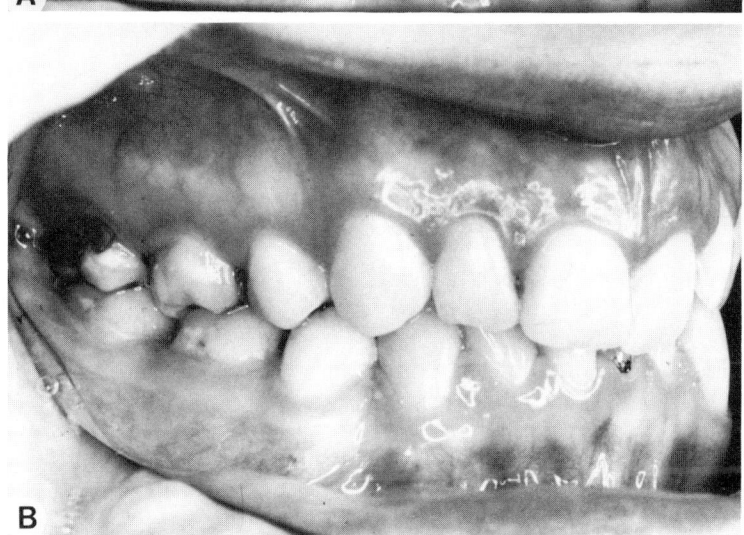

Figure 9–21. *A,* Orthodontic treatment to close the posterior open bite. Onlays remain on one premolar and one molar. Rubber bands attached to brackets are used to accelerate elongation of the lower first molar. *B,* The same patient after completion of orthodontic treatment.

Table 9–8. MEDIAN OF SUBJECTIVE SYMPTOMS AS EVALUATED BY 15 PATIENTS*

Subjective Symptoms	Before Treatment	At Follow-up
Pain at rest (median)	2	0
Pain during chewing (median)	8	0
Pain during protrusion (median)	5	0

*Using 10-cm visual analog scales with 0 and 10 as end points.

position relative to the condyle in 9 of 11 patients (82%) (Fig. 9–23) and revealed medial disc displacement with reduction in one patient and disc displacement without reduction in another patient.

PROGRESSION OF DISC DISPLACEMENT

Disc displacement seems to be a progressive disease in which displacement with reduction progresses to disc displacement without reduction and further on to degenerative joint disease.[9, 10] Little is known, however, about the progression rate and which of the patients with disc displacement with re-

Table 9-9. DISTRIBUTION (NUMBER OF PATIENTS) OF CLINICAL FINDINGS BEFORE TREATMENT AND AT FOLLOW-UP (15 PATIENTS)

Clinical Findings	Before Treatment	At Follow-up
Reciprocal clicking	15	0
Palpatory tenderness laterally over joint	8	0
Palpatory tenderness posteriorly over joint	6	0
Palpatory tenderness of insertion of temporal muscle	10	2
Palpatory tenderness of anterior portion of temporal muscle	8	0
Palpatory tenderness of superficial masseter muscle	8	2
Palpatory tenderness of medial pterygoid muscle	7	1

Table 9-10. ANAMNESTIC FINDINGS (NUMBER OF PATIENTS) BEFORE TREATMENT AND AT FOLLOW-UP (15 PATIENTS)

Anamnestic Findings	Before Treatment	At Follow-up
Intermittent locking	9	0
Use of analgesics	6	1
Sleep disturbances	6	0
Absence from work	3	0

duction have the greatest risk to progress to more advanced stages.

Three-Year Longitudinal Study

To gain more knowledge in this area, we followed 70 patients with a clinical diagnosis of anterior disc displacement with reduction over a period of 3 years.[64] Clinical examination at the end of the observation period was specifically directed toward the identification of clinical signs and symptoms of disc displacement without reduction, such as locking, limitation of opening, or deviation to the affected side at maximal mouth opening. Signs of disc displacement without reduction were found in 9% of these patients at follow-up. In an attempt to identify clinical characteristics of those patients who might have a greater risk of progression, the initial records were analyzed. In patients that initially had pronounced pain, joint tenderness, dental abrasion, and missing molar support, there was a greater tendency for the displacement to progress, compared with patients without these clinical features. These features are, however, relatively unspecific, and in the clinical setting it may be difficult to

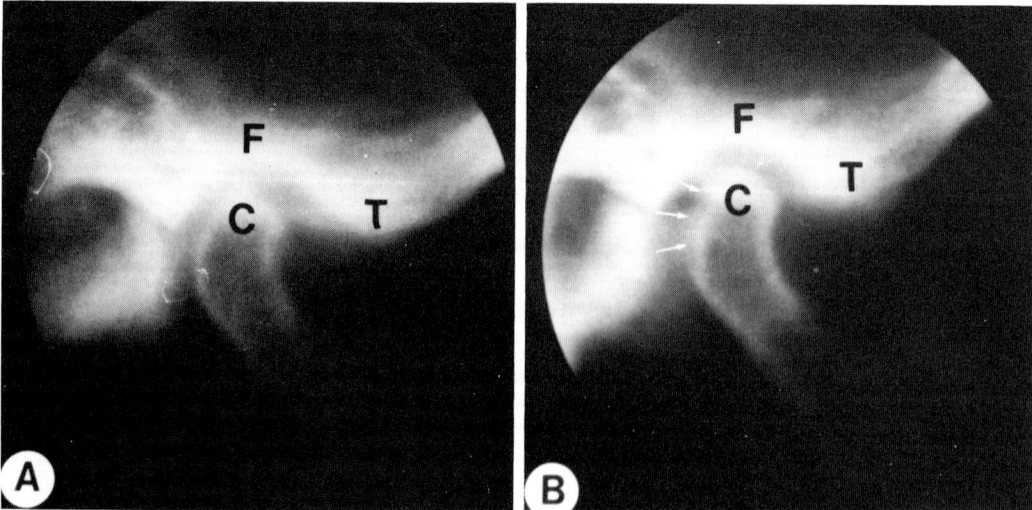

Figure 9-22. Tomograms before *(A)* and after six months of treatment *(B)* with disc repositioning onlays showing progressive remodeling on the posterior surface of the condyle after treatment *(arrows in B)*. C = condyle; F = fossa; T = tubercle.

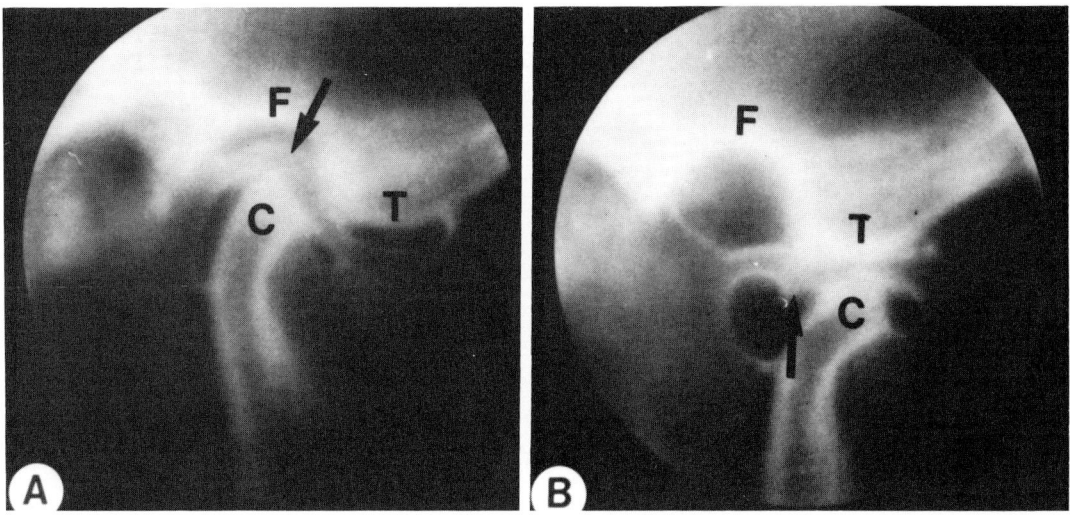

Figure 9–23. Double-contrast arthrograms obtained at rest position (A) and at maximal mouth opening (B) showing normal disc position. The posterior band of the disc (arrow) lies between the condyle (C) and the fossa (F). T = tubercle.

rely on them to identify individuals who have a greater risk of developing displacement without reduction.

Radiographic 6-Month Follow-up

In an attempt to identify further features that might be predictors of a higher risk of progression, we studied another group of patients, using radiographic criteria that might be more definitive and therefore more useful in clinical work trying to identify patients who are likely to progress.[65]

We therefore recorded clinically and arthrographically the status of 61 patients with disc displacement with reduction. The patients were followed for 6 months, and a repeated clinical examination was performed at the end of this period. Arthrography was performed on one third of the patients at this time; clinical and/or arthrographic signs of disc displacement were seen in 12 patients. An analysis of the initial arthrograms was undertaken in order to identify arthrographic criteria that were characteristic for patients with a greater risk of progression to locking. This analysis showed that the configuration of the anterior recess of the lower joint space had a tendency to be deeper (Fig. 9–24) at the initial examination in the patients who later progressed to the displacement without reduction (Table 9–11). Thus, 10 of 15 patients with a deep recess shown on the initial arthrogram progressed to displacement without reduction during the 6-month observation period. In contrast, only two of 46 patients with a shallow recess (Fig. 9–25) progressed to locking during the same observation period (see Table 9–11).

Other factors that seemed to be indicative of a greater risk of progressing to displacement without reduction were pronounced pain and disturbed joint function initially, and temporary locking (Table 9–12).

Table 9–11. RELATIONSHIP BETWEEN THE SHAPE OF THE ANTERIOR RECESS OF THE LOWER JOINT COMPARTMENT AND PROGRESSION OF DISC DISPLACEMENT WITH REDUCTION TO CLOSED LOCK (61 PATIENTS)*

	Progression to Closed Lock	No Progression to Closed Lock
Deep anterior recess of lower joint compartment	10	5
Shallow anterior recess of lower joint compartment	2	44

*$p < 0.001$ (Fisher's exact test).

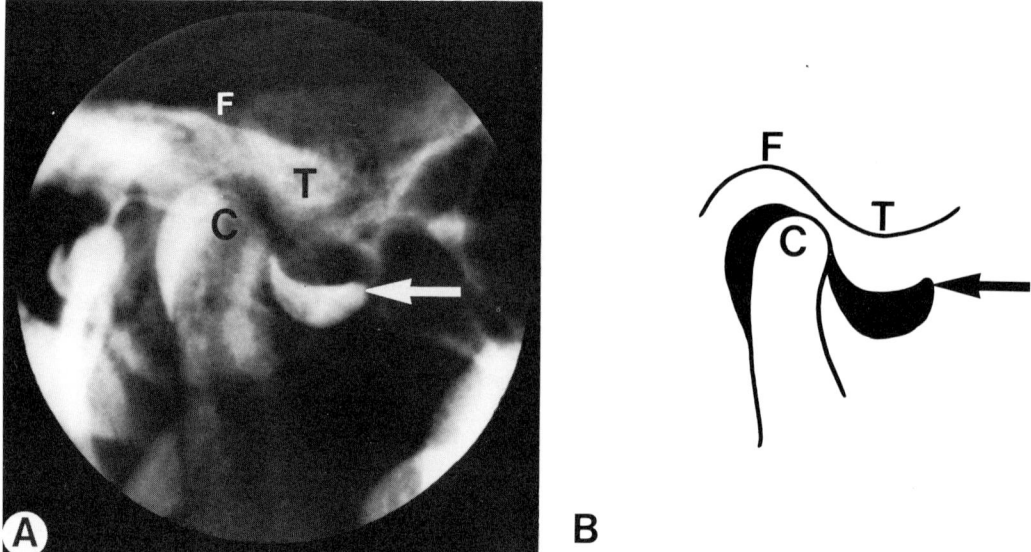

Figure 9-24. Arthrogram *(A)* and schematic drawing (B) showing a temporomandibular joint with disc displacement and deep anterior recess (arrow) of the lower joint compartment. F = fossa; C = condyle; T = tubercle.

SUMMARY AND CLINICAL CONSIDERATIONS

The results of our studies and others suggest that normalization of disc position significantly reduces pain and dysfunction in patients with disc displacement with reduction. Furthermore, disc repositioning onlays appear to be superior to the flat splint in treatment of this condition. Symptoms, however, consistently returned when the onlays were removed, even after a 6-month treatment period. This suggests that permanent maintenance of the therapeutic position is necessary for long-term success. It seems that attempts to "walk the mandible back" toward the original position include a high risk of a recurrence of disc displacement.[30, 33] Permanent reconstruction of the occlusion may be done by prosthodontics or orthodon-

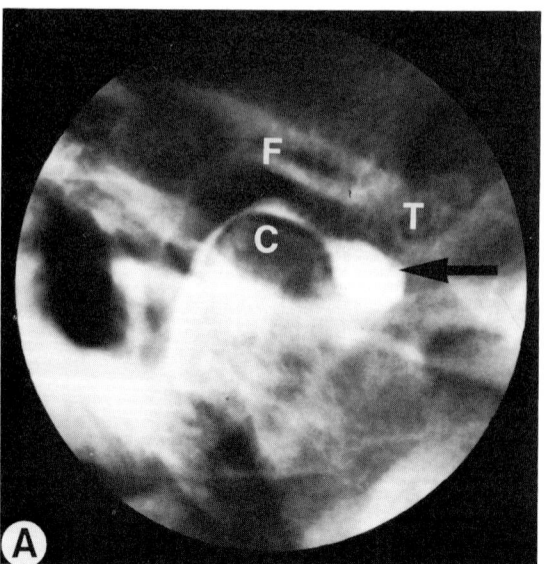
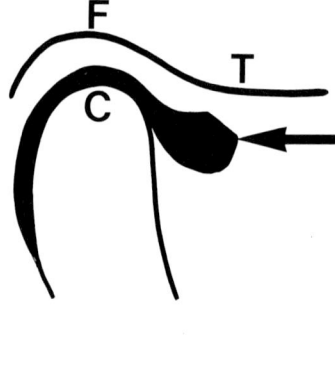

Figure 9-25. Arthrogram *(A)* and schematic drawing *(B)* showing a temporomandibular joint with disc displacement and shallow anterior recess (arrow) of lower joint compartment. F = fossa; C = condyle; T = tubercle.

Table 9-12. RELATIONSHIP BETWEEN TEMPORARY LOCKING AND PROGRESSION OF DISC DISPLACEMENT WITH REDUCTION TO CLOSED LOCK (61 PATIENTS)*

	Progression to Closed Lock	No Progression to Closed Lock
Temporary locking	12	21
No temporary locking	0	28

*$p < 0.002$ (Fisher's exact test)

tics; thus the dental treatment needed to maintain the disc in the recaptured position may sometimes be extensive. The amount of dental treatment should therefore be initially considered relative to the severity of the pain and symptoms and also relative to the possibility of no treatment or other treatment modalities in patients with mild symptoms.

The significance of the association of disc position with symptoms is emphasized by the fact that the majority of these patients previously had been unsuccessfully treated with conventional "non-disc recapturing" treatment modalities. However, the position of the disc is not the only factor responsible for the symptoms, since disc displacement is not always associated with pain.

Radiographic and clinical information can be helpful in the identification of patients who may have a higher risk of progression to closed lock.

References

1. Middleton DS: Clinical approach to derangement of the mandibular joint. J R Coll Surg Edinb 17:287-295, 1972.
2. Annandale T: Displacement of the inter-articular cartilage of the lower jaw, and its treatment by operation. Lancet 1:411, 1887.
3. Pringle JH: Displacement of the mandibular meniscus and its treatment. Br J Surg 6:385-389, 1918.
4. Wakeley CPG. The causation and treatment of displaced mandibular cartilage. Lancet 4:543-545, 1929.
5. Axhausen G: Das Kiefergelenkknacken und seine Behandlung. Dtsch Zeitschr Chir 232:238-272, 1931.
6. Goodfriend DJ: Symptomatology and treatment of abnormalities of the mandibular articulation. Dental Cosmos 75:844-852, 1933.
7. Goodfriend DJ: Symptomatology and treatment of abnormalities of the mandibular articulation. Dental Cosmos 75:947-957, 1933.
8. Goodfriend DJ: Symptomatology and treatment of abnormalities of the mandibular articulation. Case report. Dental Cosmos 75:1106-1111, 1933.
9. Wilkes CH: Arthrography of the temporomandibular joint in patients with the TMJ pain-dysfunction syndrome. Minn Med 61:645-652, 1978.
10. Wilkes CH: Structural and functional alterations of the temporomandibular joint. Northwest Dent 57:287-294, 1978.
11. Ireland VE: The problem of "the clicking jaw." Proc R Soc Med 44:363-372, 1951.
12. Farrar WB: Diagnosis and treatment of anterior dislocation of the articular disc. NY J Dent 41:348-351, 1971.
13. Farrar WB: Differentiation of temporomandibular joint dysfunction to simplify treatment. J Prosthet Dent 28:629-636, 1972.
14. Katzberg RW, Dolwick MF, Helms CA, et al: Arthrotomography of the temporomandibular joint. AJR 134:995-1003, 1980.
15. Farrar WB, McCarty Jr WL: Inferior joint space arthrography and characteristics of condylar paths in internal derangements of the TMJ. J Prosthet Dent 41:548-555, 1979.
16. Bronstein SL, Tomasetti BJ, Ryan DE: Internal derangements of the temporomandibular joint: correlation of arthrography with surgical findings. J Oral Surg 39:572-584, 1981.
17. Eriksson L, Westesson P-L: Clinical and radiological study of patients with anterior disc displacement of the temporomandibular joint. Swed Dent J 7:55-64, 1983.
18. Westesson P-L: Double-contrast arthrotomography of the temporomandibular joint: Introduction of an arthrographic technique for visualization of the disc and articular surfaces. J Oral Maxillofac Surg 41:163-172, 1983.
19. McCarty WL Jr: Diagnosis and treatment of internal derangements of the articular disk mandibular condyle. In: Solberg WK, Clark GT (eds). Temporomandibular Joint Problems. Biologic Diagnosis and Treatment. Chicago: Quintessence, 1980, pp 160-163.
20. Farrar WB, McCarty Jr WL: A clinical outline of temporomandibular joint diagnosis and treatment, 9th ed., Montgomery: Normandie 1982, pp 115-142.
21. Dolwick MF, Katzberg RW, Helms CA: Internal derangements of the temporomandibular joint: Fact or fiction? J Prosthet Dent 49:415-418, 1983.
22. Eriksson L: Diagnosis and surgical treatment of internal derangement of the temporomandibular joint. (Thesis, University of Lund.) Swed Dent J (Suppl 25): 1-49, 1985.
23. Dolwick MF, Riggs RR: Diagnosis and treatment of internal derangements of the temporomandibular joint. Dent Clin North Am 27:561-572, 1983.
24. Bollavia WD: A functional jaw device to aid in treating anterior displaced discs. J Craniomandib Pract 1:53-60, 1983.
25. Clark GT: Treatment of jaw clicking with temporomandibular repositioning: Analysis of 25 cases. J Craniomandib Pract 2:263-270, 1984.
26. Clark GT: The TMJ repositioning appliance: A technique for construction, insertion, and adjustment. J Craniomandib Pract 4:37-46, 1986.
27. Manzione JV, Tallents R, Katzberg RW, et al: Arthrographically guided splint therapy for recapturing the temporomandibular joint meniscus. Oral Surg Oral Med Oral Pathol 57:235-240, 1984.
28. Anderson GC, Schulte JK, Goodkind RJ: Comparative study of two treatment methods for internal derangement of the temporomandibular joint. J Prosthet Dent 53:392-397, 1985.

29. Hanson B, Sherman R, Ficara A: Masseter muscle silent period in patients with internal derangement of the temporomandibular joint before and after splint therapy. J Prosthet Dent 54:846–850, 1985.
30. Le Bell Y, Kirveskari P: Treatment of reciprocal clicking of the temporomandibular joint using a mandibular repositioning splint and occlusal adjustment. Proc Finn Dent Soc 81:251–255, 1985.
31. Ash MM: Current concepts in the aetiology, diagnosis and treatment of TMJ and muscle dysfunction. J Oral Rehabil 13:1–20, 1986.
32. Solberg WK: Temporomandibular disorders: management of internal derangement. Br Dent J 160:379–385, 1986.
33. Moloney F, Howard JA: Internal derangements of the temporomandibular joint. III. Anterior repositioning splint therapy. Aust Dent J 31:30–39, 1986.
34. Posselt U: Physiology of occlusion and rehabilitation. Oxford and Edinburgh: Blackwell Scientific Publications, 1962, pp 242–248.
35. Posselt U, Wolff IB: Treatment of bruxism by bite guards and bite plates. Can Dent Assoc J 29:773–778, 1963.
36. Bell WH: Nonsurgical management of the pain-dysfunction syndrome. J Am Dent Assoc 79:161–170, 1969.
37. Greene CS, Laskin DM: Long-term evaluation of treatment for myofascial pain-dysfunction syndrome: a comparative analysis. J Am Dent Assoc 107:235–238, 1983.
38. Amir A, Sakuda M, Miyazaki T: Comparative effects of muscle relaxants and occlusal bite plate in treatment of temporomandibular joint dysfunction syndrome. J Osaka Univ Dent Sch 18:1–10, 1978.
39. Carrarro JJ, Caffesse RG: Effect of occlusal splints on TMJ symptomatology. J Prosthet Dent 40:563–566, 1978.
40. Clark GT, Beemsterboer PL, Solberg WK, Rugh JD: Nocturnal electromyographic evaluation of myofascial pain dysfunction in patients undergoing occlusal splint therapy. J Am Dent Assoc 99:607–611, 1979.
41. Kopp S: Short term evaluation of counselling and occlusal adjustment in patients with mandibular dysfunction involving the temporomandibular joint. J Oral Rehabil 6:101–109, 1979.
42. Kopp S: Pain and functional disturbances of the masticatory system—a review of etiology and principles of treatment. Swed Dent J 6:49–60, 1982.
43. Beard CC, Clayton JA: Effects of occlusal splint therapy on TMJ dysfunction. J Prosthet Dent 44:324–335, 1980.
44. Magnusson T, Carlsson GE: Treatment of patients with functional disturbances in the masticatory system. A survey of 80 consecutive patients. Swed Dent J 4:145–153, 1980.
45. Kopp S, Wenneberg B: Effects of occlusal treatment and intraarticular injections on temporomandibular joint pain and dysfunction. Acta Odontol Scand 39:87–96, 1981.
46. Wedel A, Carlsson GE, Dahlström L, et al: Stabiliseringsskena eller avslappningsplåt-en jämförelse mellan två typer av bettskenor. Tandläkartidningen 4:137–144, 1981.
47. Okeson JP, Kemper JT, Moody PM: A study of the use of occlusion splints in the treatment of acute and chronic patients with craniomandibular disorders. J Prosthet Dent 48:708–712, 1982.
48. Mejersjö C, Carlsson GE: Long-term results of treatment for temporomandibular joint pain-dysfunction. J Prosthet Dent 49:809–815, 1983.
49. Magnusson T: Patients referred for stomatognathic treatment—a survey of 282 patients. Swed Dent J 8:193–201, 1984.
50. Dahlström L, Haraldsson T: Bite plates and stabilization splints in mandibular dysfunction. A clinical and electromyographic comparison. Acta Odontol Scand 43:109–114, 1985.
51. Carlsson GE: Long-term effects of treatment of craniomandibular disorders. J Craniomandib Pract 3:337–342, 1985.
52. Carlsson GE, Dahlström L, Haraldson T, et al: Diskförskjutning i käkleden. Preliminära resultat av konventionell bettfysiologisk behandling. Tandläkartidningen 78:405–409, 1986.
53. Helkimo E, Westling L: History, clinical findings, and outcome of treatment of patients with anterior disk displacement. J Craniomandib Pract 5:269–276, 1987.
54. Lundh H, Westesson P-L, Kopp S, Tillström B: Anterior repositioning splint in the treatment of temporomandibular joints with reciprocal clicking: Comparison with a flat occlusal splint and an untreated control group. Oral Surg Oral Med Oral Pathol 60:131–136, 1985.
55. Lundh H, Westesson P-L, Jisander S, Eriksson L: Disk-repositioning onlays in the treatment of temporomandibular joint disk displacement: Comparison with a flat occlusal splint and with no treatment. Oral Surg Oral Med Oral Pathol 66:155–162, 1988.
56. Westesson P-L, Lundh H: Temporomandibular joint disk displacement: Arthrographic and tomographic follow-up after six months treatment with disk repositioning onlays. Oral Surg Oral Med Oral Pathol 66:271–278, 1988.
57. Lundh H, Westesson P-L. Long-term follow-up after occlusal treatment to correct an abnormal temporomandibular joint disk position. Oral Surg Oral Med Oral Pathol 67:2–10, 1989.
58. Dahlström L, Carlsson GE, Carlsson SG: Comparison of effects of electromyographic biofeedback and occlusal splint therapy on mandibular dysfunction. Scand J Dent Res 90:151–156, 1982.
59. Tallents RH, Katzberg RW, Miller TL, et al: Arthrographically assisted splint therapy. J Prosthet Dent 53:235–238, 1985.
60. Tallents RH, Katzberg RW, Macher DJ, et al: Arthrographically assisted splint therapy: A 6-month follow-up. J Prosthet Dent 56:224–226, 1986.
61. Sved A: Changing the occlusal level and a new method of retention. Am J Orthod 30:527–535, 1944.
62. Farrar WB, McCarty Jr WL: A Clinical Outline of Temporomandibular Joint Diagnosis and Treatment, 9th Ed. Montgomery: Normandie 1982, p 121.
63. Dugal GL: Closing a minor unilateral open bite on TMJ patients. J Craniomandib Pract 1:39–41, 1982–1983.
64. Lundh H, Westesson P-L, Kopp, S: A three-year follow-up of patients with reciprocal temporomandibular joint clicking. Oral Surg Oral Med Oral Pathol 63:530–533, 1987.
65. Westesson P-L, Lundh H: Arthrographic and clinical characteristics of patients with disk displacement who progressed to closed lock during a six months' period. Oral Surg Oral Med Oral Pathol 67:654–657, 1989.

Chapter 10

IMAGING OF THE TEMPOROMANDIBULAR JOINT

*PER-LENNART WESTESSON, D.D.S., PH.D.,
RICHARD W. KATZBERG, M.D.*

The principal objective of imaging the temporomandibular joint (TMJ) is to document any clinically suspected disorders of the joint. The traditional study has been a plain film in a transcranial projection, possibly supplemented by tomography. Plain film and tomography can, however, only detect the changes in the osseous parts of the TMJ. Knowledge gathered during the last decade has demonstrated the significance of also studying the soft tissue parts of the joint, especially the position and function of the disc.[1-5] This has been made possible by the use of arthrography, computed tomography, and magnetic resonance imaging. These imaging modalities have greatly increased our understanding of the pathophysiology of the TMJ.

The purpose of this chapter is to describe the different modalities that are available for imaging the TMJ, to discuss the relative merits of each, and to present an imaging strategy that can be applied to patients with TMJ symptoms.

ANATOMY

A thorough knowledge of the anatomy of the TMJ is necessary for selection of the appropriate radiographic technique, for its interpretation and for understanding the resulting images. Therefore, a brief description of TMJ anatomy, pathology, function, and dysfunction is given.

A sagittal section of the normal TMJ is shown in Figure 10-1. The normal disc is biconcave and located with its thick posterior band superior to the condyle, the central thin zone between the condyle and articular tubercle, and the anterior thick part (anterior band) beneath the articular tubercle.[6] The disc is an oval structure with a thicker periphery and a thinner central part seen in three dimensions. The articulating surfaces are covered by a thin layer of dense fibrous tissue. The joint is surrounded by a capsule that emerges from the temporal bone, runs like a funnel inferiorly, and attaches to the neck of the condyle. In the coronal plane, the disc is crescent-shaped and attaches to the condyle medially and laterally and also to the medial and lateral capsule walls (Fig. 10-2).

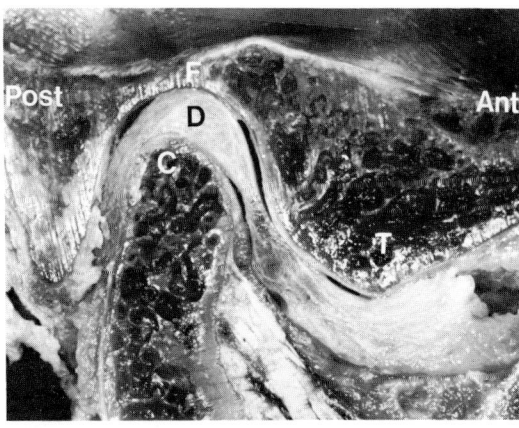

Figure 10-1. Sagittal section through the central part of a normal temporomandibular joint. The disc (D) is biconcave and located with its posterior band superior to the condyle. C = condyle; F = fossa; T = tubercle; Post = posteriorly; Ant = anteriorly.

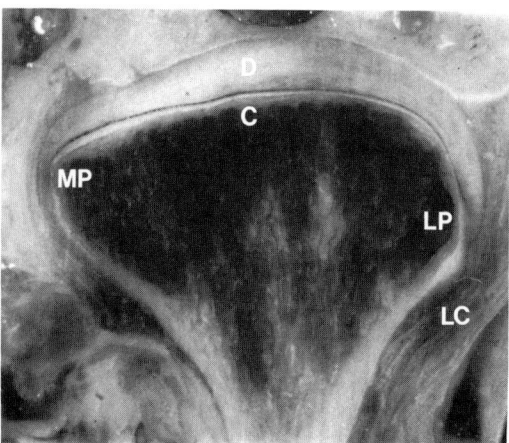

Figure 10–2. Coronal section through a normal temporomandibular joint. The medial (MP) and lateral (LP) poles of the condyles are indicated. D = disc; C = condyle; LC = lateral capsule.

FUNCTION

The function of the TMJ is complex; the upper and lower joint spaces function as two joints within the same joint capsule. This allows for great movement in relation to the size of the joint. During function there is both rotation and translation in the joint. Examples of different degrees of jaw opening in a normal TMJ are illustrated in Figure 10–3.

DISC DISPLACEMENT

Displacement of the disc is the most common finding in patients with TMJ symptoms.[1, 2, 5, 7, 8] Most commonly, the disc is displaced anteriorly, anterolaterally, or anteromedially. By definition anterior displacement implies that the posterior, thick part of the disc (posterior band) is located anterior to the condyle (Fig. 10–4). A general classification of the various types of disc displacement is shown in Table 10–1. The combination of anterior and lateral or medial displacement is termed *rotational* displacement.[9] The pure lateral or pure medial displacement is termed *sideways* displacement.[9] To further complicate the situation, the functional aspects of disc displacement multiply the combination of possible abnormalities.

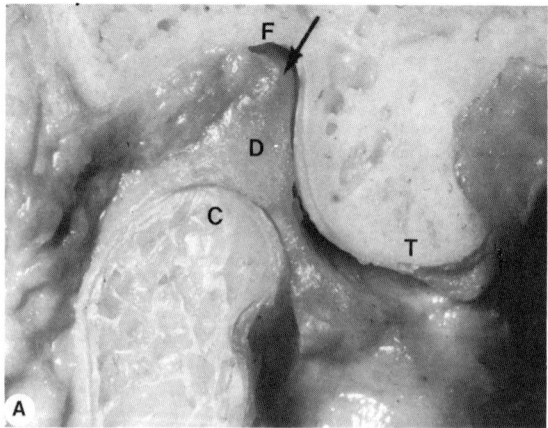

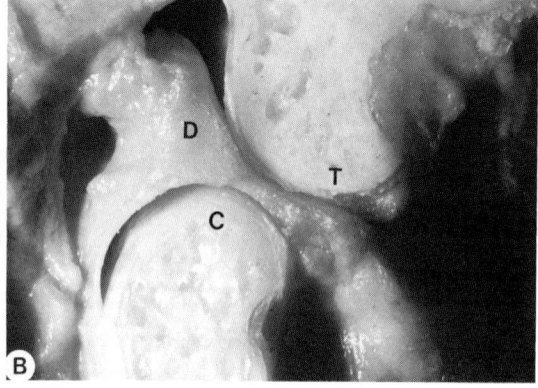

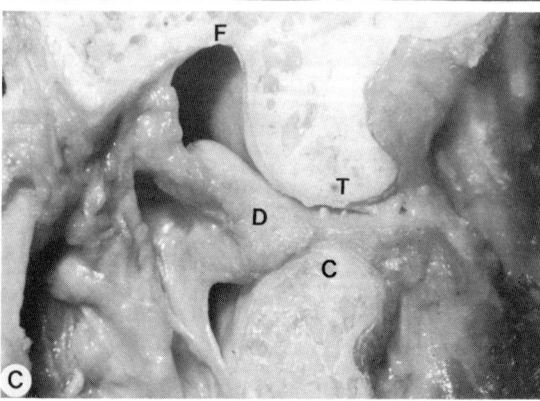

Figure 10–3. Sagittal section through the central part of a normal temporomandibular joint. *A*, Closed mouth position; *B*, half-open mouth position; *C*, full-open mouth position. Arrow indicates the posterior band of the disc. F = fossa; D = disc; C = condyle; T = tubercle.

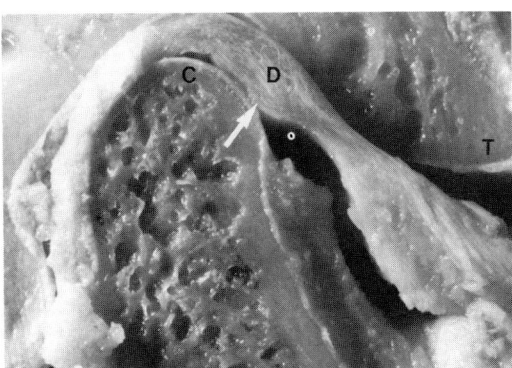

Figure 10–4. Sagittal section through the central part of a temporomandibular joint with anterior or disc displacement. The posterior band *(arrow)* of the disc is located slightly forward to the top of the condyle (C). D = disc; T = tubercle.

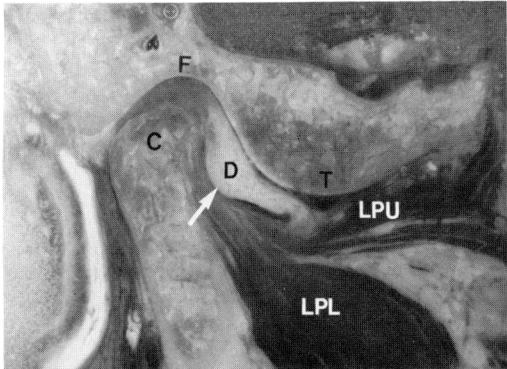

Figure 10–5. Sagittal section of temporomandibular joint showing anterior disc displacement and disc deformation. The posterior band of the disc *(arrow)* is enlarged. The upper (LPU) and lower (LPL) heads of the lateral pterygoid muscle are indicated. C = condyle; F = fossa; D = disc; T = tubercle.

The principal functional categories of internal derangement are disc displacement with reduction, which implies that the disc position normalizes during opening, and disc displacement without reduction, which implies that the disc stays in the displaced position during all mandibular movements (see Fig. 9–11). Deformation of the disc (Figs. 10–5 and 10–6) frequently is associated with disc displacement without reduction. Deformation usually starts as a thickening of the posterior band (see Fig. 10–5), and in the later stage the disc develops to biconvexity (see Fig. 10–6). The long-term result of disc displacement is a deformed, torn, or detached posterior disc attachment (Figs. 10–7 and 10–8). Perforation between the lower and upper joint spaces frequently is seen in late stage disc displacement.[5, 10, 11] Perforations usually are confined to the posterior disc attachment (see Figs. 10–7 and 10–8) and not in the disc per se. In the later stage of disc displacement without reduction, osseous changes of the condyle and temporal component may occur (see Fig. 10–8).[11] These changes consist of flattening and osteophytosis of the condyle and flattening of the temporal component.

CLINICAL EXAMINATION

Several studies have attempted to identify clinical signs and symptoms that are predictive of the status of the joint.[12–17] Joint sounds have been shown to have a positive relationship with the presence of internal derangement, but the overall accuracy for the various aspects of internal derangement has been only about 70%.[12–16] Thus there seems

Table 10–1. TERMINOLOGY FOR DESCRIBING THE POSITION OF THE DISC

Normal

Superior

Abnormal

Anterior
Anterior medial rotational displacement
Anterior lateral rotational displacement
Medial sideways displacement
Lateral sideways displacement

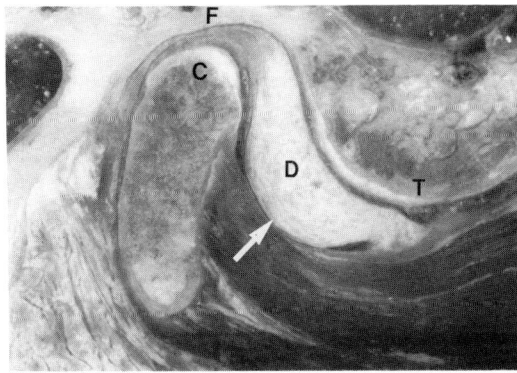

Figure 10–6. Sagittal section of temporomandibular joint showing substantial disc deformation. The posterior band of the disc *(arrow)* is considerably enlarged. C = condyle; D = disc; F = fossa; T = tubercle.

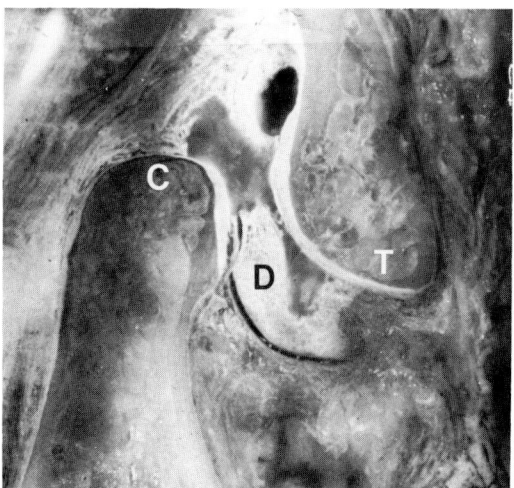

Figure 10-7. Sagittal section of temporomandibular joint showing anterior disc displacement and perforation. The perforation is located in the posterior disc attachment. The disc (D) is deformed. Osseous changes are seen in the condyle (C). The tubercle (T) is normal.

to be a need for accurate imaging to determine the intra-articular status of the joint.

PLAIN FILM RADIOGRAPHY

The most common, traditional projection of the TMJ is a transcranial projection (Fig. 10–9). This projection depicts the lateral part of the TMJ with the glenoid fossa, articular tubercle, and condyle, whereas the central

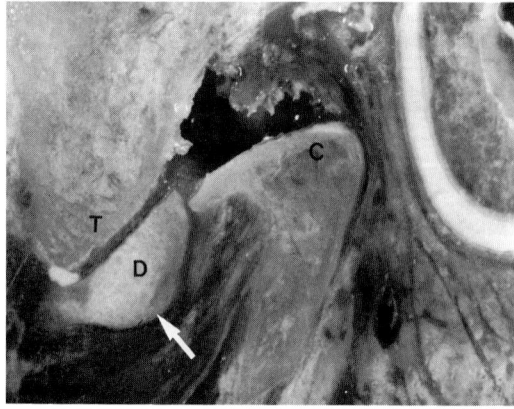

Figure 10-8. Sagittal section of temporomandibular joint with advanced degenerative changes. The disc (D) is anteriorly displaced and deformed (arrow). The condyle (C) demonstrates flattening and an anterior osteophyte. The tubercle (T) is also flattened.

and medial parts of the joint are not clearly demonstrated. To compensate for this limitation, a transmaxillary projection (Fig. 10–10) or transorbital projection may be used. The combination of the two projections has been shown to be superior to only one projection, because more osseous changes are detected.[18] Another possibility in plain film imaging of the TMJ is a transpharyngeal projection (Fig. 10–11).

TOMOGRAPHY

The next step in imaging might be tomography, which provides sectional images of the joint in the sagittal or coronal plane. Sagittal tomography is performed most commonly (Fig. 10–12). Tomography is accomplished by moving the x-ray tube and the film in opposite directions during exposure. Thereby, structures outside the tomographic plane will be blurred, whereas structures within the tomographic plane will be clearly reproduced; tomography for this reason has the risk of providing false-negative diagnoses. The tomographic layer is about 3-mm thick when using hypocycloidal tomography. Usually, about five sections are obtained to cover the medial-lateral dimension of the TMJ. More information about the osseous anatomy of the TMJ can be gained from tomography than from a transcranial projection.[19]

ARTHROGRAPHY

The traditional modality for imaging the soft tissue of the TMJ has been arthrography, which can be defined as radiography after injection of a contrast medium into the joint space. The first systematic attempt to evaluate the TMJ arthrographically was undertaken by Nørgaard during the 1940s.[20, 21] The technique was, however, considered difficult and was adopted by only a few clinicians until the end of the 1970s, when Wilkes' description of anterior disc displacement as a common cause of TMJ pain and dysfunction appeared in the literature.[1, 2] Following his publications, interest in arthrography of the TMJ increased substantially, and several articles were published that described the usefulness of arthrography.[3, 10, 22, 23] Later, several techniques for arthrography were de-

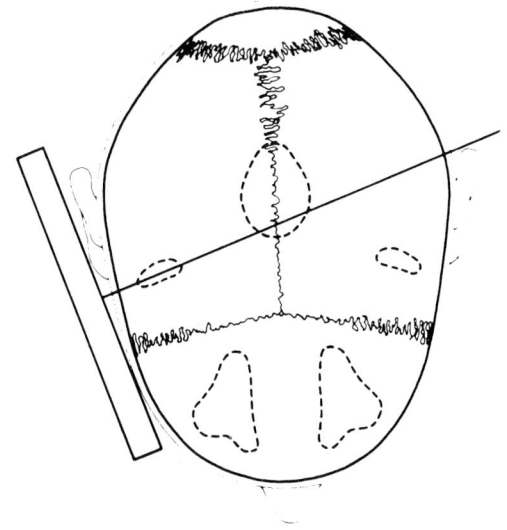
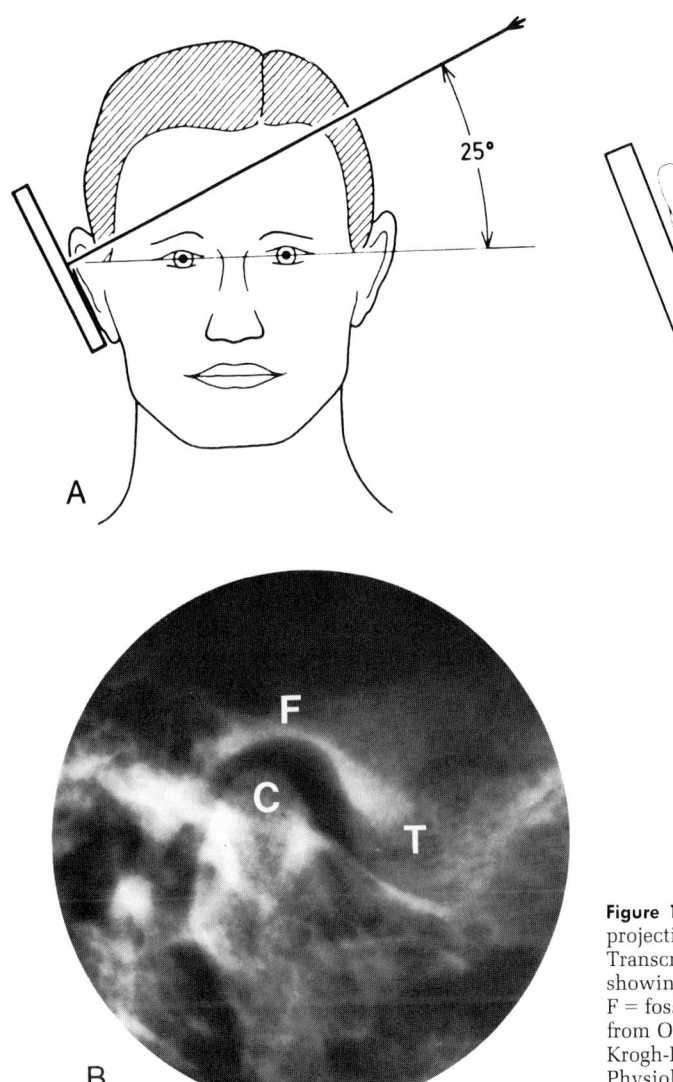

Figure 10–9. A, Schematic drawings of transcranial projection of right temporomandibular joint. B, Transcranial radiograph of temporomandibular joint showing normal osseous components. C = condyle; F = fossa; T = tubercle. (A reprinted with permission from Omnell K-Å, Lysell S: Roentgendiagnostics. In Krogh-Poulsen W (ed): Stomatognathic Function and Physiology, Vol. 2. Copenhagen: Munksgaard, 1987, pp 141–153.)

scribed, such as the single-contrast lower compartment technique (Fig. 10–13)[3] and dual-space double-contrast arthrotomography (Fig. 10–14).[4, 10, 23]

Indications and Contraindications

The major indication for arthrography is to assess the soft tissues of the TMJ—essentially the position, function, and configuration of the disc—in patients presenting with pain and mechanical symptoms that suggest internal derangements (Table 10–2). Arthrography may also be indicated for a patient with diffuse facial and head pain, in whom differential diagnosis is essential. Frequently, this patient has not responded to any therapy. Arthrography can also be employed for determining the mandibular position in which the disc is in correct relationship to the condyle. This position may be selected for protrusive splint therapy.[24, 25]

Contraindications for arthrography are mainly infections in the preauricular region that could contaminate the TMJ (see Table 10–2). A previous reaction to contrast medium is a relative indication, and other modal-

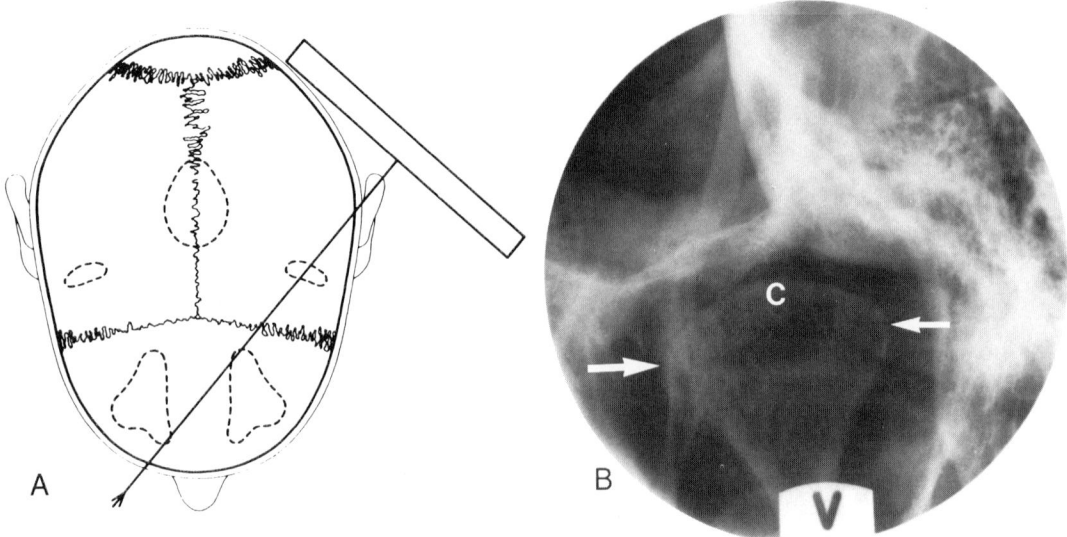

Figure 10–10. *A,* Schematic drawing of transmaxillary projection of left temporomandibular joint. *B,* Transmaxillary radiograph of temporomandibular joint. Arrows indicate the medial and lateral poles of the condyle (C). (*A* reprinted with permission from Omnell K-Å, Lysell S: Roentgendiagnostics. *In* Krogh-Poulsen W (ed): Stomatognathic Function and Physiology, Vol. 2. Copenhagen: Munksgaard, 1987, pp 141–153.)

ities, such as MRI, should be considered for these patients. Bleeding disorders and anticoagulation medication are other relative contraindications for arthrography (anticoagulation can be temporarily discontinued or decreased prior to the procedure).

Equipment

A fluoroscopic table or a C-arm with an x-ray tube and an image intensifier is useful for TMJ arthrography (Fig. 10–15). The patient is positioned on his or her side, with the

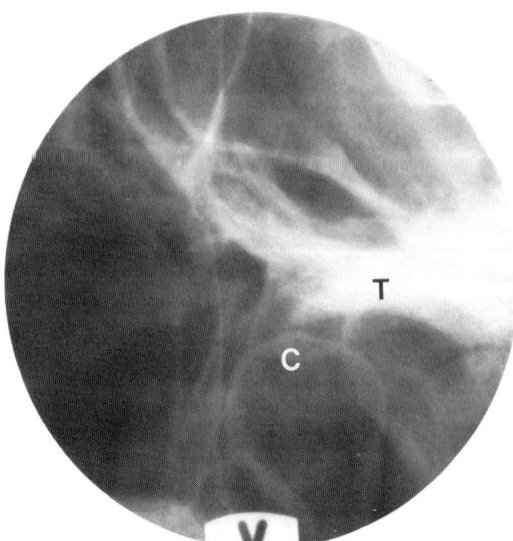

Figure 10–11. Transpharyngeal radiograph of temporomandibular joint. The osseous structure of the condyle (C) is normal. T = anterior part of the tubercle. (Courtesy of Arne Petersson.)

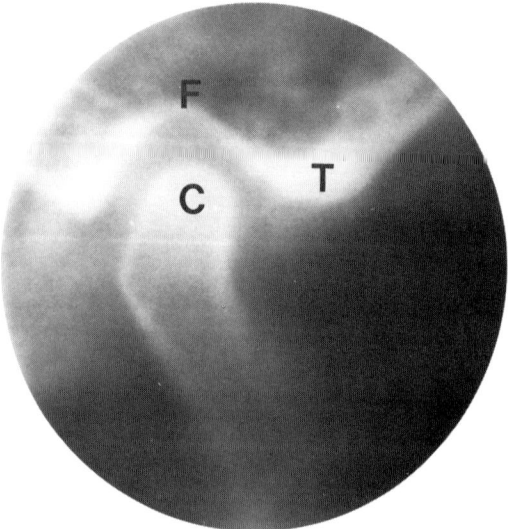

Figure 10–12. Sagittal tomogram of a temporomandibular joint without evidence of osseous disease. C = condyle; F = fossa; T = tubercle.

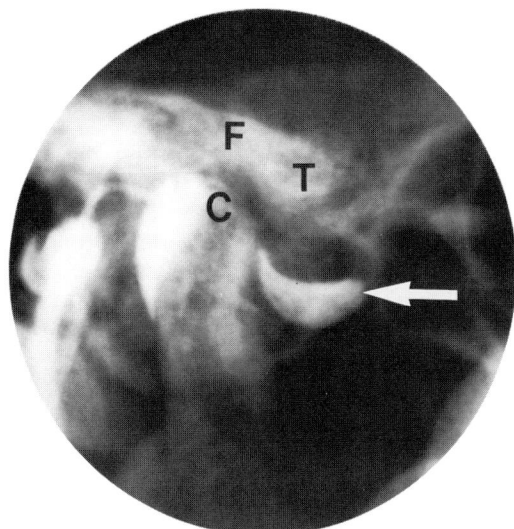

Figure 10–13. Transcranial arthrogram with contrast medium in the lower joint space. The lower joint space is enlarged *(arrow)*, suggesting anterior disc displacement. C = condyle; F = fossa; T = tubercle.

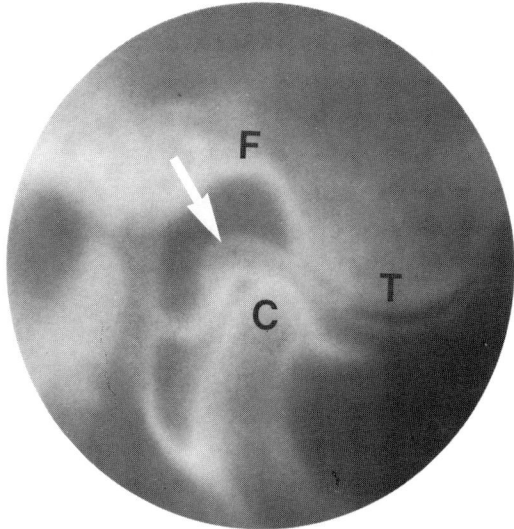

Figure 10–14. Dual-space double-contrast arthrotomogram obtained at half-open mouth position. The disc is located superior to the condyle; the arrow indicates the position of the posterior band. C = condyle; F = fossa; T = tubercle.

head oriented so that the side under examination is located superiorly. In this way, the head is slightly tilted and a transcranial projection is obtained. The image is optimized by change in the position of the head during fluoroscopy.

Techniques

Arthrography can be performed either as single-contrast lower compartment arthrography[3] or as dual-space double-contrast arthrotomography.[4, 10, 23] The techniques for

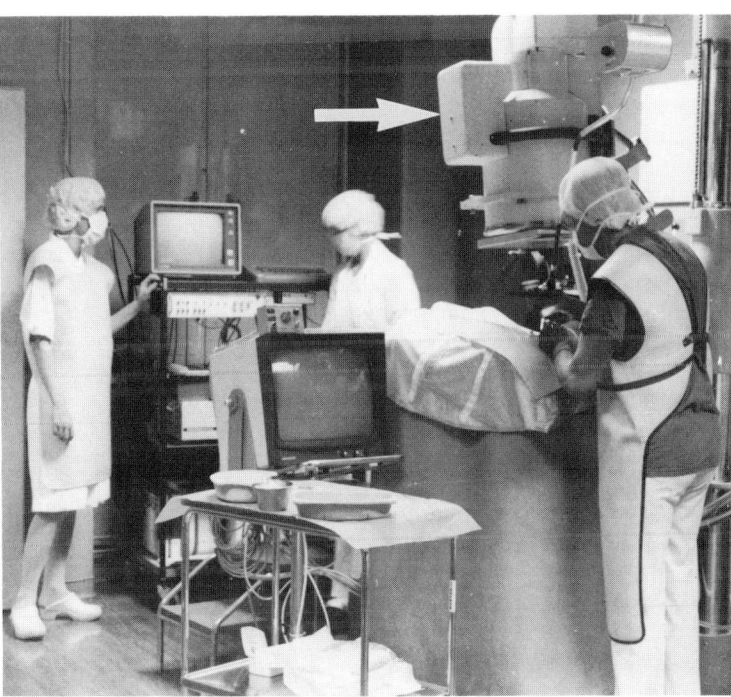

Figure 10–15. Equipment for temporomandibular joint arthrography. Arrow indicates image intensifier above the patient's head.

Table 10-2. INDICATIONS AND CONTRAINDICATIONS FOR ARTHROGRAPHY

Common Indications

Assess position, function, and configuration of the disc
Different diagnosis in patients with diffuse facial and head pain
Establish jaw position for protrusive splint therapy

Infrequent Indications

Diagnosis of loose bodies in the joint spaces
Evaluation after trauma
Aspiration of joint fluid
Intra-articular injections

Contraindications

Infections in the preauricular area
Allergy to contrast medium
Bleeding disorders
Anticoagulation medication

the different examinations vary slightly and thus are described separately.

Single-Contrast Arthrography

For a single-contrast examination, the posterior aspect of the condyle is identified by using a metal marker on the surface of the skin during fluoroscopy. Utilizing local anesthesia, the lower joint space is punctured with a 23- or 25-gauge ¾-inch scalp vein needle, and contrast medium (Omnipaque, 300 mg iodine/ml) is injected under fluoroscopic control. The amount of contrast medium is determined by observing the injection during fluoroscopy. Approximately 0.2 to 0.5 ml is sufficient for visualization of the lower joint space (Fig. 10-16). The free flow of contrast medium around the condyle is an indication of correct joint puncture. Simultaneous filling of the upper joint space suggests perforation and requires injection of another 0.5 ml of contrast medium.

The needle is withdrawn, and images at closed mouth and maximal mouth opening are obtained. Additional images may be obtained at positions where abnormalities are clearly seen. When the diagnosis is not clear, injection of contrast medium into the upper joint space also is recommended for a more detailed delineation of the disc (Fig. 10-17). This can be done by withdrawing the needle half way out and redirecting it into the fossa region until bone contact is obtained.

Double-Contrast Arthrography

For dual-space double-contrast arthrotomography, the patient is positioned as for a single-contrast examination and the joint spaces are punctured in a similar manner. Thus the lower joint space is punctured in its posterior recess and the upper joint space is punctured in the glenoid fossa or along the posterior slope of the articular tubercle. Catheters (Angiocath, 0.8 mm × 25 mm, The Desert Co., Sandy UT 84070) are preferable because they can remain in the joint spaces during the examination, thereby permitting injection and aspiration of contrast medium. The same amount of contrast medium is injected as for a single-contrast study. After studies of joint function, the contrast medium is aspirated, and new extension tubes filled with air are attached to the catheters. The patient is moved from the fluoroscopic table to the tomograph unit, air is injected into both upper and lower joint spaces (Fig. 10-18), and double-contrast arthrotomograms are obtained. Usually about 0.5 to 1 cc of air is injected into the upper and lower joint spaces simultaneously (see Fig. 10-18). The optimal amount of air is determined by the resistance to injection.

Arthrograms are obtained at the rest position and at maximal mouth opening. Additional images may be obtained at certain positions that are optimal for documentation of abnormalities. A book cassette, with five or

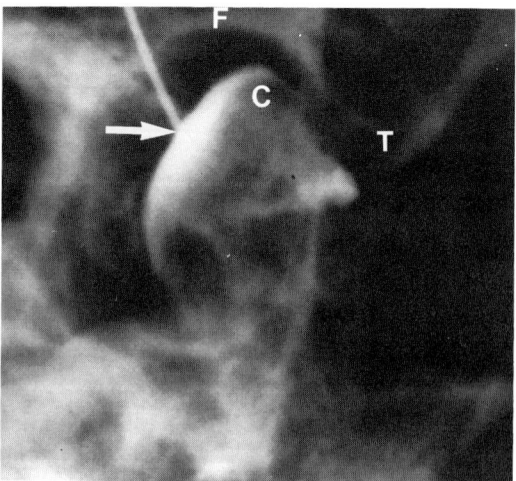

Figure 10-16. Single-contrast arthrogram with injection of contrast medium into the lower joint space. Arrow indicates the position of the needle in the lower joint space. C = condyle; F = fossa; T = tubercle.

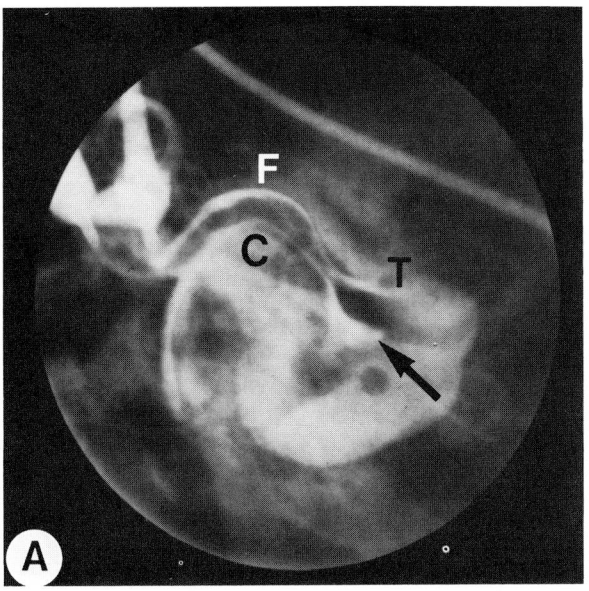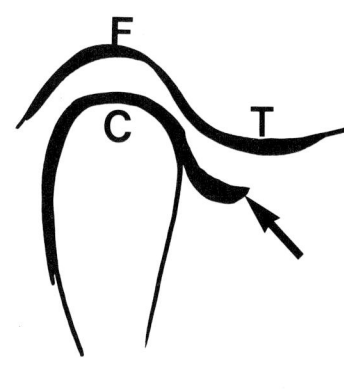

Figure 10–17. Transcranial arthrogram *(A)* and schematic drawing *(B)* with contrast medium in upper and lower joint spaces of a normal superior disc position. The disc is biconcave, located with its posterior thick part superior to the condyle. The configuration of the anterior recess *(arrow)* of the lower joint compartment is a reflection of the configuration of the anterior band of the disc. C = condyle; F = fossa; T = tubercle.

seven films for simultaneous tomography (Fig. 10–19), has been found to be time-saving and reduces radiation doses.

Arthrographic Findings

The normal TMJ is characterized arthrographically by the posterior, thick part of the

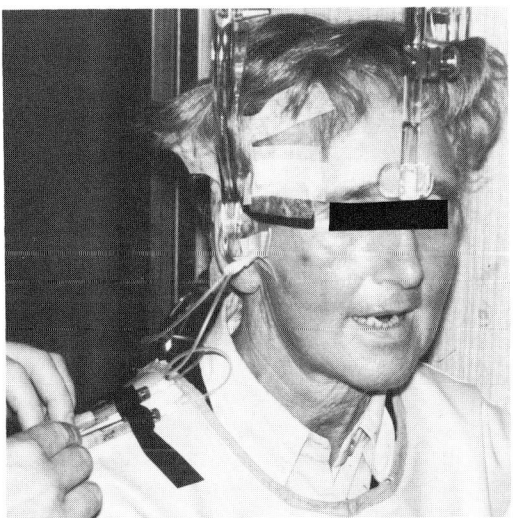

Figure 10–18. Injection of air into the right temporomandibular joint in dual-space double-contrast arthrotomography. The patient is sitting in the tomographic unit with his head positioned by the use of a head holder.

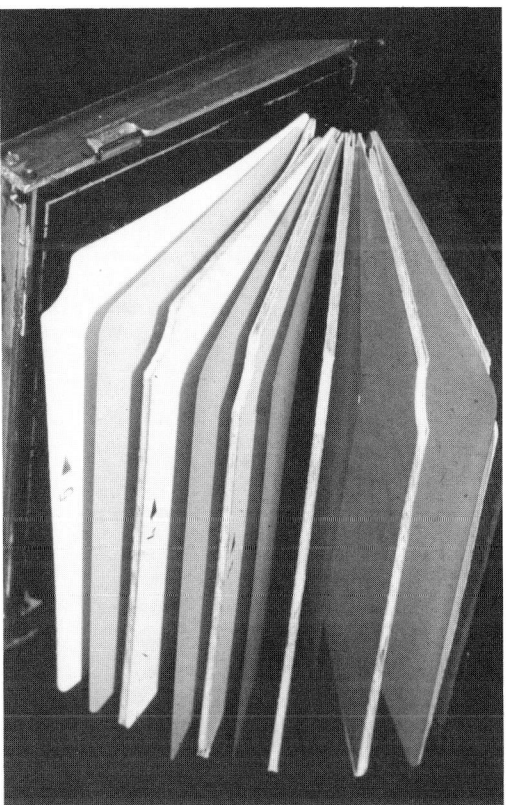

Figure 10–19. Book cassette set with five films and five pairs of intensifying screens for simultaneous tomography.

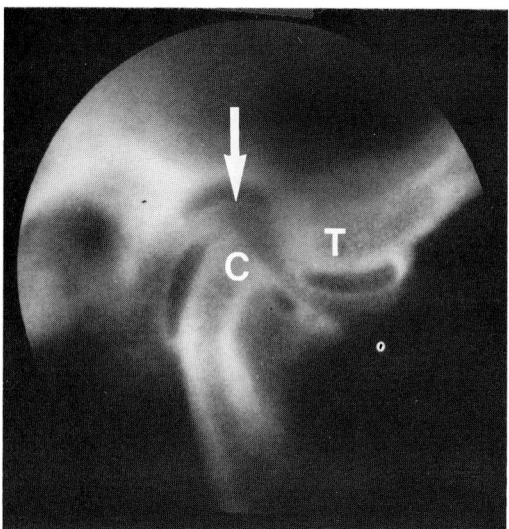

Figure 10–20. Double-contrast arthrotomogram of normal temporomandibular joint. The disc *(arrow)* is located superior to the condyle (C). T = tubercle.

disc (posterior band) lying superior to the condyle in the closed mouth position (Fig. 10–20). In the single contrast, lower space arthrogram, the normal joint is characterized by having a relatively small anterior recess (see Figs. 10–16 and 10–17). There is, however, a substantial variation of the dimension of the lower joint space in normal TMJs, and this recess could be relatively large even though the disc is located superiorly (Fig. 10–21).[26]

The pathologic change most frequently seen during arthrography is displacement of the disc.[1, 2, 4, 7, 10, 23] This implies that the posterior band of the disc is not located superior to the condyle but is displaced anteriorly, medially, or laterally. In the single-contrast arthrogram, anterior displacement is characterized by enlargement of the anterior recess of the lower joint space (Figs. 10–22 and 10–23). In disc displacement with reduction, the disc position is normalized during opening (see Fig. 10–22), whereas in disc displacement without reduction, the disc remains in the displaced position during all mandibular movements.

Medial or lateral displacement of the disc may be more difficult to demonstrate with arthrography.[27] However, sometimes the sagittal arthrograms demonstrate a horizontal contrast medium margin projecting over the lower part of the mandibular condyle (Fig. 10–24). This has been interpreted as a sign of sideways disc displacement.[28] However, a systematic study on cadavers comparing arthrographic and cryosectional findings has shown that medial and lateral disc displace-

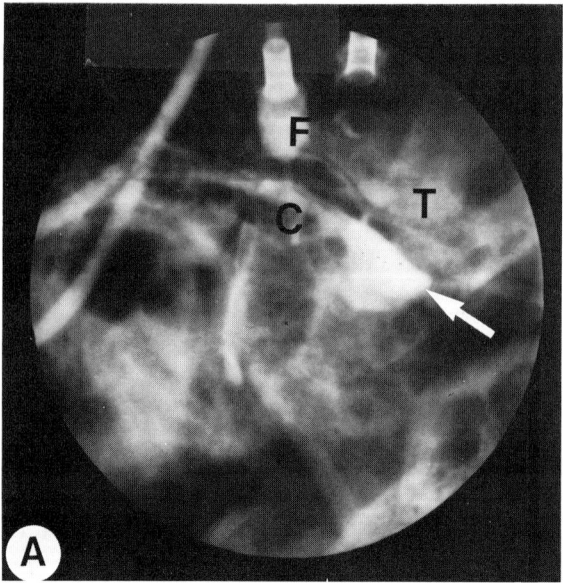 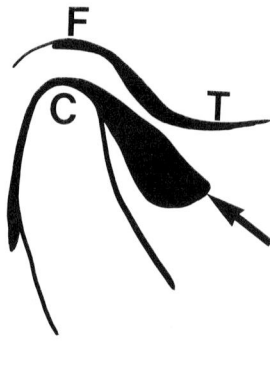

Figure 10–21. Transcranial arthrogram *(A)* with contrast medium in upper and lower joint spaces and schematic drawing *(B)* of a temporomandibular joint with normal superior disc position. The disc is biconcave and located with the posterior band superior to the condyle. The anterior recess of the lower joint space *(arrow)* is large. F = fossa; C = condyle; T = tubercle.

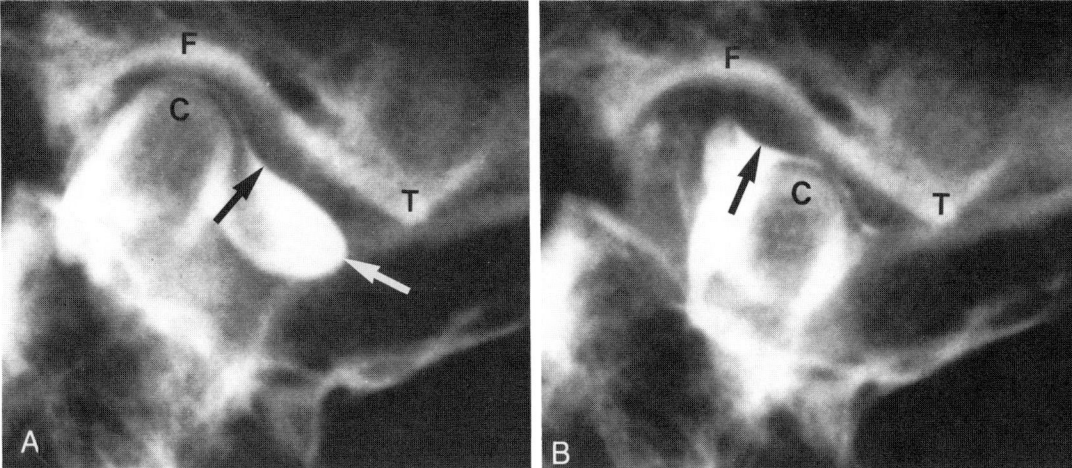

Figure 10–22. *A,* Transcranial arthrogram obtained at closed mouth position. The anterior recess of the lower joint space *(white arrow)* is enlarged suggesting anterior disc displacement. Black arrow indicates the position of the posterior part of the disc. C = condyle; F = fossa; T = tubercle. *B,* Same temporomandibular joint at half-open mouth position, showing that disc position has become normal. Arrow indicates the position of the posterior band. C = condyle; F = fossa; T = tubercle.

ment may be both under- and over-diagnosed with arthrography.[27] The clinical significance of medial or lateral displacement is not fully understood, but studies have suggested that the clinical presentations of these patients are similar to those with anterior disc displacement.[9]

Disc deformation frequently is seen in joints with displacement without reduction (Figs. 10–25 and 10–26).[8, 11] The most common deformation is enlargement of the posterior band of the disc that eventually results in a biconvex disc.

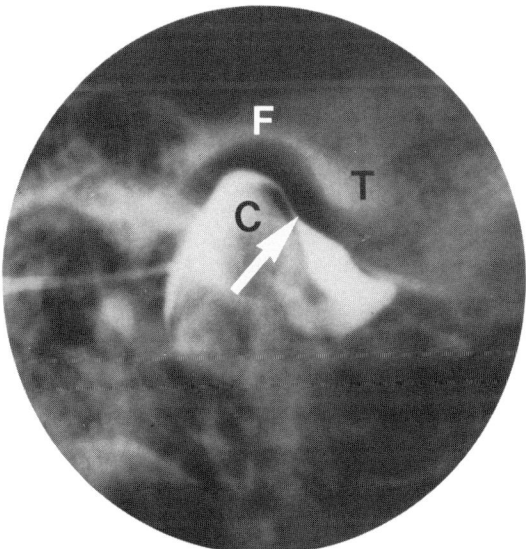

Figure 10–23. Single-contrast lower joint compartment arthrogram. The disc is anteriorly displaced and located with its posterior band *(arrow)* anterior to the condyle. The configuration of the joint spaces suggests a biconcave configuration of the disc. C = condyle; F = fossa; T = tubercle.

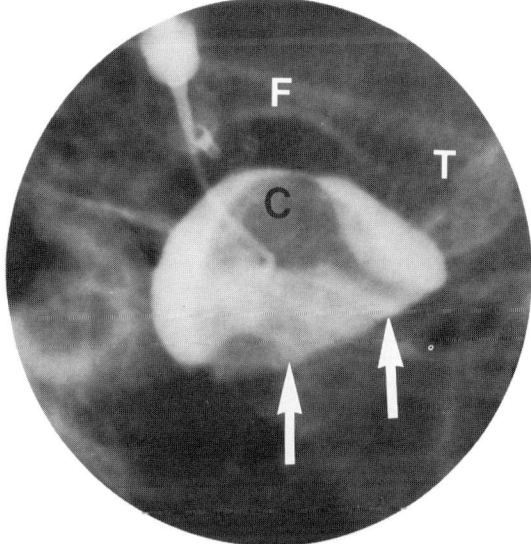

Figure 10–24. Transcranial arthrogram with contrast medium in lower joint space. The horizontal contrast medium margin *(arrows)* crossing over the lower part of the condyle (C) suggests a medial disc displacement. F = fossa; T = tubercle.

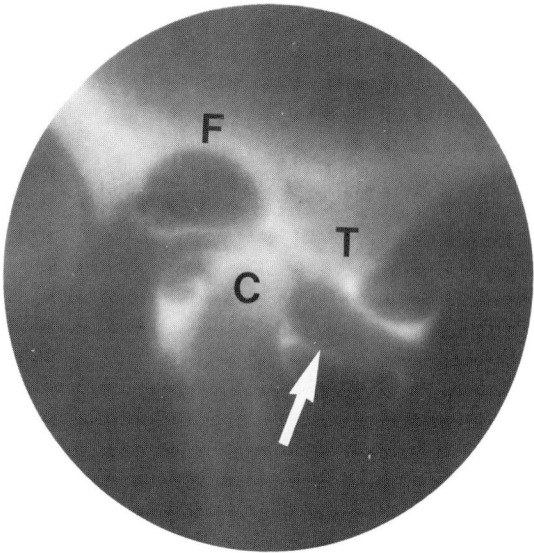

Figure 10–25. Double-contrast arthrotomogram of temporomandibular joint with anterior disc displacement. The disc *(arrow)* is deformed. C = condyle; F = fossa; T = tubercle.

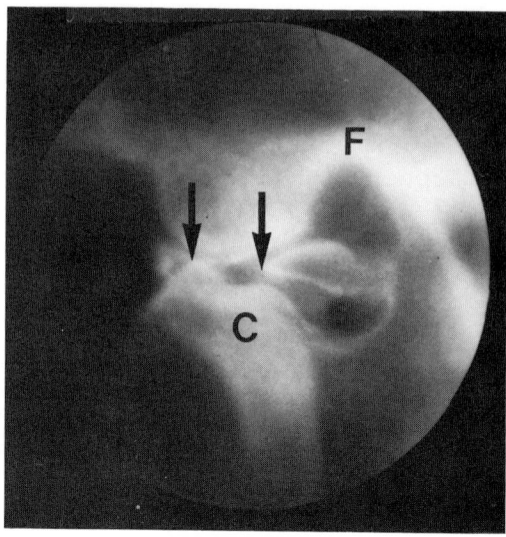

Figure 10–27. Double-contrast arthrotomogram showing perforation of the disc. C = condyle; F = fossa; T = tubercle.

Overflow of contrast medium from the lower to the upper joint space suggests perforation (Fig. 10–27). Perforation occurs most frequently in joints with disc displacement without reduction.[5, 8, 10, 11] Only rarely are perforations seen in joints with reducing discs or in discs in normal superior position.[5, 8, 10, 11] Morphologically, perforations are located in the posterior disc attachment and, more uncommonly, in the disc per se.

Adhesions are another pathologic entity that in a few instances can be diagnosed by the use of dual-space double-contrast arthrotomography (Fig. 10–28).

Complications of Arthrography

Serious complications following TMJ arthrography are uncommon. The TMJ is quite resistant to infection, and no incidence of infection following arthrography has been reported.[29] Transient palsy of the facial nerve may result from local anesthesia. Slight discomfort for 1 or 2 days after the study is sometimes encountered and, if necessary, is treated by anti-inflammatory agents. Reactions to contrast media are unusual but have occurred.[30]

Comparison of Double-Contrast with Single-Contrast Arthrography

The principal advantage of double-contrast over single-contrast arthrography is an improved visualization of the disc and joint compartments (Fig. 10–29). The accuracy in the determination of the position of the disc

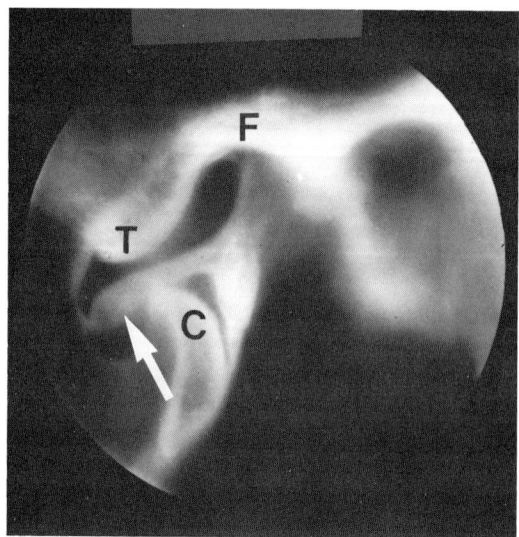

Figure 10–26. Double-contrast arthrotomogram of temporomandibular joint with anterior displacement and deformation of the disc. The biconvex disc *(arrow)* is anterior to the condyle at this half-open mouth position. C = condyle; F = fossa; T = tubercle.

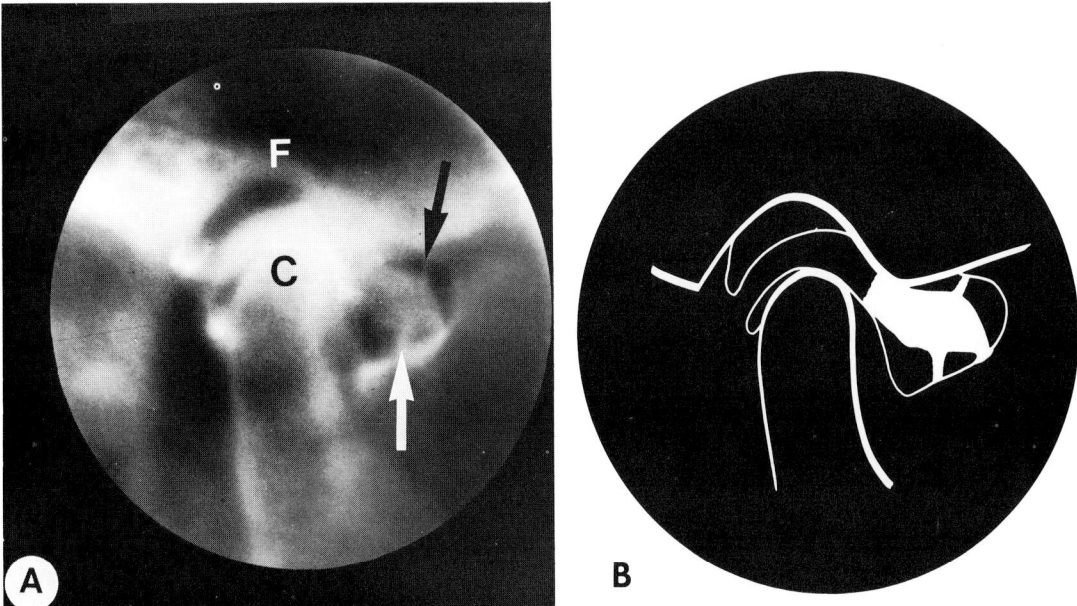

Figure 10–28. Double-contrast arthrotomogram *(A)* and schematic drawing *(B)* of a temporomandibular joint with anterior disc displacement and adhesions. There are adhesions *(arrows)* between the disc and the capsule anteriorly. C = condyle; F = fossa.

has been about the same for both types of studies.[31] A systematic comparison of the two techniques has revealed that videotape recording of lower joint space single-contrast arthrography is superior in demonstrating joint dynamics, and that dual-space double-contrast arthrotomography is superior in demonstrating the soft tissue anatomic features of the joint.[31] The clinical presentation of the patient should determine whether sin-

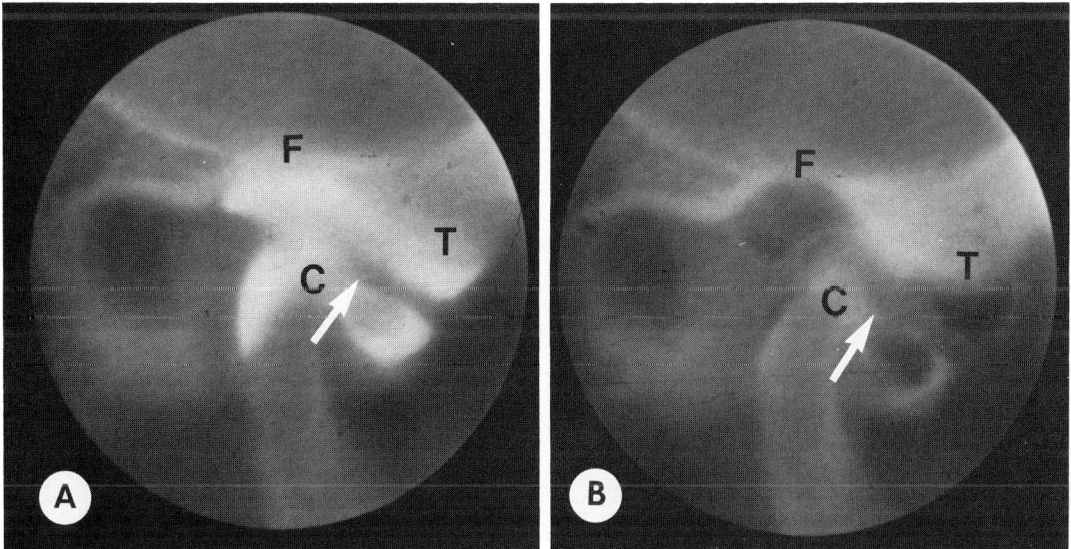

Figure 10–29. Comparison of single- *(A)* and double-contrast *(B)* arthrotomograms of the same temporomandibular joint. The disc is anteriorly displaced. Arrows indicate the location of the posterior band. The double-contrast arthrograms provide greater details of the articulating surfaces of the configuration of the disc and the posterior disc attachment. C = condyle; F = fossa; T = tubercle.

gle-contrast or double-contrast arthrography should be performed. If joint dynamics is of primary concern, single-contrast arthrography is recommended, but if information about joint morphology such as the amount of disc deformation and the extension of the joint compartments is more important for diagnosis and treatment planning, the double-contrast technique is recommended. Magnetic resonance imaging is an alternative examination technique that provides information similar to that provided by double-contrast arthrotomography and requires less examiner skill.

COMPUTED TOMOGRAPHY

Arthrography of the TMJ may sometimes be a technically difficult procedure for the inexperienced operator, and computed tomography (CT) is a noninvasive alternative that provoked a great deal of interest soon after its development. Direct sagittal (Fig. 10–30) and reconstructed axial images have been reported to be successful for the demonstration of disc displacement and osseous disease.[32–34] The use of CT has, however, decreased rapidly during the past few years with the evolution of magnetic resonance imaging (MRI) with surface coils. MRI appears to offer superior differentiation of soft tissues;[34] CT, however, is the best imaging modality for detection of osseous anatomy. CT and MRI views of the same TMJ, shown in Figure 10–31, demonstrate the superior soft tissue resolution of MRI. A comparison of MRI with CT is presented in Table 10–3.

Computed Tomographic Findings

A normally positioned disc is usually not directly depicted in the CT scan. Instead, indirect signs, such as position of the lateral pterygoid fat pad and the absence of radiopacity anterior to the condyle and inferior to the tubercle, are indicators of a normal disc position. When the disc is anteriorly displaced, it appears in the CT scan as a radiopacity anterior to the condyle (see Fig. 10–30). The configuration of the disc cannot be determined from CT scans because the resolution of the soft tissue is not sufficient for this purpose. The depiction of the disc by CT scanning is dependent upon the dimension of the disc per se. Thus, if the disc is thin and small, usually it is not possible to demonstrate it with CT. On the other hand, if the disc is large, it is more easily depicted by CT scanning. Comparisons of CT scanning and cryosections are shown in Figures 10–31 and 10–32.

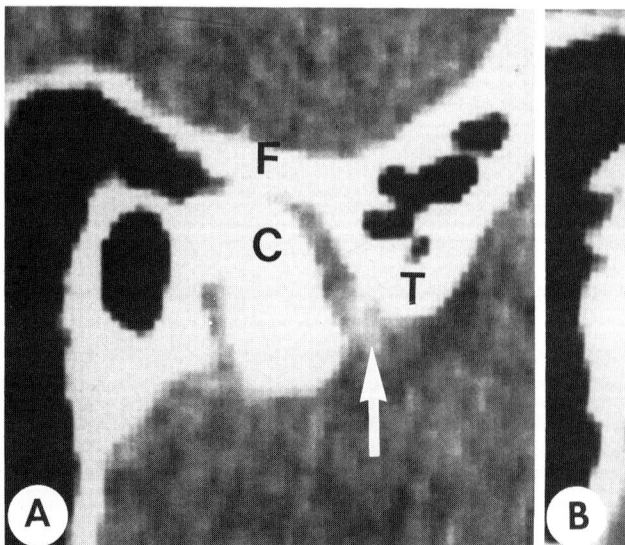 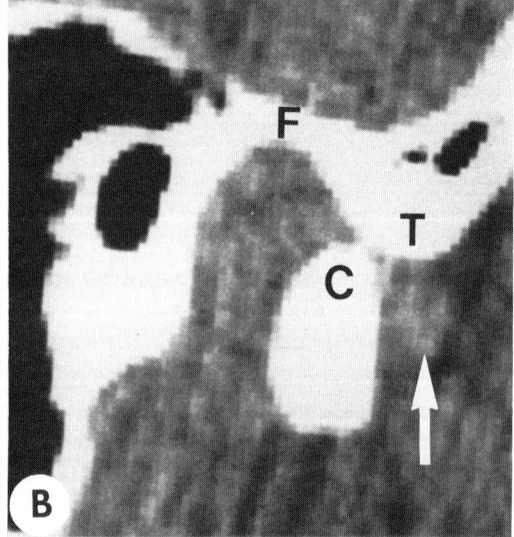

Figure 10–30. *A,* Direct sagittal computed tomography scan of a temporomandibular joint with anterior disc displacement. Arrow indicates the image of the disc. C = condyle; F = fossa; T = tubercle. *B,* The same temporomandibular joint at maximal mouth opening, showing anterior disc displacement without reduction. Arrow indicates the image of the disc. C = condyle; F = fossa; T = tubercle.

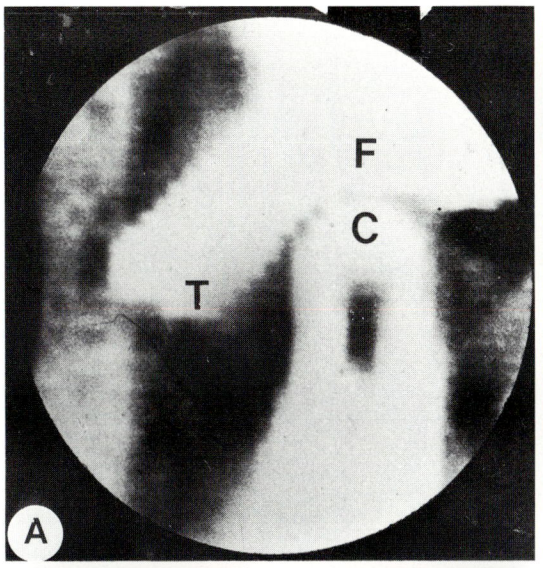
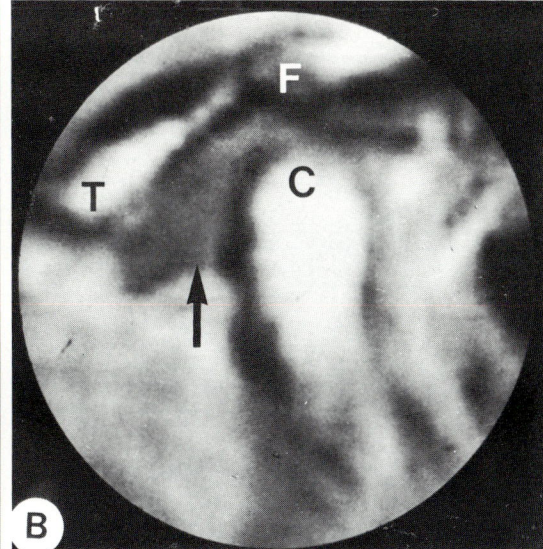
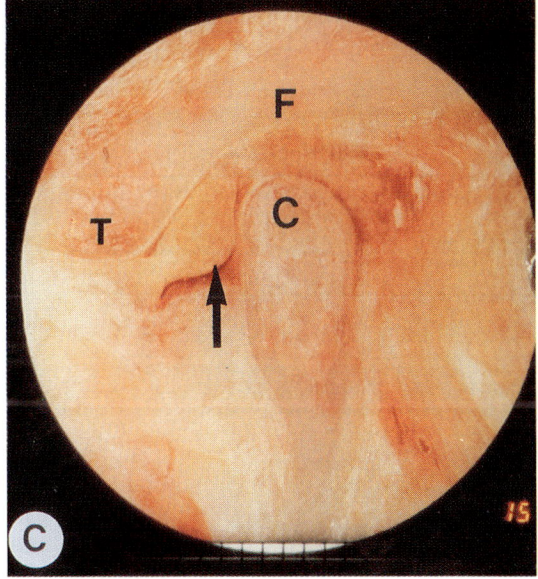

Figure 10–31. *A*, Computed tomography scan of temporomandibular joint showing normal osseous structures. *B*, Magnetic resonance scan of the same temporomandibular joint showing the disc *(arrow)* anterior to the condyle, suggesting disc displacement. *C*, Corresponding cryosection of the same temporomandibular joint confirming anterior displacement and deformation of the disc. Arrow indicates the position of the posterior band of the disc. C = condyle; F = fossa; T = tubercle.

MAGNETIC RESONANCE IMAGING

Soon after it evolved as an imaging modality, MRI was applied to the TMJ.[30, 36–41] The most important advantage of MRI over other imaging modalities is the absence of radiation. Details of the physical principles of MRI are beyond the scope of this discussion and have been described elsewhere.[42–44]

The objective of MRI of the TMJ is to detect soft tissue abnormalities in the joint itself and in the surrounding structures. An advantage of MRI over arthrography is the capability of studying soft tissue structures outside the joint capsule (see Fig. 10–31).

Table 10–3. ADVANTAGES AND DISADVANTAGES OF MAGNETIC RESONANCE IMAGING COMPARED WITH COMPUTED TOMOGRAPHY

Advantages

No ionizing radiation
Fewer artifacts from dense bone and metal clips
Imaging in multiple planes without moving the patient
Superior anatomic detail of soft tissues

Disadvantages

High initial cost
Special site planning and shielding
Claustrophobia in magnet
Inferior image of hard tissues

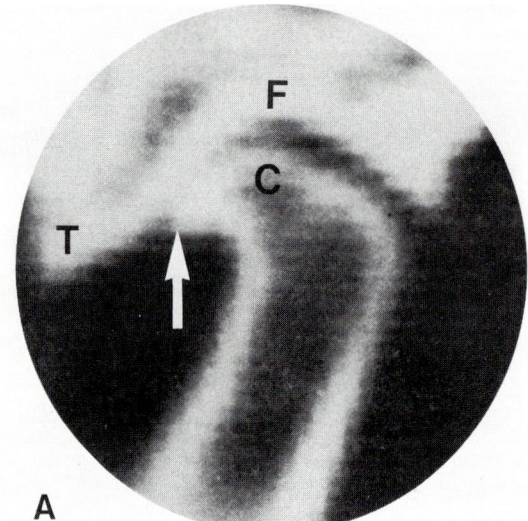 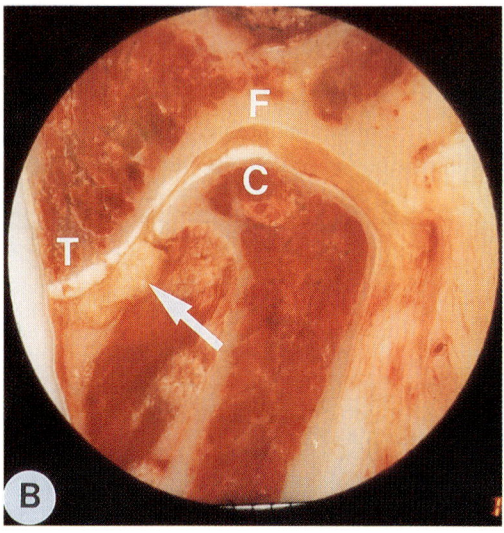

Figure 10–32. *A*, Computed tomography scan of a temporomandibular joint with extensive osseous changes. There is an osteophyte anteriorly on the condyle *(arrow)*. *B*, Corresponding cryosection of the same temporomandibular joint confirming the extensive osseous changes and showing the disc to be anteriorly displaced and deformed. There is a perforation of the posterior disc attachment. C = condyle; F = fossa; T = tubercle.

Indications, Contraindications, and Scanning Technique

MRI is an alternative imaging method to arthrography and the indications are the same. Contraindications for MRI are, however, different and are outlined in Table 10–4.

As with other imaging modalities the standard plane of imaging is sagittal. A suggested technique for a high field strength system is shown in Table 10–5. We use a dual–surface coil technique for bilateral imaging,[45] which is time-saving because both joints can be examined at the same time. Images are obtained in the sagittal plane with the mouth closed and opened, and in the coronal plane with

Table 10–4. CONTRAINDICATIONS FOR MAGNETIC RESONANCE IMAGING

Absolute

Cerebral aneurysm clips
Cardiac pacemakers

Relative

Claustrophobia or uncooperative attitude
Pregnancy
Metallic prosthetic heart valves
Ferromagnetic foreign bodies in critical locations (e.g., eye)
Implanted stimulator wires for pain control

No Contraindications

Metallic prostheses
Orthodontic fixed appliances

Table 10–5. SCANNING PARAMETERS FOR MAGNETIC RESONANCE IMAGING

		Image		
Parameter	Axial Localizer	Corrected Sagittal Closed	Corrected Sagittal Open	Corrected Coronal
TR	300	2000	1000	2000
TE	16	20/80	20/80	20/80
NEX	0.5	0.5	1	0.5
Matrix	256 × 128	256 × 192	256 × 192	256 × 192
Scanning time	25 sec	3 min; 52 sec	2 min; 8 sec	3 min; 52 sec

Slice thickness = 3 mm; 0 to 0.5 mm between slices. Scanning time for complete bilateral TMJ examination = 11 to 13 min; table time = approximately 30 min.

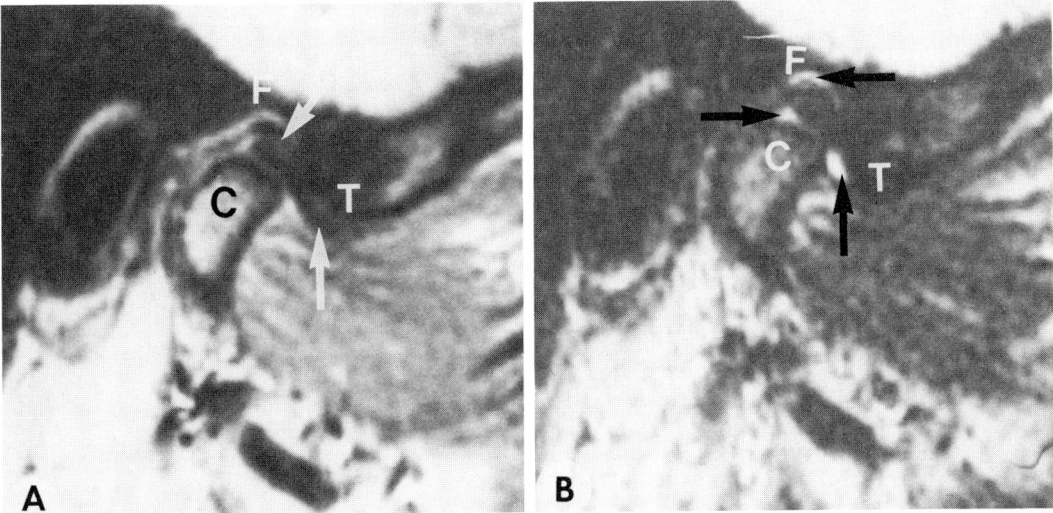

Figure 10–33. *A*, Magnetic resonance (MR) scan of a temporomandibular joint with superior disc position. The disc *(arrows)* is biconcave and is located with its posterior band superior to the condyle (TR = 2200; TE = 20). *B*, T_2 weighted MR scan (TR = 2200; TE = 80) of same temporomandibular joint. High-signal areas *(arrows)* in areas corresponding to the lower joint space suggest the presence of joint fluid. The patient presented with pain from the right temporomandibular joint and a lateral open bite on the right side. C = condyle; F = fossa; T = tubercle.

the mouth closed and opened. Disposable plastic syringes of variable sizes are used as bite blocks to stabilize the mandible during the open mouth scans. T1 or proton density images are standard for delineating the anatomy. T2-weighted images may be helpful for documenting fluid in the joint spaces (Fig. 10–33).[38, 46, 47] A protocol for scanning parameters on a high field strength magnet is shown in Table 10–5.

Normal Findings

MR images of the normal TMJ demonstrate the disc to be located superior to the condyle (Fig. 10–34), with the central thin part be-

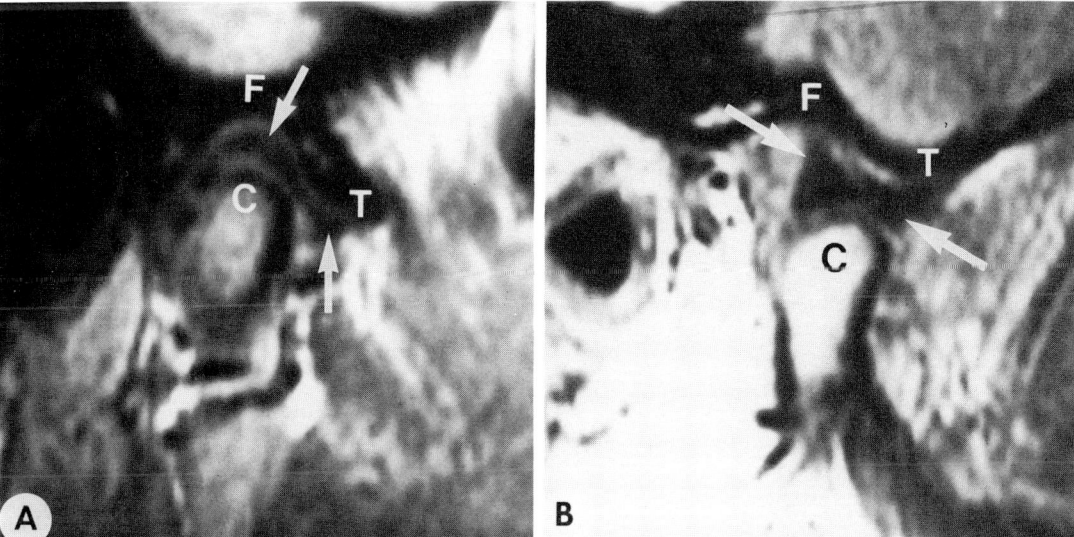

Figure 10–34. *A*, Magnetic resonance (MR) scan of a temporomandibular joint with disc in normal superior position. Arrows indicate the location of the posterior and anterior bands of the disc. *B*, MR scan of the same temporomandibular joint at half-open mouth position. The disc *(arrows)* is located in a normal position between the condyle and the temporal component. C = condyle; F = fossa; T = tubercle.

tween the condyle and the articular tubercle.[48] Owing to the low signal intensity of the fibrous connective tissue of the disc, it is clearly distinguished from the surrounding tissues that have a brighter signal. The cortex of the condyle has no signal but it is well depicted because of the relatively bright signal intensity from the articulating surface and the synovial tissues. The posterior disc attachment has a brighter signal compared with the disc, and it is therefore possible to distinguish the posterior attachment from the disc. MRI is the only imaging technique (except for arthroscopy) that can distinguish the disc from its posterior attachment. In the coronal plane, the disc has a crescent appearance, with the medial and lateral aspects of the disc located close to the medial and lateral poles of the condyle (Fig. 10–35).

In the open mouth scans, the central, thin part of the disc is seen lying between the tubercle and the condyle (Fig. 10–34B). The posterior band of the disc is clearly behind the condyle, and the superior anterior part of the condyle is articulating against the anterior band of the disc.

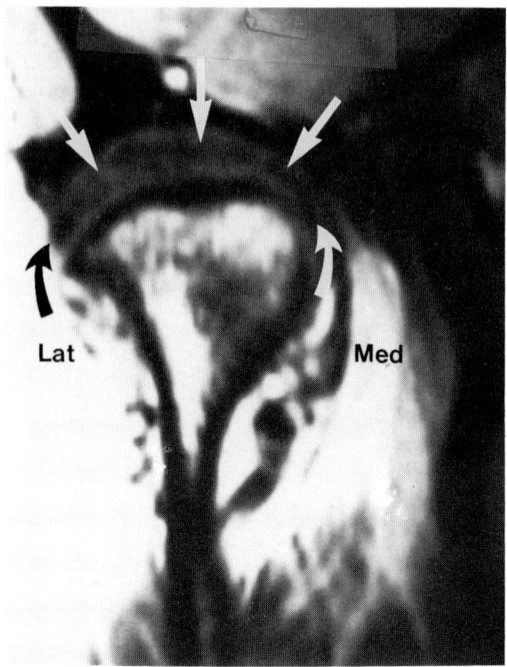

Figure 10–35. Coronal magnetic resonance scan of a temporomandibular joint with superior disc position. Straight arrows indicate the disc; curved arrows indicate the medial and lateral attachments of the disc to the capsule. Lat = laterally; Med = medially.

Abnormal Findings

Similar to arthrography, displacement of the disc is the most frequent abnormality seen in MRI of patients presenting with TMJ pain and dysfunction. The most common displacement is found in the anterior, anterior medial, and anterior lateral directions. In sagittal MR images, the disc is located anterior to the condyle in the closed mouth position (see Fig. 10–34). In disc displacement with reduction (Fig. 10–36) the position of the disc is normalized during mouth open-

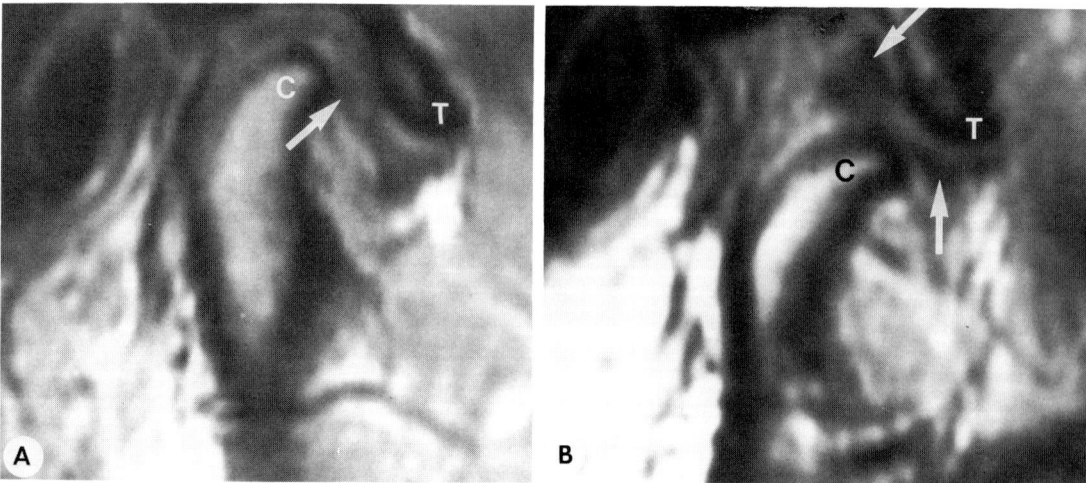

Figure 10–36. *A,* Magnetic resonance (MR) scan of a temporomandibular joint with anterior disc displacement. The posterior band *(arrow)* of the disc is located anterior to the condyle in this closed mouth scan. *B,* The same temporomandibular joint after reduction of disc position. The disc is now in a superior position, with the anterior and posterior bands *(arrows)* located anterior and posterior, respectively, to the condyle. C = condyle; T = tubercle.

ing; in disc displacement without reduction, the disc remains anterior to the condyle during all mandibular movements (Fig. 10–37). Displacement in the lateral (Fig. 10–38) and medial (Fig. 10–39) directions are visualized with MRI using the coronal plane. Deformation of the disc is a sequel to a disc displacement, and a characteristically increased dimension of the posterior band is the first sign of disc deformation (Fig. 10–40). In the later stage of disc displacement, the disc may develop a biconvex configuration (Fig. 10–41). Perforations are not really diagnosable by MRI, but in cases with extensive hard tissue changes and a very thin joint space, perforation is likely to be present (Fig. 10–42).

Some later publications have suggested that MRI of the TMJ has the potential to provide information about the condition of the bone marrow of the mandibular condyle.[49] Thus, if the central area of the condyle (bone marrow) has a low signal (Fig. 10–43) and appears black on the MR image, this is claimed to be pathologic and a sign of avascular necrosis of the condyle. More research, including histologic correlation, is needed to understand the pathophysiology of avascular necrosis of the mandibular condyle. However, it is clear that MRI may provide insight into the biology of the bone marrow of the mandibular condyle that is not possible with other imaging modalities. Soft tissue tumors in or around the joint area also can be demonstrated with MRI (Fig. 10–44).

POST-TREATMENT IMAGING

Imaging after treatment is indicated when the patient continues to have symptoms that might be caused by intra-articular pathology. Before the development of MRI, arthrography was the traditional method for this purpose; however, this procedure may be difficult to perform after surgery because of narrowing of the joint spaces and because of intra-articular adhesions (Fig. 10–45). For this reason, MRI is usually the preferred technique for examining the TMJ after treatment (Figs. 10–46 and 10–47).[29, 50, 51]

MRI can be helpful to determine if surgery was able to correct a displacement of the disc and to demonstrate that surgically placed implants are in the correct position with or without surrounding granulation tissue (see Figs. 10–46 and 10–47). Postsurgical fibrosis of the joint capsule also can be demonstrated by MRI (Fig. 10–48).

DIAGNOSTIC ACCURACY OF ARTHROGRAPHY, COMPUTER TOMOGRAPHY, AND MAGNETIC RESONANCE IMAGING

The accuracy of single- and double-contrast arthrography, CT, and MRI has been investigated in experimental studies using fresh autopsy specimens.[31, 35, 36, 52–54] All techniques have demonstrated high accuracy

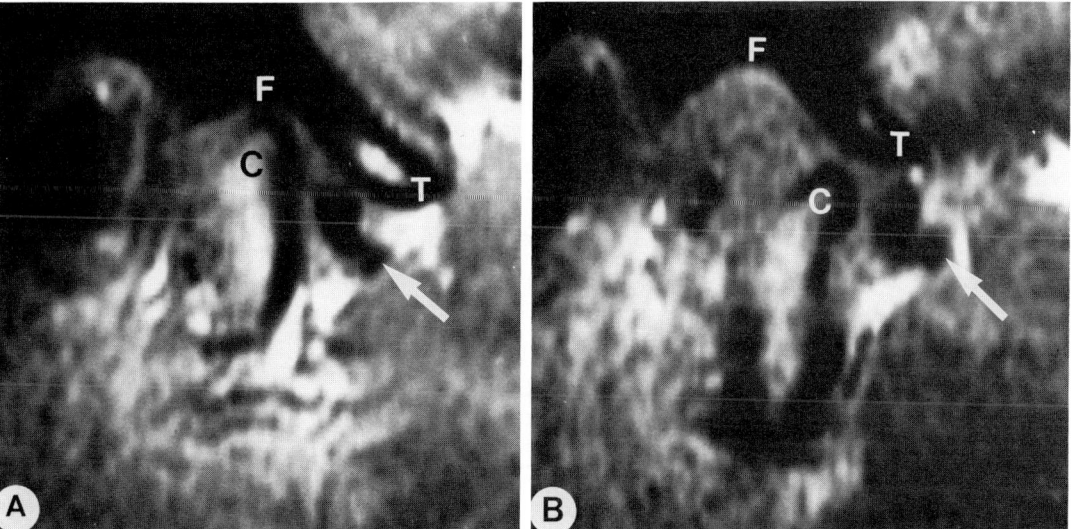

Figure 10–37. *A,* Magnetic resonance (MR) scan of a temporomandibular joint with anterior disc displacement. The anteriorly displaced disc *(arrows)* has a low signal. *B,* The same temporomandibular joint at maximal mouth opening. The disc *(arrow)* remains anterior to the condyle, suggesting disc displacement without reduction. C = condyle; F = fossa; T = tubercle.

134 ■ 10 Imaging of the Temporomandibular Joint

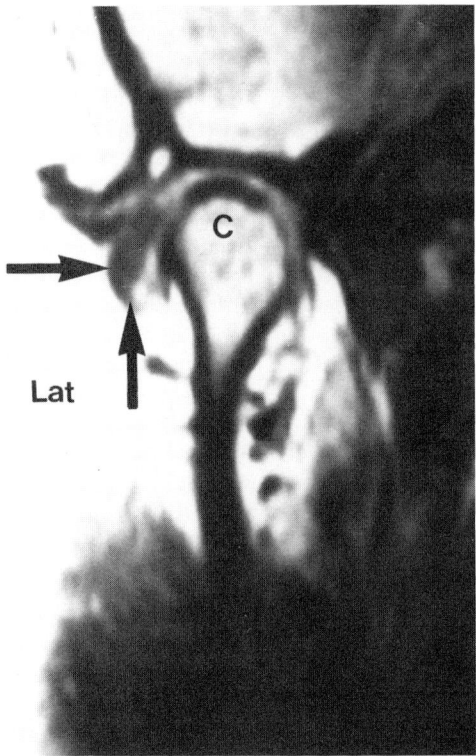

Figure 10–38. Coronal magnetic resonance scan showing lateral displacement of the disc. The disc *(arrows)* is located laterally to the condyle (C). Lat = laterally.

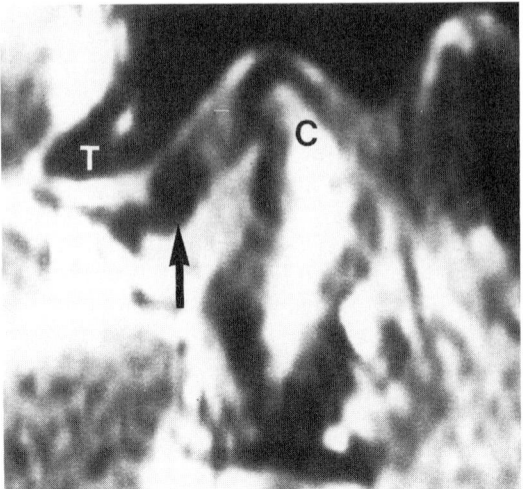

Figure 10–40. Magnetic resonance scan showing anterior displacement and deformation of the disc. There is enlargement of the posterior band *(arrow)* of the disc. C = condyle; T = tubercle.

(Table 10–6). Double-contrast arthrography provides information about position and configuration of the disc, whereas the single-contrast technique mainly demonstrates its position and functioning. CT probably is the most accurate technique for demonstration of

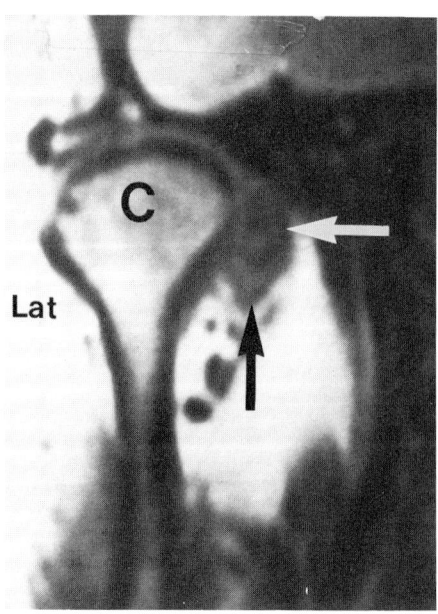

Figure 10–39. Coronal magnetic resonance scan showing medial displacement of the disc *(arrows)*. C = condyle; Lat = laterally.

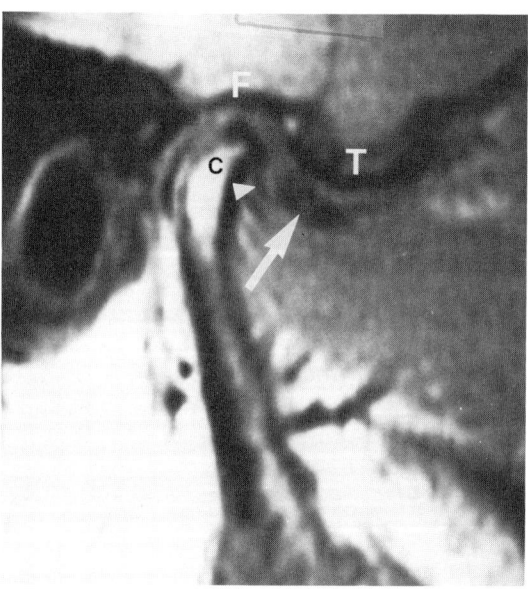

Figure 10–41. Magnetic resonance scan showing anterior displacement and deformation of the disc. The disc is biconvex *(arrow)*. The attachment of the lateral pterygoid muscle is thickened *(arrowhead)*. C = condyle; F = fossa; T = tubercle.

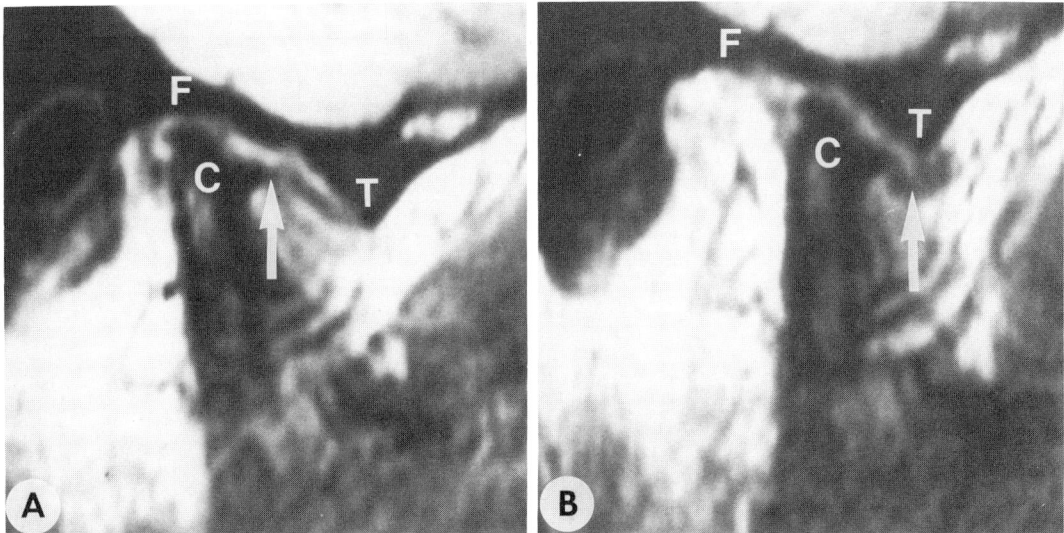

Figure 10–42. *A*, Magnetic resonance scan of a temporomandibular joint with extensive degenerative changes. The condyle is flattened and has an anterior osteophyte *(arrow)*. The temporal component is irregular, and the tubercle is flattened. *B*, The same temporomandibular joint at maximal mouth opening. The disc *(arrow)* is deformed anterior to the condyle. C = condyle; F = fossa; T = tubercle.

the disc's osseous components, whereas MRI provides information about its configuration and position in both the sagittal and coronal planes.

The values for diagnostic accuracy quoted in Table 10–6 were acquired in experimental studies with optimal imaging conditions, and it is reasonable to believe that they would have been lower in a clinical setting. These values are, however, relevant for the comparison of the techniques because they were obtained under the same conditions. In

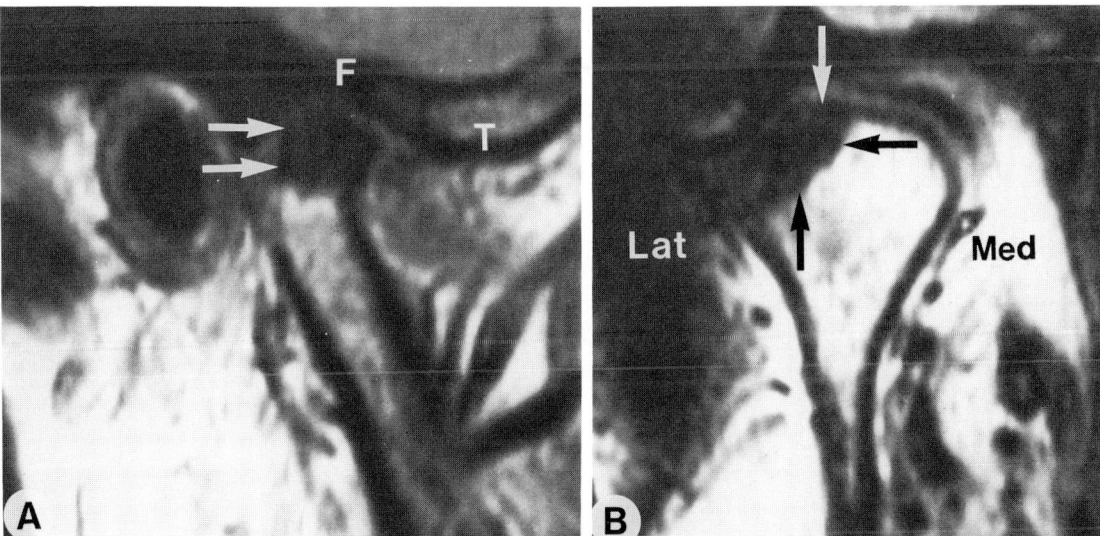

Figure 10–43. *A*, Magnetic resonance (MR) scan of temporomandibular joint in which the superior part of the condyle demonstrates a low-signal intensity *(arrow)*. F = fossa; T = tubercle. *B*, Coronal MR scan of the same temporomandibular joint. The low-signal area in the condyle *(arrows)* is located in the lateral third of the condyle. Lat = laterally; Med = medially.

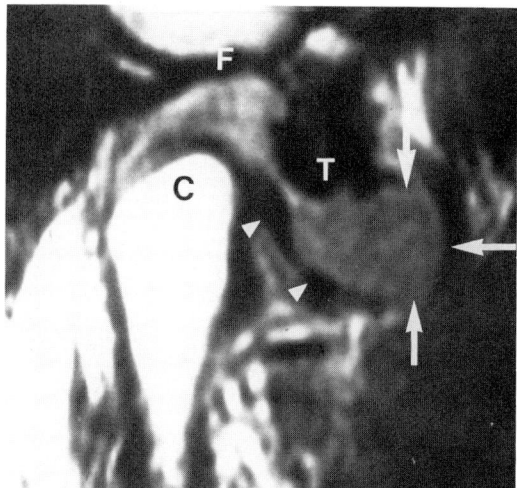

Figure 10–44. Magnetic resonance scan of temporomandibular joint with an intra-articular tumor. The rounded mass expanding the upper joint space *(arrows)* suggests an intra-articular tumor; the histologic diagnosis was chondromatosis. The disc *(arrowheads)* is displaced anteriorly and inferiorly. C = condyle; F = fossa; T = tubercle.

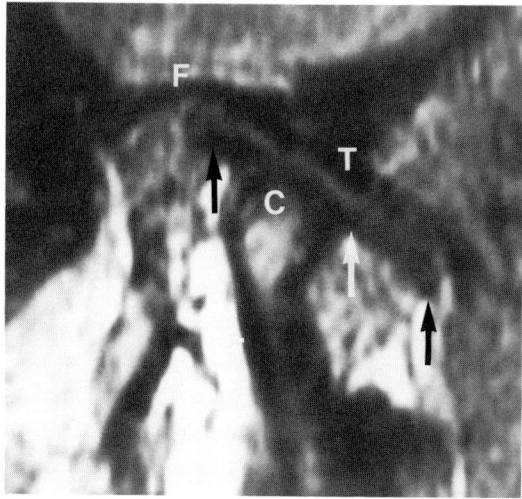

Figure 10–46. Postsurgical magnetic resonance scan of temporomandibular joint with implant. The implant *(arrows)* is in proper position, and there is no evidence of granulation tissue around it. C = condyle; F = fossa; T = tubercle.

a clinical setting, on the other hand, information about clinical symptoms may help to improve the diagnostic accuracy. Therefore, it is believed that the values in Table 10–6 represent a good estimate of the accuracy of these imaging modalities.

RADIONUCLIDE IMAGING

Radionuclide imaging of the TMJ may be a valuable screening test for osseous disease.[55, 56] This technique, which can be performed with a minimal radiation dose to the

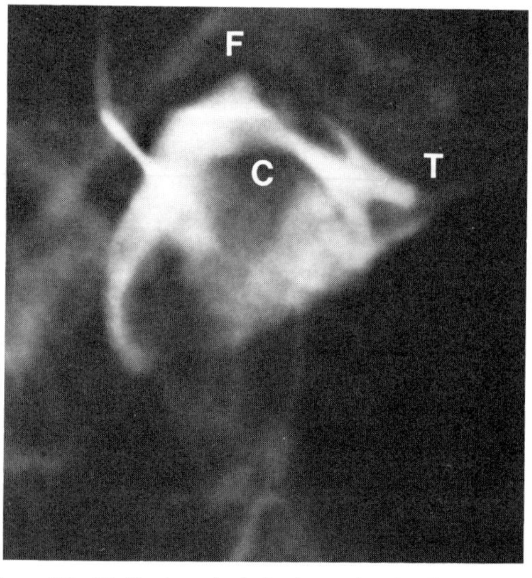

Figure 10–45. Postsurgical single-contrast arthrogram of a temporomandibular joint. The joint spaces are narrowed and show peripheral adhesions. A remnant of the disc is seen between the condyle (C) and temporal component. F = fossa; T = tubercle.

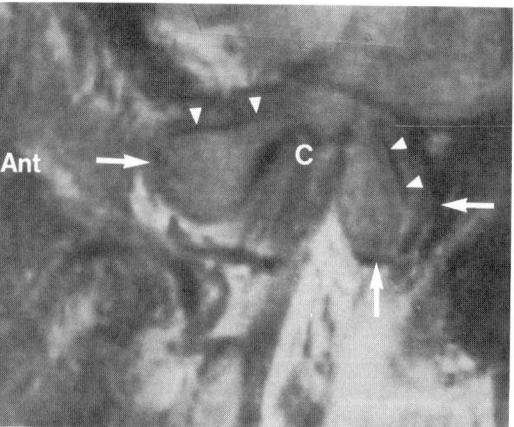

Figure 10–47. Postsurgical magnetic resonance scan of temporomandibular joint with a Silastic implant *(arrowheads)*. The implant is broken and displaced. There is an extensive amount of granulation tissue *(arrows)* surrounding the implant and the condyle (C). The condyle shows degenerative changes.

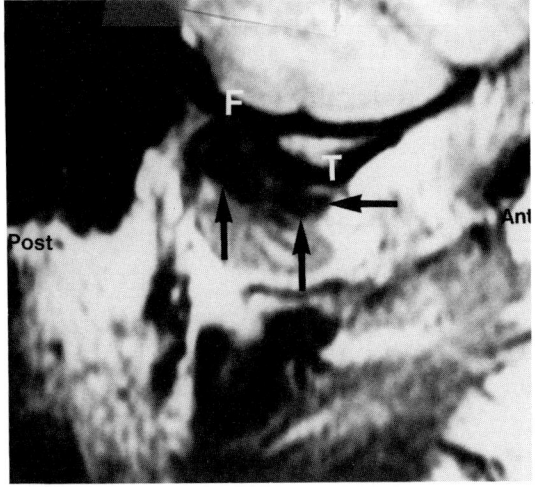

Figure 10–48. Postsurgical magnetic resonance scan showing tissue with low-signal intensity (arrows) in the joint area. This was interpreted as fibrosis of the joint capsule. F = fossa; T = tubercle; Post = posteriorly; Ant = anteriorly.

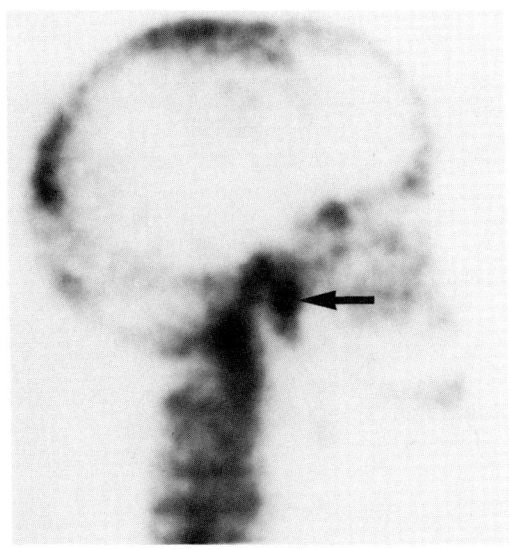

Figure 10–49. Radionuclide imaging of patient with condylar hyperplasia showing increased uptake in the area of the mandibular condyle (arrow).

Table 10–6. ACCURACY OF DIFFERENT FORMS OF IMAGING

Imaging Modality	Accuracy			
	Number of Joints	Disc Position	Disc Configuration	Perforation
Single-contrast arthrography[53]*	58	84%	NA[†]	97%
Dual-space double-contrast arthrotomography[52]	48	92	92%	100%
Computed tomography[35]	15	67%	NA	NA
Magnetic resonance imaging				
Study 1[36]	15	73%	60%	NA
Study 2[54]	39	85%	NA	NA

*Superior numbers refer to publications listed in references.
[†]NA = Not applicable.

patient, can detect not only disease and remodeling of the TMJ but also other pathologic conditions in and around the TMJ that may produce symptoms (Fig. 10–49).

SELECTION OF IMAGING METHOD

The first step in imaging a patient presenting with TMJ pain and dysfunction might be a plain film or panoramic radiography. If greater details are necessary, tomography should be used. These images are not diagnostic for internal derangement, and a negative finding does not rule out pathologic changes of the soft tissues.

The next level of imaging should be focused on soft tissue imaging. Here the choice is between MRI and arthrography or CT. Studies have shown that CT is inferior to MRI in the detection of soft tissue abnormalities, and CT does not, therefore, represent a competitive modality. The capability of multiplanar imaging and the possibility of medial and lateral displacement of the disc, the absence of radiation, and less need for examiner skill are factors that should direct the decision toward MRI. For postsurgical imaging, MRI is definitively the imaging modality of choice.

Therefore, in most clinical symptomatic presentations, MRI is the preferred imaging modality for TMJ disorders.

If the functional component of symptoms is of primary concern, arthrography is the procedure of choice. Arthrography can depict clearly the dynamics of the TMJ, and mandibular position with a normal condyle disc relationship can be established for the initiation of protrusive splint therapy.

References

1. Wilkes CH: Structural and functional alterations of the temporomandibular joint. Northwest Dent 57:287–294, 1978.
2. Wilkes CH: Arthrography of the temporomandibular joint in patients with the TMJ pain-dysfunction syndrome. Minn Med 61:645–652, 1978.
3. Farrar WB, McCarty WL Jr: Inferior joint space arthrography and characteristics of condylar paths in internal derangements of the TMJ. J Prosthet Dent 41:548–555, 1979.
4. Westesson P-L: Double-contrast arthrography and internal derangement of the temporomandibular joint. Swed Dent J [Suppl No 13], 1–57, 1982.
5. Wilkes CH: Internal derangements of the temporomandibular joint. Arch Otolaryngol 115:469–477, 1989.
6. Rees LA: The structure and function of the mandibular joint. Br Dent J 96:125–133, 1954.
7. Katzberg RW, Dolwick MF, Helms CA, et al: Arthrotomography of the temporomandibular joint. AJR 134:995–1003, 1980.
8. Eriksson L, Westesson P-L: Clinical and radiological study of patients with anterior disc displacement of the temporomandibular joint. Swed Dent J 7:55–64, 1983.
9. Katzberg RW, Westesson P-L, Tallents RH, et al: Temporomandibular joint: MR assessment of rotational and sideways disc displacements. Radiology 169:741–748, 1988.
10. Westesson P-L: Double-contrast arthrotomography of the temporomandibular joint: Introduction of an arthrographic technique for visualization of the disc and articular surfaces. J Oral Maxillofac Surg 41:163–172, 1983.
11. Westesson P-L, Bronstein SL, Liedberg JL: Internal derangement of the temporomandibular joint: Morphologic description with correlation to joint function. Oral Surg Oral Med Oral Pathol 59:323–331, 1985.
12. Roberts CA, Tallents RH, Espeland MA, et al: Mandibular range of motion versus arthrographic diagnosis of the temporomandibular joint. Oral Surg Oral Med Oral Pathol 60:244–251, 1985.
13. Roberts CA, Tallents RH, Katzberg RW, et al: Clinical and arthrographic evaluation of the temporomandibular joint. Oral Surg Oral Med Oral Pathol 62:373–376, 1986.
14. Roberts CA, Tallents RH, Katzberg RW, et al: Clinical and arthrographic evaluation of the location of temporomandibular joint pain. Oral Surg Oral Med Oral Pathol 64:6–8, 1987.
15. Roberts CA, Tallents RH, Katzberg RW, et al: Comparison of internal derangements of the TMJ with occlusal findings. Oral Surg Oral Med Oral Pathol 63:645–650, 1987.
16. Roberts CA, Tallents RH, Katzberg RW, et al: Comparison of arthrographic findings of the temporomandibular joint with palpation of the muscles of mastication. Oral Surg Oral Med Oral Pathol 64:275–277, 1987.
17. Anderson GC, Schiffman EL, Shellhas KP, Fricton JR: Clinical vs. arthrographic diagnosis of TMJ internal derangement. J Dent Res 68:826–829, 1989.
18. Petersson A, Nanthaviroj S: Radiography of the temporomandibular joint utilizing the transmaxillary projection. A comparison of the information obtained with the oblique lateral transcranial projection versus the transmaxillary projection. Dentomaxillofac Radiol 4:76–83, 1975.
19. Omnell K-Å, Petersson A: Radiography of the temporomandibular joint utilizing oblique lateral transcranial projections. Comparison of information obtained with standardized technique and individualized technique. Odontol Revy 26:77–92, 1976.
20. Nørgaard F: Artrografi af kaebeleddet. Preliminary report. Acta Radiol 25:679–685, 1944.
21. Nørgaard F: Temporomandibular arthrography. [Thesis] Copenhagen: Munksgaard, 1947.
22. Bell KA, Walters PJ: Videofluoroscopy during arthrography of the temporomandibular joint. Radiology 147:879, 1983.
23. Westesson P-L: Arthrography of the temporomandibular joint. J Prosthet Dent 51:535–543, 1984.
24. Manzione JV, Tallents R, Katzberg RW, et al: Arthrographically guided splint therapy for recapturing the temporomandibular joint meniscus. Oral Surg 57:235–240, 1984.
25. Tallents RH, Katzberg RW, Miller TL, et al: Arthrographically assisted splint therapy. J Prosthet Dent 53:235–238, 1985.
26. Westesson P-L, Eriksson L, Kurita K: Temporomandibular joint: Variation of normal arthrographic anatomy. Oral Surg Oral Med Oral Pathol. In press.
27. Liedberg J, Westesson P-L, Kurita K: Sideways and rotational displacement of the temporomandibular joint disk: Diagnosis by arthrography and correlation to cryosectional morphology. Oral Surg Oral Med Oral Pathol. In press.
28. Khoury MB, Dolan E: Sideways dislocation of the temporomandibular joint meniscus: The edge sign. AJNR 7:869–872, 1986.
29. Katzberg RW: Temporomandibular joint imaging. Radiology 170:297–307, 1989.
30. Westesson P-L, Manzione JV: Contrast media reaction associated with TMJ arthrography. AJR 154:1344, 1990.
31. Westesson P-L, Bronstein SL: Temporomandibular joint: Comparison of single and double contrast arthrography. Radiology 164:65–70, 1987.
32. Helms CA, Morrish RB, Kircos LT, et al: Computed tomography of the meniscus of the temporomandibular joint: Preliminary observations. Radiology 145:719–722, 1982.
33. Manzione JV, Seltzer SE, Katzberg RW, et al: Direct sagittal computed tomography of the temporomandibular joint. AJNR 3:677–679, 1982.
34. Thompson JR, Christiansen EL, Hasso AN, Hinshaw DB. The temporomandibular joint: High-resolution computed tomographic evaluation. Radiology 150:105–110, 1984.

35. Westesson P-L, Katzberg RW, Tallents RH, et al: CT and MRI of the temporomandibular joint: Comparison with autopsy specimens, AJR 148:1165–1171, 1987.
36. Westesson P-L, Katzberg RW, Tallents RH, et al: Temporomandibular joint: Comparison of MR images with cryosectional anatomy. Radiology 164:59–64, 1987.
37. Roberts D, Schenk J, Joseph P, et al: Temporomandibular joint: Magnetic resonance imaging. Radiology 155:829–830, 1985.
38. Harms SE, Wilk RM, Wolford LM, et al: The temporomandibular joint: Magnetic resonance imaging using surface coils. Radiology 157:133–136, 1985.
39. Helms CA, Gillespy T III, Sims RE, Richardson ML. Magnetic resonance imaging of internal derangement of the temporomandibular joint. Radiol Clin North Am 24:189–192, 1986.
40. Katzberg RW, Bessette RW, Tallents RH, et al: Normal and abnormal temporomandibular joint: MR imaging with surface coil. Radiology 158:183–189, 1986.
41. Manzione JV, Katzberg RW, Tallents RH, Bessette RW. Magnetic resonance imaging of the temporomandibular joint. J Am Dent Assoc 113:398–402, 1986.
42. Bradley WC, Newton TH, Crooks LE: Physical principles of nuclear magnetic resonance. *In* Newton TH, Potts DG (eds.): Advanced Imaging Techniques. San Francisco: Cavadell Press, 1983, pp 15–61.
43. Bottomley PA, Hart HR, Edelstein WA, et al. NMR imaging spectroscopy system to study both anatomy and metabolism. Lancet 2:273–274, 1983.
44. Edelstein WA, Bottomley PA, Hart HR, Smith LS. Signal, noise, and contrast in nuclear magnetic resonance imaging. J Comput Assist Tomogr 7:391–401, 1983.
45. Hardy CJ, Katzberg RW, Frey RL, et al: Switched surface coil system for bilateral MR imaging. Radiology 167:835–838, 1988.
46. Schellhas KP, Wilkes CH: Temporomandibular joint inflammation: Comparison of MR Fast Scanning with T_1- and T_2-weighted imaging techniques. AJR 153:93–98, 1989.
47. Schellhas KP, Fritts HM, Heithoff KB, et al: Temporomandibular joint imaging: MR fast scanning. J Craniomandib Pract 6:209–216, 1988.
48. Kaplan PA, Tu HK, Williams SM, Lydiatt DD: The normal temporomandibular joint: MR and arthrographic correlation. Radiology 165:177–178, 1987.
49. Schellhas KP, Wilkes CH, Fritts HM, et al: MR of osteochondritis dissecans and avascular necrosis of the mandibular condyle. AJNR 10:3–12, 1989.
50. Kneeland JB, Ryan DE, Carrera GF, et al: Failed temporomandibular joint prosthesis: MR imaging. Radiology 165:179–181, 1987.
51. Schellhas KP, Wilkes CH, Fritts HM, et al: Temporomandibular joint: MR imaging of internal derangements and postoperative changes. AJNR 8:1093–1101, 1987.
52. Westesson P-L, Rohlin M: Diagnostic accuracy of double contrast arthrotomography of the temporomandibular joint: Correlation with postmortem morphology. AJNR 5:463–468, 1984.
53. Westesson P-L, Bronstein SL, Liedberg J: Temporomandibular joint: Correlation between single contrast videoarthrography and postmortem morphology. Radiology 160:767–771, 1986.
54. Hansson LG, Westesson P-L, Eriksson L, et al: Comparison of MR imaging of the temporomandibular joint: Images of autopsy specimens made at 0.3 T and 1.5 T with anatomic cryosections. AJR 152:1241–1244, 1989.
55. Collier DB, Carrera GF, Messer EJ, et al: Internal derangement of the temporomandibular joint: Detection by single photon emission computed tomography. Radiology 149:557–561, 1983.
56. Katzberg RW, O'Mara RE, Tallents RH, Weber DA: Radionuclide imaging and single photon emission computed tomography in suspected internal derangement of the temporomandibular joint. J Oral Maxillofac Surg 42:782–787, 1984.
57. Omnell K-Å, Lysell L: Roentgendiagnostics. *In* Krogh-Poulsen W (ed): Stomatognathic Function and Physiology, Vol 2. Copenhagen: Munksgaard, 1978, pp 141–153.

Section III
Arthroscopy of the Temporomandibular Joint

Chapter 11
ARTHROSCOPIC ANATOMY, HISTOLOGY, AND VISUAL FIELDS IN THE TEMPOROMANDIBULAR JOINT

KEN-ICHIRO MURAKAMI, D.D.S., PH.D.

Precise, safe arthroscopic puncture requires an understanding of the topographic anatomy of the temporomandibular joint (TMJ) components and adjacent tissues. Moreover, to obtain valuable pathologic information through arthroscopic examination, the ability to recognize details of regional TMJ anatomy is mandatory. Thus, knowledge of arthroscopic anatomy and histology is fundamental in performing diagnostic arthroscopy; the recognition of exact visual fields through each puncture is necessary to begin the arthroscopic examination. Based on careful diagnostic arthroscopy of the TMJ, appropriate operative arthroscopy can be accomplished.

In this chapter, from the point of view of clinical arthroscopy, gross and arthroscopic anatomy of the TMJ and related histologic features are reviewed. Arthroscopic visual fields and subdivisions of the joint compartments are described.

GROSS ANATOMY

The TMJ is a synovial joint between the temporal bone and the mandible and has upper and lower joint cavities with an intervening articular disc. The upper joint cavity is the temporodiscal interspace, bounded above by the continuous articular surface covering the articular eminence and the mandibular fossa, below by the covering on the superior surface of the articular disc, and elsewhere by the synovial membrane. The inferior joint cavity is the condylodiscal interspace, bounded above by the covering of the undersurface of the articular disc, below by the articular surface of the mandibular condylar head, and elsewhere by the synovial membrane (Fig. 11–1A and B).

The articular disc separates the joint space into upper and lower joint cavities. These two cavities communicate freely with each other only in pathologic conditions such as

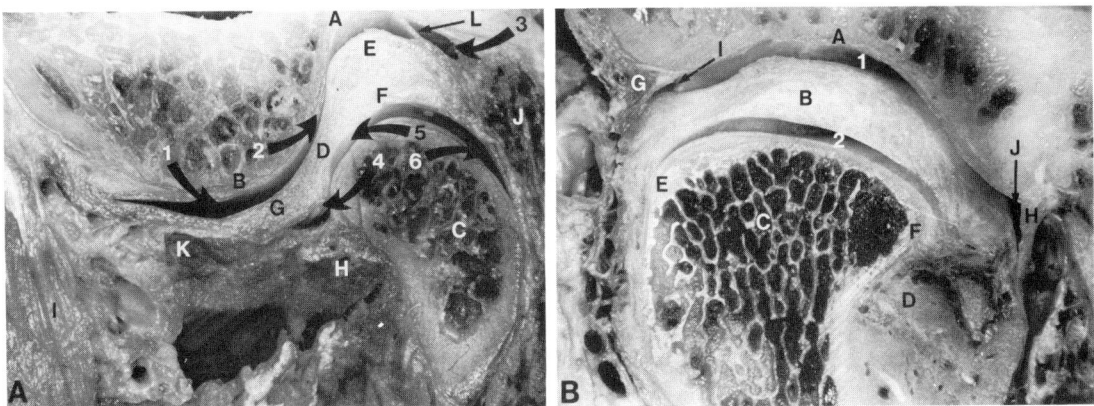

Figure 11-1. *A,* Sagittal section of the left temporomandibular joint. Upper joint cavity: 1 = anterior synovial recess; 2 = intermediate space; 3 = posterior synovial pouch. Lower joint cavity: 4 = anterior synovial pouch; 5 = intermediate space; 6 = posterior synovial pouch. A = mandibular fossa; B = articular eminence; C = condylar head; D = intermediate portion of articular disc; E = discal eminence (highest portion of the posterior band); F = discal fossa (lowest portion of the posterior band); G = flat portion (anterior portion of the anterior band); H = inferior belly of the lateral pterygoid muscle; I = masseter muscle; J = retrodiscal tissue; K = interwoven junction of the lateral pterygoid muscle to the articular disc and articular capsule; L = tongue-like synovial plica. *B,* Frontal section of the right temporomandibular joint. 1 = upper joint cavity; 2 = lower joint cavity; A = mandibular fossa; B = articular disc; C = condylar head; D = lateral pterygoid muscle; E = lateral pole; F = medial pole; G = lateral capsule with synovial lining; H = medial capsule with synovial lining; I = lateral paradiscal groove (sulcus); J = medial paradiscal groove (sulcus). (Reprinted with permission from Murakami K, Hoshino K: Regional anatomic nomenclature and arthroscopic terminology in human temporomandibular joints. Okajimas Folia Anat 58:745–760, 1982.)

perforation and rupture of the articular disc. The lateral pterygoid muscle inserts into the anteromedial aspect of the disc–condyle complex; some muscle fibers are interwoven into the fibrous connective tissues of the anterior portion of the articular disc. The articular disc blends posteriorly with the retrodiscal pad (see Fig. 11–1*A*).

The TMJ is enclosed by the articular capsule; some portions of the capsule are not readily identifiable. The lateral capsule is reinforced by the lateral ligament, which is a broad, flat, thin strong band. This ligament attaches above the lower border of the zygomatic arch and the articular tubercle and is directed backward toward the lateroposterior aspect of the condylar neck. The medial capsule is very thin, covering a narrow area because the medial rim of the temporal component of the TMJ protrudes downward to the level of the medial pole of the mandibular condyle (see Fig. 11–1*B*). As mentioned previously, the anterior and posterior portions of the articular capsule are not identifiable because of their fusion with the articular disc and adjacent tissues in each site. The inner surface of the articular capsule is lined by synovial membranes.

The anatomic structure of the TMJ is very simple, whereas the articular functions are highly complex. Normally, the upper and lower portions of each joint function simultaneously but independently. The upper joint cavity serves for gliding and the lower for hinge joint movement. During jaw movement, the position of the disc changes but its shape does not. Instead, the synovial membrane around the periphery of the articular disc alters its shape morphologically, becoming either compressed or stretched during jaw movements (Fig. 11–2*A* and 2*B*). In this sense, the TMJ may be considered as consisting of two independent joints in a single craniomandibular articulation.

ARTHROSCOPIC ANATOMY

Physiologically, the joint cavity has no real volume in itself; the articulation functions solely within synovial fluid. Therefore, prior to the arthroscopy, a fluid medium must be injected into the joint cavity under pressure in order to distend the intra-articular space. This unavoidable procedure makes anatomic relationships somewhat unnatural, a fact that

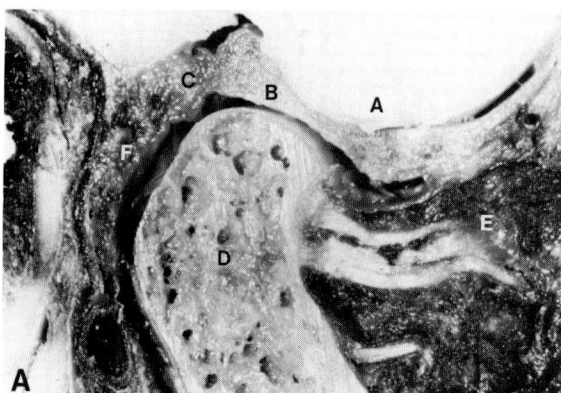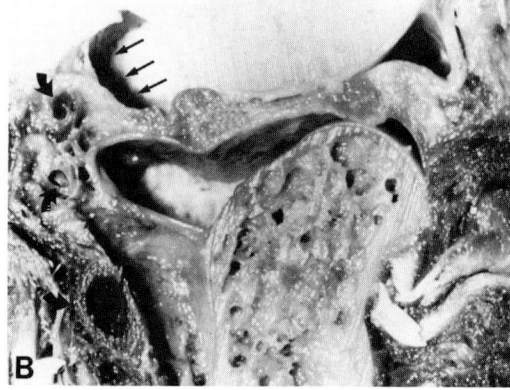

Figure 11–2. Sagittal sections of the right temporomandibular joint during closing *(A)* and opening *(B)*. During opening, the disc translates forward and the synovial membrane stretches anteriorly along with the posterior attachment *(long straight arrows)*. During this translation the venous plexus is easily identified due to dilatation of the retrodiscal capillaries *(short curved arrows)*. A = articular eminence; B = articular disc; C = posterior attachment; D = condyle; E = lateral pterygoid muscle; F = retrodiscal tissue.

must be kept in mind when arthroscopic features are interpreted. The average volume of the upper joint cavity is about 2 to 3 ml, and this maximal volume will be achieved in the open position of the mandible. The volume of the lower joint cavity is 1 to 1.5 ml.

Both the upper and the lower joint cavities may be divided into subcompartments, not only for regional anatomic description but also for arthroscopic descriptive purposes. The inner surfaces of each joint cavity are lined by an avascular articular tissue and the synovial membrane. Therefore, the joint compartments can be subdivided into the intermediate (intra-articular) spaces and the synovial pouches (recesses).

Arthroscopically, each compartment in the upper and lower joint cavities is characterized by individual and specific anatomic features and pathologic disorders.

Upper Joint Cavity

In the upper joint cavity, the posterior synovial pouch, intermediate space, and anterior synovial recess are arthroscopically defined. Osseous landmarks consist of the highest contour of the mandibular fossa and the apex of the articular eminence; these landmarks are helpful in identifying the subcompartments (Fig. 11–3). In the most lateral and medial portion of the upper joint cavity, two paradiscal synovial grooves (sulci) are formed.

Upper Posterior Synovial Pouch

An important anatomic landmark in this area is the synovial membrane characterized by a soft appearance and located in the posterior aspect of the upper posterior synovial pouch (Fig. 11–4*A* and *B*). From the lateral aspect, a number of folds are observed on the surface of the synovial membrane in the most

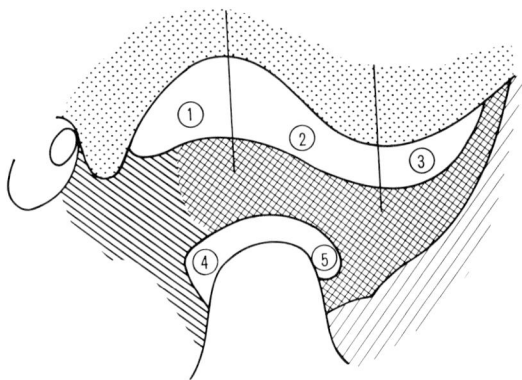

Figure 11–3. Schematic representation of regional arthroscopic anatomic subdivisions of the right temporomandibular joint cavity (sagittal view). The dividing landmarks are the height of the mandibular fossa, the apex of the articular eminence, and the most superior portion of the condyle. 1 = upper posterior synovial pouch; 2 = intermediate space; 3 = upper anterior synovial recess; 4 = lower posterior synovial pouch; 5 = lower anterior synovial pouch. (Reprinted with permission from Murakami K: Arthroscopic anatomy of the TMJ. Oral Maxillofac Surg Clin North Am 1:69–77, 1989.)

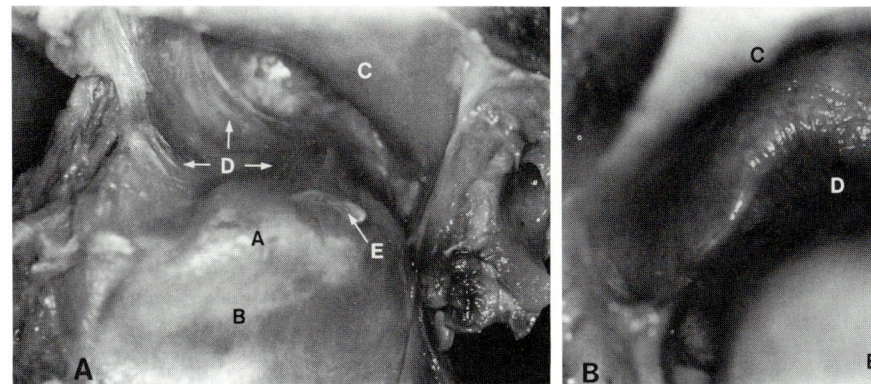

Figure 11–4. *A*, Upper posterior synovial pouch of the right temporomandibular joint and *B*, upper posterior synovial pouch of the left temporomandibular joint, both opened from the front. A = discal eminence (highest portion of posterior band); B = intermediate portion of articular disc; C = articular eminence; D = synovial membrane in upper posterior synovial pouch; E = synovial plica. (Reprinted with permission from Murakami K: Arthroscopic anatomy of the TMJ. Oral Maxillofac Surg Clin North Am 1:69–77, 1989.)

posterior portion (Fig. 11–5); these disappear when the disc slides anteriorly. Translucent vascular patterns are seen through the posterior attachment and are reflected upward posteriorly to the mandibular fossa, where the attachment blends and joins to the articular surface (Figs. 11–4*B* and 11–6).

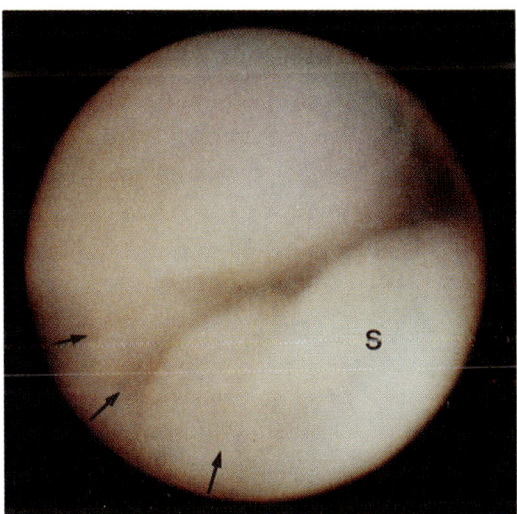

Figure 11–5. Arthroscopic photographs of the upper posterior synovial pouch of the right temporomandibular joint (left is posterior). Synovial folds (*arrows*) were formed by the synovial membrane (S) of the posterior attachment during closure of the mandible. (Reprinted with permission from Murakami K, Hoshino K: Regional anatomic nomenclature and arthroscopic terminology in human temporomandibular joints. Okajimas Folia Anat 58:745–760, 1982.)

The synovial membrane is composed histologically of two layers: superficial and deep. The former is composed of a few rows of synovial lining cells; the latter is a vascular, loose connective tissue containing a great number of short, fine collagen and elastic fibers. The surface of the synovial membrane wrinkles somewhat and often forms folds. Deep to the two layers of the synovial membrane is loose, vascular connective tissue containing abundant blood vessels. The deep subsynovial connective tissue blends into the fibrous tissue of the articular disc and into the retrodiscal pad (Fig. 11–7).

The arthroscopic appearance of the synovial membrane is usually distinguishable from that of the articular surfaces, although their boundary is not clear-cut. The anterior portion of the synovial membrane in the posterior synovial pouch ends just behind the posterior band of the articular disc (Fig. 11–8). Histologically, it seems that the synovial membrane covers the area outside of the circumference of the surface of the articular disc and lines the posterior attachment toward the posterior aspect (Fig. 11–9).

The synovial membrane's response to inflammation may be mild to severe synovitis, detectable in several inflammatory conditions in the TMJ.

The position plus form of the posterior attachment is one of the diagnostic landmarks of disc displacement, with or without reduction. In irreducible anterior disc displacement, the posterior attachment be-

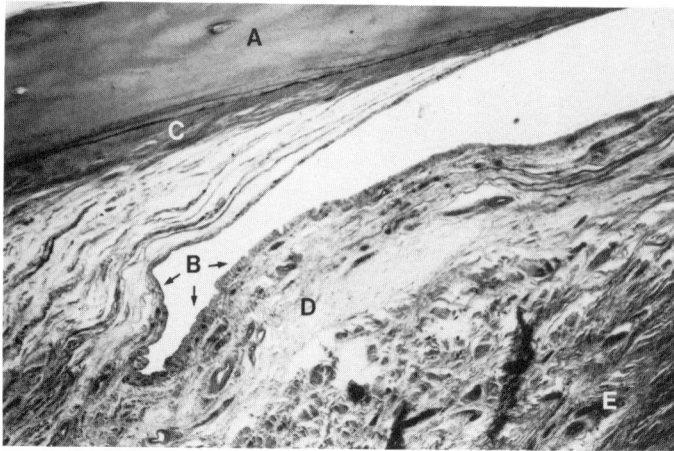

Figure 11–6. Photomicrograph of a sagittal section of the right upper posterior synovial pouch. A = mandibular fossa; B = synovial membrane; C = connective tissue; D = vascular subsynovial tissues; E = posterior attachment (upper stratum of the bilaminar zone).

Figure 11–7. Photomicrograph of synovial membrane. The superficial layer of the synovial membrane is composed of synovial lining cells (*arrows*). The deeper, vascular loose connective tissue layer contains short and fine collagenous and elastic fibers (*asterisks*). The subsynovial connective tissue is loosely formed by thick collagen fibers (A) and contains many capillaries (B). Loose connective tissue in the retrodiscal tissue is seen at C.

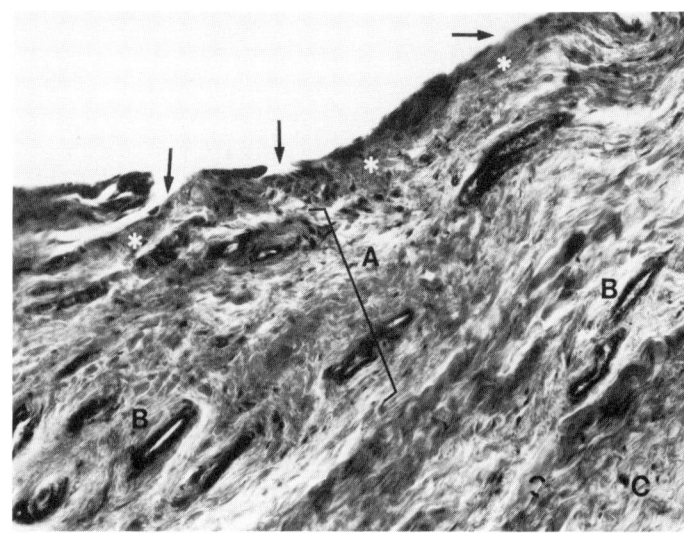

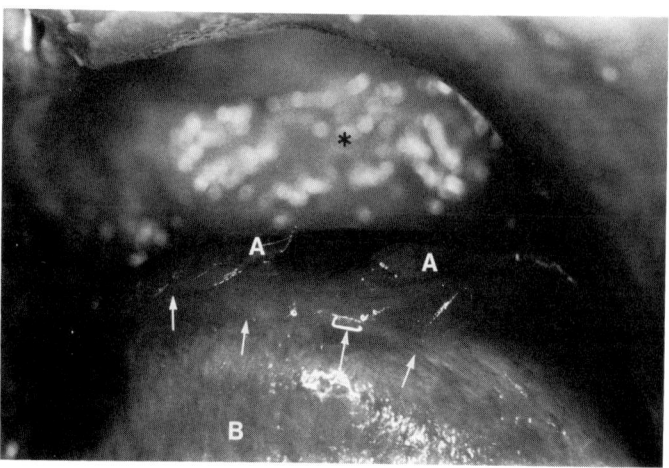

Figure 11–8. Anatomic specimen showing the transitional area (*arrows*) between the synovial membrane (A) in the opened posterior synovial pouch (*asterisk*) and the articular surface of the disc (B), at the intermediate space; frontal view.

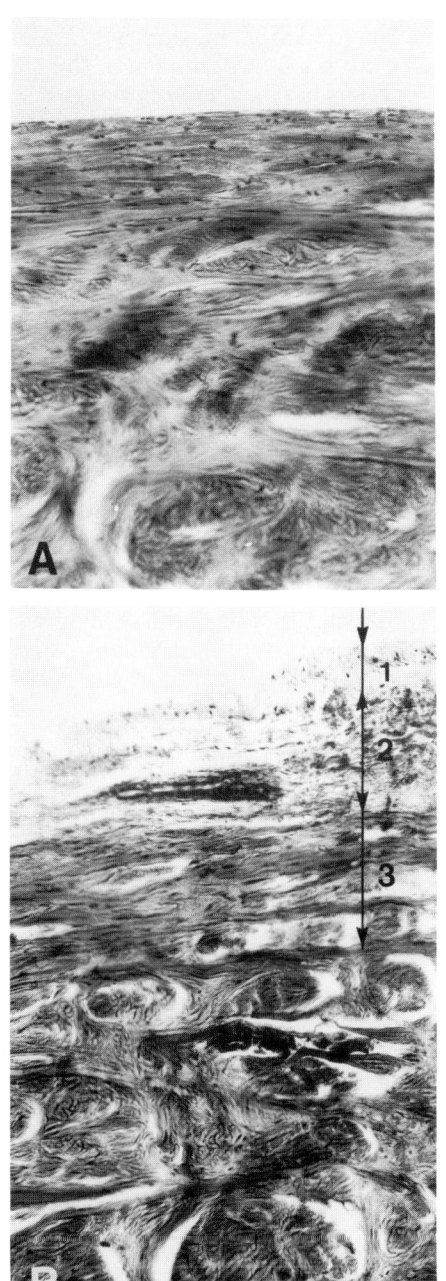
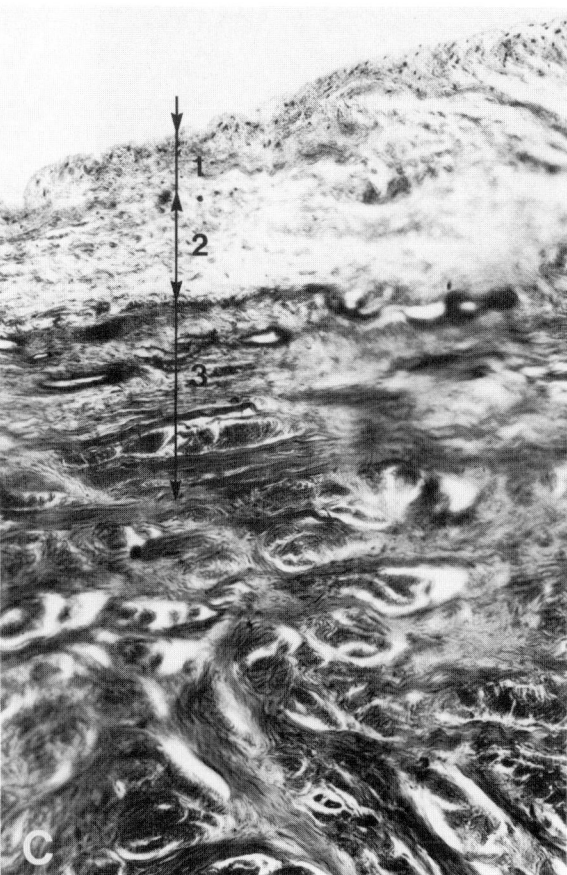

Figure 11–9. Photomicrographs of the transitional area between the synovial membrane and the disc surface. Anterior is to the reader's left. *A*, The articular disc surface consists of dense fibrous tissues with some scattered fibrocartilage cells. *B*, The synovial membrane (1) and subsynovial tissues (2) cover the surface of the disc (3). *C*, Toward the posterior portion, the subsynovial tissue contains thickened, short, fine collagen fibers with vascularity (2); the surface of the synovial membrane (1) shows wrinkles; and the fibrous tissues of the disc become loose (3). (Reprinted with permission from Murakami K, Hoshino K: Histological studies on the inner surfaces of the articular cavities of human temporomandibular joints with special reference to arthroscopic observations. Anat Anz 160:167–177, 1985.)

comes stretched, with disappearance of the accumulated synovial folds. In certain cases of chronic displacement, the posterior attachment appears similar to a "real disc"; the structure is avascular, whitish, and bright. This pseudo-disc, formed from remodeling of the retrodiscal tissue, has a softer appearance than the normal articular disc, and rupture or perforation of this tissue is occasionally encountered in the advanced pathology of internal derangement.

Intermediate Space

This intermediate space is located in the central articulating zone in the upper joint cavity. Through the arthroscope, the articular surface of the posterior slope of the articular

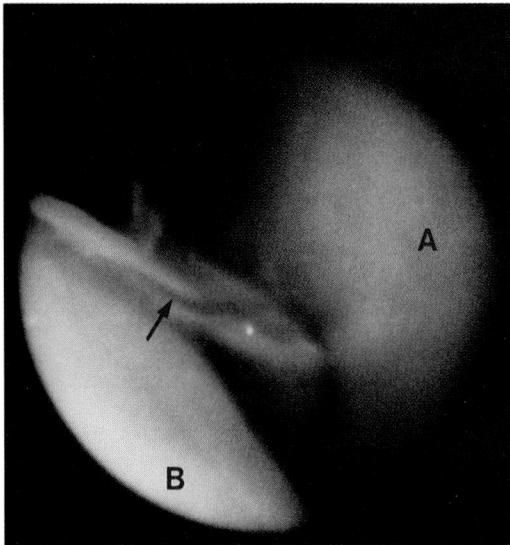

Figure 11–10. Arthroscopic photograph of the intermediate space in the right temporomandibular joint. A = articular surface of the posterior slope of the articular eminence; B = upper articular surface of the disc. Synovial plica protrudes into the space from the posterior synovial pouch (*arrow*).

formed by reflection of the synovial-lined capsule onto the superior edge of the articular disc (Fig. 11–12). The articular disc itself is loosely attached to the capsule but tightly attached to the mandibular condyle (Fig. 11–13), so that smooth anteroposterior translation of the normal disc is observed arthroscopically during jaw opening.

Histologically, the articular surface of the temporal component is essentially fibrocartilage and is composed of three layers. The connective tissue layer lines the superficial zone; the fibrocartilaginous layer is between the superficial connective tissue lining and the deepest layer, which is transitional to the bony tissues (Fig. 11–14).

The articular disc is essentially dense fibrous tissue containing scattered chondrocytes. In the intermediate portion of the articular disc, the collagen fibers run parallel to the anteroposterior axis of the disc; however, in certain circumstances, the fibrous bands may lose their direction and the articular disc itself becomes composed of looser connective tissue (Fig. 11–15).

eminence and the upper surface of the articular disc are not difficult to define (Fig. 11–10). The structures are close to each other, and their surfaces appear whitish, smooth, shiny, and avascular (Fig. 11–11). The whitish upper surface of the articular disc slides forward during jaw opening. In the most medial and lateral portions of the upper joint cavity, the synovial grooves (sulci) are

Early articular degenerative change in the TMJ observed via arthroscopy is well recognized as being secondary to fibrillation on the articular cartilage, particularly on the posterior slope of the articular eminence. Severe arthrotic change is defined as destruction of the smooth articular surface or exposure of the subchondral bone. Perforation of the articular disc is found in some cases of severe arthrosis.

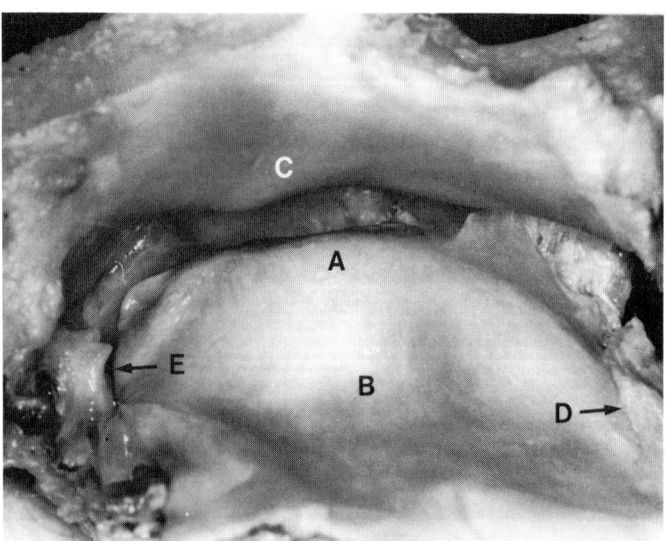

Figure 11–11. Superior surface of the disc in the left upper joint cavity viewed from the front. A = discal eminence; B = flat portion of the disc; C = eminence; D = lateral paradiscal groove; E = medial paradiscal groove.

11 Arthroscopic Anatomy, Histology, and Visual Fields in the Temporomandibular Joint ■ 147

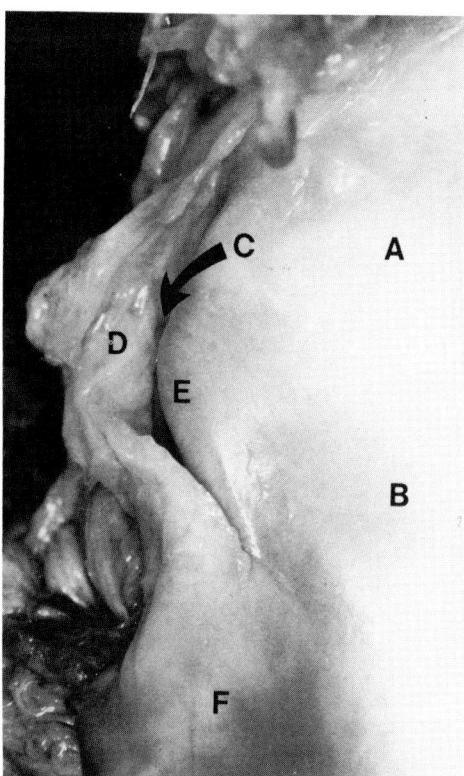

Figure 11–12. Lateral paradiscal groove viewed from above. A = discal eminence; B = flat portion of the disc; C = groove; D = synovial membrane lining lateral capsule; E = disc, which is tightly attached to lateral condylar pole; F = synovial membrane of anterior synovial recess.

Upper Anterior Synovial Recess

The lower prominence of the articular eminence and the synovial membrane anteromedial to it, partly lined by the inner wall of the capsule, are the visual anatomic landmarks of this area (Fig. 11–16). Occasionally, the pterygoid shadow (the texture of the fibers of the lateral pterygoid muscle) is detected through the synovial membrane. The articular eminence and synovial membrane adjacent to the anterior aspect of the articular disc closely oppose each other (Fig. 11–17). When the jaw opens, this recess enlarges sec-

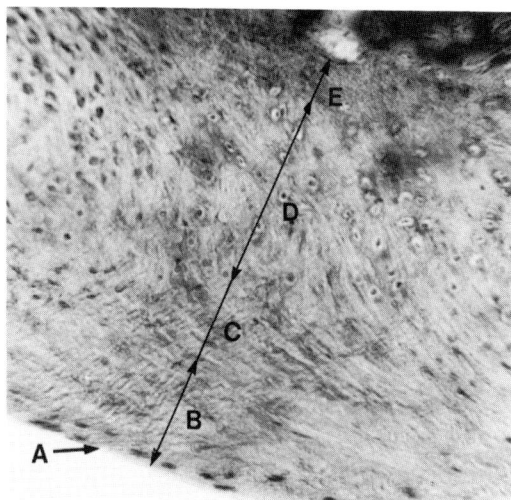

Figure 11–14. Photomicrograph of surface cartilage on the articular eminence. A = surface connective tissue covering; B = superficial lamina (proliferative zone) with collagen fibers parallel to the surface; C = intermediate lamina (transitional zone); D = deep lamina (cartilage); E = deepest layer, transitional to the bone. (Reprinted with permission from Murakami K, Hoshino K: Histological studies on the inner surfaces of the articular cavities of human temporomandibular joints with special reference to arthroscopic observations. Anat Anz 160:167–177, 1985.)

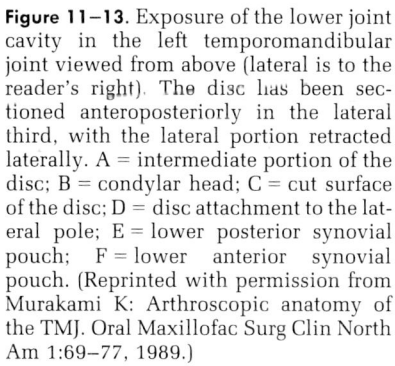

Figure 11–13. Exposure of the lower joint cavity in the left temporomandibular joint viewed from above (lateral is to the reader's right). The disc has been sectioned anteroposteriorly in the lateral third, with the lateral portion retracted laterally. A = intermediate portion of the disc; B = condylar head; C = cut surface of the disc; D = disc attachment to the lateral pole; E = lower posterior synovial pouch; F = lower anterior synovial pouch. (Reprinted with permission from Murakami K: Arthroscopic anatomy of the TMJ. Oral Maxillofac Surg Clin North Am 1:69–77, 1989.)

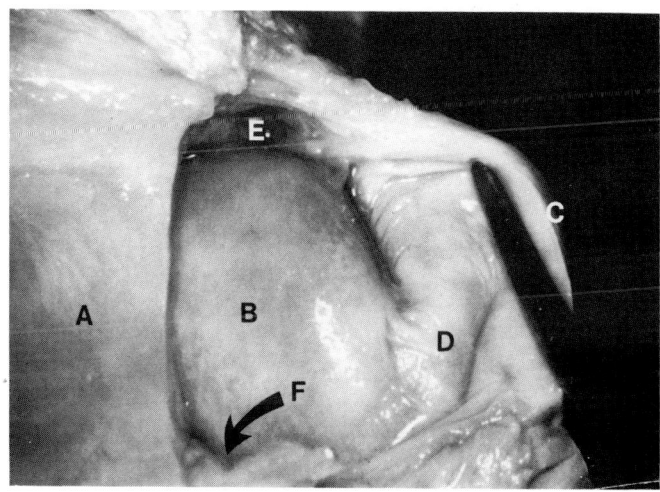

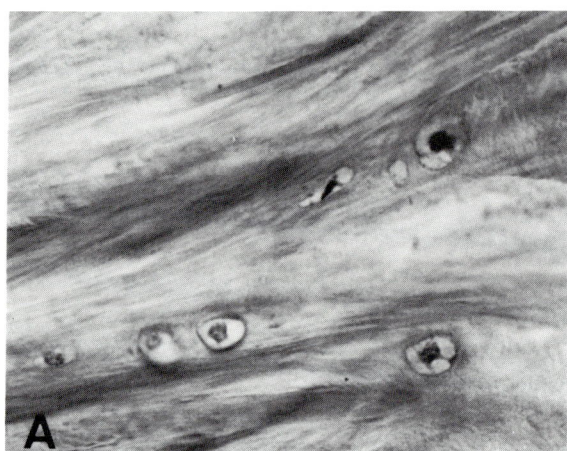
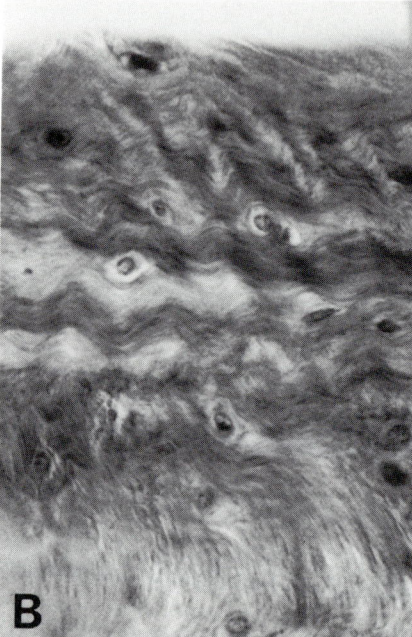

Figure 11–15. Photomicrograph of the articular disc. In the densely packed intermediate portion of the disc (*A*), single or paired spherical chondrocytes are scattered. In the posterior band of the disc (*B*), collagen fibers are wavy and loosely packed. Chondrocytes also can be seen in the interstitial tissue.

ondary to the anterior translation of the disc (see Fig. 11–2*B*).

Inflammatory responses of synovial congestion, hyperemia, and synovitis can be observed in this recess. In acute anterior disc displacement, this compartment increases in volume and, via the relative narrower intermediate space, an expanded anterior recess develops and can be recognized. In contrast, in patients with persistent closed locked disorders and arthrosis, mild to severe fibrous adhesions are detected in this recess; as a result, the compartment volume is significantly smaller.

Visual Fields in the Upper Joint Cavity

By lateral puncture, using an inferolateral approach and aiming the arthroscopic trocar toward the posterior slope of the articular eminence, the posterior synovial pouch is the first compartment to be seen. Following appropriate intra-articular manipulation of the arthroscope, the anterior synovial recess and the intermediate space can be seen (Fig. 11–18). It is difficult to see the medial paradiscal sulcus and lateral aspect of the joint cavity. Occasionally, when using this approach, the anterior slope of the articular eminence is also out of the visual field. The anterolateral puncture, aiming the tip of the trocar toward the anterior slope of the articular eminence, increases the possibility of observing the anterior slope of the eminence and part of the medial sulcus. To visualize

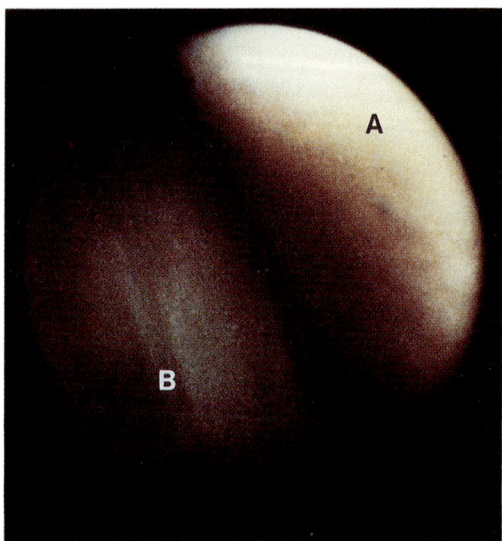

Figure 11–16. Arthroscopic photograph of the left upper anterior synovial recess (left is anterior). A = eminence; B = synovial membrane lining the anteromedial capsule. Fibers of the lateral pterygoid muscle can be seen through the membrane.

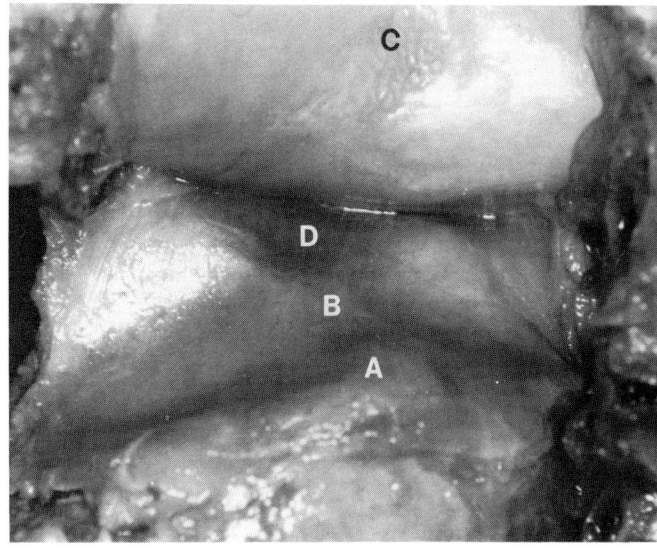

Figure 11–17. Left upper anterior synovial recess opened from behind (right is medial). A = discal eminence; B = discal flat portion; C = eminence; D = synovium. (Reprinted with permission from Murakami K: Arthroscopic anatomy. *In* Sanders B, Murakami K, Clark G (eds): Diagnostic and Surgical Arthroscopy of the Temporomandibular Joint. Philadelphia: WB Saunders, 1989.)

the lateral part of the joint compartments as well as the lateral sulcus, the endaural portal must be used.

Lower Joint Cavity

The lower joint cavity is very narrow in comparison to the upper joint cavity. As in the upper joint cavity, the anterior and posterior synovial pouches are identifiable, separated by the intermediate space between the condyle and disc (see Fig. 11–3). The arthroscopic and regional anatomy of this joint cavity has been described; the clinical significance of lower joint compartment arthroscopy has not been established.

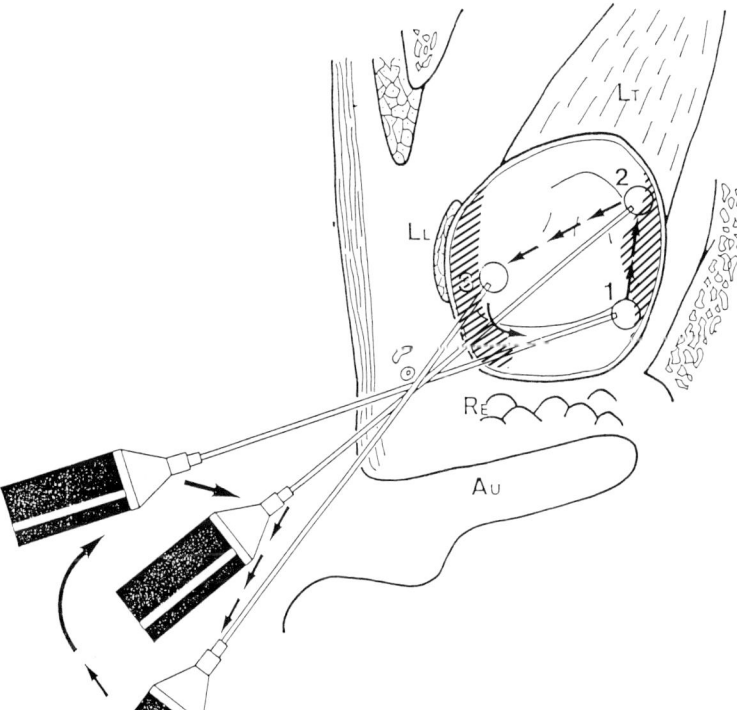

Figure 11–18. Schematic visual field of the upper joint cavity by inferolateral puncture viewed from above. Shadow images indicate areas difficult to observe. Systematic arthroscopic observation begins at the posterior synovial pouch (1), proceeds to the anterior synovial recess (2), and returns to the intermediate portion (3) toward the posterior. Au = auditory canal; Re = retrodiscal pad; Ll = lateral ligament; Lt = lateral pterygoid muscle.

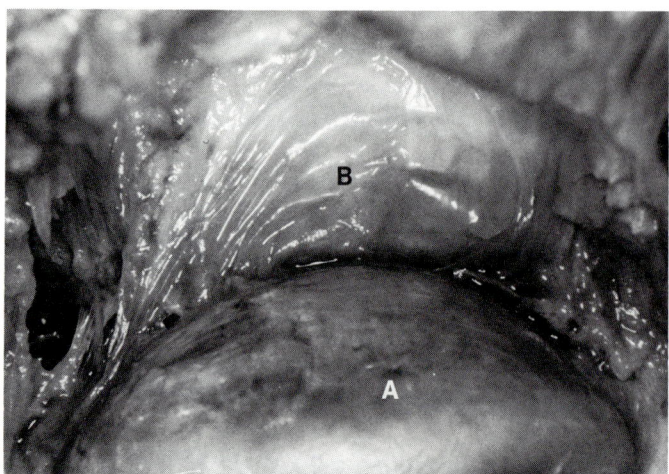

Figure 11-19. Right lower posterior synovial pouch opened from the front (right is medial). A = posterior condylar surface; B = synovial membrane attached deeply on the condyle, with numerous folds on its surface. (Reprinted with permission from Murakami K, Hoshino K: Regional anatomic nomenclature and arthroscopic terminology in human temporomandibular joints. Okajimas Folia Anat 58:745-760, 1982.).

Lower Posterior Synovial Pouch

The lower posterior synovial pouch is larger than the lower anterior synovial pouch. The posterior surface of the mandibular condyle is broadly facing the synovial membrane (Fig. 11-19). In the deepest portion of this pouch, the posterior surface of the condyle and the synovial membrane covering the retrodiscal pad interface closely. The synovial membrane of the posterior portion of the pouch appears more vascular because of the blood vessels in the retrodiscal pad deep to the synovial lining. The retrodiscal pad is a cushion for the condyle (see Fig. 11-2). Actually, the retrodiscal pad expands in the mandibular fossa with condylar translation, secondary to extreme venous pooling in the retrodiscal tissues (see Fig. 11-2B). Arthroscopically, the synovial membrane in this area appears softer and more cushion-like (Fig. 11-20), reflecting the contour of the underlying retrodiscal pad. Viewed from this synovial pouch, the intermediate space between the condyle and the undersurface of the disc is visible anteriorly (Fig. 11-21).

The retrodiscal pad is simply loose areolar tissue composed of connective and adipose tissues, abundant arteries, and venous plexus (Fig. 11-22).

Lower Anterior Synovial Pouch

The lower anterior synovial pouch consists of the mandibular condyle and the lower anterior undersurface of the articular disc (Fig. 11-23 and 11-24). This compartment has the least space in the TMJ. The synovial membrane is observed in the lower anterior aspect of this pouch (Fig. 11-25). The synovial reflection upward toward the undersurface of the articular disc from the floor of this pouch is similar to that in the upper posterior synovial pouch; however, the surface of the synovial membrane appears less flexible than in the other synovial pouches. The synovial membrane that lines this pouch is also identifiable histologically (Fig. 11-26), but

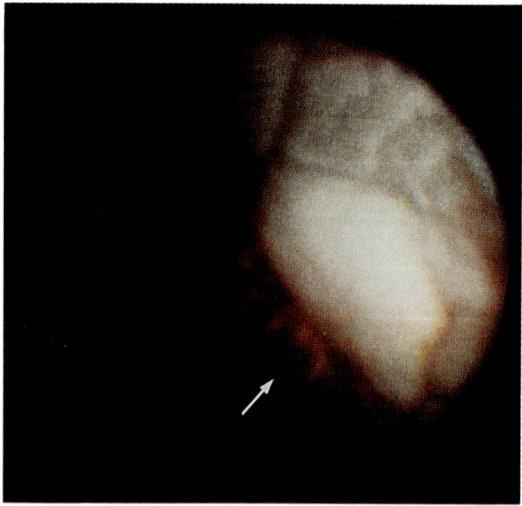

Figure 11-20. Arthroscopic photograph of synovial membrane in the left lower posterior synovial pouch (right is posterior). The cushion-like appearance of the synovial folds is defined and capillaries are noted (arrows). (Reprinted with permission from Murakami K: Arthroscopic anatomy. In Sanders B, Murakami K, Clark G (eds): Diagnostic and Surgical Arthroscopy of the Temporomandibular Joint. Philadelphia: WB Saunders, 1989.)

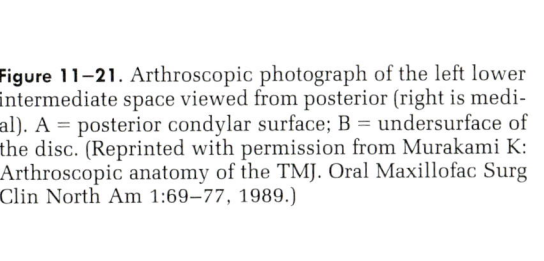

Figure 11–21. Arthroscopic photograph of the left lower intermediate space viewed from posterior (right is medial). A = posterior condylar surface; B = undersurface of the disc. (Reprinted with permission from Murakami K: Arthroscopic anatomy of the TMJ. Oral Maxillofac Surg Clin North Am 1:69–77, 1989.)

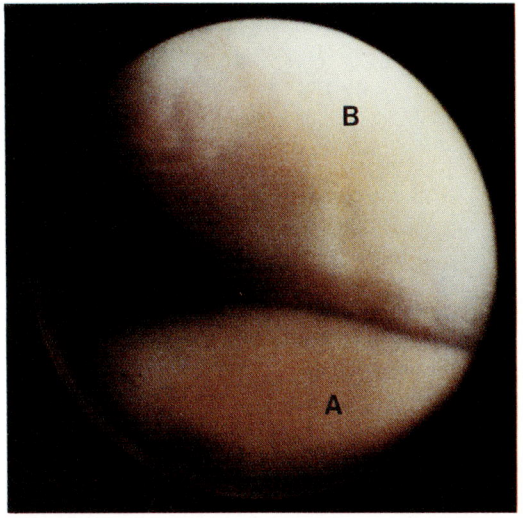

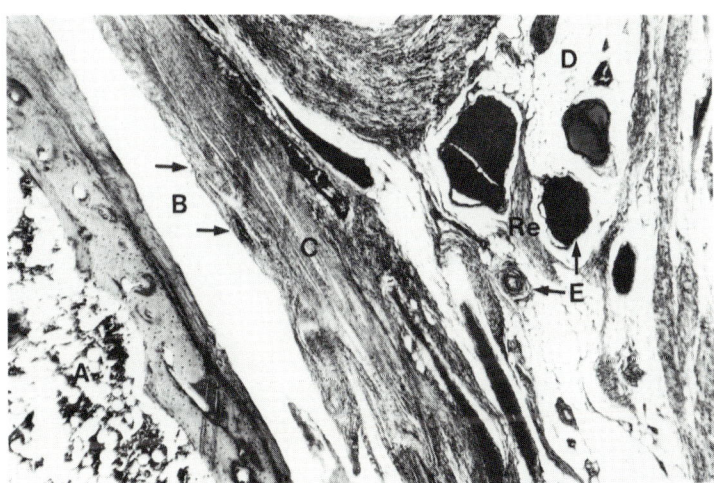

Figure 11–22. Photomicrograph of a sagittal section of the retrodiscal tissue and the posterior surface of the condyle. A = condylar head; B = synovial lining; C = connective tissue bundles intervening between the synovial membrane and the retrodiscal pad (Re). This pad is composed of adipose tissue (D) and venous plexus and small arteries (arrows, E) in the loose interstitial fibrous tissue. (Reprinted with permission from Murakami K, Hoshino K: Histological studies on the inner surfaces of the articular cavities of human temporomandibular joints with special reference to arthroscopic observations. Anat Anz 160:167–177, 1985.)

Figure 11–23. Sagittal sectional anatomy of the left temporomandibular joint, anterior portion. 1 = upper anterior synovial recess; 2 = lower anterior synovial pouch; A = articular eminence; B = disc; C = condyle; D = synovial plica. (Reprinted with permission from Murakami K: Arthroscopic anatomy. In Sanders B, Murakami K, Clark G (eds): Diagnostic and Surgical Arthroscopy of the Temporomandibular Joint. Philadelphia: WB Saunders, 1989.)

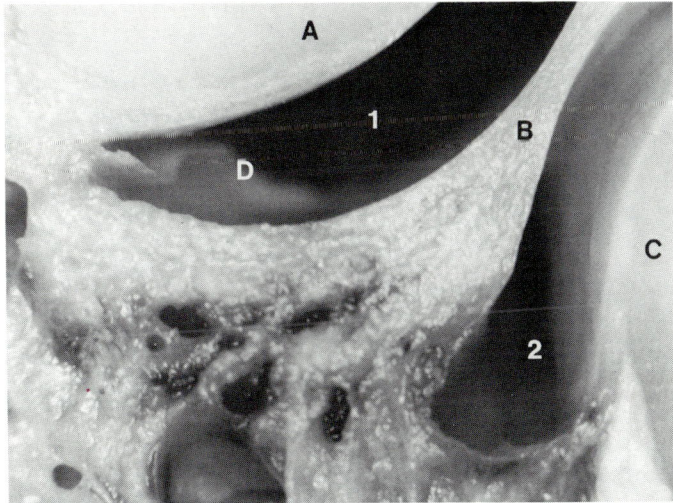

152 ■ 11 Arthroscopic Anatomy, Histology, and Visual Fields in the Temporomandibular Joint

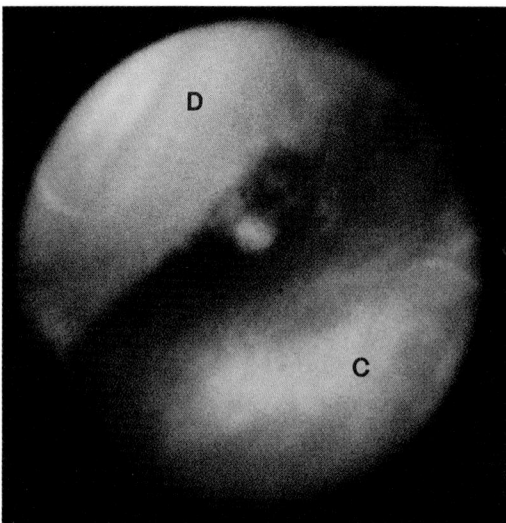

Figure 11–24. Arthroscopic photograph of the left lower anterior synovial pouch (left is anterior). Dissection showed disc displacement. C = condyle; D = disc undersurface. (Reprinted with permission from Murakami K: Arthroscopic anatomy. *In* Sanders B, Murakami K, Clark G (eds): Diagnostic and Surgical Arthroscopy of the Temporomandibular Joint. Philadelphia: WB Saunders, 1989.)

Figure 11–25. Synovial lining (*arrow*) in the lower anterior synovial pouch. Anterior portion of the disc, interwoven with the sphenodiscal portion of the lateral pterygoid muscle, is retracted upward, having been released from the anterior aspect of the condyle. A = anterior aspect of the condyle; B = undersurface of the disc (discal fossa); C = sphenodiscal portion of the lateral pterygoid muscle.

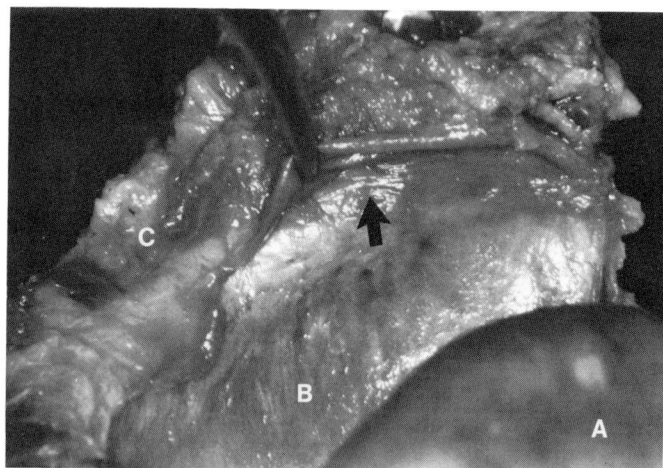

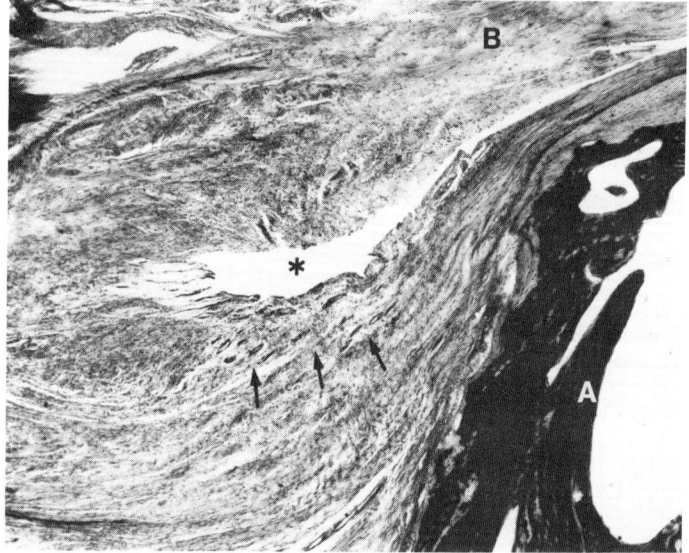

Figure 11–26. Histology of a sagittal section of the lower anterior synovial pouch (*asterisk*). The surface of the pouch is lined by thin synovial membrane covering subsynovial tissue that contains capillaries (*arrows*). A = mandibular condyle; B = articular disc. (Reprinted with permission from Murakami K: Arthroscopic anatomy. *In* Sanders B, Murakami K, Clark G (eds): Diagnostic and Surgical Arthroscopy of the Temporomandibular Joint. Philadelphia: WB Saunders, 1989.)

one observes less vascularity in the synovial membrane as well as in the subsynovial tissues.

The lower anterior synovial recess can be detected anatomically where it separates the two portions of the lateral pterygoid muscle. The floor of this recess is observed on the lower portion of the lateral pterygoid muscle, which is attached to the pterygoid fovea on the anterior aspect of the condylar neck. Some fibers of the upper portion of the lateral pterygoid muscle are interwoven into the anterior aspect of the articular disc.

ACKNOWLEDGMENT

Anatomic illustrations in this chapter were carried out primarily in the Department of Anatomy at the Kyoto University Faculty of Medicine, in collaboration with Dr. Kazumasa Hoshino.

Suggested Reading

Heffez L, Blaustein D: Diagnostic arthroscopy of the temporomandibular joint. Part I: Normal arthroscopic findings. Oral Surg 64:653–670, 1987.

Holmlund A, Hellsing G: Arthroscopy of the temporomandibular joint. An autopsy study. Int J Oral Surg 14:169–175, 1985.

Liedberg J, Westesson P-L: Diagnostic accuracy of upper compartment arthroscopy of the temporomandibular joint: Correlation with postmortem morphology. Oral Surg 62:618–624, 1988.

Moses JJ, Poker ID: Temporomandibular joint arthroscopy: The endaural approach. Int J Oral Maxillofac Surg 18: 347–351, 1989.

Murakami K, Hoshino K: Regional anatomic nomenclature and arthroscopic terminology in human temporomandibular joints. Okajimas Folia Anat 58:745–760, 1982.

Murakami K, Hoshino K: Histological studies on the inner surface of the articular cavities of human temporomandibular joints with special reference to arthroscopic observations. Anat Anz 160:167–177, 1985.

Murakami K, Ito K: Arthroscopy of the temporomandibular joint. *In* Watanabe M (ed): Arthroscopy of Small Joints. Tokyo: Igaku-Shoin, 1985, pp 128–139.

Westesson P-L, Eriksson L, Liedberg J: The risk of damage to facial nerve, superficial temporal vessels, disc and articular surfaces during arthroscopic examination of the temporomandibular joint. Oral Surg 62:124–127, 1986.

Chapter 12

DIAGNOSTIC AND OPERATIVE ARTHROSCOPY OF THE TEMPOROMANDIBULAR JOINT

A. Operating Room Protocol

MOHAN THOMAS, D.D.S., F.A.C.D.

Temporomandibular joint (TMJ) arthroscopy is usually done on an outpatient basis in an arthroscopic facility in a hospital setting, with the patient under general anesthesia via a nasoendotracheal intubation. A large, special facility is recommended for TMJ surgery because arthroscopic procedures are very equipment-dependent, and the surgeon and supporting staff need room to maneuver while concentrating on performing intricate maneuvers in the small, restricted space of the TMJ. It is essential that the surgeon have complete freedom in this environment and that the surgical team be well trained in the latest arthroscopic methods. It is best when members of the arthroscopy team work together frequently, which will enable them to achieve better results.[1]

The surgeon should assume a leadership role in creating the proper operating room (OR) environment, in order to maximize skills, while ensuring proper patient care.[1] The arthroscopic surgical team should be formed on a volunteer basis, with input and consultations from experienced arthroscopists.

A good relationship between the surgeon and the patient is essential. The surgeon must discuss the possibility of the necessity of an open joint procedure with the patient prior to surgery.[1]

To perform arthroscopic surgery requires great skill and patience.[1] Surgeons should always operate at a level slightly below their ability, such that if unforeseen complications arise they will be able to handle them. The primary goal of the surgeon should be the care, comfort, and treatment of the patient.

Every patient should be given preoperative and postoperative verbal and written instructions that discuss medications, wound care, dressing changes, expectations from the procedure, anticipated follow-up visits, and physical therapy (see Appendix).[1] During the postoperative follow-up visits, the surgeon should elicit patient feedback.

The demeanor and attitude of supporting hospital personnel are also important. A professional demeanor and attitude should always be maintained by support personnel as well as the surgical team.

In regard to the arthroscopic equipment, it should always be handled with utmost care.[1]

All members of the surgical team must know how to use the arthroscopic equipment and how to correct any problem that may arise during its use. This ability is important, in order to ensure smooth diagnostic and surgical procedures.

The patient, under general anesthesia via nasoendotracheal intubation, is prepared and draped in the usual manner as for a TMJ arthrotomy procedure. The patient's mouth is covered with a plastic drape so that the assistant surgeon may place the thumb intraorally or employ one of the devices used in the manipulation of the mandible (see Chapter 12 B for illustration of mandible manipulator), in order not to contaminate the surgical field by entering the oral cavity.[2]

The surgeon usually stands opposite the side of the TMJ to be operated on. The anesthesiologist should be positioned well off to the side of the surgical table in order that the surgeon and assistant surgeon may have access to operate and exchange positions during right and left TMJ arthroscopies. It is essential that the surgeon, assistant surgeon, and scrub nurse have a direct view of the TV monitor (Fig. 12-1). The arthroscope and video cassette recorder (VCR) camera should be at the head of the table in a sterile draped basin within the surgeon's reach. The placement of all necessary surgical instruments must allow for proper positioning of cables, electrical cords, suction tubing, and anesthesia circuit tubing, all of which have to be positioned exactly for ease of use. A diagram of the proper positions for the equipment cabinet, anesthesia machine, light source, back table, and Mayo stand is provided in the appendix of this text.

SUGGESTIONS FOR SETUP OF MAYO STAND AND BACK TABLE
MAYO STAND

- 10-cc Aspirating syringe—local anesthetic with vasoconstrictor
- 10-cc Aspirating syringe—fluid for joint distension (e.g., lactated Ringer's, normal saline)
- Inflow cannulas
- Trochars and obturators: sharp, pyramidal, and blunt
- Outflow cannulas
- 15-gauge, 1½-inch needles
- 18-gauge spinal needle
- 1.7-mm 0-degree arthroscope
- 2.7-mm 30-degree arthroscope
- Outflow tubing (IV extension tube)
- Inflow tubing (IV extension tube)

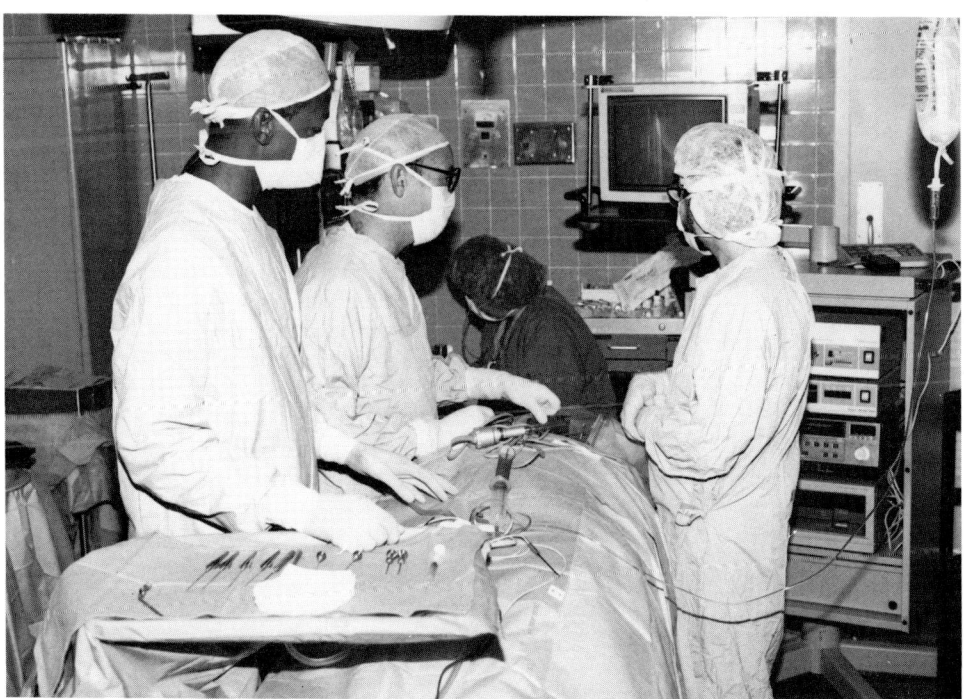

Figure 12-1. Operating room setup. (Courtesy of Dr. Michael Koslin.)

- Marking pen
- 20-cc Syringe for joint lavage and irrigation

HEAD OF THE TABLE

- Basin—light cable, video camera
- Light source
- Cabinet
  High resolution video monitor
  Video tape recorder
  Video camera control unit
  Color video printer (Sony UP-5000/UP-5000W)

SUGGESTIONS FOR TMJ ARTHROSCOPY—MEDICATIONS, INSTRUMENTS, AND SUPPLIES

Medications

- Cefazolin (Ancef) 1 gm IV or equivalent
- Methylprednisolone (Solu-Medrol) 125 mg IV
- Droperidol IV, 1.25–2.5 mg, 15 minutes before end of case
- Betamethasone 5 ml in 10 cc syringe with B-D #5181 spinal needle, 22-gauge, 3½-inch long (Becton Dickinson & Co., Franklin Lakes, NJ)
- Viscoelastic solution—2 doses

Instruments and Supplies

- Arthroscope—2.7 mm
- 2 Cannulas—2.9 mm
- Sharp trochar
- Blunt obturator
- Video camera
- VCR
- Monitor
- Light source and cable
- Electrocautery with Concept, Inc., #8321 straight electrode and #8322 90-degree hook electrode (Concept, Inc., 11311 Concept Blvd., Largo, FL 34643)
- Electrocautery machine (Valley Lab)
- ASP Irrigation System #900-001 (Apple Medical Corp., 93 Nashaway Rd., Bolton, MA 01740)
- Dyonics small joint shaving system
- Dyonics 2.9-mm turbowhisker blade
- 2 Angiocath needles—16-gauge, 2-inch (Desert Medical)
- 2 Ethicon J-869 2-0 Vicryl sutures with CP-2 cutting needles
- 2 Ethicon 682 5-0 silk sutures with FS-2 cutting needles
- Large scissors with 2-inch blades
- Dean angular scissors—5-inch
- 2 Curved mosquito hemostats
- Suture needle holder—6-inch
- Dyonics golden magnetic retriever
- Magnetic retriever with suction—3.0-mm (Acufex #011503, Acufex Microsurgical, Inc., Norwood, MA)
- Dyonics small, hooked probe
- Metal 6-inch ruler with mm scale
- Sterile marking pen
- Extension tubing
- IV bag tubing set (cut off bulbous end and remove stop wheel)
- 4 Towel clamps
- Dyonics suction punch instrument
- McCain serrated biopsy forceps (#01-6640, Walter Lorenz Surgical Instruments, Inc., Jacksonville, FL 32218)
- McCain arthroscopic scissors, blunt (#01-6662, Walter Lorenz Surgical Instruments, Inc., Jacksonville, FL 32218)
- Adson forceps
- 10-cc control syringe with 10-ml 2% lidocaine (Xylocaine) with 1:100,000 epinephrine
- Package of 5 peanut dissectors
- Mineral oil in medicine glass or cup
- 6 Towels
- 2 Packages of 4" × 4" sponges
- 8 2" × 2" Sponges
- Bacitracin ointment
- Razor with blade
- Plastic tape—1-inch and 2-inch
- 2 Steri-Drapes with 2" × 3" oval opening (#1030)
- 2 2-Hour Super VHS video tapes
- Bilateral TMJ arthroscopy drape (#3983 Microtek Medical Inc., Columbus, MS 39704) (Fig. 12–2).

References

1. Johnson LL: Arthroscopic Surgery: Principles and Practice, 3rd Ed. St. Louis, CV Mosby, 1986, pp 138–143.
2. Sanders B, Murakami K-I, Clark GT: Diagnostic and Surgical Arthroscopy of the Temporomandibular Joint. Philadelphia, WB Saunders, 1989, pp 39, 44–46.

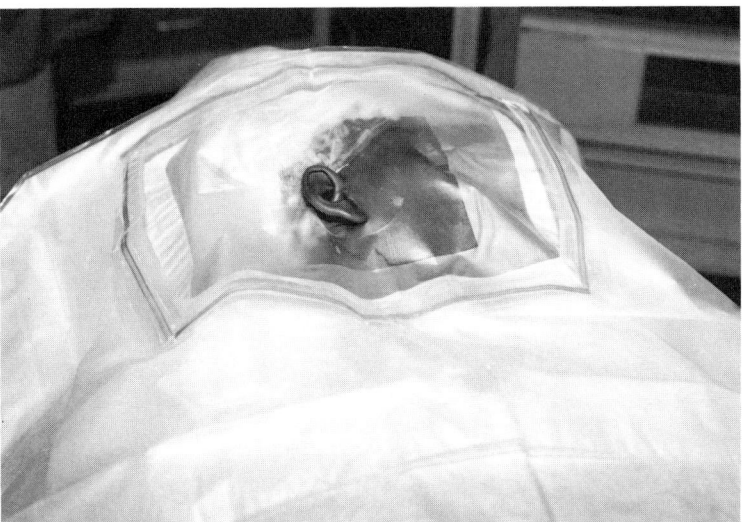

Figure 12–2. The temporomandibular drape. (Courtesy of Dr. Michael Koslin.)

B. Instrumentation (Optical and Surgical)

MOHAN THOMAS, D.D.S., F.A.C.D.
CHRISTOPHER LANE, D.D.S.

The development of the arthroscope began in the 1970s by Casscells, Jackson, and Abe who introduced diagnostic arthroscopy to North America. Following these pioneers, O'Connor in 1974 employing his own design, performed partial menisectomies with an operative arthroscope. Subsequently, motorized instrumentation was introduced by Lanny Johnson.

The arthroscope is a cylinder that conducts light and transmits an image back to the eye. The concept of arthroscopy is simplistic in nature. During arthroscopy, one is actually photographing the joint. The camera is the scope, and the object photographed is within the joint space. A more in-depth discussion of the arthroscope proper is presented in Chapter 3.

The telescopic systems of arthroscopy fall into three categories: traditional lens systems, self-scope lens systems, and rods-lens systems. Rigid endoscopy is exemplified by the traditional lens systems and the rods-lens systems. The self-scope lens systems are somewhere between rigid endoscopy and fiberoptic endoscopy.[1]

In the rods-lens systems, there is a series of glass cylinders separated by smaller areas of air. This is the opposite of a thin-lens system. Conventional lens systems are characterized by a series of thin lenses divided by cylinders of air that transmit light toward the arthroscopist's eye.

Modern arthroscopes contain a variety of diameter sizes, such as the Storz rods-lens arthroscopes available in 1.7-mm and 2.2-mm diameters, capable of providing optical clarity. In the Dyonics rods-lens endoscope, the diameters available are 1.7 and 2.2 mm. Larger diameter arthroscopes are recommended for operative procedures (Fig. 12–3).[1,2]

The field of view is either perceived or actual. In the apparent or perceived view, the diameter of the image is visualized at the ocular end of the arthroscope. The actual field of view is the measured angle of view that is seen arthroscopically. The images

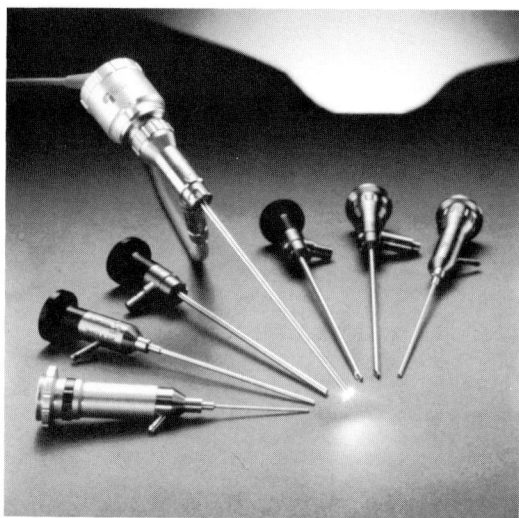

Figure 12-3. Arthroscopes and videoscopes. (Courtesy of Smith and Nephew Dyonics, Inc.)

seen on the TV screen can affect the apparent view, when coupled with the arthroscope. Varied sizes of images are related to the size and placement of the lens.

The angle of inclination equals the angle of projection at the objective end of the arthroscope. The angle of incline can be either straight or angled. The most common angles of inclination in operative arthroscopy are 30, 70, 90, and 120 degrees. The 30-degree angle of inclination is utilized most often for the surgical approach of arthroscopy. When using the more upright angles, orientation is more difficult to obtain. The 70-degree angle of inclination is selected commonly for posterior viewing via the transcondylar approach.[2]

SURGICAL INSTRUMENTATION AND APPLICATIONS

Hand Instrumentation

Probe. The probe is considered to be the "extension of the arthroscopist's fingers." The probe is a dull right angle hook, used both diagnostically and operatively in arthroscopy. It is the safest instrument in triangulation techniques. The instrument may be employed for probing perforations, determining the extent and depth of tears, as well as evaluating the consistency of both the retrodiscal tissue and the articular disc.

The probe can be utilized in a diagnostic fashion to ascertain the attachment of articular cartilage to subchondral bone and to determine the presence of chondromalacia and adhesions. If the size of the probe is known, one is able to estimate the extent of the lesion.[2]

Spinal Needles. The spinal needle can be inserted as an outflow portal for diagnostic arthroscopy and can be used for subsynovial placement of steroids under arthroscopic control. Spinal needles can be effective for placement of traction sutures through the disc in relocation procedures. These needles can direct placement of operative portals and determine accessibility of various instruments in diseased areas. The needles are available in 3- to 6-inch lengths. The 18-gauge needle is able to be manipulated without bending.

Switching Sticks. Switching sticks are 9.0-inch rods with a diameter of 2.0 mm. They maintain the position in the arthroscopic portals so that wider layer cannulas can be exchanged without reintroducing trocars or obturators. K-wire can be used in the same fashion.

Knives. The retrograde knife combines a probe's shape with a sharp blade angled at 90 degrees. It can be used to shave redundant tissue and remodeled retrodiscal tissue. The retrograde knife is especially helpful in inaccessible areas. It may be useful for anterior release of the disc as described by McCain. This particular knife must be utilized carefully in a sawing fashion to avoid indiscriminate removal of adjacent tissue.

The banana knife is slightly curved and has a smooth or serrated blade with pointed tips and sharp edges. It is used predominantly to contour the disc or to excise the area of grade III chondromalacia.

The angled knife possesses a V-shaped cutting edge, which angles downward 45 to 90 degrees, and may be used to lyse adhesions and areas of chondromalacia. Care should be taken not to injure articular surfaces with this type of knife.[1,2]

Ring Curettes. The ring curette is a circular instrument, sharp on both inclined sides, that allows debridement of articular surfaces. The curette is mainly used in grade III and IV chondromalacia. It should be utilized carefully so as to prevent damage to the articular cartilage. The best application of the ring curette is in a light, sweeping motion. This motion enables the curette to sever the loose cartilaginous fragments and to smooth the articular surfaces.[1,2]

Forceps and Suction Punch. The forceps and suction punch are available in a variety of sizes and shapes. The forceps are upbiting or downbiting, with either blunt-nosed or flat tips. The forceps can be curved, flat, or angled 45 to 90 degrees to the right or left. The forceps are chosen primarily to excise any type of soft tissue, such as synovium, disc, or scar tissue.

The biopsy (grasping) forceps obtain tissue samples. The basket forceps are very helpful in contouring the free edges of perforations and are available in several sizes.

The Dyonics suction punch or punch forceps, a debriding instrument, is available in both 2.5 and 3.4 mm sizes. The suction punch is similar to the basket forceps in that it has a grasping forceps with a cutting edge. The punch attaches to the suction device, whereby it removes resected accumulated soft tissue from the joint and collects it in a trap. The collected tissue can then be submitted for pathologic examination to substantiate clinical disease. This debriding instrument is recommended only for use under arthroscopic control. The practitioner should watch the video screen when working with this instrument. The suction punch is excellent for the management of intra-articular pathology and managing degenerative joint diseases, such as rheumatoid arthritis, chondromalacia, and other arthropathies (Fig. 12–4).[1,2]

Scissors. Scissors are used to cut tissue that has been pinched under tension. Three basic blade types are available: hook, plain, and serrated. Although some blades are straight and angled 20 degrees to the right or left, others are curved to the right or left 60 degrees. Scissors are employed to cut synovial plicas and to cut the edge of perforations. The disc can be released anteriorly utilizing the scissors as described by McCain. When beginning the cut at the free edge, it is important to place the closed scissors under and parallel to the free edge of the disc. The scissors should be opened and rotated 45 degrees so that the cutting surfaces are above and below the free disc edge. The angle of the cut can be better controlled utilizing this method.

Bone File. The bone file is a straight instrument with a single cut tip and straight teeth

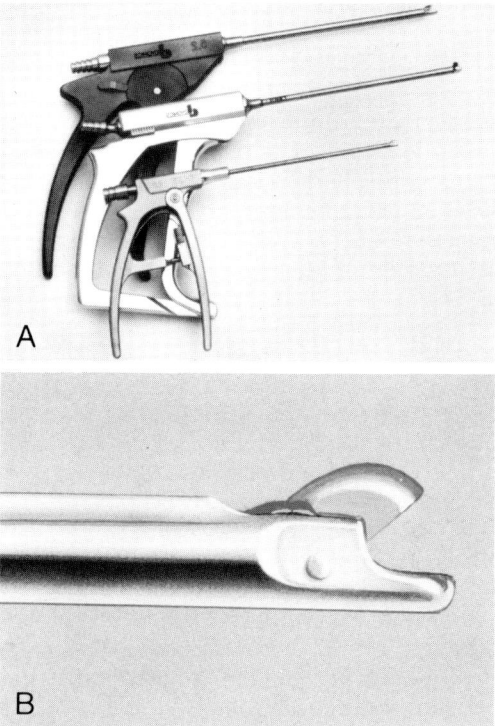

Figure 12–4. *A,* Suction punches. *B,* Closeup of a suction punch end. (Courtesy of Smith and Nephew Dyonics, Inc.)

on one side. It is used to smooth articular surfaces in grades III and IV chondromalacia that are inaccessible to the shaver and to loosen cartilaginous fragments on the articular surfaces. Initially, large fragments can be trimmed with a curette and, afterwards, smoothed with the bone file.[1,2]

First Assistant. The first assistant, available from Leonard Medical, is a pliable tension arm that is attached to the side of the operating table, while the other end holds the arthroscope in place. This provides an extra secure "arm" in operative arthroscopy, thereby reducing operator fatigue and increasing productivity. The first assistant is infinitely adjustable, instantly lockable, vacuum powered, and steam autoclaved. The tension arm may be adjusted to carry additional weight, such as video cameras.[1]

Golden Retrievers. The golden retriever is a rod about 2.0 mm in diameter, which can be introduced through the cannula to apply magnetic force to remove metal fragments from joints arthroscopically. These rods can also retrieve instruments should they break in the joint space.[2]

Motorized Instruments

Cartilage Shaver. The cartilage shaver is a hollow fenestrated tube utilizing a rotating two-edged cylindric blade that spins within the hollow tube. The blade, driven by a motor, is controlled by a foot pedal. Adequate motor power and close tolerance between the inner two-edged blades and the outer tube are important for proper function of the shaver. The shaver is most commonly applied in local or general synovectomy and in removal of scuffed articular cartilage and meniscal fragments or multiple cartilaginous loose bodies. Several configurations of cartilage shavers are available: end cutting, safe-sided, turbo, whisker, and abrader (Fig. 12–5).[1,2]

Other Instruments

Mandible Manipulator. The mandible manipulator, available from Leonard Medical, is a hand-held device that is custom-fitted to the mandible. The device functions to simulate jaw movements and distracts the jaws, which allows increased intra-articular space for operative arthroscopy. The device is custom-fitted via trays and rubber impression materials. The mandible manipulator may be steam autoclaved, gas sterilized, or soaked in disinfectant (Fig. 12–6).

Disc Suturing Device. The disc suturing device or "suture stick" (Concept, Inc.) can be used to pass sutures through the articular disc; a spinal needle can be used as well. This device can be effectively employed for relocation of the articular disc as well as for traction procedures (Fig. 12–7).

TECHNIQUES AND PITFALLS

1. The proper selection of instrumentation is essential. Instrument selection is furthermore based on the size of the cannula.
2. The proper usage, care, and cleaning of instruments are important. Suggestions include the following:
   a. Grasp small pieces of tissue to avoid breakage of instruments
   b. Avoid instruments with shearing pins outside the joint
   c. Avoid direct contact with other instruments
   d. Avoid ultrasonic cleaners
   e. Routinely lubricate and clean arthroscopes.
3. Sterilization of Instruments
   See the manufacturer's instructions.[1,2]
   a. All instruments should be precleaned prior to sterilization. Adapters and telescopes should be cleaned with a mild detergent and water. Ocular and

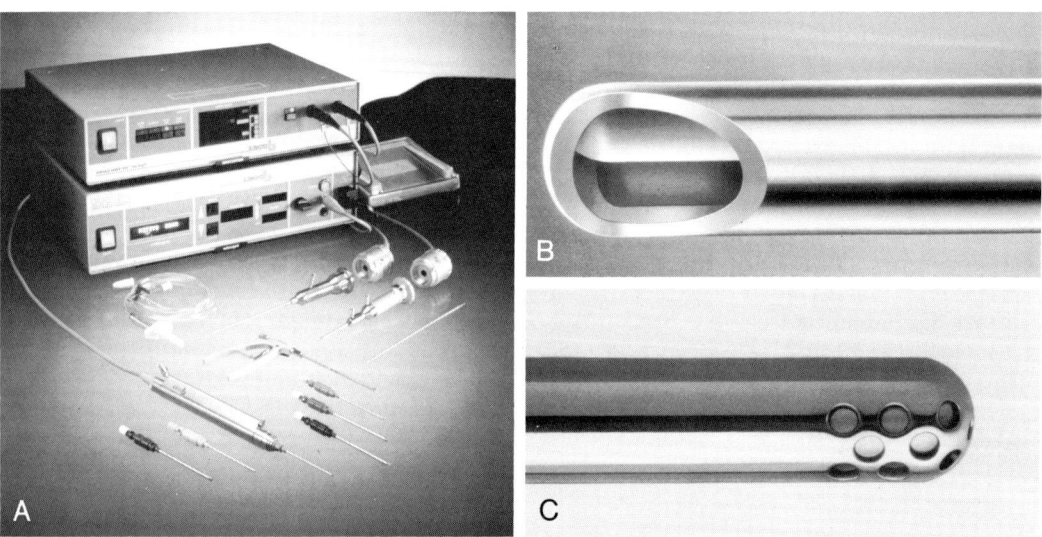

Figure 12–5. *A*, Motorized shaving unit and a variety of blades. *B*, Side-cutting blade. *C*, Turbo whisker blade. (Courtesy of Smith and Nephew Dyonics, Inc.)

B. Instrumentation (Optical and Surgical) ■ 161

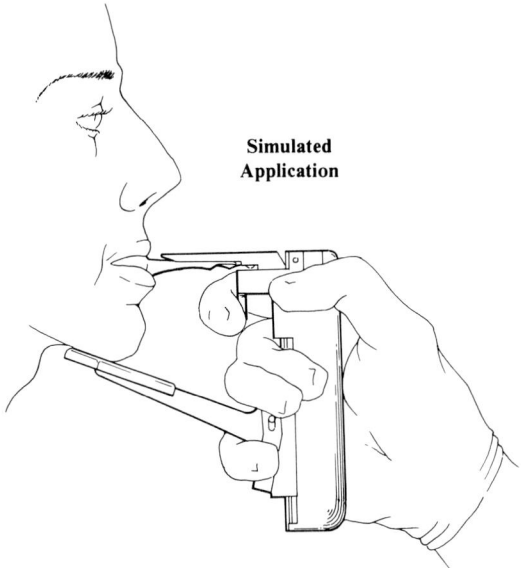

Figure 12–6. Simulated application of the mandible manipulator. (Courtesy of Leonard Medical, Inc.)

objective lenses should be cleaned with 70% isopropyl alcohol and dried with compressed air or a soft cloth. Stopcocks should be oiled with a silicone spray.
b. Metal instruments, such as trocars and cannulas, require conventional high-pressure steam autoclaving.
c. Arthroscopes should be sterilized with ethylene oxide gas. Generally, a mandatory aeration period of 12 to 24 hours is needed with this technique. Repeated high pressure steam sterilization leads to deterioration of the adhesive seals on the lens. Differential thermal expansion can damage parts of the arthroscope. Some arthroscopes can be autoclaved; check with the manufacturer's instructions. A cold sterilant can also be used. Activated gluteraldehyde (2%) in a 15-minute soak is effective. The soak should not exceed 20 minutes because of potential damage to the patient's tissues, the surgeon's eyes, and the instrument itself.
d. The fiberoptic cables and video cameras can only be cold sterilized, unless the manufacturer specifies otherwise. Another method of care for these instruments is "bagging" or draping them in sterile plastic wrapping, depending on the manufacturer's instructions.

References

1. Shahriaree H, Ericksen C: Arthroscopic instrumentation, sterilization and photography. *In* O'Connor's Textbook of Arthroscopic Surgery. Philadelphia: JB Lippincott, 1984, pp 20, 23–26, 31–36.
2. Parisien S, Dzenis P: Development of Modern Arthroscopic Techniques. Principles of Arthroscopic Instrumentation. New York, McGraw-Hill, 1989, pp 47–64.

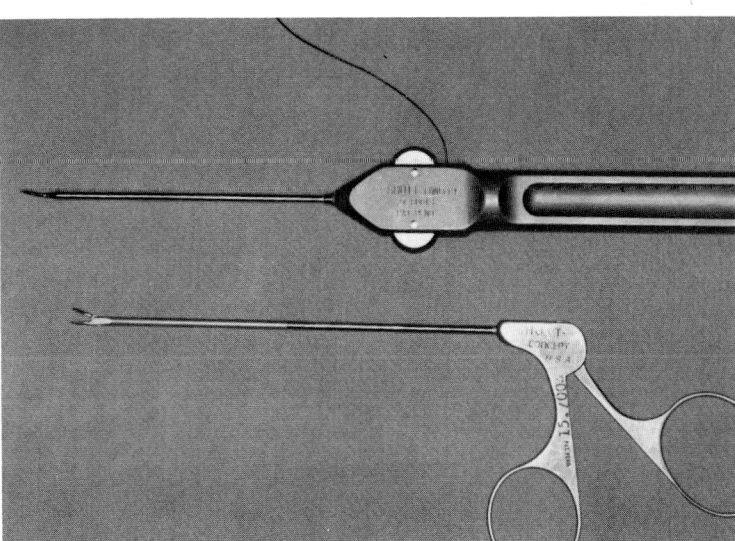

Figure 12–7. Suture stick and grasping forceps.

□ C. Documentation

MOHAN THOMAS, D.D.S., F.A.C.D.
CHRISTOPHER LANE, D.D.S.

Sophisticated photographic methods and color TV systems have become indispensable developments for arthroscopic surgery. The arthroscopic image on the TV screen allows the entire surgical team to view the procedure and thus work together more efficiently. One major advancement that led to the use of color TV in arthroscopy was in the work of Watanabe and Takeda. In 1976, they worked diligently to develop a new color TV system suitable for small joint arthroscopy.[1] Watanabe was successful in creating a highly sensitive, high quality color TV system in 1978. This achievement was a logical outcome of the original development of a clinical arthroscopic TV system for the knee, developed in 1975 by John McGinty.[2]

Accurate documentation of temporomandibular joint (TMJ) arthroscopic procedures requires that detailed handwritten notes and dictated operative notes be completed immediately after the procedures have been completed. Forms have been designed for recording operative findings and postoperative patient instructions (see Appendix). The time interval between the procedure and the actual documentation of the procedure is critical to the accuracy of the documentation.[3] Drawings, diagrams, and charts further aid the arthroscopic surgeon in the preciseness of the document. From a medicolegal standpoint, there can never be overdocumentation of a case. Thus, an arthroscopic surgeon has a multitude of techniques available to aid in the most accurate documentation of cases, including computer-generated records, still photography, TV, and still video recording and retrieval.

The communication of methods and results in arthroscopic surgery naturally requires the means to permanently record findings. A photographic record is of great value to the diagnostician and surgeon. The selection of method of photographing the image should depend on how the information is to be used. Documentation of diagnostic and surgical findings offers a permanent visual record of the procedure, helps to increase acceptance from maxillofacial practitioners for new arthroscopic surgical procedures, and serves as an excellent diagnostic medium to determine if conventional surgery is required.[3-5]

Still photography in arthroscopic surgery generates slides for teaching, research, and publication. However, it is not a practical method for case documentation due to difficulty in identifying specific slides, increase in surgical time, length of developing time, and cumbersome nature of equipment. For still photography the following equipment is recommended: rod-lens telescope, 35mm camera, xenon light source, through-the-lens (TTL) sync cable, lenses with adapters (Fig. 12-8), articulated teaching attachments (two-, three-, and four-joint are available; Fig. 12-9), tripod or stabilizing arm, fiber optic light cables, data back system, and motor drive. Equipment is available from several vendors, including Karl Storz, Endoscopy-America, Inc., Culver City, CA.

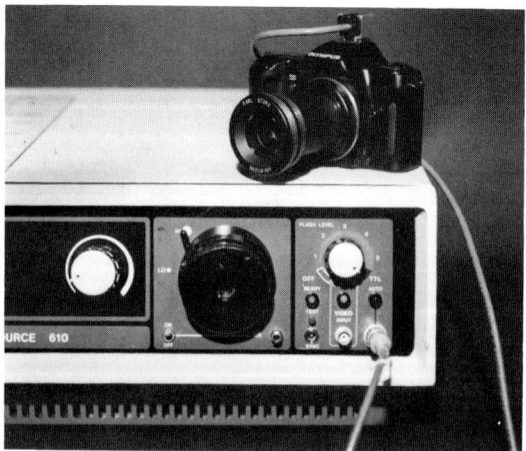

Figure 12-8. A 35mm camera with adapter for intraarticular photography and a xenon light source. (Courtesy of Karl Storz, Culver City, CA.)

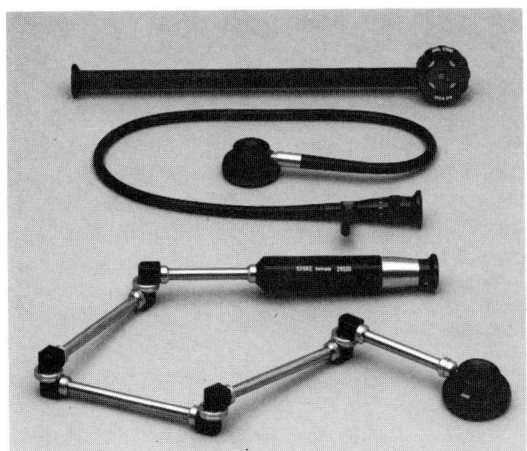

Figure 12-9. Articulated teaching attachments with possibility of multiple viewing while maintaining sterility. (Courtesy of Karl Storz, Culver City, CA.)

The light source is crucial in still photography. A 150-watt tungsten bulb will produce a dull, dark, yellow picture with the best of the large arthroscopes.[4] The xenon light source, e.g., Karl Storz 610 Xenon Flash Generator and Light Source (see Fig. 12-8) provides brighter images with better color rendition than halogen light.

Video recording has definite advantages over conventional slide photography for accurate documentation. Modern video tape equipment makes it possible to document arthroscopic procedures while the image is simultaneously viewed for operative purposes.[2,3,5,6] With the advent of Super VHS video tapes, the images obtained and stored for retrieval are incredible. There is no waiting time for developing the video tape, therefore a more accurate record can be organized and viewed immediately.

COLOR MONITORS

The newer video monitors have lines of resolution as high as 400 and have thus made viewing the true-to-life images both encouraging and extremely gratifying. We recommend color monitors with the maximum lines of resolution capable of exhibiting Super VHS video tape format.

CHARACTER GENERATOR

Through character generators, labeling of video tapes (name, date, procedure) has been made possible. This labeling further ensures the accuracy of records.

STILL VIDEO RECORDING

With the advent of still video recording (Sony MVR-5600/5600AM Still Video Recorder, Sony Medical Electronics, Sony Corp. of America, Park Ridge, NJ), it is now possible to capture, store, and retrieve up to 50 black and white or color images on a 2-inch Sony Mavipak disk. This system eliminates film processing, offers hands-free control, and is efficiently stored on floppy disks for simple presentation and economical distribution.

COLOR VIDEO PRINTERS

Several video printers are available, such as the Sony UP-5000/UP-5000W Color Video Printer (Sony Medical Electronics, Sony Corp. of America, Park Ridge, NJ) (Fig. 12-10A) and the Polaroid FreezeFrame Video Image Recorder (Polaroid Corp., Cambridge, MA) (Fig. 12-10B). With the advent of this new technology, we are now able to generate instant photographs or slides on the "fly" (while the tape is being recorded or played) as well as from material stored on video tapes and floppy disks.

Through the use of video image recording, the surgeon and the operating team are able to observe the arthroscopic images on the video monitor and maintain a permanent record of the procedure on video tape. The photographs and slides generated from the printers prove useful for enhancing case presentation to fellow surgeons and patients, as well as excellent images for the purpose of referral.

References

1. Watanabe M, Ito K, Fujii S: Equipment and procedures. *In* Watanabe M (ed): Arthroscopy of Small Joints. Tokyo: Igaju-Shoin Ltd., 1985, pp 1-30.
2. McGinty JA: Photography in arthroscopy. American Academy of Orthopedic Surgeons. Symposium on Arthroscopy and Arthrography of the Knee. St. Louis: CV Mosby, 1978.
3. Johnson LL: Documentation. *In* Arthroscopic Surgery, Principles and Practice, 3rd Ed. St. Louis: CV Mosby, 1986, pp 246-323.

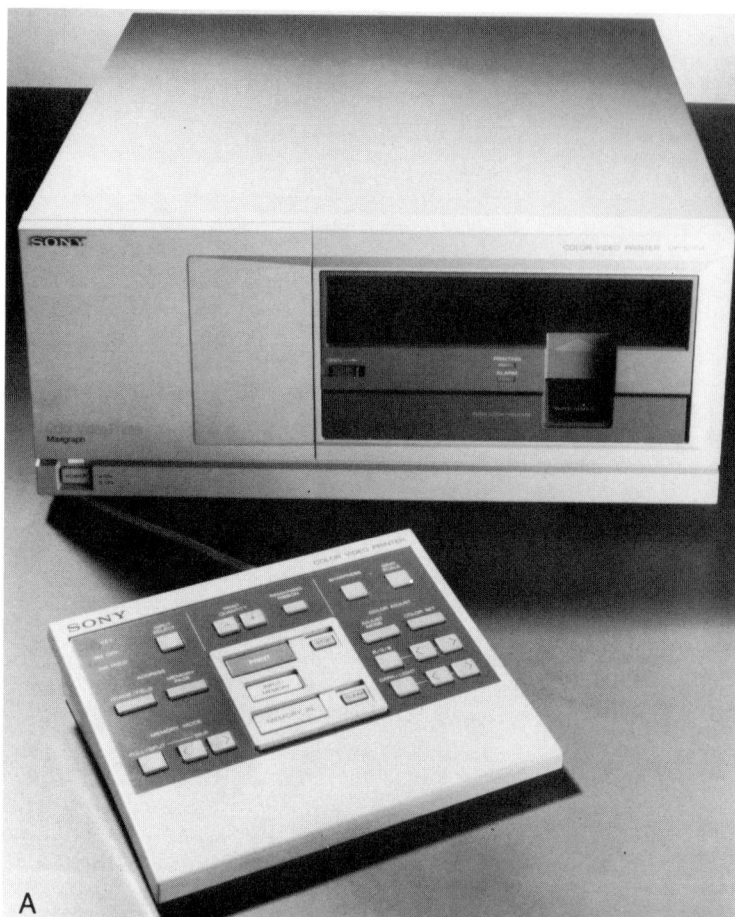
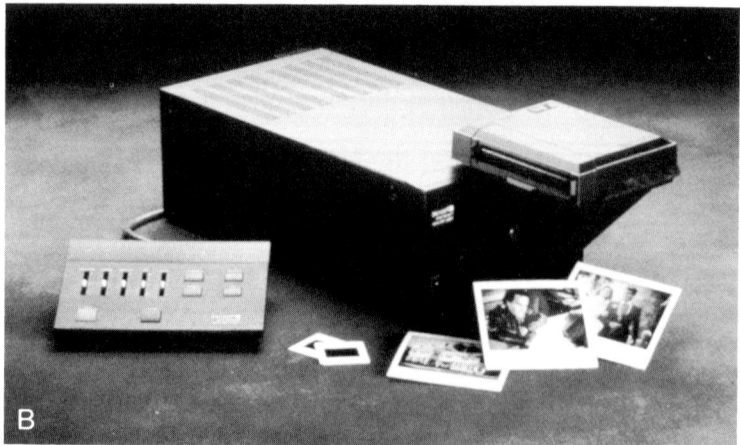

Figure 12–10. *A*, Color video printer. (Courtesy of Sony Medical Electronics, Park Ridge, NJ.) *B*, Color video printer capable of generating both prints and slides. (Courtesy of Polaroid Corp., Cambridge, MA.)

4. Blaustein DI, Heffez LB: Arthroscopic instrumentation, sterilization, and photography. *In* Arthroscopic Atlas of the Temporomandibular Joint. Philadelphia: Lea & Febiger, 1990, pp 31–46.

5. Jackson DW, Ovadia DN: Video arthroscopy: present and future developments. Arthroscopy 2:108, 1985.

6. Eriksson E: Problems in recording arthroscopy. Orthop Clin North Am 10:735, 1979.

D. Surgical Procedures and Techniques

SIDNEY L. BRONSTEIN, D.D.S., M.SC.D., F.A.C.D.

From the outset in the development of temporomandibular joint (TMJ) arthroscopy, determination was evident by those especially interested in this modality to seriously question, earnestly discuss, vigorously debate, and then, finally, clearly propose certain general indications for diagnostic and operative arthroscopy. Over a period of about 2 years these indications were formulated, improved, and modified; now, through their application in several thousands of cases, they have proved to be eminently workable in clinical practice.

Diagnostic arthroscopy needs to be considered as a data-gathering modality, adding extra information to a thorough history, clinical examination, and diagnostic imaging work-up.[1] Operative arthroscopy has now proved to be a significantly useful therapeutic modality for a multitude of articular problems.[2-4]

DIAGNOSTIC ARTHROSCOPY

The surgical staging classification for internal joint derangement devised by Clyde Wilkes has proved to be a highly useful method by which to divide the various signs and symptoms of this disorder into stages with clinical significance.[5] (See Chapter 14, Table 14–1.) Wilkes recognized that the presenting clinical manifestations of dysfunctional TMJ disease varied directly with the duration of symptoms and with the pathologic changes that had been produced within the joint, in a characteristic manner, and in a progressive fashion. He concluded that internal joint derangement is the basic pathophysiologic change responsible for the clinical picture currently labeled "TMJ syndrome" and the like.[6] Wilkes originally presented and discussed these stages categorized into clinical, radiologic, and anatomic divisions;

Table 12–1. TREATMENT RESULTS CORRELATED WITH STAGE OF DISEASE

Stage (No. of Cases)	Results				
	Excellent	Good	Fair	Poor	Worse
Early/Intermediate (42)	34	5 [1]	2	1 [1]	
Intermediate (32)	21	4	1	6 [4]	
Late/Intermediate (4)	1	2		1 [1]	
Late (26)	13	4		7 [6]	2 [2]
Status Post-Repair (14)	2	7 [1]	3 [1]	2	
Status Post-Implant (8)	3	3 [1]		2 [2]	

Figures in brackets denote cases progressing to open surgery.

recently an arthroscopic category correlated with these original divisions has been developed.[7] (See Table 14–2.) This additional staging criterion has been utilized to study clinical progress and outcomes of operative TMJ arthroscopy. It appears that as the stage of disease progresses, arthrotomy is required more often to manage the disorder, indicating that a more guarded prognosis for success must be given the patient showing later stage disease (Table 12–1).

The general indications for diagnostic arthroscopy of the TMJ, as developed and outlined by the International Study Group for TMJ Arthroscopy, are as follows:

1. Unexplained, persistent pre-auricular and/or TMJ pain.
2. Enhancement or confirmation of diagnostic findings for surgical treatment decisions in cases of hypermobility, hypomobility, and painful or otherwise noxious clicking.
3. Local tumor invasion into the TMJ.
4. Systemic arthritides or arthropathies involving the TMJ.

These indications require specific, individualized application based on numerous diagnostic decisions encountered in TMJ practice. When faced with the decision whether or not to perform arthrotomy, it might be useful to employ diagnostic arthroscopy to observe and confirm a clinical diagnosis of advanced, late-stage degenerative joint disease, or the procedure might be expanded to obtain a synovial or articular surface biopsy to further assess the joint status. As an example, Figure 12–11A and B shows the microscopic appearance of biopsy tissue obtained to aid in diagnosing recurrent postsurgical pain. Proliferative tissue was discovered, the joint was debrided, and tissue was sampled. Pathologic examination diagnosed the starch granuloma pictured here. Figures 12–11C and E depict tissue obtained through postsurgical arthroscopic evaluation. Silicone elastomer particles were identified 2 years after an implant had been placed and were removed as planned 3 months later. Thus, diagnostic techniques can provide the clinician with much helpful information relative to treatment of the postarthrotomy or postarthroscopy joint (see Fig. 12–11E and F).

Following direct acute joint trauma, hemarthrosis or subsynovial injury with hemorrhage may be prominent. Berger, in a paper presented at the Third International Symposium on TMJ Arthroscopy, reported on 65 patients (70 joints) who had had acute trauma. These patients underwent arthroscopy shortly after the time of the injury and, in some cases, after fracture fixation was removed. Berger reported the following arthroscopic findings: (1) post-fixation disc displacement, 60%; (2) subsynovial hemorrhage, 95%; (3) hemarthrosis, 70%; (4) abrasions of disc and fibrocartilage, 65%; (5) rupture of the medial capsule, 22%; and (6) disc perforation, 10%. This type of injury can be confirmed through diagnostic arthroscopy and, indeed, would also benefit therapeutically from the lavaging used during that procedure.

OPERATIVE ARTHROSCOPY

Certain historical characteristics of each patient's TMJ disorder and the peculiarities of each of these individuals' clinical progress require consideration when one is contemplating operative intervention:

1. The major source of the patient's pain and dysfunction should be articular and constitute a significant disability for the patient.
2. Appropriate nonsurgical therapy applied over a reasonable period of time should have been unsuccessful in providing an acceptable degree of relief of the patient's disabling symptoms.
3. Any myofascial pain symptoms should be under successful management.
4. Stress management should have been instituted, if necessary, and be at least in a maintenance phase before any operative arthroscopic treatment is initiated.

Indications for operative arthroscopy also require bases supported by the existence of significant clinical criteria such as (1) intolerable pain with normal jaw function; (2) mechanical dysfunction manifested, for example, as hypermobility, hypomobility, and noxious clicking; and (3) confirmatory imaging studies such as tomography, arthrography, and magnetic resonance imaging examination. The general indications include the following:

D. Surgical Procedures and Techniques

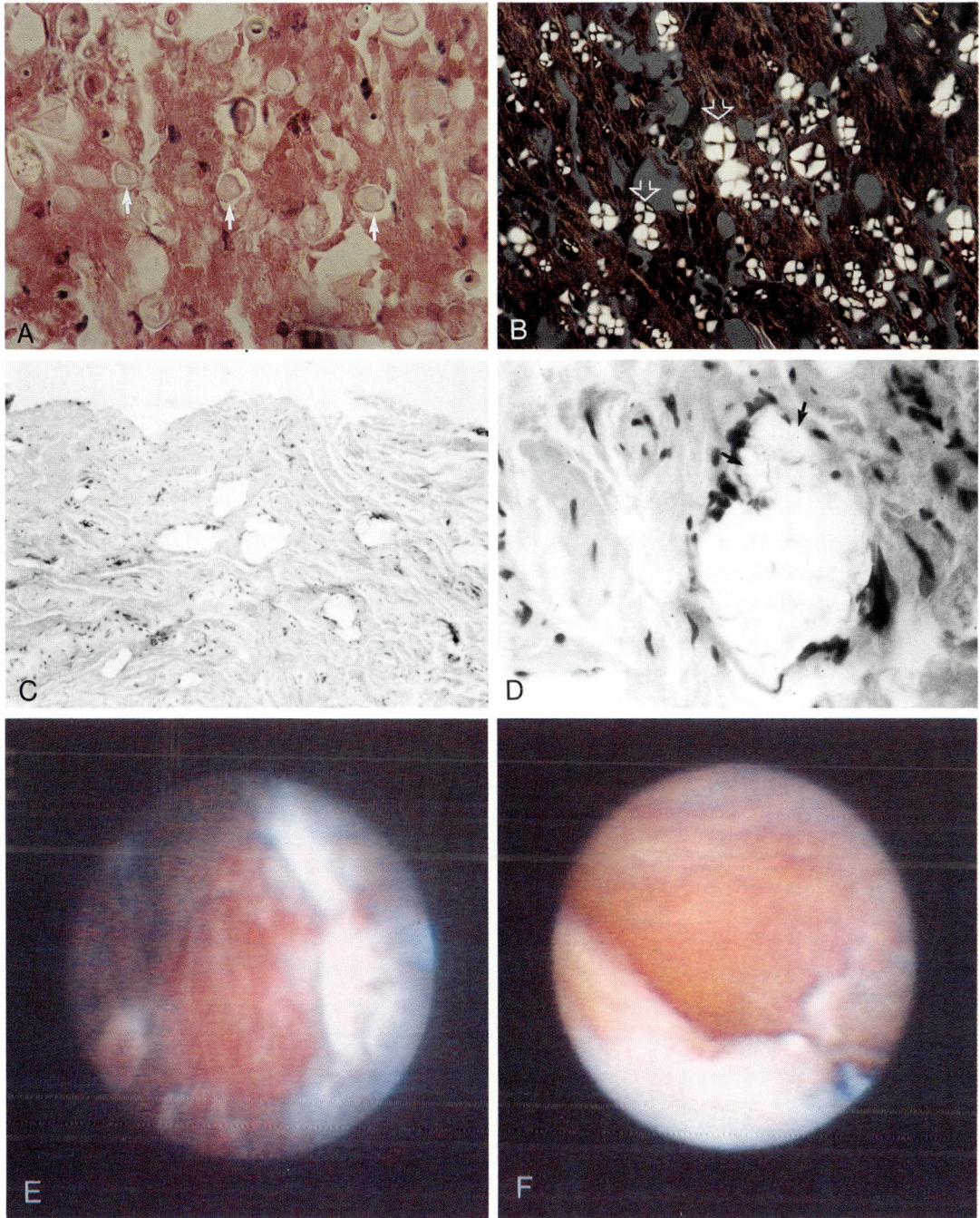

Figure 12-11. Standard light microscopy (A) and polarized light microscopy (B) revealing the classic Maltese cross appearance of starch granules (*arrows*); low-power (C) and high-power (D) photomicrographs of biopsy tissue displaying retained silicone elastomer particles (*arrows*); fossa and eminence (E) and disc (F) of the right temporomandibular joint showing areas of reactive tissue of C and D.

1. Internal joint derangement or arthropathy that is refractory to other management and that constitutes a significant disability to the patient.

2. Joint disease requiring biopsy.
3. Synovitis.
4. Adhesions.
5. Degenerative joint disease.

Acute joint macrotrauma can be direct (e.g., motor vehicle accidents, athletic injury, or battery) or indirect (e.g., acceleration/deceleration injuries or whiplash). This type of trauma may cause capsular stretching, ligament strain, or severe bilaminar zone compression, and it is noted clinically and primarily as painful decreased ranges of motion (ROM), especially opening. This dysfunctional state may be characterized pathophysiologically by an anteromedially displaced disc, acute adhesive capsulitis, capsular fibrosis, or traumatic synovitis, any or all of which can limit joint movement. Such intraarticular pathology then becomes responsible for the progressive obstructive and degenerative phenomena characterizing internal joint derangement.

Chronic microtrauma produced by hyperfunctional or parafunctional jaw forces classically produces an extended progressive clinical state of decreasing ranges of motion, refractory to nonsurgical treatment, in which pain becomes significant. The articular pathology of this painful hypomobility includes chronic anterior disc displacement with or without reduction or with intermittent reduction, chronic synovitis, advanced chondromalacia, degenerative joint disease, and osteoarthritis.

Numerous clinical TMJ arthropathies and disorders are amenable to operative arthroscopic treatment. Conditions that heretofore were usually treated by open surgery can now be managed with an equal or better degree of success by arthroscopy. The surgical trauma is less severe, the postsurgical course is milder, the healing is faster, and the patient regains function more rapidly. Morbidity has been noted to be much less than with open surgery, although complications still occur and must be avoided.

ARTHROSCOPIC TECHNIQUES

The major equipment necessary for standard-of-care arthroscopy has been identified and listed in Chapter 2. In addition to the arthroscope (the various types are described in detail in Chapter 2) a high-intensity light source and a state-of-the-art video camera and monitor are required. Documenting electronic equipment such as a video recorder and a character generator are extremely useful. The ability to take photographs with a video printer or a 35-mm still camera can provide excellent educational material for patients, students, and colleagues. The addition of a power source for debriding and shaving joint tissues is also helpful (Fig. 12–12).

Basic instrumentation for joint entry consists of blunt and sharp trocars and cannulas, or sheaths. These sheaths have inside diameters essentially equal to the diameters of the trocars but slightly larger than the diameters of the scopes; this allows the flow of lavaging fluid around the scope after it is placed within the sheath. Cannulas are designed to have a sideport for the attachment of the fluid tubing and are usually calibrated with a series of marks at 5-mm intervals to measure the depth that the cannula extends into the joint (Fig. 12–13). Hand instrumentation for use in operative TMJ arthroscopy, being primarily a smaller version of the instruments originally developed for the larger joints, has developed exceedingly rapidly over the past few years. Blunt or hooked arthroscopic probes (Fig. 12–14) become "extensions of the arthroscopist's finger"[9] to palpate joint surfaces; determine consistency of adhesions;

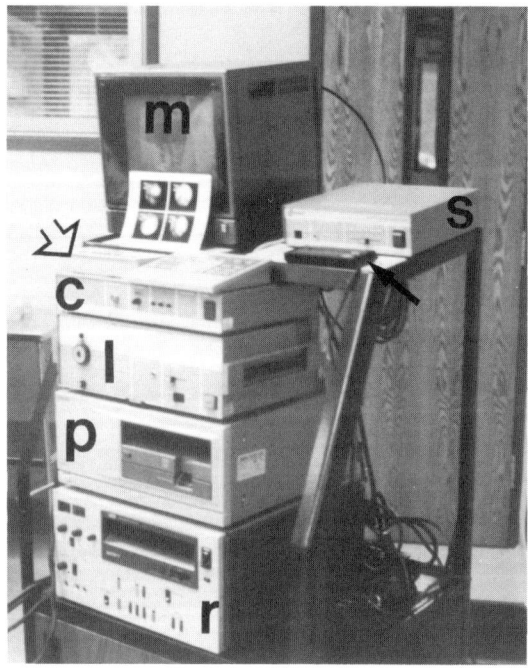

Figure 12–12. The arthroscopic cart. Closed arrow indicates character generator; open arrow indicates remote control for recorder. m = monitor, s = power source for shaver; remote c = camera; l = light source; p = video printer; r = recorder.

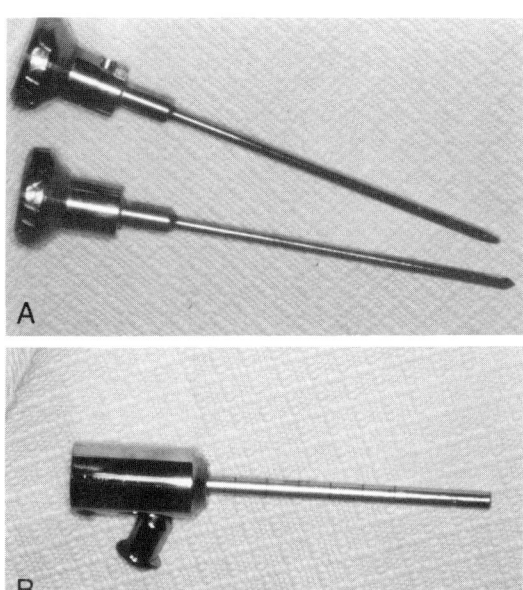

Figure 12-13. Instrumentation for joint entry. *A*, Sharp and blunt trocars; *B*, cannula with 5-mm markings and a side port for attachment of fluid tubing.

release small areas of blood clots, synovial proliferations, fibroses, and adhesions; and outline perforations (Fig. 12-15). Occasionally, the blunt trocar can be utilized to perform some of these procedures; it is especially helpful for separating sheetlike synovial adhesions in the anterior synovial pouch of the superior joint compartment.

Small instruments based on the design of the Penfield neurosurgical dissector or Freer

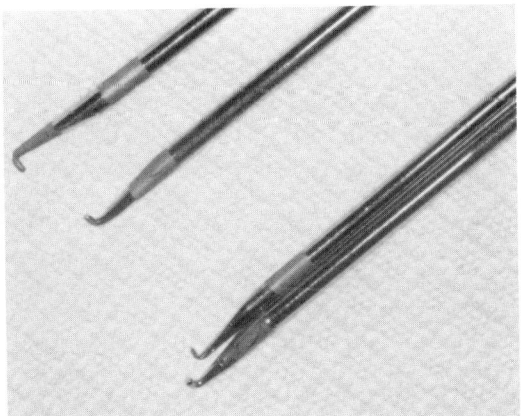

Figure 12-14. An assortment of small hooked probes. The instrument at the bottom of the photograph is hollow to allow simultaneous irrigation if it is used without a sheath. The markings on the others measure 5 mm.

elevator have been developed to aid in reducing a displaced disc after it has been mobilized. This type of instrument allows the operator to visualize the disc being moved posteriorly as the attachment is positioned down and behind the condyle (Fig. 12-16). The attachment can then be electrically cauterized or chemically sclerosed to help retain the ligament in the new position. Small disposable electrocautery probes are available in either monopolar (coagulating) or bipolar (cutting) configurations, already protected by a nonconductive coating for use within the joint.

Most manufacturers now provide biopsy forceps, grasping forceps, and scissors to allow tissue samples to be harvested for histopathology or for severing well-formed fibrotic adhesions (Fig. 12-17). These forceps are available with either finger-hole horizontal handles or vertical finger compression handles. Other instruments at the arthroscopist's disposal, but used less frequently, are curettes, bone files, and a variety of knives (Fig. 12-18).

A suggested operating room set-up for equipment and personnel is diagrammed in Appendix VII. Both the surgeon and assistant must be able to view the monitor easily (Fig. 12-19A). Although it is useful for the instrument nurse to see the monitor and be aware of the progress of the case, that individual also must be watching the outflow and irrigating solution reservoir to prevent any untoward complications from lack of irrigating fluid for the joint or from extravasation of fluid into the subcutaneous tissues (see Fig. 12-19B). At other times, the instrument nurse may be required to adjust suction when it is being applied with the power shaver or suction forceps.

Sterile draping is accomplished as in other surgical procedures; the use of special TMJ arthroscopy drapes facilitates this procedure, and actually it may be less expensive than using individual draping items. After shaving the indicated pre-auricular area up to the level of the helix of the ear, the hairline is prepared with tincture of benzoin to aid in the adherence of the drapes to the skin. Using a plastic drape with one self-sticking edge (see Fig. 12-19C), the patient's hair above and behind the ear is isolated to prevent contamination. The plastic drape can be prepped exactly as the skin is prepped.

Fluids utilized for joint lavage must be

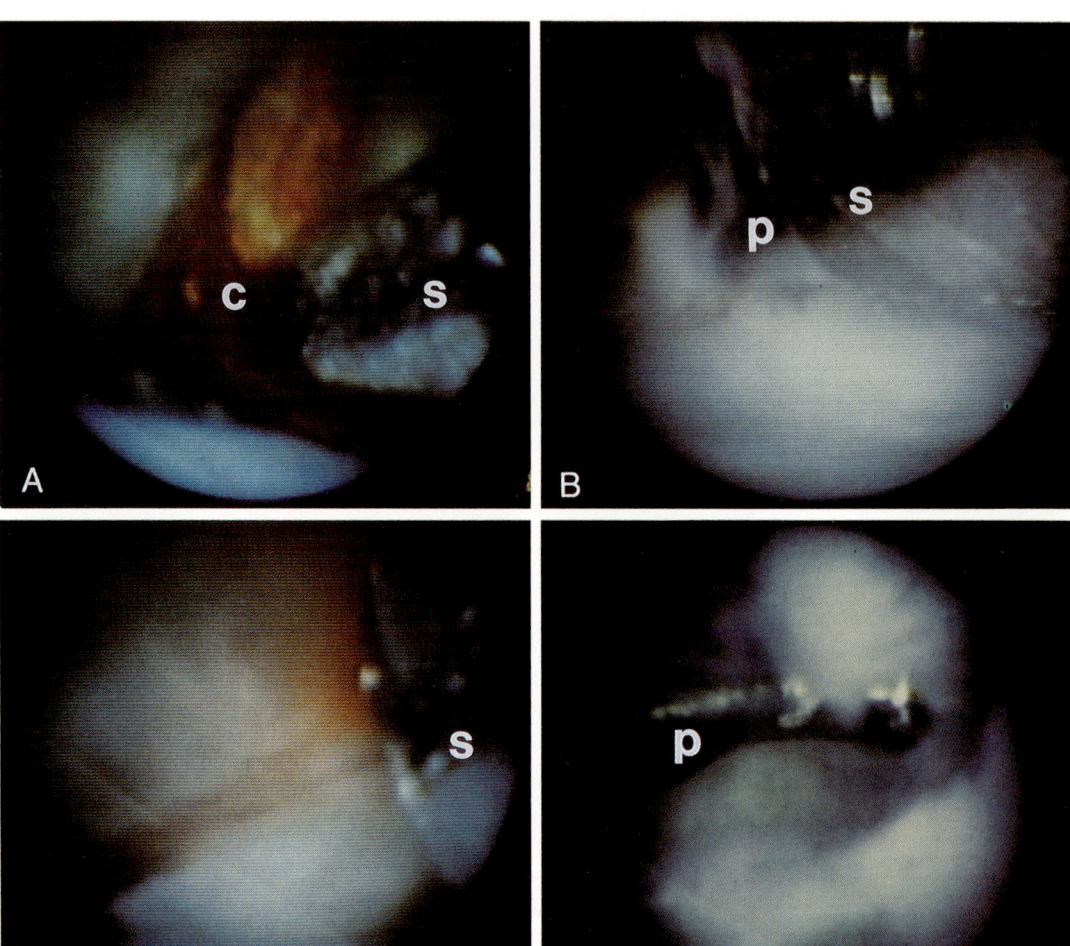

Figure 12–15. *A*, A sheath (s) placed against a small blood clot (c); *B*, a hooked probe (p) protruding from the sheath (s), loosening the clot and allowing it to be irrigated from the temporomandibular joint (TMJ); *C*, the original area in *A*, now free of clot; *D*, a probe (p) testing the consistency of the articular covering on the eminence in a different TMJ.

chosen with care to reduce or prevent osmotic changes in the cells of the articulating surfaces, to provide good visibility, and to support electrocautery, electrosurgery, or laser. The solution most often chosen for lavage is lactated Ringer's solution, as it seems to support cartilage metabolism better. A non-ionized solution such as sterile water must be used for monopolar cautery. Physiologic saline cannot be used for cautery because it is ionized; in addition, it inhibits proteoglycan synthesis. Distilled water, being very hypo-osmolar, causes severe swelling and nuclear changes in the synovial cells of the articular surfaces, as well as in the superficial chondrocytes; it also inhibits proteoglycan synthesis. Glycine, 1.5%, has been shown to be useful and safe for urologic cautery, but it can cause surface tissue and cellular changes because of its hypo-osmolarity. An iso-osmolar glycerol-based proprietary solution, currently undergoing clinical trials, has been well tested in animal models and has proved safe for lavage and cautery.[10]

After skin preparation and patient draping are completed, arthroscopy is initiated with insufflation into the superior joint space of 3 ml of fluid to distend the joint and provide simpler entry of instruments into the space. The initial entry point can be determined by various methods; each utilizes known landmarks that can be located by measurement or

D. Surgical Procedures and Techniques ■ 171

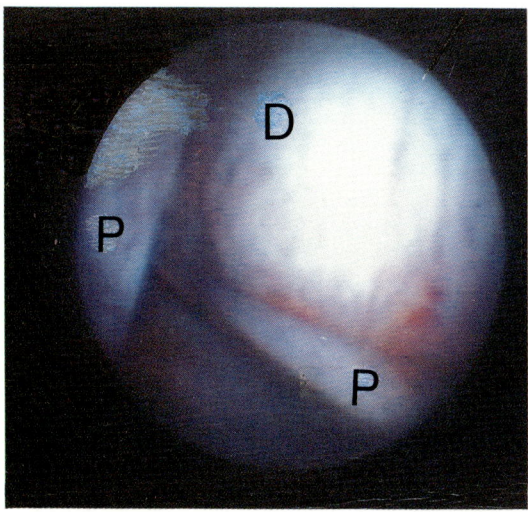

Figure 12–16. Arthroscopic photograph showing the instrument repositioning the posterior attachment (P) and disc (D); behind and below the condylar head (C).

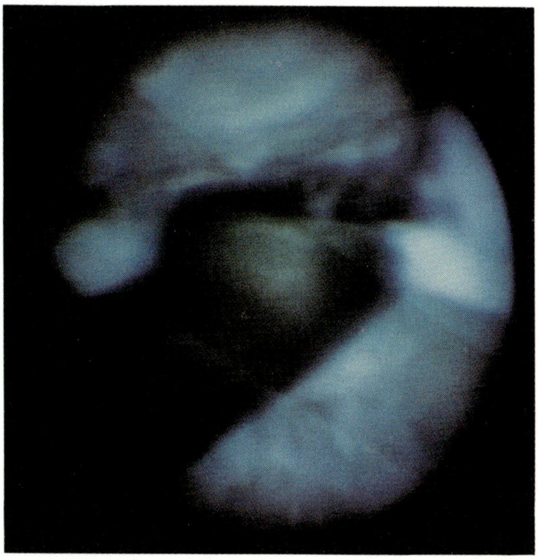

Figure 12–18. A curette being utilized to loosen and remove tissue from the eminence.

can be palpated to indicate the puncture site. Measured landmarks for joint entry have been reported in the literature by Holmlund and Hellsing.[11] By means of a cadaver study, they were able to locate a point of entry along a line drawn from the point of the tragus of the ear to the lateral canthus of the eye. This site was measured at about 10 mm anterior to the tragus and 2 mm inferior to the line (Fig. 12–20). This portal also corresponds to the inferolateral entry of Murakami and Ono[12] and the posterior superior entry described by Moses.[13] It is sometimes very useful to check one landmark against the other, as some condyles may be much more posteriorly or anteriorly positioned than normal. Thus, the main portion of the superior joint space may present farther from or closer to the entry portal than is usual. The zygomatic arch and glenoid fossa usually can be palpated very easily, except in those patients with excessive tissue thickness covering these structures.

There are several important anatomic structures in the entry areas, especially the temporal branch of the facial nerve and the auriculotemporal branch of the trigeminal nerve; close attention to the landmarks described here will, in most patients, prevent complications involving these structures. Branches of the facial vein will also be encountered but seldom cause significant bleeding problems.[14, 15]

While the surgical assistant moves the mandible, the surgeon is able to palpate the condylar head as it is alternately protruded and seated. Many surgeons will then use a sterile skin-marking pen to mark the entry points on the tragal–canthal line or to outline the fossa and condyle and enter the joint just

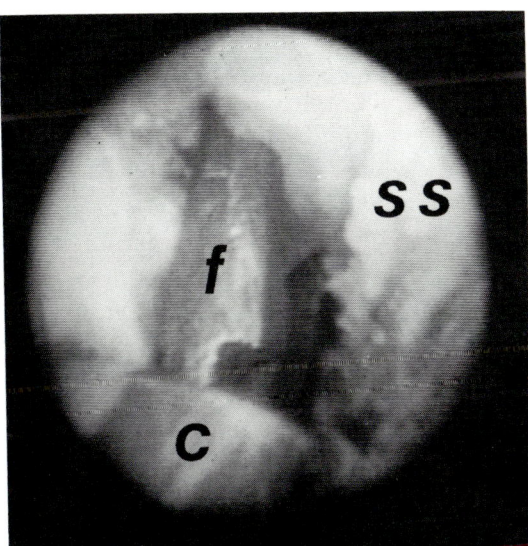

Figure 12–17. Arthroscopic photograph showing tissue (ss) being obtained with forceps (f) through the cannula (c). (Reprinted with permission from Bronstein SL: Starch synovitis of the TMJ treated by arthroscopic debridement: A case report. J Craniomandib Disord Fac Oral Pain 2[1]:10, 1988.)

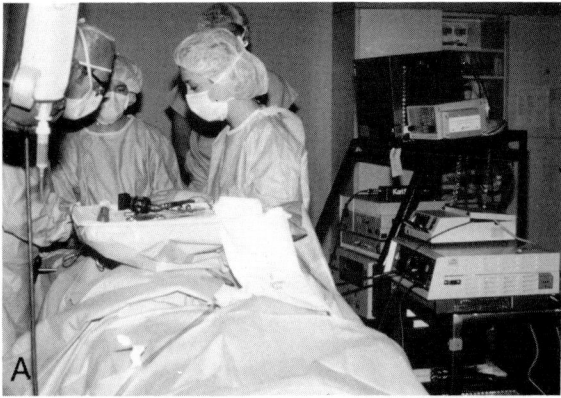
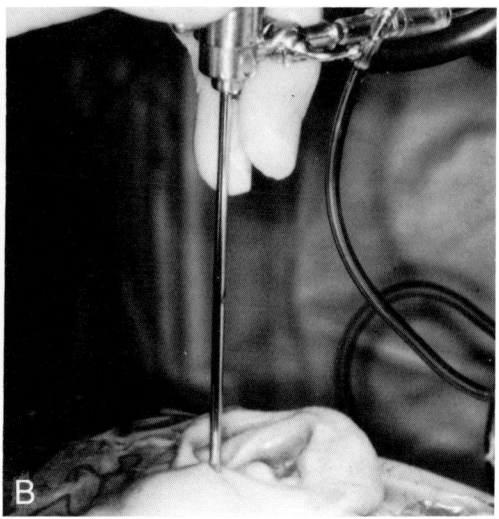
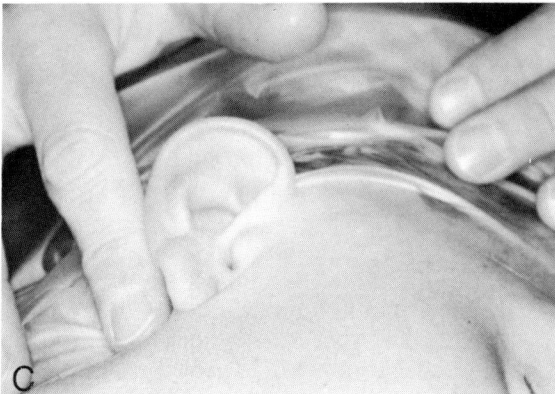

Figure 12-19 A, Operating team performing arthroscopy. The monitor will be moved more toward the head of the table for easier viewing. B, Subcutaneous fluid extravasation. This should be monitored by a member of the operating team as the surgery progresses. C, Draping to isolate the surgical field from the hairline.

posterior to the height of the condyle (Fig. 12-21).

A 3-cc syringe with a 27-gauge needle is recommended for joint insufflation. This will not leave a large needle track through which fluid may escape, and the small volume available will not allow the surgeon to inadvertently overdistend the space and possibly produce fluid extravasation into the subcutaneous tissues.

The arthroscopist must direct the needle toward the posterior slope of the articular eminence, combining a mind's-eye picture of the joint anatomy with tactile information as the needle positioning proceeds (Fig. 12-22). After the posterior slope of the eminence is contacted and it is determined that the needle is indeed in the joint space, the fluid is slowly injected. The operator will notice the hydraulic effect of a fluid column falling and rising within the syringe as pressure is applied and then released during the insufflation; the assistant will sense the mandible being depressed during this procedure. Following distention of the superior compartment, joint entry for the arthroscope is gained through the same portal; using the same path enhances clean entry without penetrating the retrodiscal tissues.

McCain[16] has described a technique whereby the sharp trocar, in its sheath, is placed through the skin, with or without a

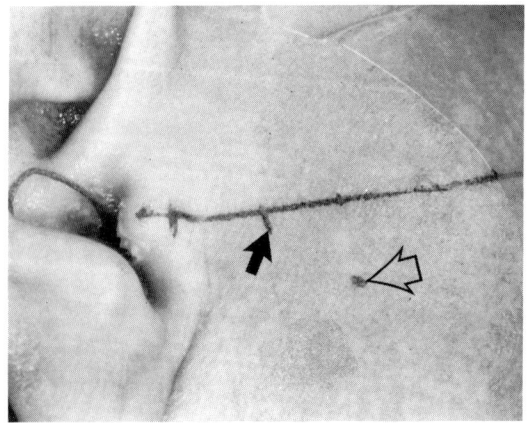

Figure 12-20. The tragal-lateral canthus line showing the 10.2 mm entry location (*solid arrow*), and the 20.10 mm site for a second portal (*open arrow*).

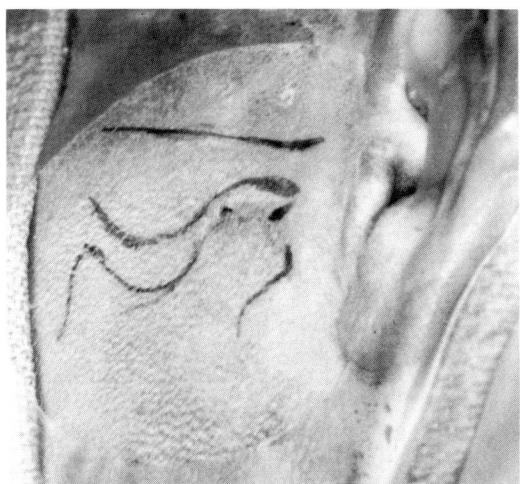

Figure 12–21. The outline of the temporomandibular joint (TMJ) marked on the skin after palpating the TMJ, with the posterior and anterior entry points indicated.

small stab incision, at the site described above. The trocar is advanced, using an axially rotating motion, toward the inferior border of the zygomatic arch, 10 degrees horizontally outward from the skin and 10 degrees below the tragal–canthal line. Once the inferior border is contacted, the trocar is moved deeper, in a swiveling motion, along the bony surface to penetrate the lateral capsule, much like using a periosteotome to raise a mucoperiosteal flap. Soon after this maneuver is initiated, penetration of the capsule and entry into the joint will be recognized as a slight "snap" is felt. The blunt trocar is then substituted for the sharp one and is advanced into the superior joint space until the posterior slope of the eminence is contacted. Gentle probing with the end of the blunt trocar will allow the surgeon to sense the bony surface anatomy of the upper joint space (Fig. 12–23). It is well to point out at this time that the roof of the glenoid fossa is quite thin, averaging 0.9 mm,[14] and may easily be penetrated if care is not exercised. Likewise, the junction of the bony and cartilaginous auditory canals is an area where penetration into vital structures may be encountered.[16]

At this time, the arthroscope may be placed to confirm successful joint entry (Fig. 12–24). An outflow needle may be placed anterior to the cannula to establish the lavaging system (Fig. 12–25). Once the scope is in place, after having been focused and white-balanced outside the joint, the upper compartment can be examined and evaluated. It is important to develop a systematic method and technique for accomplishing this, so that with each patient the surgeon will be sure to examine the color, texture, surface, and general appearance of all the specific joint tissues, as well as the position of the disc. For example, one can begin at the upper posterior synovial pouch, examining the posterior attachment, oblique protuberance, and syno-

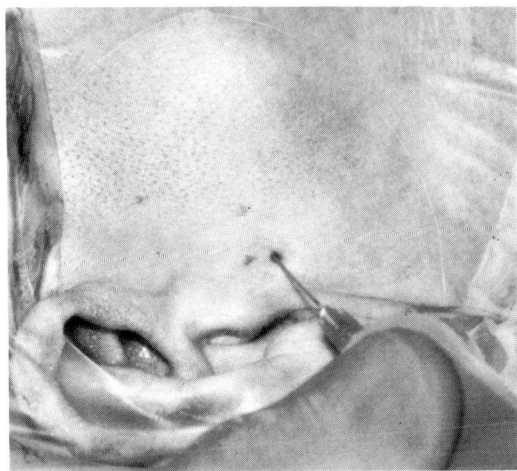

Figure 12–22. Needle inserted at the posterior or inferolateral entry point to insufflate the temporomandibular joint with irrigating fluid. Note the angle of insertion to aim for the posterior slope of the eminence.

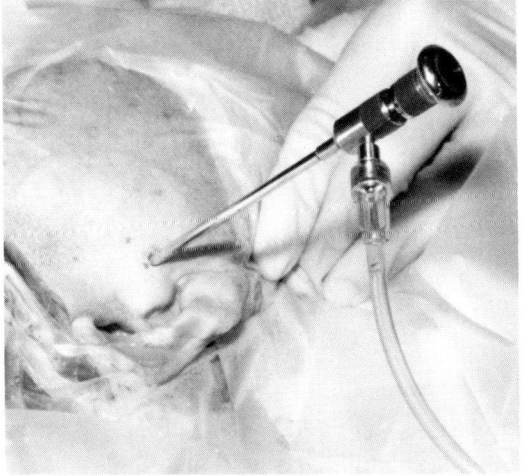

Figure 12–23. The blunt trocar in its sheath is now in position in the temporomandibular joint, and the fluid tubing has been placed in the sideport. The entry is the same as in Figure 12–12.

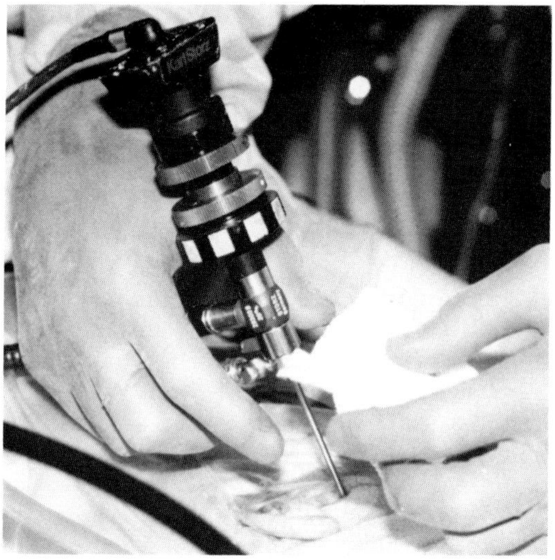

Figure 12–24. The arthroscope has been placed to confirm temporomandibular joint (TMJ) entry. At this time the TMJ could be evaluated without placing an outflow portal, but with very judicious use of lavaging fluid to prevent extravasation into the tissues.

vium. Then the fossa roof and slope of the eminence may be evaluated, along with the superior surface of the disc, moving from posterior to anterior. Disc roofing can be determined during this time.[18] During this portion of the initial evaluation, the joint will be held in the open and forward position by the assistant. As the operator prepares to advance the scope farther anteriorly, the scope must be withdrawn slightly to advance along the lateral trough or lateral paradiscal groove. The assistant will need to slowly close and retrude the mandible to allow the anterior pouch to open and be entered. A typical triangular space is formed between the apex of the eminence and the anterior portion of the disc when this movement is accomplished. The scope can then be placed into the anterior synovial pouch and the tissues evaluated. Another useful maneuver at this time is to close off the outflow and distend the joint with fluid so that the space will be enlarged and easier to enter.

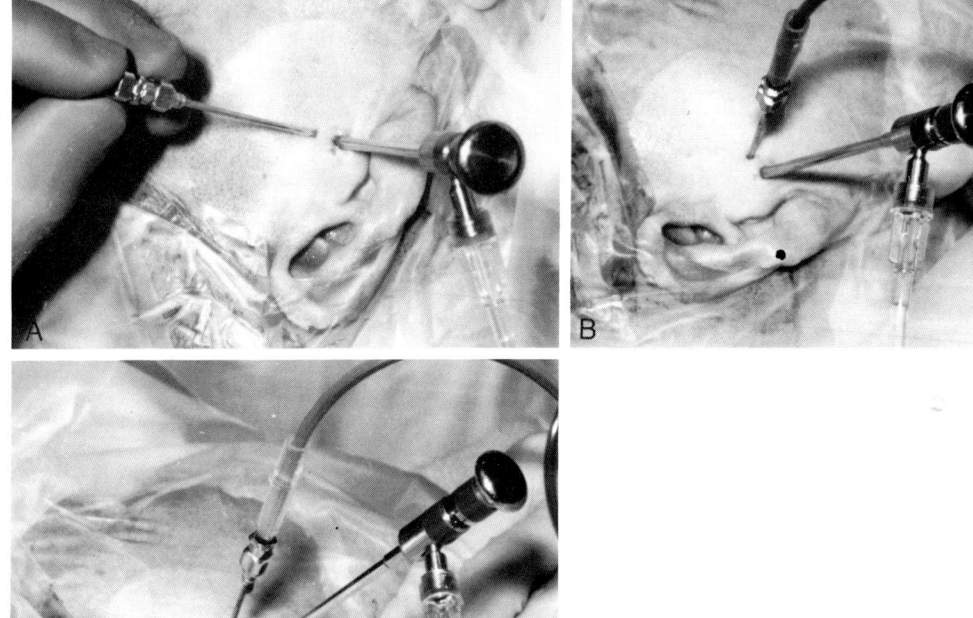

Figure 12–25. *A*, An outflow needle is being placed anteriorly to the first entry. *B*, The temporomandibular joint (TMJ) is being lavaged of blood. *C*, The TMJ is now showing clear fluid outflow.

The conditions of the bony and disc surfaces—appearance, tissue color of the synovial pouches, presence of ridges or fibrillations of the fibrocartilage, vascularity of the synovium medial drape of the capsule, medial and lateral paradiscal grooves—all need to be evaluated to establish a diagnosis. The size of the anterior recess also must be assessed, to correlate with the preoperative imaging regarding disc displacement and its potential for reducibility. The disc must be carefully inspected laterally to determine the presence of a perforation. If a perforation is present, the condylar head should be examined and the inferior joint space entered for evaluation.

The technique described above is known as the single portal technique and is generally adequate for diagnostic evaluation (see Fig. 12–14). An outflow may not be required if care is taken to limit the amount of fluid entering the joint. The modified single portal method, using a larger-gauge outflow needle placed farther anteriorly along the tragal–canthal line, is also quite useful (see Fig. 12–15). The outflow needle occasionally can be visualized with the scope and used to achieve lysis of small adhesions anteriorly.

A true double-portal technique requires the placement of another arthroscopic cannula anteriorly so that the scope and the surgical instruments can be interchanged alternately, anteriorly and posteriorly, to accomplish the required surgical procedures. The cannulas then become alternately the inflow and outflow portals (Fig. 12–26).

The double-portal technique is required if triangulation procedures are to be used. Triangulation allows direct visualization of the working cannula and the instruments inserted through it for surgery. To develop skill at triangulation takes many hours and experience with many cases. Just a very small amount of positional discrepancy between the scope and the working cannula will prevent visualization of the surgical instrument. To make this procedure easier, an angled lens should be used; usually a 15- to 30-degree arthroscope is necessary. With this type of lens, the joint can be visualized easily merely by rotating the arthroscope, keeping the camera oriented to the 6 o'clock–12 o'clock positions, and viewing the joint space through 360 degrees. Once the second cannula is located and triangulated, both instruments must be moved in unison throughout the joint, keeping the working instrument in view as the surgery is being performed in the anterior and posterior pouches.

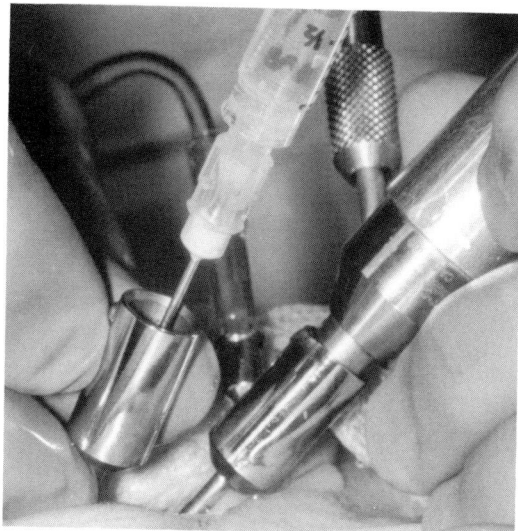

Figure 12–26. Double-portal technique is shown. The cannula to the right houses the arthroscope, and the one to the left shows a spinal needle being used in the working portal to inject sclerosing solution into the oblique protuberance.

The endaural portal, which has been described elsewhere in this text, is also a useful portal for viewing the lateral and medial paradiscal grooves, for retrieving broken instruments, and for accomplishing lateral capsular release procedures. It is, however, subject to certain complications that both the operator and patient must fully understand.

OPERATIVE PROCEDURES

Establishing a working diagnosis prior to initiating definitive surgical treatment is mandatory. Operative procedures that have been developed to treat specific clinical entities are discussed here.

Arthrocentesis

Arthrocentesis is simply lavage of the joint and is often done without actually viewing the joint space. It may be accomplished under local anesthesia as an office procedure, with the addition of sedation. Its purpose is to clear the joint of certain tissue debris, blood, and pain mediators that are believed to be by-products of inflammation occurring within the joint.[19] An inflow needle or arthroscope is required as one portal, and a larger-gauge outflow needle (18 to 16 gauge) as the other. Copious lavaging solution such as lactated Ringer's can then be lavaged through the system. Arthrocentesis can be very effective in certain inflammatory conditions such as acute capsulitis or traumatic synovitis.

Lysis of Adhesions and Joint Lavage (L/L)

Lysis of adhesions (adhesiolysis) and joint lavage (abbreviated L/L for "lysis and lavage") is probably the most common procedure being done today for the relief of painful hypomobility. The objectives of adhesiolysis include the elimination of adhesive restriction of the disc and lateral capsule, the enhancement of translatory movement by the removal of this restriction, and the improvement of condylar mobility. During these lysis maneuvers, a lavaging solution is utilized to wash out microscopic debris left from the breakdown of the articular surfaces, to irrigate the joint cavity of enzymes that are released from granulocytes of the inflammatory process, and to stimulate the normal lubricating properties of the synovial membrane. Its initial use was reported by Sanders and Buoncristiani[3] and was performed as an indirect ablation of superior compartment adhesions and release of a "suction-cup effect." Generally a blunt trocar or blunt probe is utilized to accomplish adhesiolysis; however, other instruments can also be utilized, depending on the development and tenacity of the adhesions. As the mandible is manipulated during the procedure the assistant often reports a sudden release of the hypomobility as the adhesions are separated.

Lysis, Lavage, and Disc Reduction or Manipulation (L/L/R; L/L/M)

With the objective of anatomically repositioning the displaced disc that is contributing to hypomobility, some arthroscopists are attempting disc reduction under direct visualization. After disc mobilization is accomplished by adhesiolysis and anterior release, the surgeon utilizes a small Penfield or Freer design blunt dissector to reposition the posterior attachment backward in the joint space. While doing this one can observe the disc being reduced posteriorly, sliding over the condylar head (see Fig. 12–6). The surgeon then further positions the retrodiscal tissue inferiorly and behind the condylar head as the condyle and disc are seated in the fossa. In some cases this maneuver is successful in retaining the retrodiscal tissue in this location; it may remain there if the patient follows instructions to limit jaw movements for a few weeks to no more than 20 mm, and to increase jaw function very slowly after that.

Lysis, Lavage, Reduction, and Sclerosis or Coagulation (L/L/R/S; L/L/R/C)

Because many arthroscopists question whether the disc actually stays reduced, the disc reduction technique has been modified to include procedures that induce scarring in the posterior attachment, by electrocoagulation or laser or by the injection of a sclerosing solution, after the attachment is seen to be in the desired location (see Fig. 12–6). This method seems to be effective, but at this time there have been no studies proving the efficacy of this modification.[20-23]

Biopsy

Being able to establish a diagnosis through biopsy procedures is always gratifying, because it provides the surgeon with a known clinical entity for which a proper medical or surgical treatment can be chosen. Clinical conditions such as rheumatoid arthritis, psoriatic arthritis, synovial chondromatosis, and neoplastic lesions can be diagnosed by pathologic examination of a good tissue sample. Triangulation techniques allow this to be done directly, and the recently improved instrumentation makes it possible. Basket forceps and powered shavers can be used to obtain adequate tissue for pathologic examination (Fig. 12–27; also see Fig. 12–35B).[24]

Lysis, Lavage, and Joint Debridement (L/L/D)

Late-stage and postarthrotomy joints are often affected by extensive and exuberant

D. Surgical Procedures and Techniques ■ 177

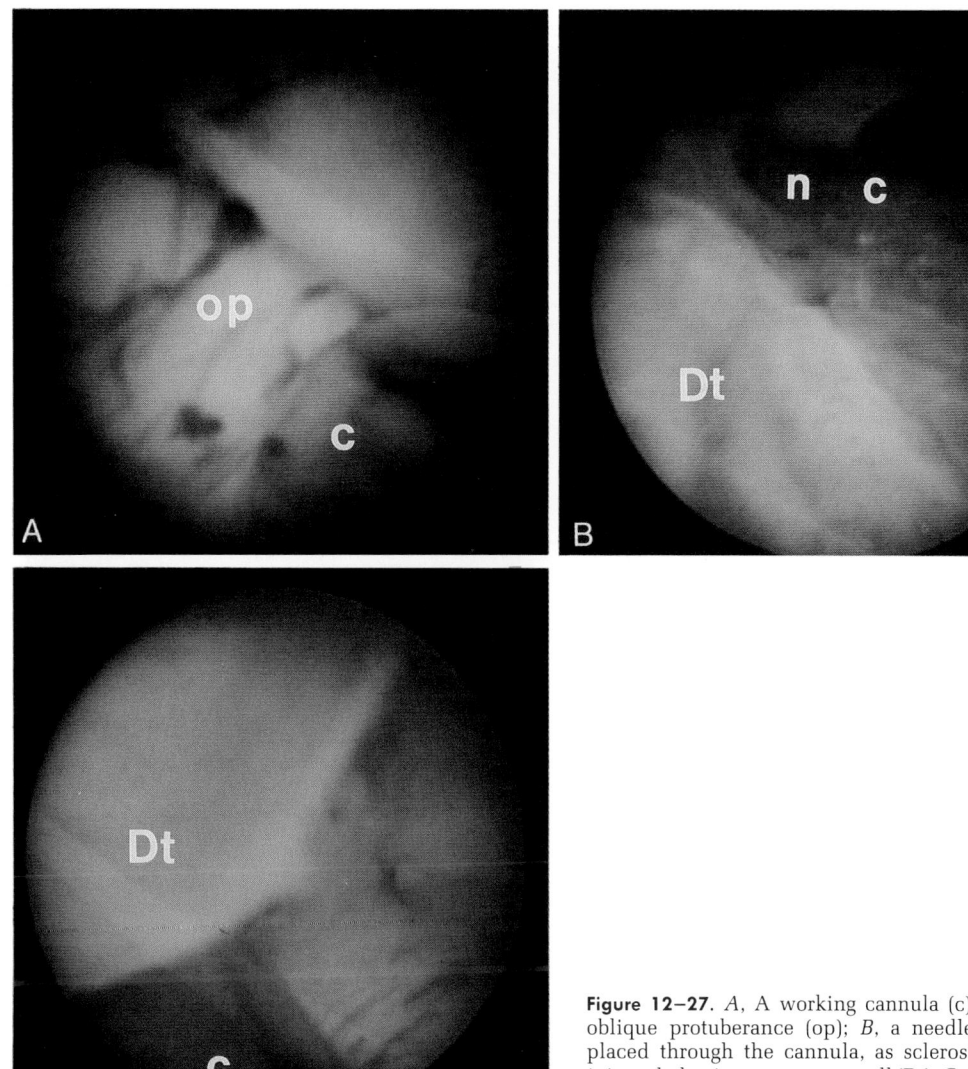

Figure 12–27. *A*, A working cannula (c) is seen at the oblique protuberance (op); *B*, a needle (n) has been placed through the cannula, as sclerosing solution is injected, the tissues start to swell (Dt). *C*, As the injection progresses, the tissues continue to swell with fluid and fill the area.

proliferative synovitis. In many cases the normal joint configuration cannot be discerned. The spaces become completely filled with tissue that has formed in response to long-standing joint disease or to postsurgical scarring or fibrosis, or as a foreign-body giant cell reaction to alloplastic implant material. Other disorders such as long-standing inflammatory conditions and tumors may also cause joint space obturation, and fibrous ankylosis may obliterate the joint compartments. To remove or break up this tissue and to enhance joint mobility, specially designed suction forceps and powered shavers and abraders have been developed. It is probably impossible to clean the joint as adequately as can be done by arthrotomy, but in many cases joint function can be improved and joint pain decreased satisfactorily without opening the joint. The tissues removed from the joint by suction are collected in traps in the suction containers and submitted for examination.[18]

Anterior Release

An extremely important part of successful arthroscopic surgery of the TMJ, as has been alluded to throughout this chapter, is to increase the mobility of the disc to promote painless, normalized joint function. Increasing mobility is dependent on lysis of adhesions, especially in the anterior synovial pouch, and opening of the anterior recess on the anterior slope of the eminence. McCain[16] has developed a procedure wherein the anterior attachment of the lateral pterygoid muscle is released using electrosurgery to allow the disc to be brought posteriorly and positioned in an anatomically normal situation over the condylar head. The posterior attachment is then located behind the condyle and coagulated on its superior lamina to maintain that position by scarring. Some of these cases are placed in short-term intermaxillary fixation immediately postsurgically.

The use of sclerosing solution injected into the oblique protuberance has been advocated and developed by Merrill[20] to produce the same effect as electrocoagulation or laser scarring; he injected 0.25 to 0.5 ml of 1% Sotradecol, along with 0.25 to 0.50% bupivacaine, to produce the necessary sclerosis and scarring for maintenance of the disc in its new position (see Fig. 12–27).

Lateral Capsule Release

This maneuver was developed by Moses to its present state as a means of freeing the capsule in treating lateral impingement syndrome. The procedure is described in detail elsewhere in Chapter 13B.

EXAMPLES OF ARTHROSCOPIC APPLICATION: CASE HISTORIES

The cases that follow were selected to exemplify the several indications for diagnostic and/or operative arthroscopy. Pertinent history and clinical findings are discussed, along with the chosen operative procedure.

Diagnostic Clarification

Evaluation of the TMJ through intra-articular observation or to obtain a biopsy specimen utilizes both applications of arthroscopy to clarify diagnosis and/or to determine treatment options.

Case 1

B.S., a 47-year-old woman, was seen with bilateral pre-auricular pain, bilateral persistent severe pain in the masseter and cervical muscles, and bilateral temporal headaches after prolonged chewing. Her pain and discomfort decreased if she moved the mandible forward.

Past history revealed that the patient had had bilateral TMJ disc repair arthroplasty approximately 5 years previously, followed by a rather uneven postoperative course.

The following preoperative ROM data were obtained: opening of 35 mm, right lateral of 8 to 10 mm, left lateral of 3 to 5 mm, and protrusive excursion of 5 mm. Bilateral reciprocal clicks and crepitus were noted. Both joints were tender on palpation.

Arthrography was interpreted as bilateral adhesive capsulitis with right-sided condylar thinning. Left bony morphology was normal.

Superior compartment arthroscopy was performed in the right TMJ, and extensive proliferative fibrotic tissue was seen in the joint compartment, on the disc, and attached to the capsule (Fig. 12–28). Joint debridement and lateral capsular release provided no intraoperative increase in disc mobility.

Immediate right arthrotomy was initiated. At joint entry, the proliferative fibrosis was confirmed. Very little disc tissue could be identified and what remained was adherent to the superior aspect of the condylar head. Osteoarthrotic changes were present in the fossa, on the eminence, and on the condyle. Subsequent left arthrotomy revealed similar findings.

Case 2

D.M., a 34-year-old woman, presented with bilateral TMJ pain and apertognathia that had developed spontaneously over the previous 12 to 18 months. A maxillary orthosis placed by her orthodontist to control the joint pain had been ineffective.

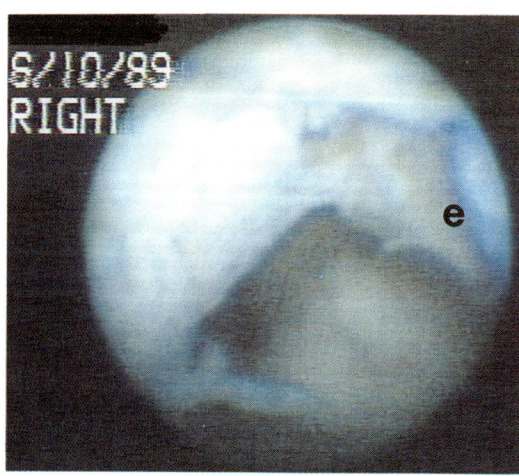

Figure 12–28. Arthroscopic photograph of extensive postarthrotomy fibrosis. e = eminence.

Crohn's disease, which was in remission after successful medical and surgical treatment, was pertinent in her past medical history. All test findings for other inflammatory arthritic conditions, including a specialty consultation for rheumatoid arthritis, were negative.

Opening ROM was 40 mm, including an open bite of about 3 to 4 mm; right lateral was 15 mm, left lateral was 10 mm, and protrusive excursion was 5 to 6 mm. Bilateral crepitus was noted. The patient said that the noises were becoming louder.

Radiography showed decreased condylar height and flattening bilaterally, with marked destruction of the condylar heads. Subchondral sclerosis of the fossae was seen (Fig. 12–29A–D). Bone scans revealed increased metabolic activity in the joint areas.

Arthroscopy was chosen to clarify the diagnosis. Biopsy samples of the right superior compartment (Fig. 12–29E) and the left inferior compartment (Fig. 12–29F) indicated a diagnosis of nonspecific fibrosis. Although the specimens were diagnostic, they did not lend themselves to satisfactory photomicroscopy.

Hypomobility

Management of hypomobility secondary to internal joint derangement with nonreducible anterior disc displacement, to dysfunction produced by a non-disc etiology such as metabolic arthritis or synovial chondromato-

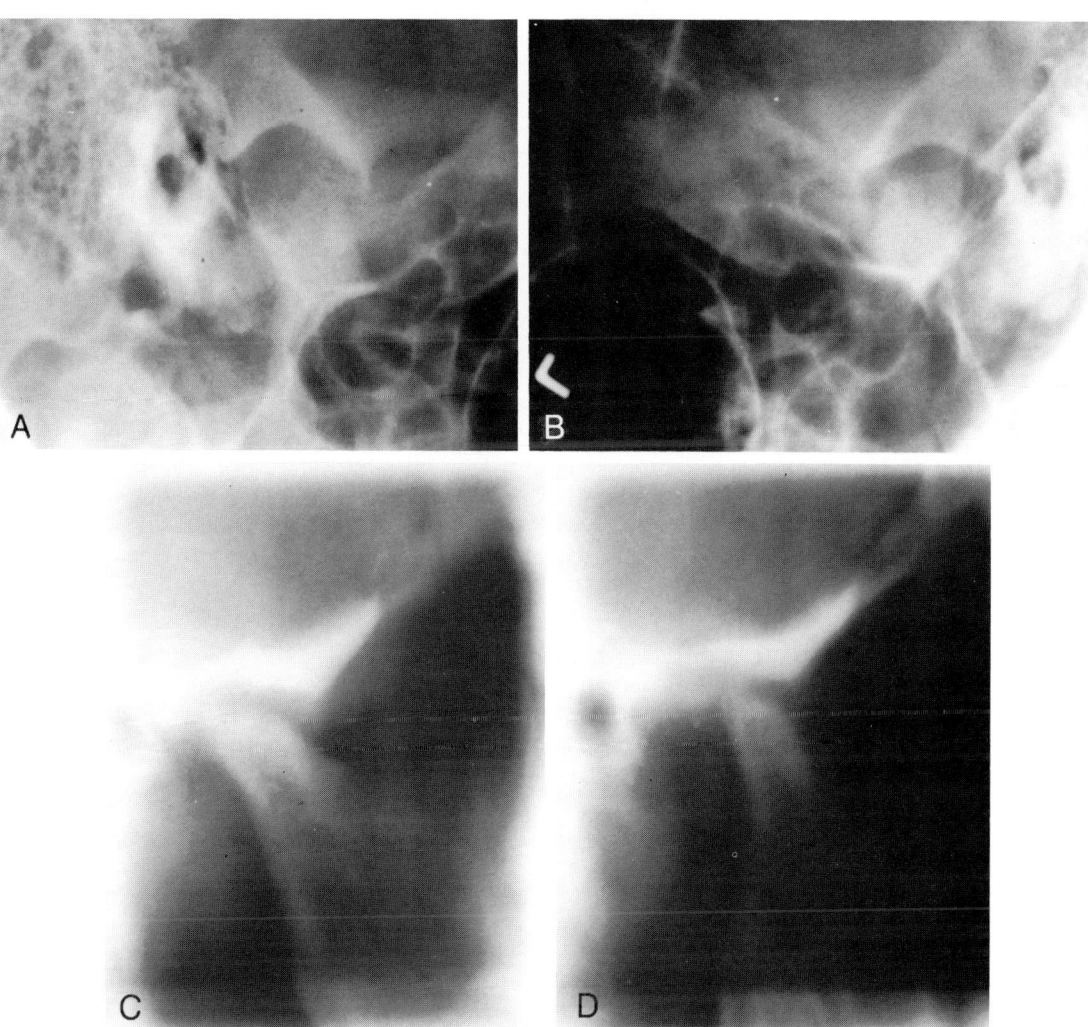

Figure 12–29. Plain films of the right (*A*) and left (*B*) temporomandibular joints (TMJ) depict severe erosion and loss of bone substance seen on initial examination. Tomograms of the right TMJ in the closed (*C*) and open (*D*) mouth positions conform bony loss in the condyle and sclerosis of the fossa and eminence.

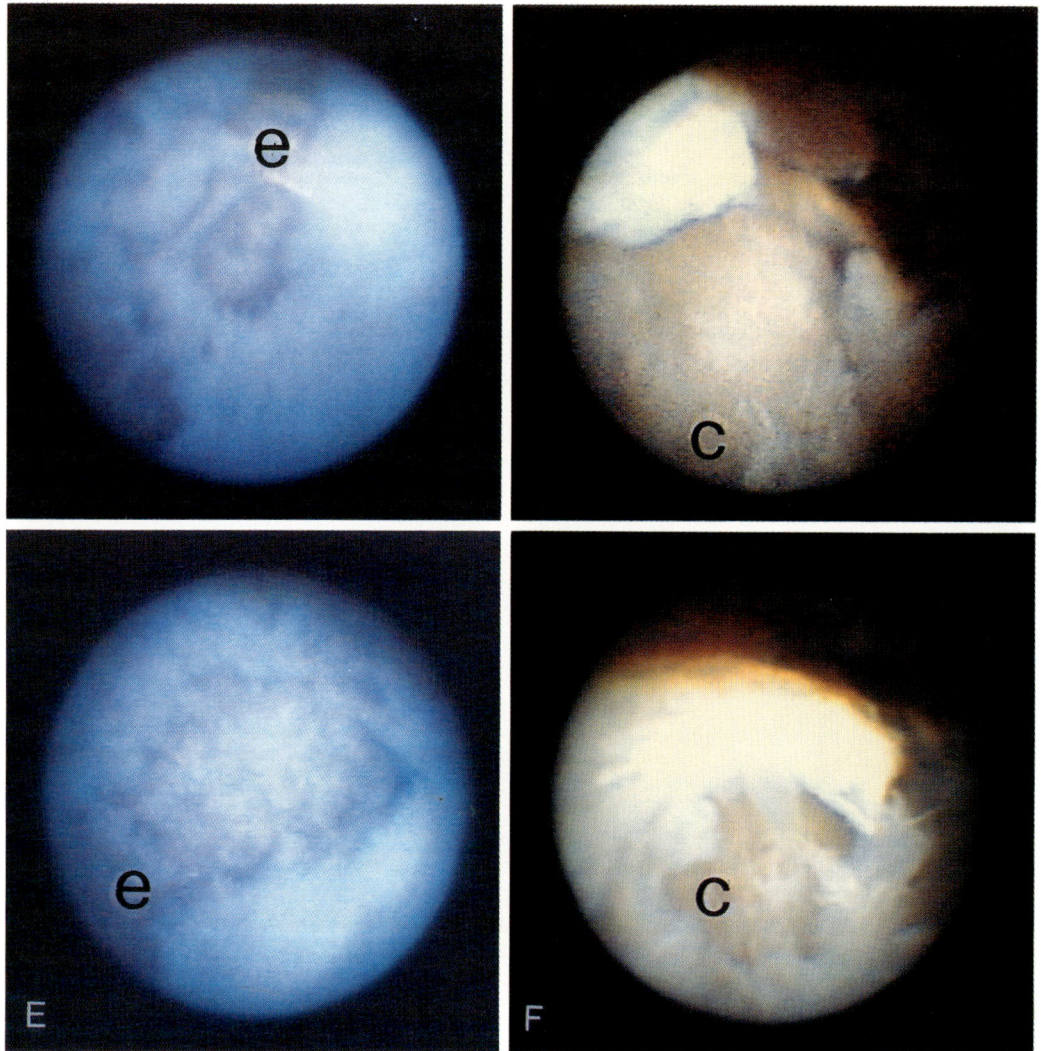

Figure 12-29 *Continued E* and *F* Arthroscopic photographs of the right superior compartment (*E*) and the left inferior compartment (*F*) display the fibrotic tissue overlying the bony surfaces. e = eminence; c = condyle.

sis, or to painful clicking or crepitation associated with reducible disc displacement, has shown an excellent response to arthroscopic intervention.

Case 3

D.P., a 16-year-old girl, sought treatment for locking that had occurred spontaneously 2 weeks prior to being seen. This locking had occurred once previously, lasting about 30 minutes, 2 months earlier, while she was snorkeling. There was a history of chronic gum chewing.

The patient reported pain with opening. History also revealed a click for about the past 5 months; however, this had ceased with the onset of locking.

Clinical examination revealed a maximal incisal opening of 25 mm, right lateral of 8 mm, left lateral of 10 mm, and protrusive excursion of 5 mm. A left deviation on opening was noted. No pain, tenderness, or clicking was found.

Right arthrography was normal; left arthrography showed anterior disc displacement with incomplete reduction, but with normal disc morphology.

Left arthroscopy confirmed anterior disc displacement with about 5 to 10% condylar roofing in the closed position. There was surface irregularity in the posterior synovial pouch, along with hyperemic synovitis. Traumatic synovitis with subsurface hematoma was identified in the medial fossa wall and in the anterior synovial pouch. Low-grade chondromalacia was seen on the apex of the articular eminence. Some of this tissue was removed for biopsy and was reported as fibrocollagen and synovium without evidence of inflammation (Fig. 12–30).

The disc was reduced, increasing condylar roofing from 5 to 10% to approximately 90%; the oblique protuberance and lateral posterior attachment were then sclerosed with 0.25 ml of 1% Sotradecol and 0.5 ml of 0.25% Marcaine.

Case 4

S.B., a 54-year-old woman, was referred with left TMJ pain of 9 years' duration. A severe episode of pain, while eating, had occurred 1 month prior to her appointment. At that time she experienced immediate jaw locking and has heard a grating noise ever since. She reported being a severe bruxer.

ROM showed opening of 25 mm, right lateral of 8 mm, left lateral of 12 mm, and protrusive excursion of 6 mm. A left deviation was seen on opening. The left TMJ was tender on palpation. Crepitus was noted.

Magnetic resonance imaging revealed left anteromedial disc displacement and disc deformation.

Left arthroscopy was performed; subsurface hyperemia and synovitis with hyperemia were seen throughout the fossa, posterior attachment, and eminence. The discal synovium was well vascularized and possibly hyperemic. A perforation was noted laterally, but the underlying condylar fibrocartilage appeared normal (Fig. 12–31). A partial fibrosynovial pseudowall was found in the anterior synovial pouch, which also was involved with a severe hyperemic response and synovitis.

The pseudowall adhesion was lysed, the edges of the perforation were debrided, and the joint was thoroughly lavaged. An increase in joint mobility was subsequently noted.

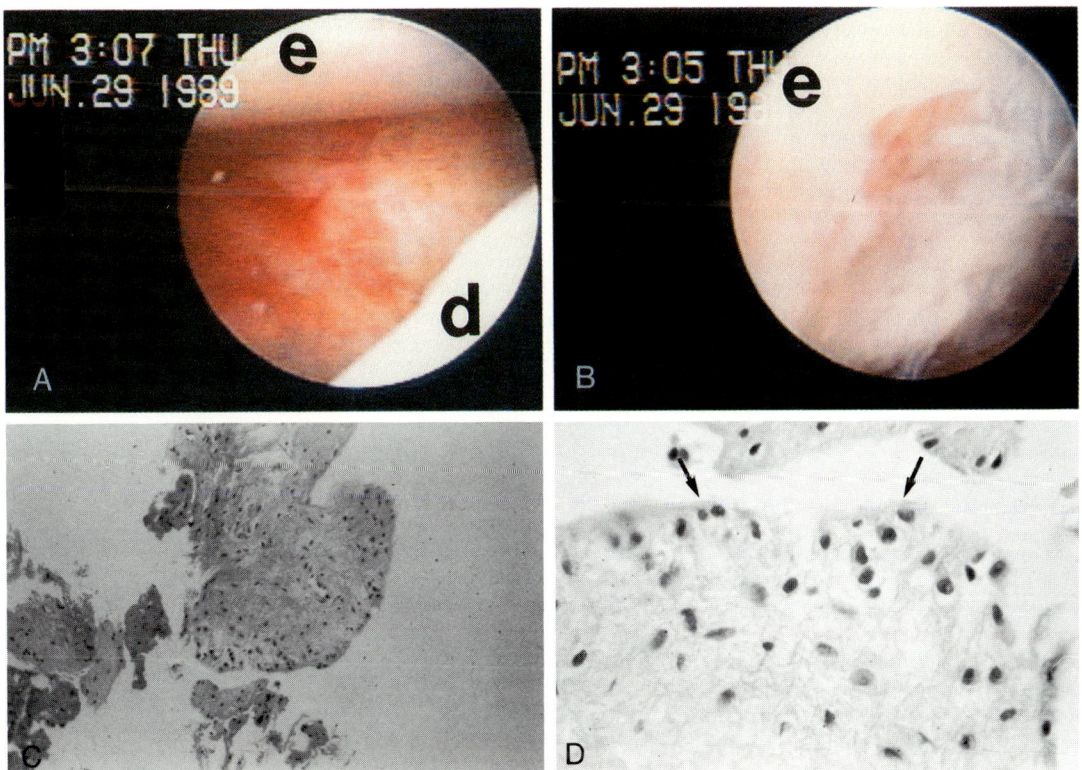

Figure 12–30. *A,* Subsynovial hyperemia in the left anterior synovial pouch; *B,* low-grade chondromalacia on the eminence; low-power (*C*) and high-power (*D*) photomicrographs of the biopsy from the eminence area. The synovial membrane is designated by arrows. e = eminence; d = disc.

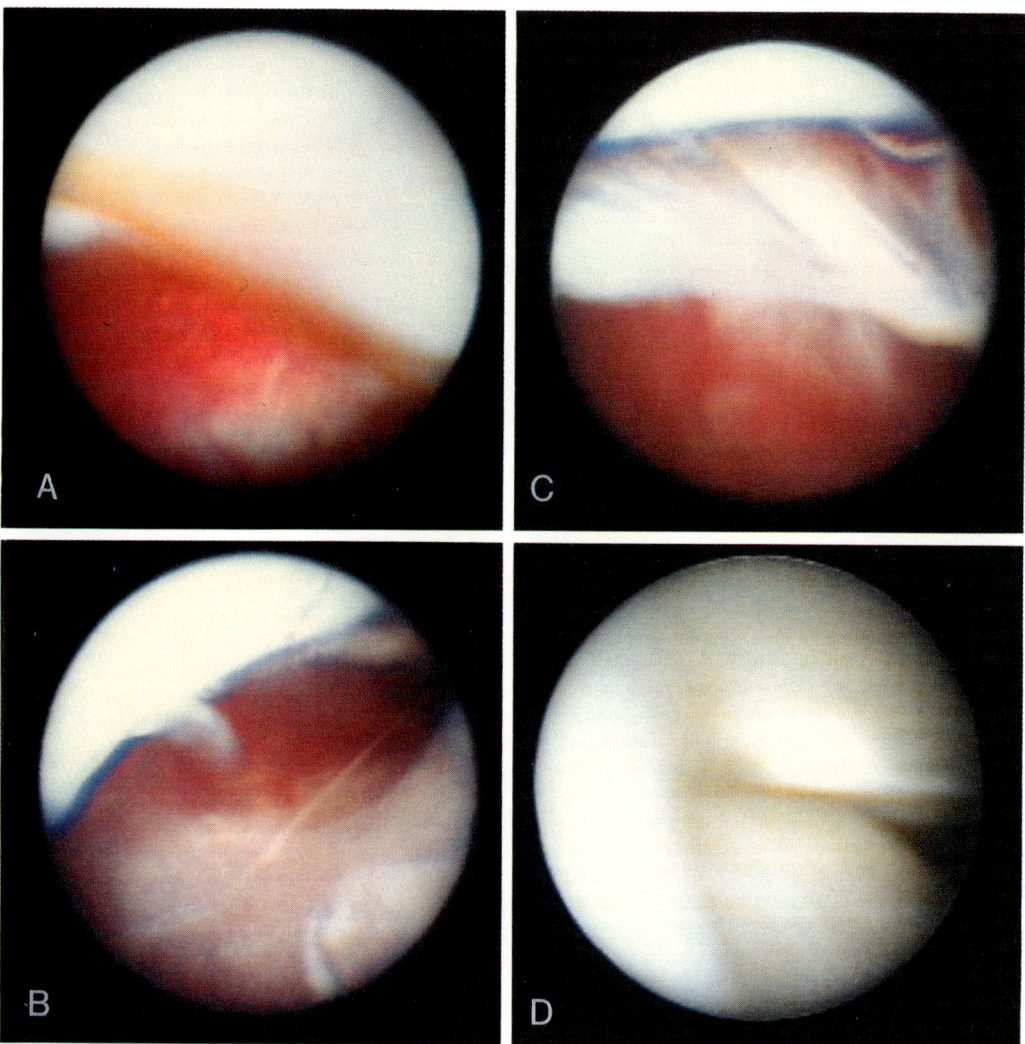

Figure 12-31. Left temporomandibular joint. Involvement of the medial portion of the superior compartment (*A*) and the anterior synovial pouch (*B*) with hyperemia; *C*, disc perforation; *D*, partial fibrosynovial pseudowall adhesion in the anterior pouch.

Case 5

N.M., a 15-year-old girl, suffered acute, very severe locking while eating, 10 days prior to being examined, and could absolutely not separate her teeth, even to the extent of inserting the thickness of a piece of paper between them. She reported jaw aching of 2 weeks' duration and occasional clicking in the past. Two other episodes of locking had occurred during the past year. She gave a further history of having been hit recently on the left side of the face with a softball.

Bilateral joint pain on attempted opening was noted (left greater than right), plus left masseter tenderness. ROM was zero in all excursions.

Magnetic resonance imaging showed bilateral anterior disc displacement with some lateral displacement on the left; because there was no translation at all, open-mouth or dynamic studies were not possible.

The patient was given intravenous midazolam, 15 mg, and morphine sulfate, 4 mg, over 25 minutes, in an attempt to improve jaw mobility. An opening of only 10 mm, lasting about one-half hour, was gained.

The patient was scheduled for the operating room, at which time she was intubated using a flexible laryngoscope. Mandibular mobility was then easily gained manually. Arthroscopy was performed and 100% roofing, normal joint surfaces and recesses, and normal synovium were noted (Fig. 12–32).

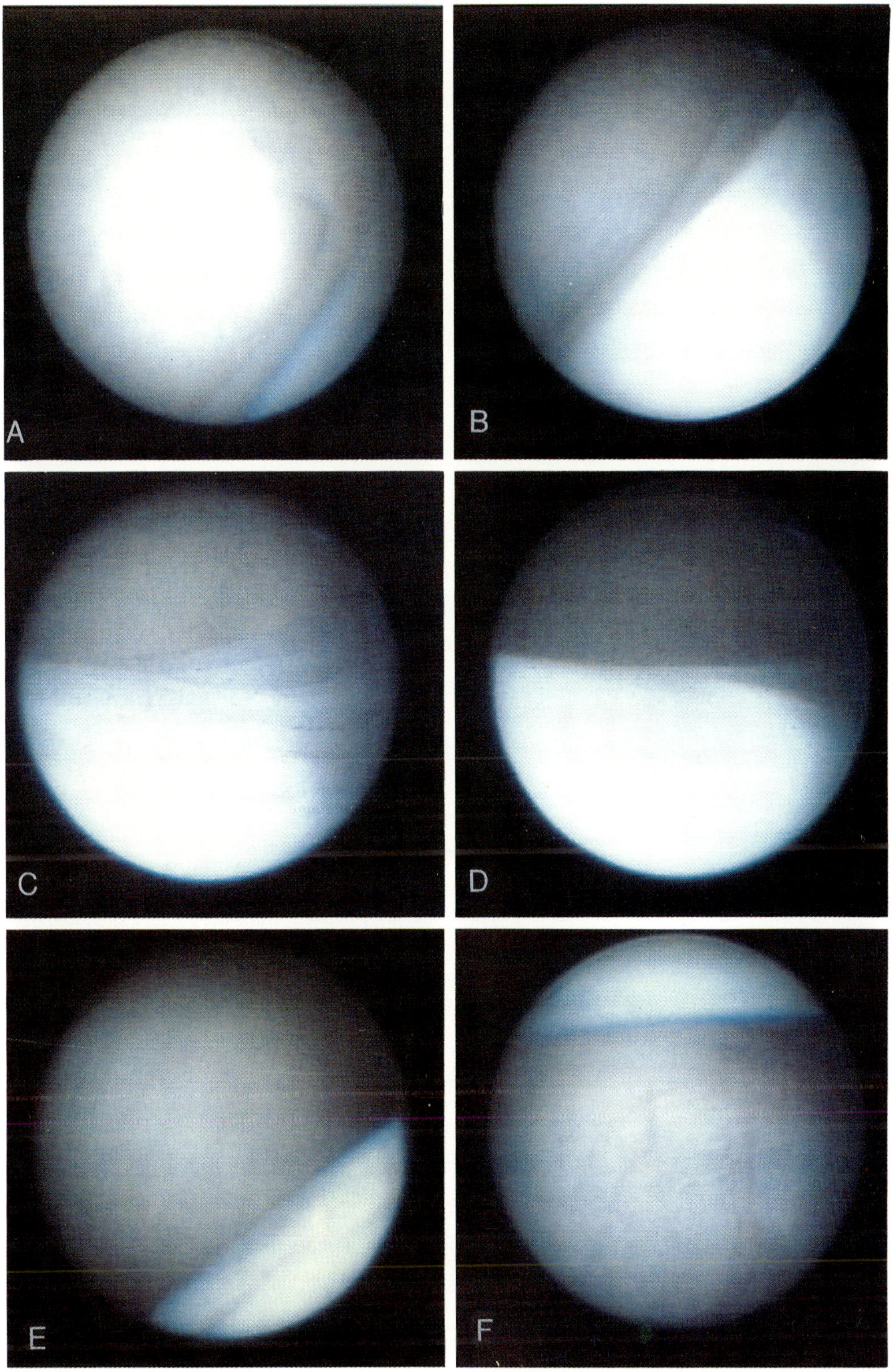

D. Surgical Procedures and Techniques ■ 183

Figure 12–32. *A* through *F* represent sequential views of the left temporomandibular joint, beginning from the posterior synovial pouch and finishing in the anterior synovial pouch (posterior is to the right). *A*, top of posterior attachment; *B*, lower portion of attachment; *C*, junction of disc and attachment; *D*, intermediate zone of disc; *E*, anterior slope of disc; *F*, anterior synovial pouch.

Postoperative magnetic resonance imaging showed a completely normal joint with normal translation. No further locking has been reported. The actual etiology of this incident remains unidentified.

Case 6

N.Z., a 26-year-old woman, presented with right-sided popping and clicking, pain on chewing, ear pain, and stuffiness, all of which increased with jaw function. Pertinent history included fracture of the left parasymphyseal region and loss of maxillary anterior teeth in an automobile accident. Six months after the accident, the patient's TMJ symptoms became significant while she was riding a trail bike over bumpy terrain.

Examination showed a maximal incisal opening of 30 mm, right lateral of 8 mm, left lateral of 8 mm, and protrusive excursion range of 4 mm. The right joint and all muscles of mastication were tender. Protrusive jaw positioning lessened the joint pain.

Magnetic resonance imaging diagnosed anterior disc displacement with reduction on the right side; the left joint was radiographically normal.

On arthroscopy, areas of patchy traumatic synovitis with pseudowall adhesions were noted, especially in the anterior pouch. The right joint showed a well-formed pseudowall in the lateral portion of the pouch (Fig. 12–33).

Lysis and lavage were chosen to treat this patient.

Hypermobility

Arthroscopic treatment of disc hypermobility and painful dysfunction with normal ROM has produced only moderate success. Sclerotherapy may provide improvement in these cases.

Case 7

C.J., a 44-year-old woman, sought treatment for jaw popping, jaw pain that was exacerbated by yawning and dental work, and joint pain with function. She had an acute lock for the week prior to her appointment. History revealed 4+ bruxism; she had been using a Hawley appliance for this for many years.

On clinical examination, jaw opening measured 40 to 52 mm; right lateral, left lateral, and protrusive excursion were within normal limits. There were late opening, bilateral, and reciprocal clicks and a translatory eminence popping with subluxation at wide opening.

A reducible anterior disc displacement on the right, with possibly a medial or lateral component as well, was seen on arthrograms. The left joint was very difficult to enter and diagnosis was inconclusive.

Right arthroscopy revealed a large, sheetlike anterior synovial pouch pseudowall along with anterior and medial disc displacement. This pseudowall was lysed; the disc was mobilized and then reduced. Sclerosing injections, as described in Case 3, were then placed in the retrodiscal tissues (see Fig. 12–17). Left arthroscopy showed anterior and medial disc displacement, bilaminar redundancy, lateral adhesive capsulitis, and an anterior pouch pseudowall. It was not possible to reduce this disc for sclerosing; however, it was mobilized as much as possible to promote normal joint function. Follow-up to date has shown much improved joint function.

Joint Debridement

Postsurgical debridement of the TMJ can be accomplished with motorized shavers and sharp hand instruments. This may provide relief of painful, dysfunctional symptoms. Occasionally, however, repeat arthroscopy is required in these cases.

Case 8

G.H., a 30-year-old woman, presented in 1987 with severe hypomobility (right worse than left) that had been increasing slowly over the past 2 years. In April of 1985, she had undergone bilateral disc removal arthroplasty utilizing planned temporary silicone elastomer implants.

Following the history taking and physical examination, arthrography was performed; however, this was unsuccessful on the right side because no joint space could be found; on the left side, adhesions and osteophytosis were diagnosed.

At surgery, bony ankylosis of the right joint was diagnosed and treated accordingly. The left joint was arthroscoped, and extensive proliferative fibrosis was discovered (Fig. 12–34A). The joint was debrided and mobility of the condyle was improved, employing motorized shavers and hand instruments (Fig. 12–34B and C).

Trauma

Traumatic capsulitis and synovitis, evinced by hemarthrosis, synovial hyper-

D. Surgical Procedures and Techniques ■ 185

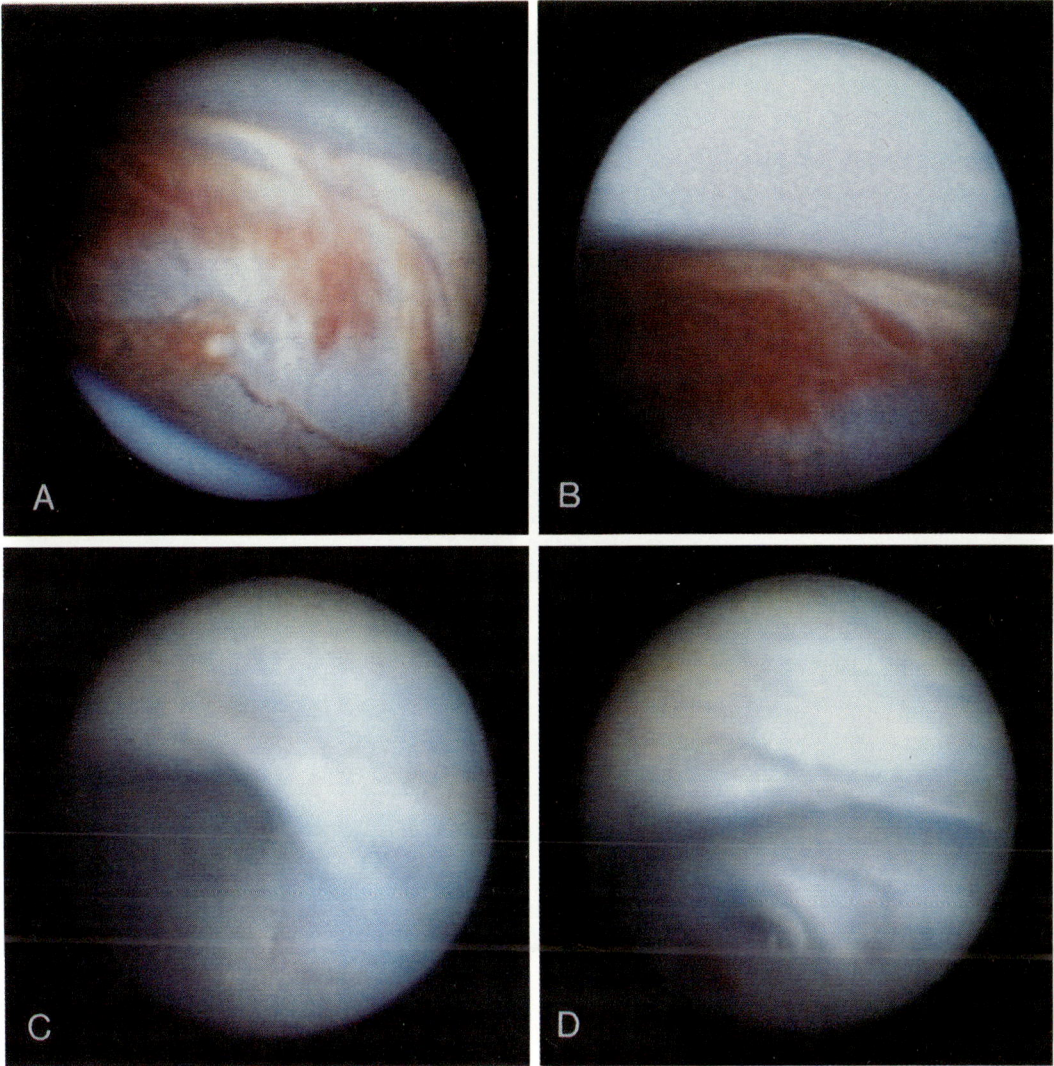

Figure 12–33. Patchy hemorrhagic synovitis in the medial portion of the left superior compartment (*A*) and in the anterior pouch (*B*). *C* and *D*, Well-formed fibrous pseudowall in the lateral portion of the anterior pouch of the right superior compartment.

emia, synovial adhesions, or fibrosis, respond favorably to operative arthroscopy. Early treatment appears to produce the most favorable results. In a study describing treatment success utilizing lysis and lavage procedures, Porter and Zeitler[4] reported a 90% success rate in patients treated within 6 months of the onset of pain.

Case 9

K.D., a 13-year-old girl, described right TMJ hypomobility of several weeks' duration. This occurred secondary to habitual biting on the cap of a pen, when a "popping" on the right side was immediately heard, followed by joint pain and headache on that side. The patient also had a history of multiple traumatic episodes during athletic endeavors and of chronic gum chewing.

Clinical examination revealed jaw opening of 40 mm, right lateral of 10 mm, left lateral of 8 mm, and protrusive movement of 6 mm. There was opening deviation to the right.

Arthrographic studies were interpreted as showing right anterior disc displacement without reduction and left anterior disc displacement with reduction.

Arthroscopy was performed on the right TMJ. Anterior disc displacement with less than

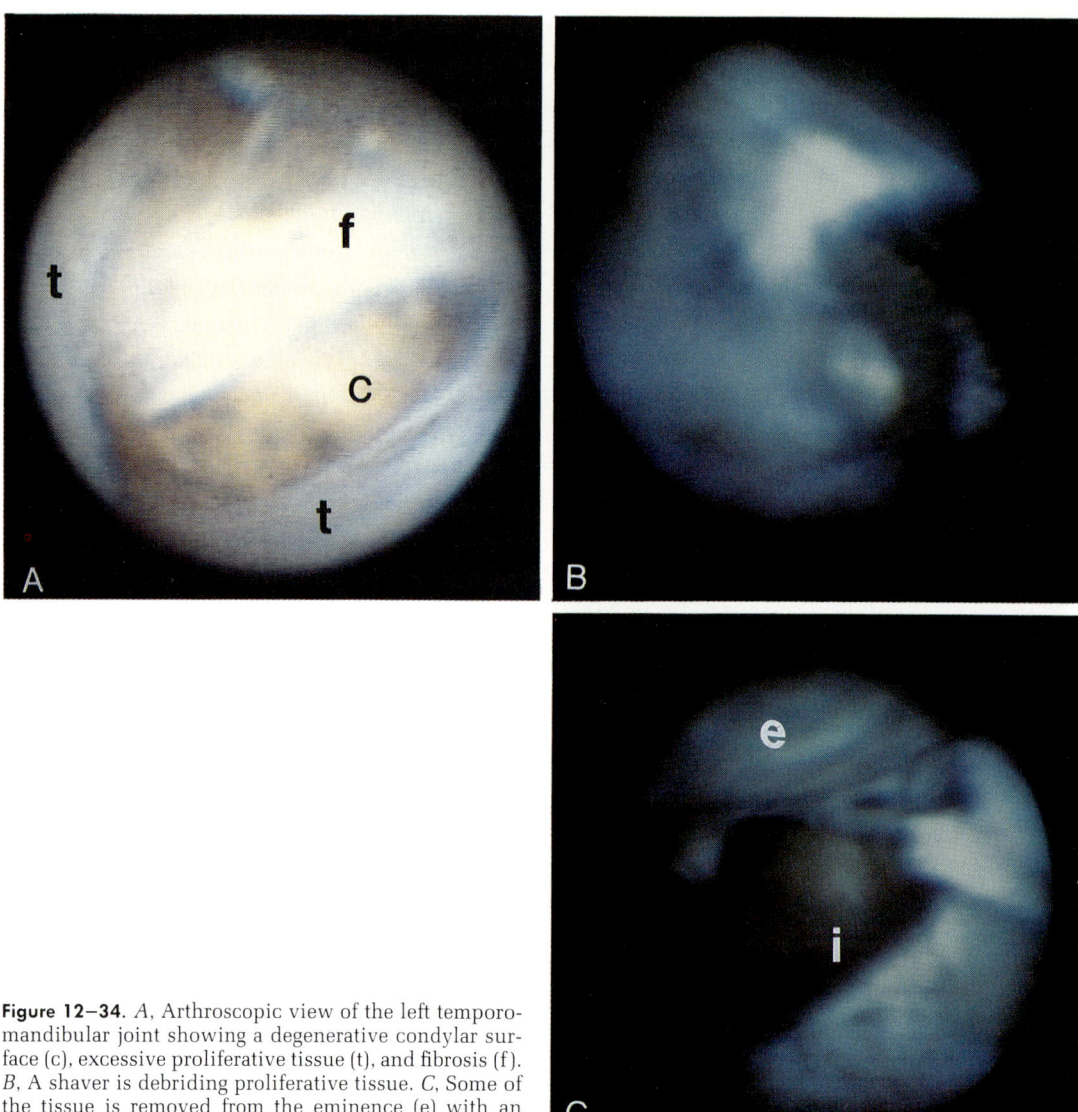

Figure 12-34. *A*, Arthroscopic view of the left temporomandibular joint showing a degenerative condylar surface (c), excessive proliferative tissue (t), and fibrosis (f). *B*, A shaver is debriding proliferative tissue. *C*, Some of the tissue is removed from the eminence (e) with an arthroscopic curette (i).

25% condylar roofing was noted. Rather extensive articular surface changes, adhesive capsulitis, and a well-formed, sheetlike anterior pouch adhesion were found (Fig. 12-35). The adhesion was lysed, utilizing hooked and blunt probes. The loose proliferative tissue fragments were removed by lavage.

SUMMARY

Arthroscopy provides valuable information that can confirm details of a patient's joint pathology. Thus, important diagnostic information is obtained utilizing a relatively innocuous, minimally invasive technique. A suitable treatment procedure can be selected in an attempt to correct the arthropathy. It is important to remember, however, that criteria must be established for the choice and application of each procedure, and followed rigorously, to avoid abuse of this modality.

References

1. Dolwick MF: Introductory Chapter. *In* Sanders B, Murakami K-I, Clark G (eds): Diagnostic and Surgical Arthroscopy of the Temporomandibular Joint. Philadelphia: WB Saunders, 1989, pp 1-3.

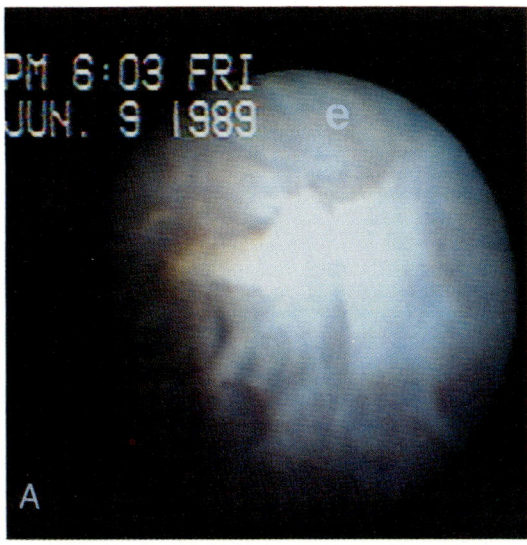 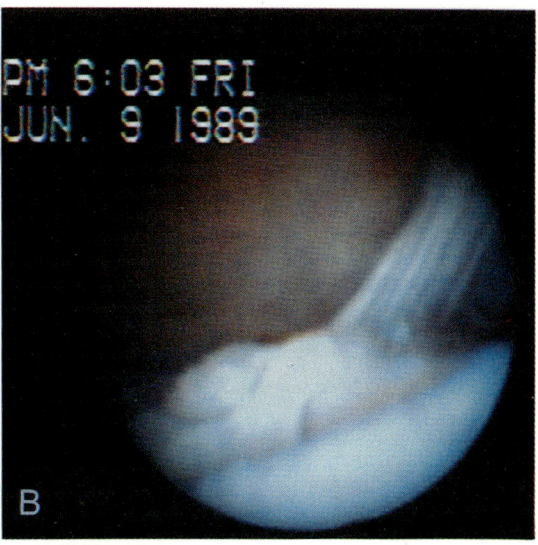

Figure 12–35. *A*, Articular surface degeneration, possibly chondromalacia, in the fossa and on the posterior slope of the eminence (e); *B*, a sheetlike adhesion in the anterior synovial pouch.

2. Dolwick MF, Nitzan DW: Temporomandibular joint arthroscopic lavage and lysis of adhesions: Preliminary report. New York: Third International Symposium on TMJ Arthroscopy, 1988.
3. Sanders B, Buoncristiani R: Diagnostic and surgical arthroscopy of the temporomandibular joint: Clinical experience with 137 clinical procedures over a 2-year period. J Craniomandib Disord 1:202–213, 1987.
4. Porter B, Zeitler D: A retrospective study of the therapeutic success of TMJ arthroscopic surgery. New York: Third International Symposium on TMJ Arthroscopy, 1988.
5. Wilkes CH: Internal derangements of the temporomandibular joint. Arch Otolaryngol Head Neck Surg 115:469–477, 1989.
6. Bronstein SL: Diagnostic and operative arthroscopy: Historical perspectives and indications. Maxillofac Surg Clin North Am. 1(1):59–68, 1989.
7. Bronstein SL: Diagnostic and surgical staging in the practice of TMJ arthroscopy. Proceedings, Arthroscopic Workshop, Pacific Clinical Research Foundation, La Jolla, California, September, 1989.
8. Berger J: Arthroscopic findings of acute temporomandibular joint trauma. New York: Third International Symposium on TMJ Arthroscopy, 1988.
9. Shahriaree H, Ericksen C: Arthroscopic instrumentation. *In* Shahriaree H (ed): O'Connor's Textbook of Arthroscopic Surgery. Philadelphia: JB Lippincott, 1984, p 23.
10. Fox JM, Ferkel RD: Use of electrosurgery in arthroscopic surgery. *In* Parisien JS (ed): Arthroscopic Surgery. New York: McGraw-Hill, 1988 pp 319–320.
11. Holmlund A, Hellsing G: Arthroscopy of the temporomandibular joint. Int J Oral Surg 14:169–175, 1985.
12. Murakami K-I, Ono T: Temporomandibular joint arthroscopy by inferolateral approach. J Oral Maxillofac Surg 15:410–417, 1986.
13. Moses J: Personal communication.
14. Greene MW, Hackney FL, Van Sickels JE: Arthroscopy of the temporomandibular joint: An anatomic perspective. J Oral Maxillofac Surg 47:386–389, 1989.
15. Westesson P-L, Eriksson L, Leidberg J: The risk of damage to the facial nerve, superficial temporal vessels, disk, and articular surfaces during arthroscopic examination of the temporomandibular joint. Oral Surg 62:124–127, 1986.
16. McCain JP: Arthroscopy of the human temporomandibular joint. J Oral Maxillofac Surg 46:648–655, 1988.
17. Van Sickels JE, Nishioka GJ, Hegewald MD, et al: Middle ear injury resulting from temporomandibular joint arthroscopy. J Oral Maxillofac Surg 45:962, 1987.
18. McCain J, de la Rua H, LeBlanc WG: Correlation of clinical, radiographic, and arthroscopic findings in internal derangements of the TMJ. J Oral Maxillofac Surg 47:913–921, 1989.
19. Quinn J: Proceedings, Third International Symposium on TMJ Arthroscopy. New York, December 1988.
20. Merrill R: Proceedings, Fourth International Symposium on TMJ Arthroscopy. Maui, Hawaii, 1989.
21. Montgomery MT, Van Sickels JE, Harms SE, Thrash WJ: Arthroscopic TMJ surgery: Effects on signs, symptoms and disc position. J Oral Maxillofac Surg 47:1263–1271, 1989.
22. Gabler MJ, Greene CS, Palacios EP, Perry HT: Effect of arthroscopic temporomandibular joint surgery on articular disk position. J Craniomandib Disord Fac Oral Pain 3:191–202, 1989.
23. Moses JJ, Sartoris D, Glass R, et al: The effect of arthroscopic surgical lysis and lavage of the superior joint space on TMJ disc position and mobility. J Oral Maxillofac Surg 47:674–678, 1989.
24. Bronstein SL: Starch synovitis of the TMJ treated by arthroscopic debridement: A case report. J Craniomandib Disord Fac Oral Pain 2:1, 9–12; 1988.

■ Chapter 13

SPECIAL APPLICATIONS
☐ A. Arthroscopic Procedures to Increase Disc Mobility

ALLEN W. TARRO, D.M.D.

In symptomatic temporomandibular joints (TMJs), the mobility of the disc is a critical factor. Disc mobility usually reflects the degree of translatory motion in the superior joint space. Decreased disc mobility may influence or be influenced by the lubrication in the joint from the synovial fluid, inflammation, and degradation of the cartilage in the joint. The exact mechanisms of these events are not fully understood. However, knowledge at the cellular and biochemical level is increasing and may explain these events and their sequence in the future. Adding to the complexity of the problem are the effects of hereditary influences, trauma-inducing stress and parafunctional habits, and individual accommodations. One example of an accommodation is the fibrous remodeling of the posterior attachment area that occurs in some TMJs.[1] This may be partly the reason why some individuals with anteriorly displaced discs do not have pain or jaw dysfunction.

In spite of the many variable factors and etiologies that may be involved, decreased disc mobility is frequently observed arthroscopically in symptomatic TMJs. One of the major treatment objectives of TMJ arthroscopy in these cases is to increase disc mobility. Disc mobility can be evaluated by observing the movement of the disc arthroscopically as the mandible is opened and closed and manipulated in various excursions. Furthermore, the relationship of the disc to the posterior slope of the articular eminence with the mandible in a closed position will show any disc displacement, if present. If the disc is displaced, the mandible is manipulated between open and closed positions with arthroscopic visualization of the disc and the posterior slope of the eminence to determine if the disc has a reducing or nonreducing displacement. As previously noted, limited mobility of the disc is a common finding with anterior disc displacement (Fig. 13–1). The disc must be carefully evaluated concerning its shape, length, and pathologic findings such as surface tears or perforations. Then, any adhesions, if present, should be lysed with blunt instruments, cut with arthroscopic scissors, or removed by a suction punch or a motorized cutting instrument. Adhesions are covered elsewhere in this text; however, a truly functional adhesion (Fig. 13–2A and B), limiting disc mobility, is presented for continuity here.

After the removal of adhesions, and if disc mobility is still limited, arthroscopic examination is focused in the anterior recess to evaluate the tissue anterior to the disc (Fig. 13–3). A blunt, hooked probe is used to palpate the tissue in this area and to remove any pseudowalls in the anterior recess, if they are present. Disc mobility is evaluated again, as the mandible is manipulated. If disc mobility remains unacceptable, some tissue anterior to the disc will be incised. This will increase disc mobility and afford a more posterior positioning of the anteriorly displaced disc. The procedure, first performed by McCain, was termed an "anterior muscle release" because some fibers of the superior head of the

A. Arthroscopic Procedures to Increase Disc Mobility

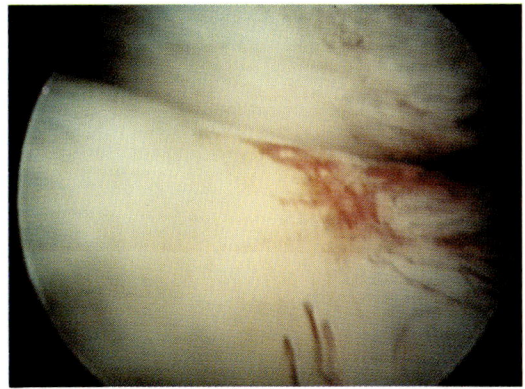

Figure 13–1. Arthroscopic view of anteriorly displaced disc: posterior attachment tissue (bottom right) is shown below the posterior slope of the articular eminence (upper right). The disc (posterior portion, bottom left) is positioned below the anterior slope of the articular eminence.

lateral pterygoid muscle were incised. In removing tissue anterior to the disc, my experience has been that, in some cases, only dense connective tissue was incised to adequately increase disc mobility. In these cases, the procedure is termed an "anterior band release."

The anterior band or muscle release procedure is performed with two cannulas in the anterior recess area. With direct arthroscopic visualization, tissue is incised anterior to the disc with arthroscopic scissors (Fig. 13–4A and B) or a 90-degree electrocautery tip used in the cutting mode (Figs. 13–5 and 13–6). The procedure is facilitated by making cannula insertions through the skin about 20 mm apart in order to approach a 90-degree triangulation with the two cannulas. It must be emphasized that the tissue incised should be anterior to the disc and performed only with clear arthroscopic visualization. The amount of tissue incised should be adequate to release the anterior hold of the disc. However, surgical discretion must be exercised so that a perforation is not made into the inferior joint space or that the disc is not completely severed from its anterior attachments. The use of arthroscopic scissors offers fine control but often produces some hemorrhage from incised blood vessels. These small bleeders should be cauterized with a straight,

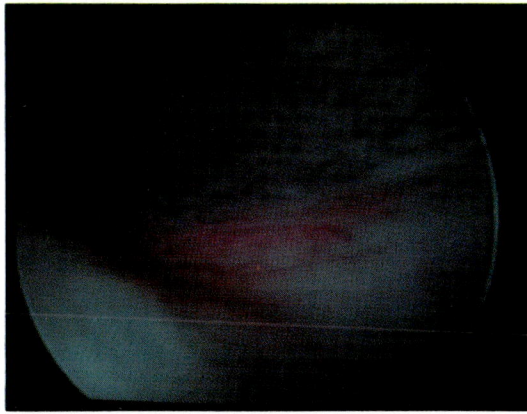

Figure 13–3. Arthroscopic view of anterior recess area; the anterior portion of the disc is shown in the lower left. Note that there is significant inflammation in the anterior recess synovium.

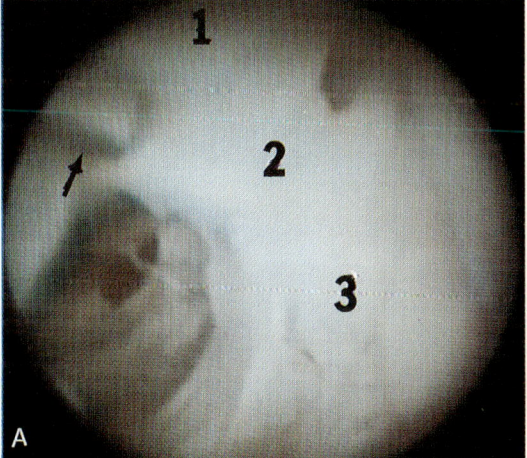
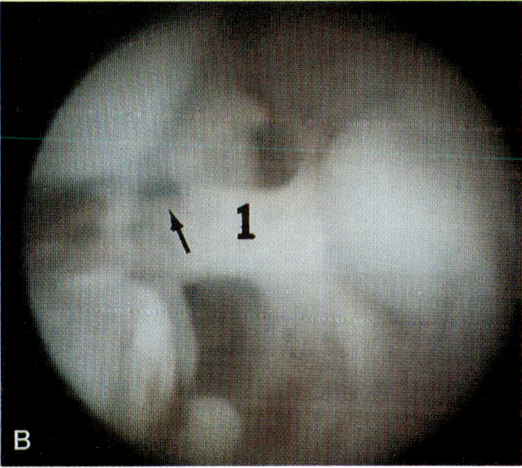

Figure 13–2. *A,* Strong adhesion (2) beginning to be stretched by probe (*arrow*). The adhesion is attaching the disc (1) to the glenoid fossa (3). *B,* Extreme stretching of adhesion (1) by probe (*arrow*) just prior to lysing the adhesion.

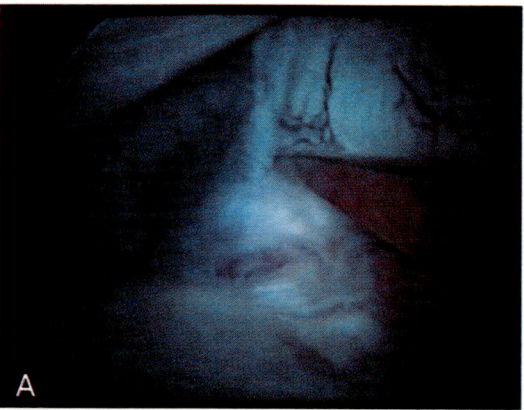

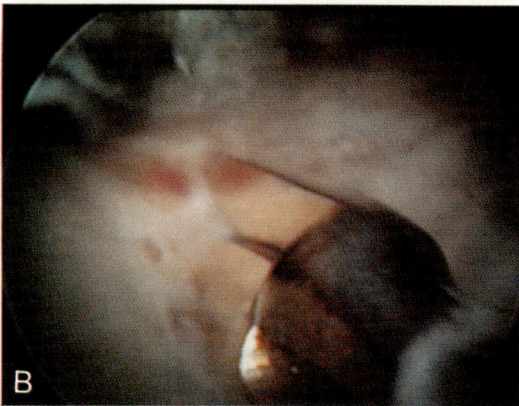

Figure 13-4. *A* and *B*, Sequence of arthroscopic photographs showing scissors incising tissue anterior to the disc to increase disc mobility. (Gold-colored scissors are the improved version of this instrument from Walter Lorenz Surgical Instruments, Inc., Jacksonville, FL.)

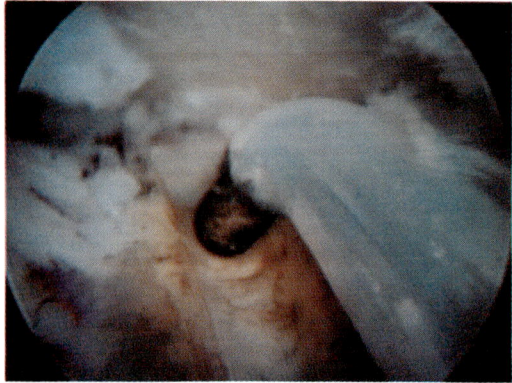

Figure 13-5. Photograph of a 90-degree angled electrocautery tip used to perform an anterior release. This view is in the anterior recess area, showing the initial trough made by the electrocautery tip. (Cautery tip by Concept, Inc., Largo, FL.)

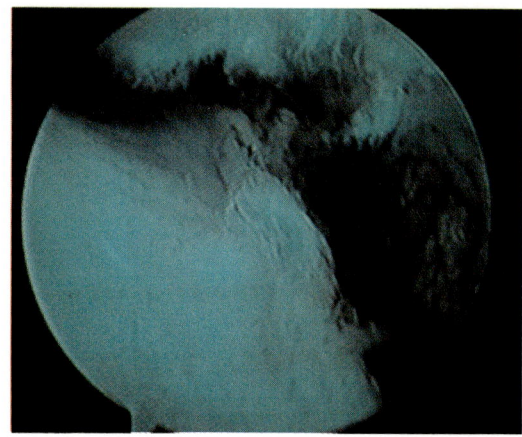

Figure 13-6. Arthroscopic view of a completed anterior release procedure performed with electrocautery (the most anterior portion of the disc is shown on the left).

blunt arthroscopic electrocautery tip in order to achieve hemostasis, which is a very important consideration in TMJ arthroscopic surgery.

Some types of arthroscopic scissors are delicate and have broken inside the joint during surgery.[2] This has occurred in my experience in two cases during arthroscopic surgery. In each case, a 3.0-mm diameter magnetic retriever with attached suction (Acufex No. 011503, Acufex Microsurgical, Inc., Norwood, MA) was employed successfully to remove the broken instrument fragment, with no joint damage. The original instruments of this type that have broken (scissors, tissue-grasping forceps, and biopsy forceps from Walter Lorenz Surgical Instruments, Inc., Jacksonville, FL) have been redesigned by the manufacturer and utilize more corrosion-resistant metals. These changes should prevent occurrence of this problem in the future. It is strongly recommended, however, that the working ends of these instruments be tested for their integrity each time before they are used.

In some cases, usually involving deep joints, it may be difficult to properly position arthroscopic scissors to incise an adequate amount of tissue anterior to the disc. In these cases, electrocautery with a 90-degree cutting tip (Concept, Inc., Largo, FL) has been utilized under continuous, high-flow irrigation to perform successfully the anterior muscle or band release procedure. In some cases, the arthroscopic scissors were used initially to incise some tissue anterior to the disc; the 90-degree electrocautery tip was then used to incise deeper tissue. It is important to incise adequately tissue on the medial aspect of this incision anterior to the disc, because many disc displacements are medial as well as anterior.

An additional consideration in disc mobility is the effect of the lateral capsule attachments. The lateral capsule release advocated by Moses involves stretching the lateral capsule and lysing some fibers with blunt instrumentation through an endaural approach.[3] Although worthy of consideration, stretching the lateral capsule is almost certainly accomplished by the movement of cannulas from the posterior to anterior recesses and vice versa during arthroscopic diagnoses and arthroscopic surgical procedures.

After procedures are performed to increase disc mobility, copious TMJ lavage through the inflow-outflow irrigation system is utilized to remove loose tissue remnants and other contaminants. The disc is then positioned posteriorly, aided by the use of a blunt, hooked probe in the retrodiscal cul-de-sac. Finally, a disc stabilizing suture technique is used to temporarily secure the more posterior position of the disc (see Chapter 13E).[4]

A pertinent question is whether posterior positioning and temporary stabilization of displaced discs are necessary when they have been increased in mobility by the various procedures previously discussed. It is apparent from my experience and the experience of a number of TMJ arthroscopists that some successful results have been attained by increasing disc mobility without posterior repositioning and stabilization of displaced discs.[5-8] Furthermore, it may not always be possible arthroscopically to "reduce" displaced discs to the "normal" position between the fibrocartilage surfaces of the glenoid fossa and condyle with 100% roofing of the disc over the articulating portion of the condyle. On the other hand, there have been cases with unacceptable results when more posterior positioning and stabilization of the displaced discs were not performed.[4] Certainly it does not seem reasonable to expect TMJ lavage alone to achieve a long-term resolution of symptoms in cases of anterior disc displacement. Lysis and lavage have been performed with good results in cases of closed lock internal derangements with adhesive capsulitis.[9] This technique also may afford successful treatment in cases involving functional adhesions that limit disc mobility. However, functional adhesions are not found in the majority of cases involving symptomatic anteriorly displaced discs. Additionally, fibrous remodeling of the posterior attachment does not occur in all TMJs. It is known that the avascular fibrocartilage of the TMJ is nourished by the synovial fluid. Whether this occurs actively or passively has not been fully determined. If the nourishment is accomplished by active compression of properly aligned articulating surfaces of the cartilage, then posterior disc positioning and stabilization are very important.

In symptomatic TMJs with decreased disc mobility and anterior disc displacement, it is the prevalent opinion of many experienced TMJ arthroscopists that a major objective is to increase the mobility of the disc. When this has been accomplished by various arthroscopic surgical procedures, it seems reasonable to position the disc posteriorly and to stabilize temporarily the more posterior position of the disc.[10] There have been no reported failures of TMJ arthroscopic treatment that have occurred solely because an anteriorly displaced disc was positioned and stabilized temporarily in a more posterior position. Furthermore, the history of medicine and dentistry has consistently shown that "form and function go hand in hand." Therefore, it seems that if the surgeon has the ability to perform these procedures,[11] there is nothing to lose and, most likely, successful results to be gained.[10]

References

1. Blaustein D, Heffez L: Diagnostic arthroscopy of the temporomandibular joint. Part II. Arthroscopic findings of arthrographically diagnosed disk displacements. Oral Surg Oral Med Oral Pathol 65:135, 1988.
2. Tarro A: Instrument breakage associated with arthroscopy of the temporomandibular joint: Report of a case. J Oral Maxillofac Surg 47:1226, 1989.
3. Moses J, Poker I: TMJ arthroscopic surgery: An analysis of 237 patients. J Oral Maxillofac Surg 47:790, 1989.
4. Tarro A: Arthroscopic treatment of anterior disc displacement: a preliminary report. J Oral Maxillofac Surg 47:353, 1989.
5. Sanders B, Buoncristiani R: Diagnostic and surgical arthroscopy of the temporomandibular joint: Clinical experience with 137 procedures over a 2-year period. J Craniomandib Disords Facial Oral Pain 1:202, 1987.

6. Tarro A: Arthroscopic diagnosis and surgery of the temporomandibular joint. J Oral Maxillofac Surg 46:282, 1988.
7. Indresano A: Arthroscopic surgery of the temporomandibular joint: Report of 64 patients with long-term follow-up. J Oral Maxillofac Surg 47:439, 1989.
8. White R: Retrospective analysis of 100 consecutive surgical arthroscopies of the temporomandibular joint. J Oral Maxillofac Surg 47:1014, 1989.
9. Sanders B: Arthroscopic surgery of the temporomandibular joint: Treatment of internal derangement with persistent closed lock. Oral Surg Oral Med Oral Pathol 62:361, 1986.
10. Tarro A: TMJ arthroscopic diagnosis and surgery: clinical experience with 152 procedures over a 2½ year period. J Craniomandib Pract. In press.
11. Merrill R: Discussion [related to an article on TMJ arthroscopic lysis and lavage]. J Oral Maxillofac Surg 48:802, 1990.

□ B. Endaural Arthroscopic Approach

JEFFREY J. MOSES, D.D.S.

Arthroscopy of the temporomandibular joint (TMJ) is gaining popularity internationally both as a diagnostic tool and as a therapeutic mode for procedures involving internal joint derangement and intracapsular dysfunctional pathology. Many of the surgical techniques proposed have yet to demonstrate scientifically substantiated results over the long term; however, the initial reports seem promising, and continuing clinical research is under way.[1,2]

The endaural approach, discussed here, gives the diagnostician and surgeon extended access to lateral and medial joint pathologies. Because many of our radiology imaging procedures cannot accurately visualize early lateral capsular synovial proliferations (see Fig. 13–10), capsular herniations (Fig. 13–7), and discal impingements (see Fig. 16–1), capsular access can become an important diagnostic tool in these and other conditions. This aids the surgeon immensely by providing alternative portals by which to achieve more effective triangulation.

Since Ohnishi[3] first described the application of arthroscopy to the TMJ, it has become a valuable tool in the management of TMJ dysfunction.[4,5] The endaural puncture was originally described by Ohnishi.[6-8] Although many techniques for entering this joint have been advocated, the four approaches described as follows have been most widely used (Fig. 13–8).

Superior Posterolateral Approach (Inferolateral).[9] In this technique, the mandible is distracted downward and forward, producing a triangular depression in the front of the tragus. This depression represents an area bordered superiorly by the glenoid fossa, anteroinferiorly by the dorsal aspect of the condylar head, and posteriorly by the external auditory canal. It is within this depression, 1 cm from the anterior aspect of the tragus, that the trocar is inserted. The tip is directed anterosuperiorly 45 degrees to all planes, aiming toward the posterior slope of the eminence. This permits placement of the trocar into the superior joint space and allows examination of the superior joint space. The areas that are difficult to visualize are the superior anterior

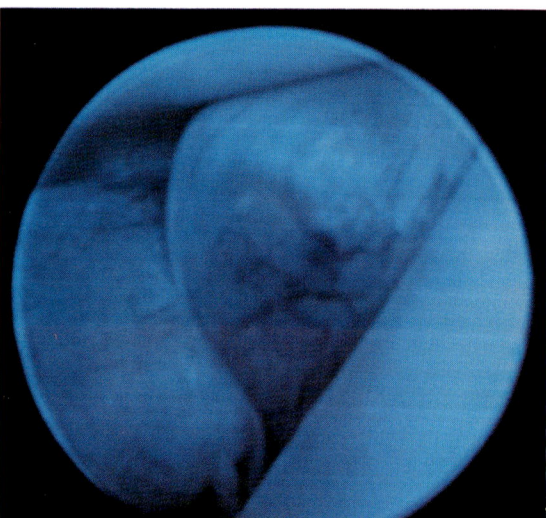

Figure 13–7. Capsular herniation noted in the medial wall of a right temporomandibular joint.

B. Endaural Arthroscopic Approach ■ 193

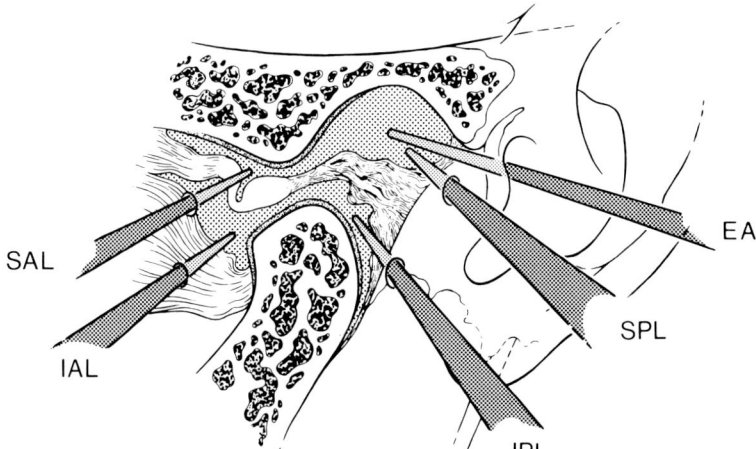

Figure 13–8. Arthroscopic approaches to the temporomandibular joint. SAL = superior anterolateral; IAL = inferior anterolateral; IPL = inferior posterolateral; SPL = superior posterolateral; EA = endaural.

synovial pouch and the medial paradiscal synovial groove.

Inferior Posterolateral Approach.[10] This is a variation of the inferolateral approach in that the trocar is directed against the lateral posterior surface of the mandibular head. The inferior posterior synovial pouch and posterior condylar surface can then be examined.

Superior Anterolateral Approach. In this technique, the trocar is directed superiorly, posteriorly, and medially along the anterior slope of the articular eminence after first locating the prominence of the lateral articular tubercle as a landmark. The mandibular condyle is distracted inferiorly and positioned posteriorly by the surgical assistant. This approach allows anterosuperior joint compartment instrumentation or visualization.

Inferior Anterolateral Approach.[10] This is a technically more difficult approach than those described previously and allows observation of the lower anterior synovial pouch. In this technique, the condylar head and articular tubercle are palpated. The trocar is then inserted at a point anterior to the lateral pole of the condylar head and immediately below the articular tubercle. This places the trocar in the lower anterior synovial pouch adjacent to the anterior aspect of the condylar head. The technique allows observation of the lower anterior synovial pouch.

ENDAURAL APPROACH—RATIONALE AND TECHNIQUE

Certain limitations have become evident using the traditional posterolateral and anterolateral arthroscopic approaches to the TMJ. This is especially true for visualization of the lateral trough and anterolateral joint space or where access for instrumentation to the medial and lateral paradiscal grooves is required. Clear visualization of these areas is impeded using the currently available 15-degree angled scopes and lateral portals.

To solve these visualization and access problems, the endaural entry portal provides clear visualization and enhances instrumentation to the medial and, especially, the lateral spaces (Figs. 13–9 and 13–10).[11] This new approach also provides better access for the retrieval of loose bodies and broken instruments. Working with the arthroscope in the endaural portal permits access to other portals for instrumentation.

In order to perform this technique, a 30-degree angled arthroscope is recommended, which increases the panoramic visualization of the joint. The off-axis viewing angulation changes as the scope is rotated and permits a more comprehensive examination of the TMJ in areas difficult to examine with the conventional 15-degree arthroscopes. In order to visualize the lateral capsule and attachment areas, it is important to obtain an arthroscope that has the visual axis oriented toward the light cord, preventing the impediment of having the light cord forced against the patient's temporal area. Because this is a deviation from the usual manufacturer's product, it must be specifically requested during the ordering process.

For the surgeon inexperienced in this technique, it is best initially to penetrate the superior joint space from the standard superior posterolateral approach. Once this has

194 ■ 13 Special Applications

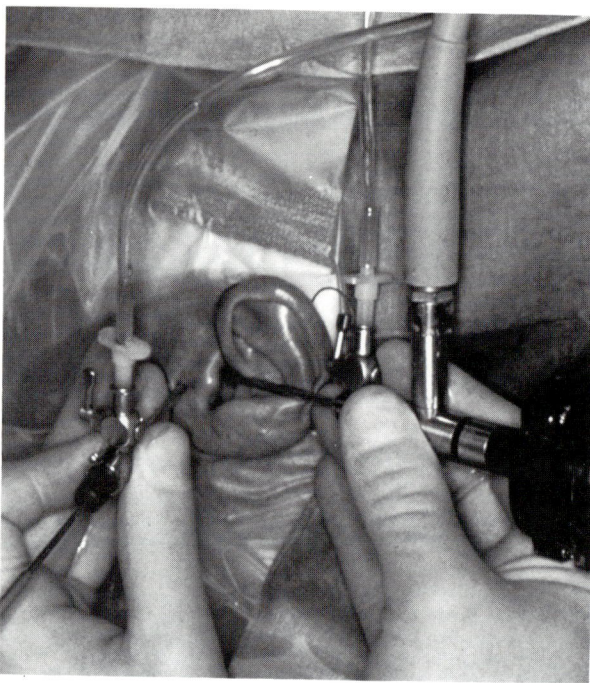

Figure 13–9. Clinical view of an arthroscope in the temporomandibular joint, which has been placed through the endaural portal. The working portal is now located in the superior posterolateral location.

been accomplished, the arthroscope is then rotated and angled superiorly, posteriorly, and laterally so that the light shines through the anterior wall of the external auditory canal (Fig. 13–11). This spot usually is located approximately 1 to 1.5 cm medial to the lateral edge of the tragus in the external auditory canal (Fig. 13–12). While the mandible is distracted downward and forward, the anterior wall of the external auditory canal is perforated with the sharp trocar and 30-degree arthroscopic cannula. The cannula and trocar are angled anterosuperiorly and slightly medially, perpendicular to the posterior slope of the articular eminence. Most important, these instruments enter into the joint above the level of the arthroscope, in order to ensure superior compartment puncture (Fig. 13–13). Penetration should be carried to a depth no greater than 1.5 cm, using the cannula markings as a guide. Visual confirmation of the penetration into the joint space can then be made using the arthroscope, which has been placed in the inferolateral portal. Additional confirmation that the endaural cannula tip lies within the superior joint space can be ascertained when removal of the trocar results in an outflow of irrigation fluid from the endaural cannula. The arthroscope, with the attached fiberoptic cable and inflow tubing, can then be removed from the inferolateral cannula and connected to the endaural cannula. The inferolateral cannula can then be sealed off with a rubber cap to prevent excessive outflow when the TMJ is being irrigated, and the cannula can be utilized as a working portal while visualization is accomplished via the endaural portal.

By rotating the arthroscope, the medial, lateral, and superior aspects of the TMJ can be examined. This approach is especially

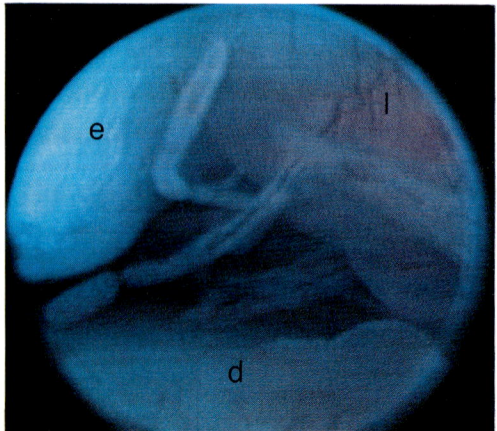

Figure 13–10. Arthroscopic view of right temporomandibular joint through an endaural portal of villonodular synovitis. e = eminence; d = disc; l = lateral capsule.

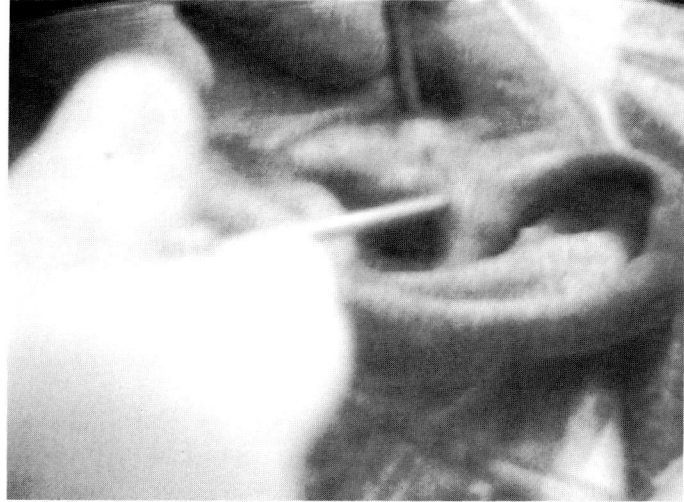

Figure 13–11. The arthroscope via the inferolateral portal is angled so that the light from the scope is transilluminated through the tragal cartilage, identifying the site for endaural puncture into the joint.

helpful in visualizing the anterolateral synovial space, which is difficult to do from either the superior posterolateral or anterolateral portal (Fig. 13–14). This technique also allows the superior posterolateral or anterolateral portal to be used for the instrumentation if necessary (Figs. 13–13 and 13–15).

As skill is acquired, direct puncture through the anterior wall of the external auditory canal into the TMJ can be performed after initial joint distention, without the need for superior posterolateral cannulation. Following the arthroscopic surgical procedure, the lateral puncture site receives pressure and round Band-Aid dressings. No sutures are necessary. The endaural puncture is difficult to dress and is left as is. Usually, if there is minimal manipulation through this portal, the cartilaginous elastic memory of the canal serves to close the puncture site. A routine otoscopic examination is always made following arthroscopy to visualize the external acoustic meatus and tympanic membrane in order to confirm that no iatrogenic damage has been caused by the procedure.

DISCUSSION

Thus far, at our facility, more than 120 patients have been treated with the endaural puncture arthroscopic technique, combined with the superior posterolateral and anterolateral techniques. To date there have been three cases of otitis externa. Each of these resolved with therapy with Cortisporin suspension, which is now prescribed prophylactically during the first 3 days after arthroscopy. It is believed that these cases were directly related to inadequate external auditory canal skin preparation. Placement of a cotton ball in the canal during the surgical skin preparation was abandoned, requiring the outer half of the canal to be prepared with cotton-tipped applicators. A small cottonoid sponge is placed after draping. To date, no complications have occurred with the procedure.

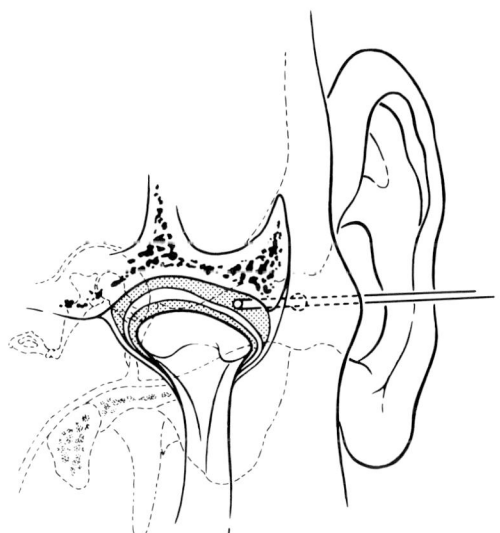

Figure 13–12. Diagram indicating approximate site of puncture for the endaural approach. Coronal section is positioned just anterior to the cartilaginous meatus and tragus.

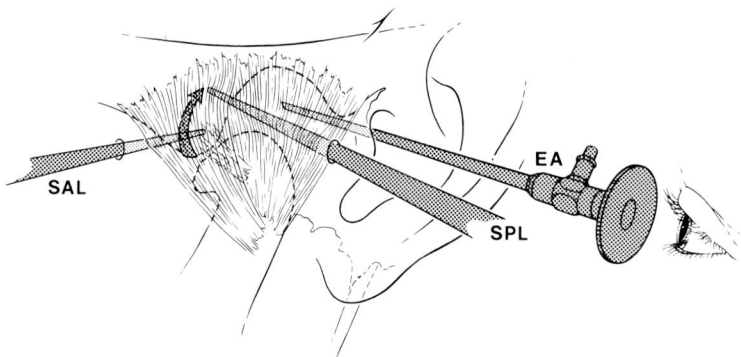

Figure 13–13. Diagram of puncture into the temporomandibular joint. The trocar and cannula (EA) are directed anterosuperiorly and medially, perpendicular to the posterior slope of the articular eminence and above the inferolateral cannula (SPL). SAL = superior anterolateral. The probes located in either of the working portals, SAL or SPL, may now be used for the lateral eminence release and the capsular stretch (see arrows).

However, there is still concern regarding abnormal anatomy, combined with the anatomic pitfalls of the bony auditory canal (Fig. 13–16A) and inadvertent damage to the tympanic membrane and ossicles. Because in some patients this bony canal may extend laterally farther than is common, the canal conceivably could be mistaken for the glenoid fossa and articular eminence, thereby leading to trocar placement into the middle ear. This has been described,[12, 13] occurring during a superior posterolateral approach. However, it has been my experience that if one starts from within the cartilaginous ear

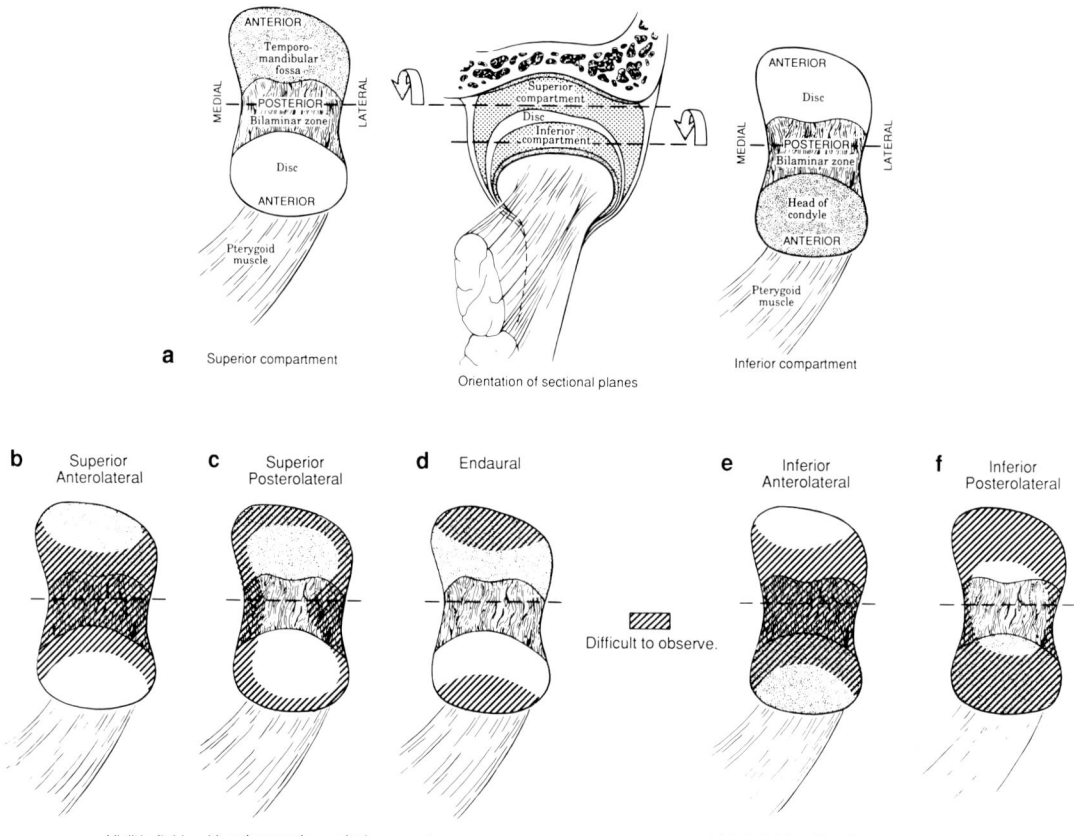

Figure 13–14. Visible fields with the various arthroscopic approaches; oriented to the left temporomandibular joint (TMJ) with the roof of the TMJ folded upward. Areas depicted with diagonal lines are difficult to observe arthroscopically.

B. Endaural Arthroscopic Approach ■ 197

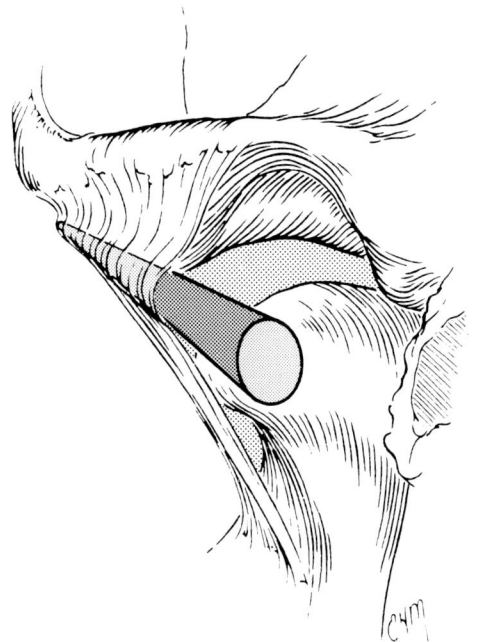

Figure 13–15. Diagram showing lateral eminence release.

canal and works one's way forward into the superior joint compartment, this is unlikely to occur. It is also suggested that the surgeon make attempts to direct the puncture more to the lateral third of the canal (Fig. 13–17), both for safety reasons and to enhance movement of the cannula along the lateral areas and throughout the TMJ. The use of an angled 30-degree arthroscope must be emphasized in order to facilitate triangulation.

SUMMARY

The endaural approach to the TMJ overcomes some of the drawbacks associated with the commonly employed superior posterolateral and anterolateral approaches (Table 13–1). The technique allows improved visualization and access to instrumentation, especially to the lateral and medial joint troughs, as well as to the anterolateral region of the superior joint space, areas difficult to access using previously described tech-

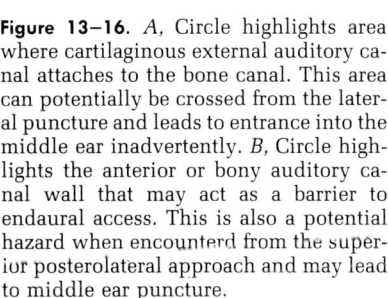

Figure 13–16. *A*, Circle highlights area where cartilaginous external auditory canal attaches to the bone canal. This area can potentially be crossed from the lateral puncture and leads to entrance into the middle ear inadvertently. *B*, Circle highlights the anterior or bony auditory canal wall that may act as a barrier to endaural access. This is also a potential hazard when encountered from the superior posterolateral approach and may lead to middle ear puncture.

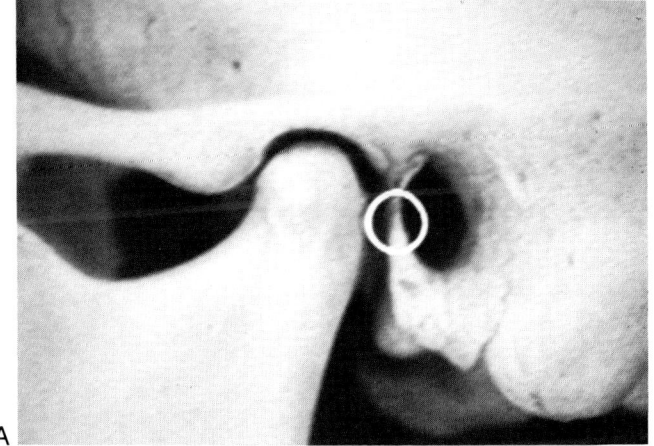

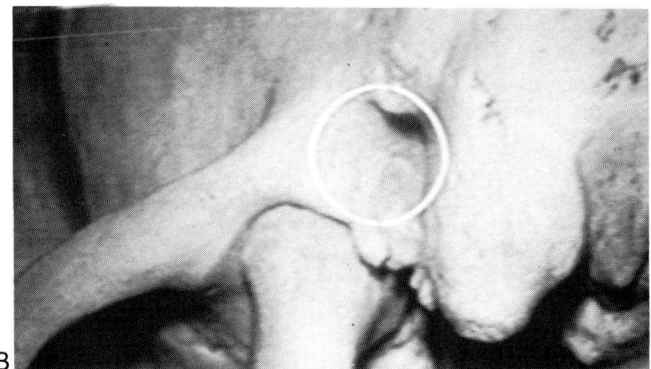

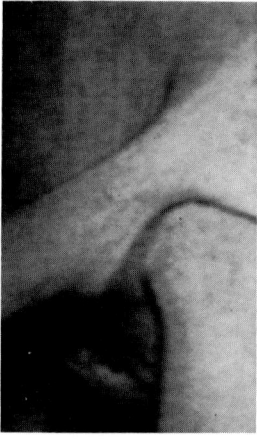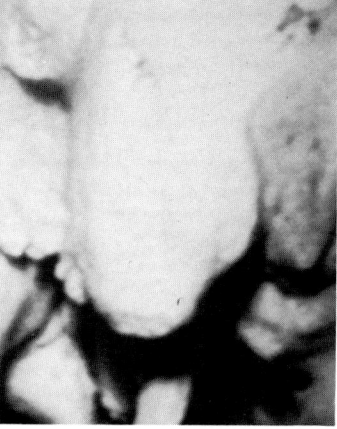

Figure 13–17. The line designates that area where the cartilaginous canal attaches to the bony canal. The endaural puncture is best attempted lateral to this line (shaded), allowing access along the lateral third of the temporomandibular joint.

Table 13–1. ADVANTAGES AND DISADVANTAGES OF THE ENDAURAL APPROACH

Advantages
1. Better visualization of medial and lateral troughs.
2. Allows an additional portal to be used for visualization or instrumentation.
3. Better access for the retrieval of broken instruments and the retrieval of loose bodies.

Disadvantages
1. Requires added instrumentation.
2. Requires increased operator skill.
3. Added puncture site increasing risk of iatrogenic intra-articular joint damage.
4. Possible increased incidence of chondritis postoperatively.

Contraindications
1. Otitis externa.
2. Abnormal anatomy of the external auditory canal.

niques. This practice has allowed better correlative observations of the lateral impingement phenomenon occurring in the lateral superior joint space. Triangulation, and therefore the type of surgery performed, and the results achieved have been greatly facilitated using the endaural approach.

References

1. Moses J, Poker I: TMJ arthoscopic surgery—an analysis of 237 patients. J Oral Maxillofac Surg 47:790–794, 1989.
2. Moses J, Poker I: Correlation studies of effects of the TMJ arthroscopic surgical lysis of superior joint compartment adhesions and lavage. J Oral Maxillofac Surg 47:674–678, 1989.
3. Ohnishi M.: Arthroscopy of the temporomandibular joint. Kokubyu Gakkai Zasshi J Japan Stomatol Soc 42:207–213, 1975.
4. Sanders B: Arthroscopic surgery of the temporomandibular joint: Treatment of internal derangement with persistent closed lock. Oral Surg 62:361–372, 1975.
5. Sanders B, Buoncristiani R: Diagnostic and surgical arthroscopy of the temporomandibular joint: Clinical experience with 137 procedures over a two year period. J Craniomandib Disord Fac Oral Pain 1:202–213, 1987.
6. Ohnishi M: Kokubyu Gakkai Zasshi J Japan Stomatol Soc 31:487–512, 1982.
7. Ohnishi M: Arthroscopy 9:43–48, 1984.
8. Ohnishi M: Proceedings of the Symposium on TMJ Arthroscopy. Southern California OMFS Foundation, 1986.
9. Murakami K, Takatoki O: Temporomandibular joint arthroscopy by inferolateral approach. Int J Oral Surg 15:410–417, 1986.
10. Watanabe M: Arthroscopy of the temporomandibular joint. In Arthroscopy of Small Joints: New York: Igaku Shoin, 1985.
11. Moses J, Poker I: Temporomandibular Joint Arthroscopy—the Endaural Approach. Int J Oral Maxillofac Surg. Submitted for publication.
12. Merrill R: Personal communication.

C. Arthroscopic Biopsy of the Temporomandibular Joint

RALPH G. MERRILL, D.D.S., M.Sc.D.

Synovial and articular surface biopsy of the temporomandibular joint (TMJ) is an important adjunct to diagnostic and operative arthroscopy. The most reliable diagnosis is accomplished through integration of information gained by history, clinical examination, radiology, observation at surgery either by arthroscopy or arthrotomy, histopathology, and synovial fluid analysis and other laboratory assays. Diagnostic arthroscopy with the judicious use of biopsy offers an excellent method to enhance the accuracy of diagnosis, which can aid in nonsurgical and surgical decisions.

Arthroscopic evaluation affords the opportunity to observe directly under magnification the pathology of the synovium, the fibrocartilage of the disc and eminence, the vasculature, and the position and form of the disc. Holmlund[1] and Merrill and co-workers[2] have confirmed a high degree of accuracy of diagnosis by arthroscopic observations and histologic evaluation. Accuracy was high for findings of synovitis and osteoarthrosis in Holmlund's studies.

In our comparison[2] of arthroscopic observations and histologic findings from biopsies in the study of 67 TMJs, arthroscopic diagnosis of intra-articular tissue abnormalities was 89.1% accurate and 100% sensitive. Pathologic changes observed in a large series of TMJs included isolated patches of inflammation, diffuse synovitis, creeping synovitis over functional articular surfaces, petechia-like subsynovial lesions, hyperemia, hyperplastic synovium, nodular synovitis, fibrillations, single and multiple fibrous adhesions, fibrosis, lateral capsular prolapse with impingement, perforations, tears, articular chondromalacia (osteoarthrosis), foreign body reactions to implant material, and chondromatosis.

More than 200 types of arthropathy have been described.[3] Most of these, particularly the more commonly encountered types such as osteoarthritis and rheumatoid arthritis, are seen clinically with synovitis. Biopsy findings of the synovial membrane by arthroscopy usually provides a diagnosis of chronic nonspecific synovitis. Biopsy can provide very useful information about the more unusual types such as villonodular synovitis and chondromatosis. The question arises whether routine biopsy is indicated when synovitis is observed arthroscopically. It certainly confirms a clinical and arthroscopic diagnosis of synovitis, which can be helpful for documentation and treatment decisions; it can aid in differentiating the source of pain as being intra-articular or extra-articular. The degree of intra-articular pain is associated with the degree of synovitis. In bilateral TMJ arthroscopy studies, the most painful side has the most significant synovitis. Cases in which synovitis is absent and disc position is normal usually have a masticatory muscle source of pain or referral of pain from other sources in the head and neck.

In the 67 TMJs in our study,[2] 31 had synovitis and 11 had synovial hyperplasia. Of the 31 TMJs with synovitis, 24 exhibited moderate to severe synovitis (Fig. 13–18), which was correlated with histopathology. The remaining seven were judged arthroscopically to have mild synovitis, but did not show synovitis histologically.

Most of the TMJs examined had delicate, single, or multiple adhesions. Dense adhesions were noted in nine, and four of these were around perforations. Biopsy revealed

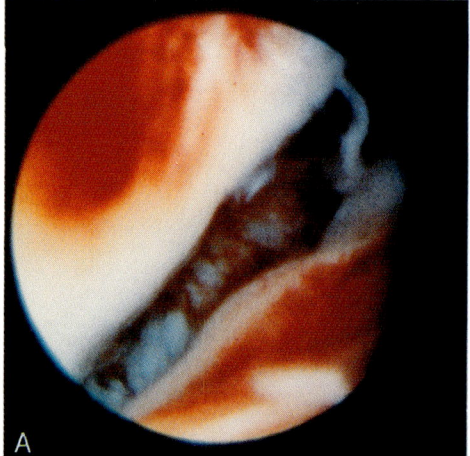

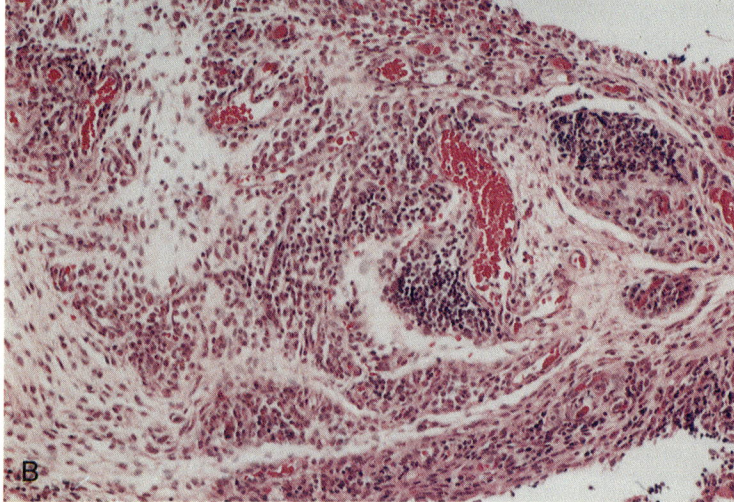

Figure 13–18. *A*, Arthroscopic view in the posterior synovial pouch of the superior temporomandibular joint compartment of severe synovitis with hyperemia, increased vascularity, and fibrous adhesions. *B*, Severe synovitis with increased vascularity, intimal cell hyperplasia, and lymphocytic and plasma cell perivascular infiltrate. (Hematoxylin and eosin; ×400.)

increased collagen fibers and hyalinization. Chondroid formation was noted in a few specimens, which could represent a precursor to bony ankylosis. Nine of the joints studied had previously placed alloplastic implants. The arthroscopic appearance of foreign-body granuloma was a reddish, vascular, friable, irregular proliferation of tissue surrounding the condyle. Histologically, foreign-body giant cells surrounded small particles of foreign material and an inflammatory infiltrate. The structure of three TMJs examined by arthroscopy were normal in appearance; biopsies in the retrodiscal synovium revealed normal histologic patterns. Arthroscopic observations of moderate to severe synovitis, hyperplastic synovium, adhesions, and foreign body granulomas were accurate. Biopsy and histologic examination of these and other questionable lesions are appropriate.

EXAMINATION AND BIOPSY PROCEDURES

A single cannula approach and a 19-gauge outflow needle are usually adequate to perform an arthroscopic diagnostic examination and biopsy of synovial and articular pathology. The "half-blind" technique described by Murakami[4] is adequate to obtain most biopsy samples with a hand instrument, such as basket forceps (Fig. 13–19). Triangulation by a double-puncture technique with the use of an anterior working cannula allows direct observation of the biopsy procedure (Fig. 13–20). The working arthroscope designed by

C. Arthroscopic Biopsy of the Temporomandibular Joint ■ 201

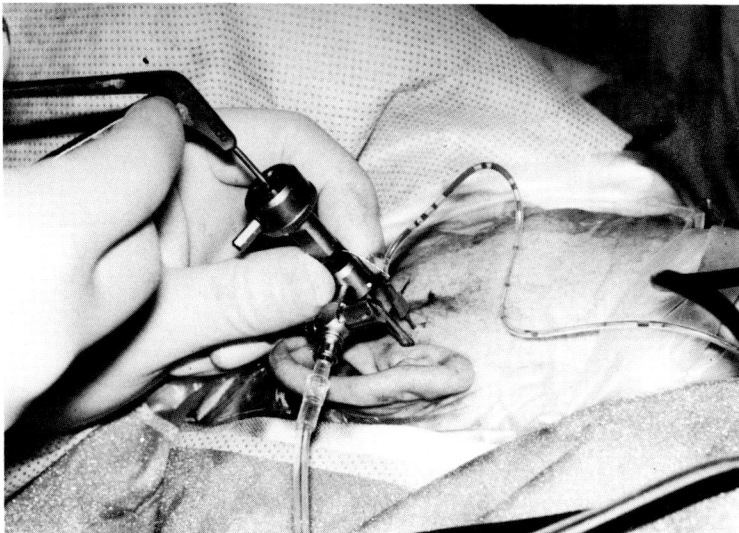

Figure 13–19. A lesion has been identified with the scope. The cannula is held stationary while the scope is removed and a basket forceps placed to take a biopsy using the "half-blind" technique.

Ohnishi[5] utilizes a single puncture and permits direct observation of the use of hand instruments.

The examination of the superior joint compartment is made in a systematic way. The assistant holds the mandible in a forward and distracted position. It is convenient to start the examination and video recording at the posterosuperior attachment of the superior lamina of the retrodiscal tissues. The retrodiscal tissue is examined first, from medial to lateral, and then the fossa, from lateral to medial. The medial capsule comes into view and is examined along the medial paradiscal groove. One then advances the arthroscope from medial to lateral, observing the posterior slope of the eminence and the posterior discal eminence or the retrodiscal tissue eminence interface if the disc is displaced. The lateral capsule, lateral articular eminence, disc, and lateral paradiscal groove are encountered next. The assistant then gently manipulates the condyle into the fossa. The arthroscope is advanced into the anterolateral pouch for examination of the area. Capsular fibrosis and pseudowall formation will at times limit this maneuver to the anterior synovial pouch. The arthroscope is retracted into the posterior pouch, as the assistant moves the condyle inferiorly and anteriorly.

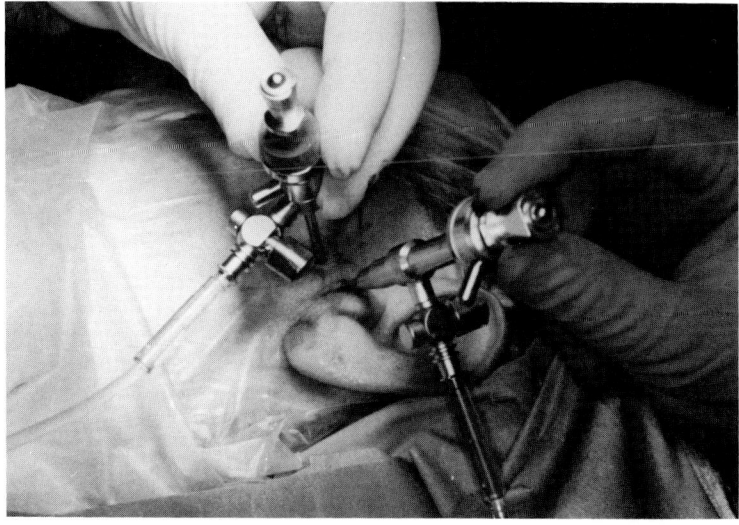

Figure 13–20. Direct visualization of the biopsy is possible by triangulation, using a double-puncture technique. A scope replaces the trocar in the posterior cannula and a basket forceps is exchanged for the trocar through the rubber cap of the anterior working cannula to obtain the biopsy.

The scope is placed near the entry point into the TMJ to examine motion and position of the disc while the assistant gently seats the condyle in the fossa and moves the condyle-disc complex forward and back across the articular eminence. Catching, interference, and degree of roofing or capping of the condyle by the disc are observed. The condyle is then distracted and positioned forward. The arthroscope is then advanced to the medial wall and into the medial paradiscal groove. The condyle is manipulated posteriorly and distracted by pressure over the molars. The arthroscope is moved next from medial to lateral within the anterior synovial pouch to observe the capsule and anterior discal tissues. Some adhesions can be lysed with this maneuver. Care must be taken to avoid damage to fibrocartilage of the eminence. Scuffing may occur with excessive force. The arthroscope is retracted again into the posterior pouch, and the condyle is moved inferior and forward. The examination is completed at this point.

Synovial pathology has been observed in the following areas: the posterior synovial pouch, medial or lateral paradiscal grooves, capsular walls, and anterior synovial pouch of the superior joint compartment. Fibrous adhesions may be seen between articular surfaces and around perforations.

The arthroscope is returned to the pathologic area where the biopsy is to be taken. A basket forceps is placed through the cannula, after the scope is withdrawn in the half-blind technique. It is important to hold the cannula directly over the pathologic tissue, without moving it after the arthroscope is removed and while taking the biopsy sample. Triangulation to obtain the biopsy through the anterior working cannula probably offers greater accuracy. This is the desired technique of most arthroscopists.

References

1. Holmlund AB: Diagnostic accuracy of TMJ arthroscopy: A comparison of findings during arthroscopy and arthrotomy. Oral Maxillofac Clin North Am 1(1):79–84, 1989.
2. Merrill, RG, Yih WY, Langan M: A histologic evaluation of the accuracy of TMJ diagnostic arthroscopy. Oral Surg Oral Med Oral Pathol. 70:393–398, 1990.
3. Huskisson EC, Hart FD: Joint Disease: All the arthropathies, 3rd Ed. Bristol: John Wright, 1978.
4. Murakami K-I, Ito K: Arthroscopy of the temporomandibular joint. In Watanabe M (ed): Arthroscopy of Small Joints. Tokyo: Igaku-Shoin, 1985, p 128.
5. Ohnishi M. Arthroscopic surgery for hypermobility and recurrent mandibular dislocation. Oral Maxillofac Clin North Am 1(1):153–164, 1989.

☐ D. Electrocautery and Fluid Mediums

*MOHAN THOMAS, D.D.S., F.A.C.D.,
CHRISTOPHER LANE, D.D.S, and
MICHAEL G. KOSLIN, D.M.D.*

The use of electrocautery in arthroscopic surgery of the temporomandibular joint (TMJ) evolved after extensive experience with electrocautery in arthroscopic surgery of the knee. Originally utilized for hemostasis, electrocautery in joint surgery has expanded to include repair of meniscal tears, lysis of synovial lesions, lateral retinacular release, and subacromial decompression. The application of electrosurgery in knee surgery arose from the need to address the problem of hemarthrosis following lateral retinacular release.[1] Today, electrosurgery has become a useful adjunct in performing a number of TMJ arthroscopic procedures, including electrosurgical anterior release (McCain technique), posterior synovial pouch cauterization, electrosurgical synovectomy, and cautery for hemostasis. We discuss here the history, principles, and pitfalls of electrocautery and offer practical suggestions.

HISTORY

William Gilbert, known as the father of electrotherapy, experimented with magnetism and electricity as early as the sixteenth century.[2] However, it was not until the 1890s that electrosurgery was actually developed by D'Arsonval.[3] Using a series of circuits consisting of two human volunteers and a 100-watt bulb, D'Arsonval passed 1 ampere of 500 kHz through the series. The bulb glowed brilliantly; also, at a frequency greater than 10,000 Hz, muscle stimulation was not produced. He was thus able to produce electrosurgical results at these levels, whereas at lower frequency levels various types of neuromuscular contractions were evoked.[3]

The popularization of electrosurgery in the United States is credited to Harvey Cushing. Cushing, in collaboration with W. T. Bovie, developed the first "spark gap generator" used to coagulate vessels intracranially.[4] Progress with electrocautery proceeded slowly because of incomplete acceptance of its usefulness, and fear of explosion from flammable anesthetic agents (prior to the 1960s).

With the advent of solid-state electrocautery units in the 1970s, there was a surge in its application to arthroscopic surgery. In 1981, Miller and colleagues[5] designed an electrosurgery system specifically for arthroscopic knee surgery. Further equipment modification and improvement have made electrosurgery an important tool for arthroscopic surgery in both orthopedic and maxillofacial surgery.

PRINCIPLES

To understand the principles of electrosurgery, a knowledge of the basic principles of electricity is necessary. Electricity is a form of energy that exhibits magnetic, chemical, mechanical, and thermal effects; it is created by interactions of positive and negative charges. Body tissues, with their electrolyte composition, are an ideal medium for the conduction of electric current.

The strength of an electric current is directly proportional to the impressed electromotive force and inversely proportional to the resistance, in the case of direct current (DC), and to the impedance, in the case of alternating current (AC). In living tissues, DC (flow in one direction) results in muscle and nerve excitation. If too much current is applied, cell death can occur.[1,6] Electrocautery utilizes AC electric energy, at a rapid rate, thereby pulling cellular ions to and fro. Although polarization will occur, a current pulse in the opposite direction will reverse the polarization.

The human body has two unique qualities that make electrosurgery possible: (1) a high-frequency electrode greater than approximately 10,000 Hz can be sent through the body without evidence of neuromuscular contraction; and (2) the tissues and fluids have a definite electrical impedance. At frequencies lower than approximately 300 Hz, the body responds with marked neuromuscular stimulation, such as occurs when being shocked from a "live" wall outlet. As the frequency increases, there is less neuromuscular response. At 10,000 Hz, the neuromuscular system no longer responds to the electrical stimuli. At higher frequencies, the body's fluids and tissues act as electrical conduction paths, owing to the presence of various ions.[7]

To illustrate how electrosurgery works in the human body, the loop principle was developed. This loop consists of a generator source, conductive cable, active electrode, patient return or dispersive electrode, and return cable to the generator.[6] As long as the loop is intact, both the patient and the surgeon are safe; however, if the loop is broken, a hazard can be created for both the patient and the surgeon.

FLUIDS IN ELECTROSURGERY

A nonconductive fluid must be used if electrosurgery is to be done. Normal saline is usually contraindicated because it has free ions in solution and is, therefore, a conductive fluid. However, within the TMJ, the conductivity of normal saline does not seem to be a problem, because of the small amounts of solutions present. Sterile water is also contraindicated because studies have shown that sterile water causes dramatic changes in the synovial surface of cells and the superficial chondrocytes, causing swelling, nuclear disruption, and in some cases destruction.[1] Reagan and co-workers[8] recommend Ringer's lactate for arthroscopy because it seems to support cartilage metabolism, unlike normal saline and sterile water. Theoretically, Ringer's lactate, a conductive fluid medium, should not be used in electrosurgical applications; however, our experience seems to support its safety in electrosurgical applications in TMJ arthroscopy.[1] A solution of 1.5% glycine also has been reported to be safe for use in electrosurgery, with minimal problems.[1] However, it has been reported that unexplainable fogging of the arthroscopic lens has occurred.

Marshall and colleagues[9] developed a solution called Arthrosol that is based on glycerol in an iso-osmotic and physiologic balance. Extensive animal laboratory testing has shown this fluid to be an ideal solution for electrosurgery in conjunction with arthroscopic surgery.

USES, PITFALLS, AND PRACTICAL CONSIDERATIONS

Electrocautery in TMJ arthroscopic surgery can be employed to cauterize bleeding points (i.e., hemostasis) (Fig. 13–21), hyperemic synovial tissue, and in the anterior and posterior pouches (as described by McCain); it also can be used for posterior cauterization in the management of hypermobility (as described by Onishi) (Figs. 13–22 and 13–23). Electrocautery in TMJ arthroscopy has

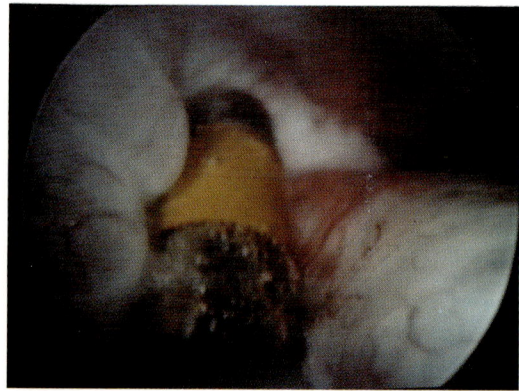

Figure 13–22. Posterior cauterization of retrodiscal tissue using the bipolar cautery tip (courtesy of Dr. Allen Tarro).

evolved over the last few years. In our experience, the optimal setting for TMJ electrosurgery is 20 to 25 watts in the coagulation mode, using the Concept monopolar cautery tip* and the Valley Laboratory cautery unit† (Figs. 13–23 and 13–24). Practitioners are advised to use cautery tips initially at lower settings, advancing to the recommended levels gradually, because of variations in the size and output of the cautery tips and generators.

Cautery tips generally are 1.5 to 2.0 mm in diameter. We recommend that electrocautery

---

*Concept Corp., Clearwater, FL.
†Valley Laboratory, Boulder, CO.

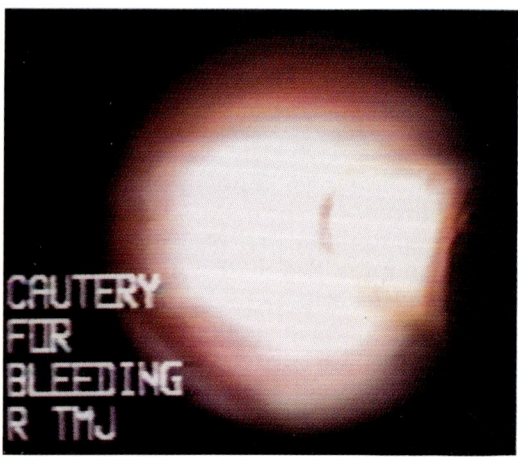

Figure 13–21. Cautery for bleeding in the right temporomandibular joint (courtesy of Dr. Robert Schwartz).

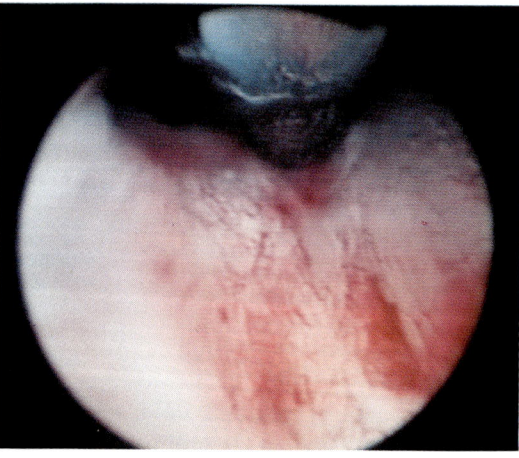

Figure 13–23. Anterior release for increased disc mobility.

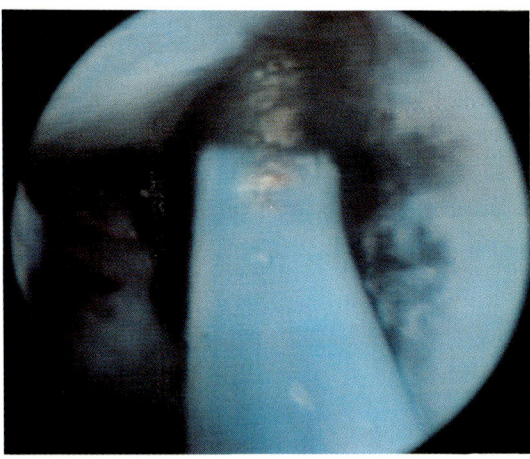

Figure 13-24. Use of the Concept Corp. disposable monopolar cautery tip (courtesy of Dr. Allen Tarro).

be utilized with caution when abrasive procedures are contemplated. Cautery tips are available in both monopolar and bipolar units. Concept monopolar cautery tips are disposable and single-use and require more energy than the bipolar tips. However, the monopolar units are isolated and programmed to seek the generator; thus, they are safer than the bipolar tips. The McCain bipolar tips‡ are reusable and require less energy than the monopolar tips, thereby being faster. The bipolar tips have a grounded unit and thus are programmed to seek ground, making them slightly less safe than the monopolar tips.

Electrocautery is not without hazards and pitfalls. Failures of electrosurgery units are primarily the results of faulty or improper connections to or from the generator, the use of a conductive fluid, or improper settings for the coagulation and cutting modes. Attention to detail can facilitate resolution of most problems. One may encounter difficulty in moving the electrode from the anterior recess to the posterior pouch. This, however, can be alleviated by proper placement of cannulas and proper puncture technique. Problems with visualization can be remedied by utilizing larger working cannulas and additional portals, if indicated. Single-use disposable, monopolar cautery tips (Concept) can lessen or prevent the complication of intra-articular loss of insulation material. A particular word of caution should be mentioned in regard to the TMJ. Because of close proximity to the midbrain and auditory apparatus, excessive heat routinely should be avoided. A study performed by Koslin, as reported at the Third International Arthroscopy Study Meeting, quantitated heat generated by arthroscopic surgery of the TMJ. Conclusions were supported and proved that heat generated during TMJ arthroscopy could be modified significantly by proper flow of irrigant and subsequently is not totally dependent on the type of electrosurgery procedure performed, the duration of the procedure, or the type of irrigant.

Disadvantages of electrosurgery in conjunction with TMJ arthroscopy include the extensive cutting/coagulation currents and the subsequent heat emitted (as previously mentioned), poor wound healing, and possible infection if extensive unnecessary tissue damage is caused by inappropriate cutting/coagulation settings.

LASERS

Electrosurgery has a definite place in the surgical armamentarium of the TMJ arthroscopist, and new applications are currently being developed. One of these is the laser. The use of the neodymium:yttrium-aluminum-garnet (Nd:YAG) laser and the KTP-532 laser in the TMJ has been reported. Pioneer work in the use of the Nd:YAG laser and its effects on cartilage in dogs has been carried out by Indresano and Bradrick. Lasers in TMJ arthroscopy for electrocauterization versus traditional electrocautery units seem to have some advantages; however, more research is necessary before endorsement.

References

1. Fox JM, Ferkel RD: Use of electrosurgery in arthroscopic surgery. *In* Parisien S (ed): Arthroscopic Surgery. New York: McGraw-Hill, 1989, pp. 315–324.
2. Krusen F: William Gilbert, the father of electrotherapy. Arch Phys Therapy 12:12, 1931.
3. D'Arsonval A: Action physiologique des courants alternatifs à grande frequence. Arch Physiol Norm Pathol 5:401, 1893.
4. Cushing H, Bovie W: Electrosurgery as an aid to the removal of intracranial tumors. Surg Gynecol Obstet 47:751, 1928.

---

‡Walter Lorenz Co., Jacksonville, FL

5. Miller G, Dickason J, Fox J, et al: The use of electrosurgery for arthroscopic subcutaneous lateral release. Orthopedics 5:300, 1982.
6. Fox J, Ferkel R, Del Pizzo W, et al: Electrosurgery in orthopaedics: I. Principles. Contemp Orthop 8:21, 1984.
7. Glover J, Benedick P, Link W: The use of thermal knives in surgery: Electrosurgery, lasers, plasma, scalpel. Curr Probl Surg 15:1, 1978.
8. Reagan B, McInerny V, Treadwell B, et al: Irrigating solutions for arthroscopy. A metabolic study. J Bone Joint Surg 65A:629, 1983.
9. Marshall GJ, Snyder SJ, Kirchen ME, et al: The effects of water, surgical saline and buffered saline on the synovia and articular cartilages of rabbit knees. Presented at the Orthopaedic Research Society Annual Meeting, Las Vegas, January, 1985.
10. Kelly H, Ward G: Electrosurgery. Philadelphia, WB Saunders, 1932.

□ E. Disc-Stabilizing Techniques

ALLEN W. TARRO, D.M.D.

Disc-stabilizing techniques are important in treating symptomatic temporomandibular joint (TMJ) hypermobility with chronic dislocation and, in my opinion, in treating symptomatic anteriorly displaced discs.[1] When an anteriorly displaced disc is placed in a more posterior position, it is vulnerable to be displaced again as the result of a variety of possible subsequent events, such as postoperative vomiting, coughing, or sneezing. If these occur in the first few weeks after surgery, the disc may again be displaced anteriorly, with possible treatment failure. It is advisable, therefore, to stabilize the posteriorly repositioned disc in order to obtain a more predictable result. A number of techniques have been devised for the purpose of stabilizing posteriorly positioned discs. These techniques also have been highly successful in treating symptomatic TMJ hypermobility.

One technique, first performed by McCain, is cauterization of the posterior attachment (Fig. 13-25). In theory, the cauterization causes scarification and a resultant tissue constriction that is supposed to hold the disc in a more posterior position. From a practical standpoint, it is very doubtful that cauterization of the posterior attachment alone would be capable of retaining the disc in a more posterior position. If cauterization of the posterior attachment is performed, it should be accompanied by high-flow irrigation and followed by copious TMJ lavage.

A technique advocated by Merrill in treating symptomatic TMJ hypermobility is the subintimal injection of sclerosing solution into the oblique protuberance in the posteromedial aspect of the joint.[2] Under arthroscopic visualization, a 3½-inch spinal needle is used through a cannula to deposit the sclerosing solution into the oblique protuberance. This technique, at least in preliminary studies, has produced successful results in resolving symptomatic TMJ hypermobility. However, reports indicate that patients experience about 3 to 5 days of pain from this procedure. Some practitioners are using intermaxillary fixation for about 3 to 4 weeks in conjunction with this technique.

Subintimal injections have also been employed to treat synovitis. Quinn has recom-

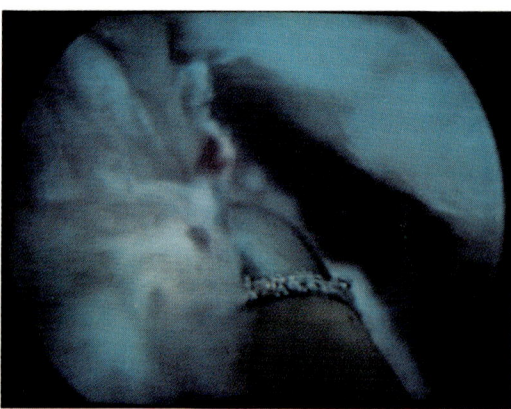

Figure 13-25. Cauterization of the posterior attachment area using a blunt, straight cautery tip. (Walter Lorenz Surgical Instruments, Inc., Jacksonville FL.)

mended the injection of 3 mg of betamethasone into the subintimal area of synovial inflammation, using a spinal needle under arthroscopic visualization (Fig. 13–26).[3] This is thought to be much more appropriate than injecting steroid into the superior joint space, which can result in degradation of proteoglycan in the articular cartilage, producing chondromalacia.

Securing the posterior positioning of a disc can be accomplished by utilizing a variety of disc-stabilizing suture techniques. One technique, utilized in over 200 TMJ arthroscopic surgery cases and described here, has significantly increased the success rate in treating cases with symptomatic anteriorly displaced discs.[1] This disc-stabilizing suture technique utilizes 2-0 Vicryl suture on a CP-1 or CP-2 needle (Ethicon J-266 and J-869, respectively, from Ethicon, Inc., Somerville, NJ) (Fig. 13–27). Small, 3-mm vertical skin incisions that were made for cannula placements are used for needle entrance and exit points in this technique (Fig. 13–28A). The choice of needle depends on the depth of the individual joint being treated. The CP-1 needle is most commonly selected. The needle is passed as deeply as possible through the superior aspect of the 3-mm vertical incision that was made for the posterior cannula placement (Fig. 13–28B). The needle passes through the lateral TMJ capsule and a lateral portion of the disc and emerges through the superior aspect of the 3-mm vertical incision that was made for the anterior cannula placement (Fig. 13–28C). Owing to the depth of the

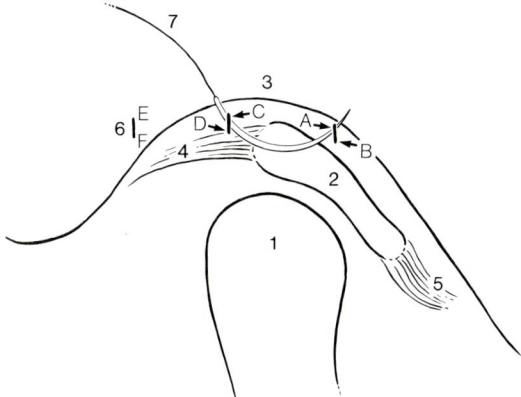

Figure 13–27. Disc-stabilizing suture technique. 1 = mandibular condyle; 2 = disc; 3 = superior aspect of glenoid fossa; 4 = posterior attachment; 5 = anterior disc attachments; 6 = third and most posterior incision; 7 = Vicryl suture with CP-1 or CP-2 needle; A = superior aspect of anterior incision; B = inferior aspect of anterior incision; C = superior aspect of middle incision; D = inferior aspect of middle incision; E = superior aspect of posterior incision; F = inferior aspect of posterior incision.

suture needle placement, it is sometimes necessary to palpate the tip of the needle with a finger over the site of emergence (Fig. 13–28D) and then to grasp the needle tip with a hemostat. The needle is withdrawn (Fig. 13–28E), completing the deep portion of this suturing technique.

Verification that the suture has captured a lateral portion of the disc is established in the following manner. A cannula and the arthroscope are placed in the superior compartment of the joint through the posterior incision. The suture strands are then pulled posteriorly (Fig. 13–28F). The disc should be observed arthroscopically to move posteriorly as the suture strands are pulled in that direction. The degree of disc movement observed arthroscopically will depend on the amount of disc mobility that was accomplished by the previously performed surgical techniques.

When the surgeon is satisfied that the suture has engaged a lateral portion of the disc, the arthroscope and cannula are removed, and the suture is completed in the following manner. A third 3-mm vertical incision is made posterior to the other two incisions and just anterior to the tragus. The suture needle is passed subcutaneously from the inferior aspect of the anterior incision (point B, Fig. 13–27) to the inferior aspect of what is now

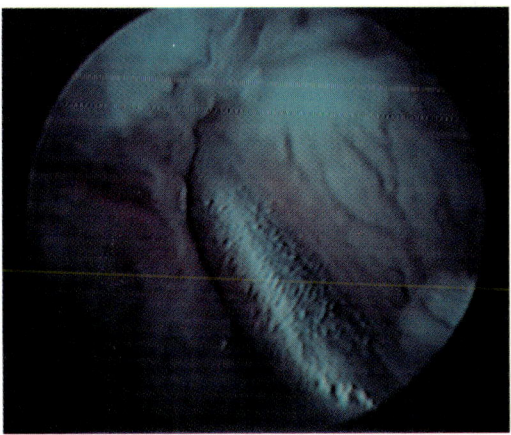

Figure 13–26. Arthroscopic view of subintimal steroid injection showing the 22-gauge spinal needle entering inflamed synovial tissue.

208 ■ 13 Special Applications

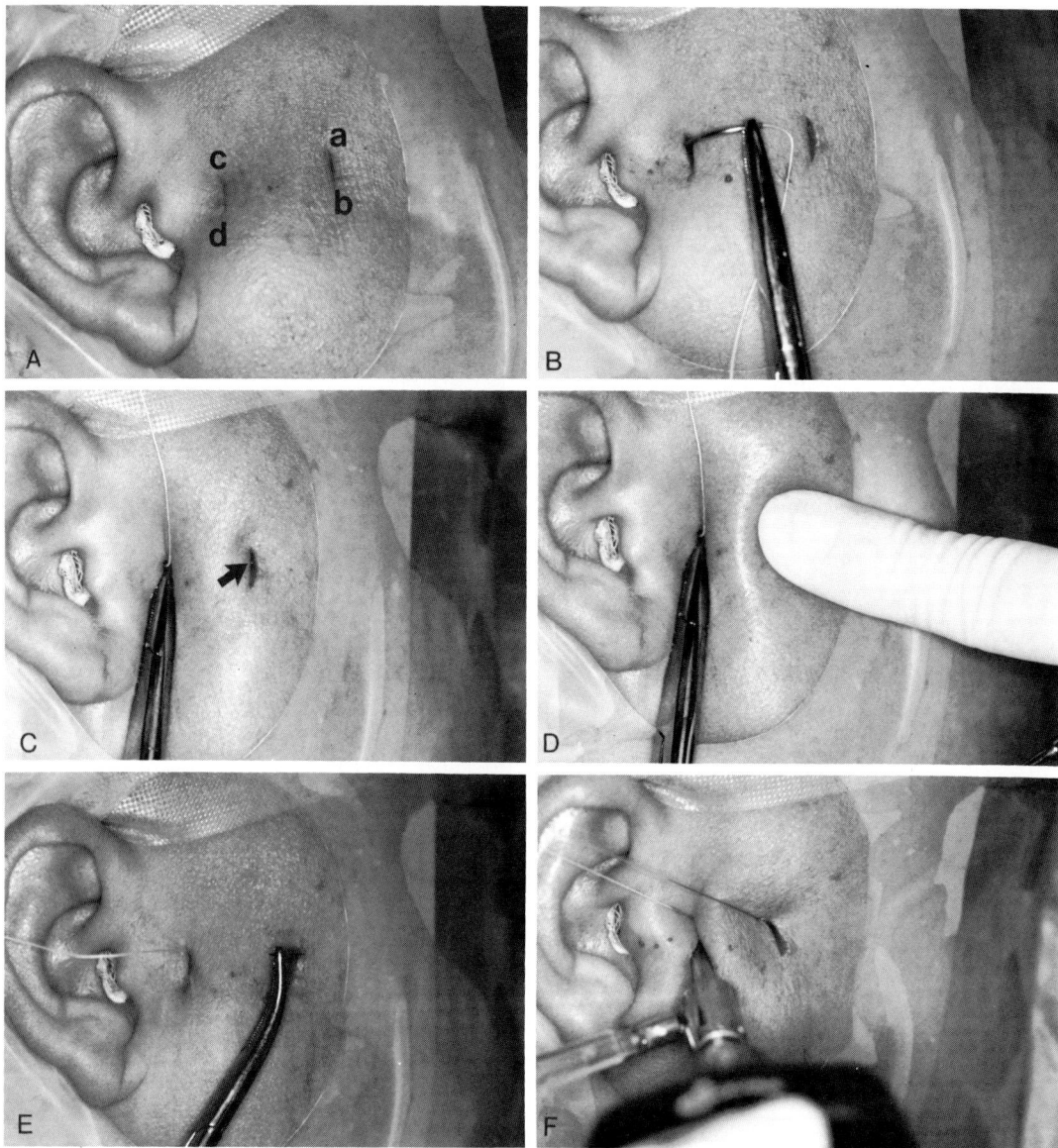

Figure 13–28. *A*, Preauricular area prior to placement of disc-stabilizing suture, showing the two skin incisions a–b and c–d that were made for cannula insertions. *B*, Initial entrance of CP-1 needle through the superior aspect of the 3-mm vertical skin incision that was made for the insertion of the posterior cannula. *C*, Placement of the deep portion of the disc-stabilizing suture technique. The tip of the needle (*arrow*) is just barely visible through the anterior incision. *D*, Surgeon using a finger to palpate the tip of the needle after placement of the deep portion of the disc-stabilizing suture technique. *E*, Use of a hemostat to grasp the tip of CP-2 needle after placement of the deep portion of the disc-stabilizing suture technique. *F*, Evaluating the movement of the disc through the arthroscope as the suture strands are pulled posteriorly and slightly laterally.

the middle incision (point D, Fig. 13–27) (Fig. 13–28*G*). The needle is now passed subcutaneously from the inferior aspect of the middle incision to the inferior aspect of the posterior incision (point F, Fig. 13–27) and then from the superior aspect of the posterior incision (point E, Fig. 13–27) to the superior aspect of the middle incision (point C, Fig. 13–27) (Fig. 13–28*H*). The suture is tied tightly, securing the disc in a more posterior position. A puckering of the skin tissue will be observed, and the 3-mm skin incisions are closed with 5-0 silk sutures (Fig. 13–28*I*).

A stronger posterior pull on the disc can be

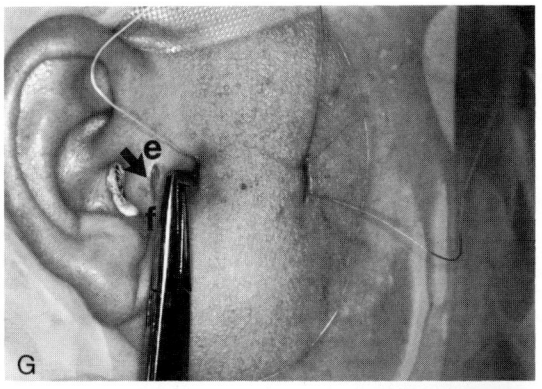
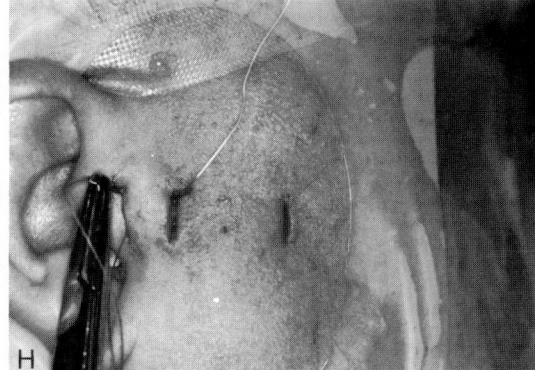
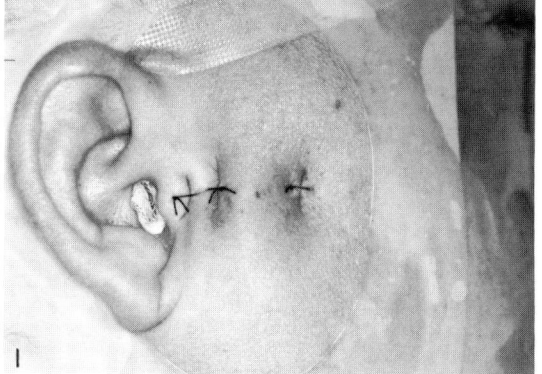

Figure 13–28. *Continued G,* Continuation of suture technique after placement of the initial deep portion by passing the suture needle subcutaneously from the inferior aspect of the anterior incision to the inferior portion of what is now the middle incision. Note that the third incision (*arrow*) has been made posterior to the first two incisions. *H,* Passing the suture needle from the superior aspect of the posterior incision subcutaneously to the superior aspect of the middle incision. *I,* Puckering of the skin tissue after tightly tying the disc-stabilizing suture and suturing the three small vertical incision sites.

achieved by passing the needle subcutaneously through some of the dense tissue in the tragus area. This tissue is just posterior to the third incision (between points E and F, Fig. 13–27). This suture, properly placed, will stabilize the disc in a more posterior and slightly lateral position. The suture material will dissolve after it has served its purpose, and any skin puckering will disappear.

Vicryl suture was selected because it has high tensile strength, and it dissolves in about 4 to 6 weeks. Experience has shown that the first 3 to 4 weeks after surgery are critical for stabilizing posteriorly positioned discs. However, it is important that a resorbable suture is selected so that after 4 to 6 weeks the disc is not tied down and adequate disc mobility is realized.

The three main advantages of this disc-stabilizing suture technique are as follows: First, it is a relatively simple procedure, once adequate experience has been gained. Second, it is a quick procedure that usually takes no longer than a few minutes to perform. Third, no complications have been attributed to this technique in the more than 200 cases.

A disadvantage is that this procedure is a blind disc suturing technique. As previously mentioned, however, the effectiveness of the technique can be evaluated by arthroscopically viewing the disc as the suture strands are pulled posteriorly, after the deep portion of the suture is placed. Moreover, open surgical verification of the effectiveness of this technique has been established during a number of TMJ arthrotomy cases.[4] After the surgical dissection was performed, the skin flap was repositioned and a suture was placed through the skin in a manner similar to that performed during TMJ arthroscopy (Fig. 13–29A). In Figure 13–29, the needle is being passed from the anterior incision area posteriorly. This is the reverse of the method used in the arthroscopic disc suturing technique. It was done in this manner in arthrotomy cases in order to see where the needle was emerging when the tissue flap was raised. In every arthrotomy case in which this procedure was performed, the CP-1 or CP-2 needle passed through a lateral portion of the disc and was adequate to pull the disc posteriorly and stabilize it in a more posterior position (Figs. 13–29B and C).

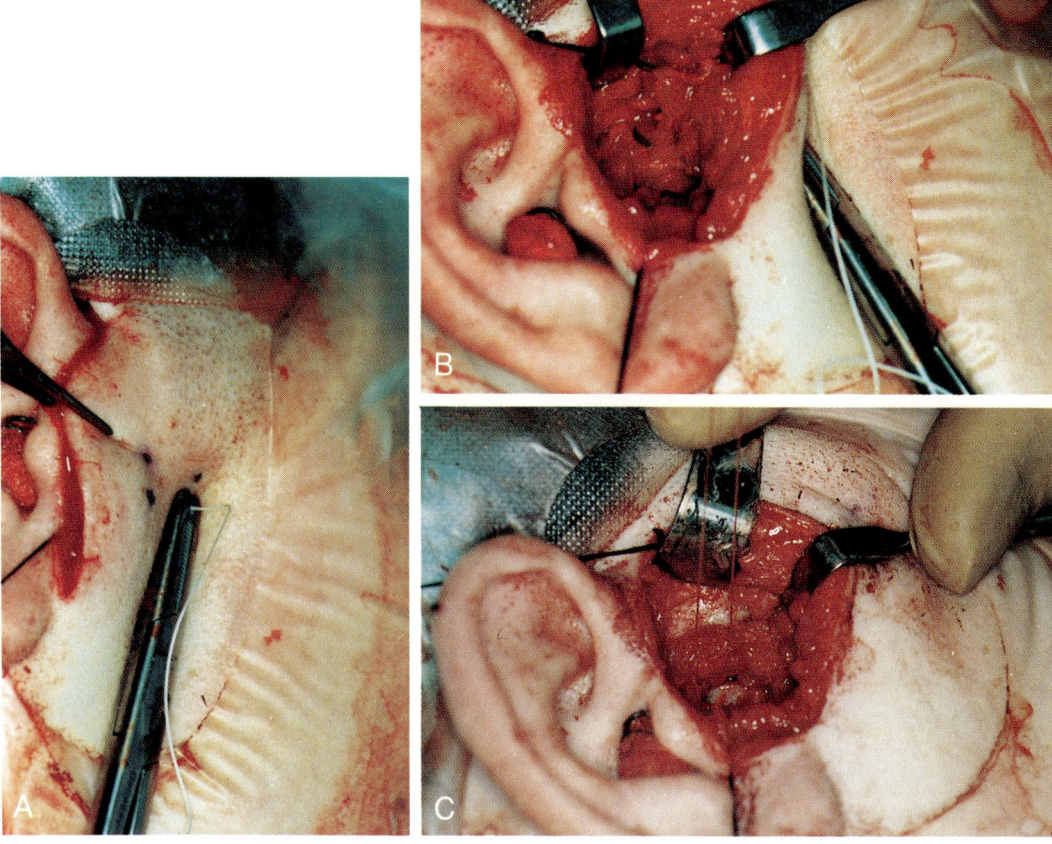

Figure 13–29. *A*, After surgical exposure of the superior and inferior joint compartments during temporomandibular joint arthrotomy, the skin flap is repositioned using a tissue forceps. Placement of the deep portion of a disc-stabilizing suture is then performed, using a technique similar to that for temporomandibular joint arthroscopy. *B*, The arthrotomy skin flap is raised, showing the tip of a CP-2 needle emerging through the lateral aspect of the disc (center and slightly left in the surgical area). *C*, The CP-2 needle is pulled through the disc tissue, and the other end of the suture is retrieved from under the skin flap, clearly showing a significant portion of the disc engaged by the suture.

Although this disc-stabilizing suture technique requires small vertical incisions, the incisions have posed no problem cosmetically, and they have served as areas of fluid venting during arthroscopic surgery.[5] This is an advantage if the irrigation inflow is too vigorously injected by the assistant or if the outflow is inadequate for a short period of time. In these instances, the venting aspect of the incisions will minimize the extravasation of fluid into the surrounding tissues.

The disc-stabilizing suture technique that has been described can be altered slightly so that it is a partially blind technique. The needle can be placed in the superior joint space and visualized arthroscopically, as it enters tissue in the joint during the initial deep needle placement.[4] This is accomplished in the following manner. After double-cannula arthroscopic surgery and the final lavage have been performed, the posterior cannula is removed, but the anterior cannula remains inserted into the superior joint space. The arthroscope is placed in the anterior cannula. The disc-stabilizing suture technique is then started by passing the needle through the superior aspect of the 3-mm vertical incision that was made for the posterior cannula placement (Fig. 13–30). The tip of the needle is passed into the posterior recess of the superior joint space. The arthroscope is then positioned so that the tip of the needle can be viewed. At this point, the needle, under arthroscopic visualization, is passed through discal tissue or tissue just posterior to the disc (Fig. 13–31). The needle is advanced

E. Disc-Stabilizing Techniques ■ 211

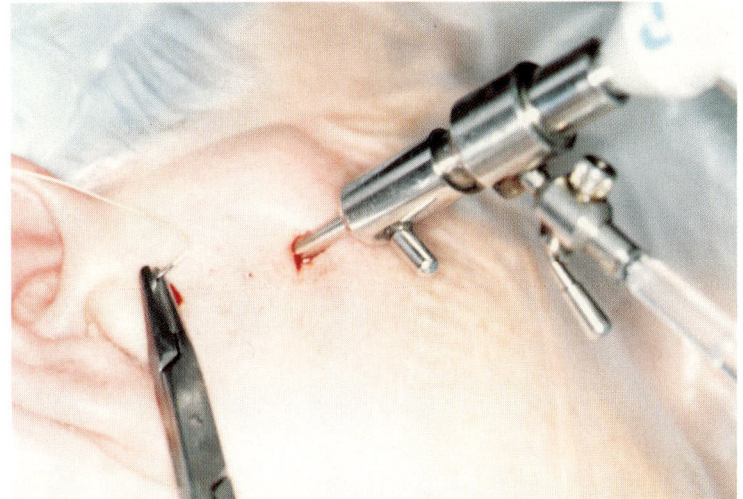

Figure 13–30. View of the right side of the face showing the insertion of the needle into the superior joint space and the arthroscope for direct visualization of the needle as it pierces tissue in the superior joint space.

anteriorly through the disc and then superiorly, until it emerges through the superior aspect of the 3-mm incision that contains the shaft of the cannula and arthroscope. The cannula and arthroscope are then removed, and the suturing technique is completed in the same manner that has been described previously for the blind technique.

Direct visualization of the needle in this technique may be more effective for some surgeons and is recommended for surgeons with limited experience in disc suturing techniques. However, it requires more manipulation and can be more traumatic. For these reasons, after considerable experience, the blind technique has been routinely used and is advocated by this author.

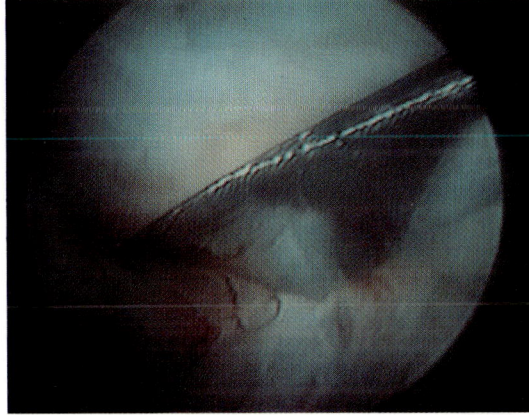

Figure 13–31. Arthroscopic view of the needle entering the tissue during the deep needle placement of the disc-stabilizing suture technique.

Other suturing techniques can be utilized to stabilize posteriorly positioned discs.[6,7] Most are partially blind techniques, like the version of the above technique that utilizes direct arthroscopic visualization of the needle. In these techniques, a needle or specialized instrument with a lumen is passed into the superior joint space. A lateral approach is most commonly used, although an endaural approach can be used. In one technique, the instrument is passed blindly through the disc from an inferolateral approach and into the superior joint space. In another technique, the instrument is passed into the superior joint space, is visualized arthroscopically, and is then passed through the disc. Suture material is passed through the lumen of the needle or specialized instrument into the superior joint space. The suture is observed through the arthroscope (Figs. 13–32 and 13–33), secured with a grasping forceps (Fig. 13–34), and removed from the joint through the cannula in which the grasping forceps was placed. The needle or specialized instrument and the cannula are carefully removed, and the suture strands are tied around a small cotton roll or through a button.

In another suturing technique, described by Ohnishi,[7] a specially designed metal awl with threaded suture material is inserted into the superior joint space. Then, under arthroscopic visualization, the awl pierces the disc and is passed posteriorly under the disc. The awl emerges through the skin behind the tragus of the ear. One strand of suture is grasped and held as the awl is withdrawn, back into

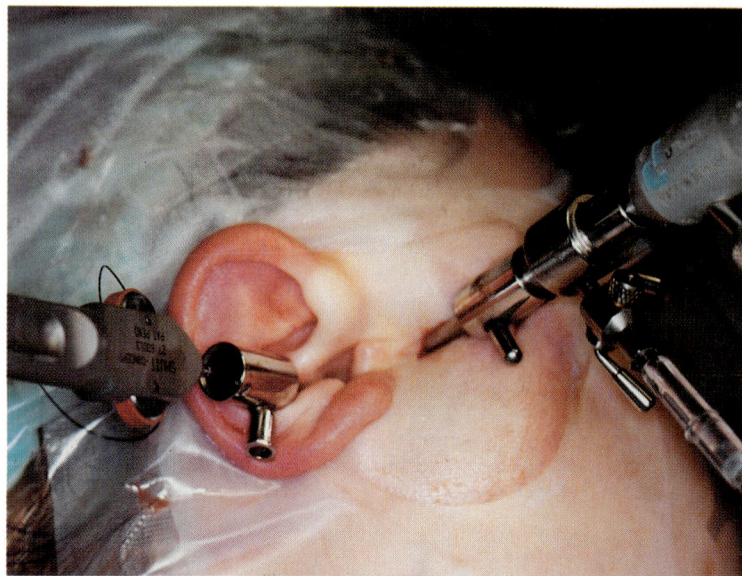

Figure 13–32. View of the right side of the face showing the Shutt suturing instrument inserted into the joint via the endaural approach, and the arthroscope inserted through a lateral approach. (Shutt instrument from Shutt Medical Technologies, Inc., a subsidiary of Concept, Inc., Largo, FL.)

the superior joint space. The awl then is passed posteriorly over the disc and again emerges through the skin behind the tragus of the ear. The second suture strand is grasped, and finally the two suture strands are tied around a small cotton roll, securing the disc in a more posterior position. The suture is usually removed in about 10 days.

Partially blind suturing techniques and the technique in which both the entrance and exit points of the disc puncture are visualized arthroscopically may prove to be of considerable value in TMJ arthroscopic surgery.

They can, however, be traumatic, time-consuming, and quite difficult to perform. Moreover, there are no published data regarding the results of their use in specific TMJ arthroscopy cases. More time and experience are needed to evaluate their effectiveness.

It must be stressed that in performing disc-stabilizing techniques in cases with anterior disc displacement, the effectiveness of these procedures is directly related to disc mobility. In these cases, creating a relaxing incision anterior to the disc (an anterior muscle or band release) is usually critical. It probably is of little value to pull a disc posteriorly if the disc is under significant tension. This has been shown by the relatively high failure rate associated with open TMJ disc plication surgery that did not incorporate relaxing incisions anterior to the disc.

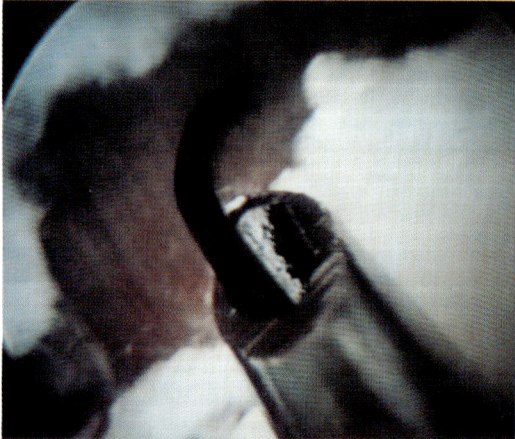

Figure 13–33. Arthroscopic view of the tip of the Shutt suturing instrument and suture material in the superior joint space after piercing the disc.

References

1. Tarro A: Arthroscopic treatment of anterior disc displacement: a preliminary report. J Oral Maxillofac Surg Clin North Am 47:353, 1989.
2. Merrill R: Mandibular dislocation and hypermobility. Oral Maxillofac Surg Clin North Am. 1, 1989.
3. Quinn J: Pathogenesis of TMJ chondromalacia and arthralgia. Oral Maxillofac Surg Clin North Am. 1, 1989.
4. Tarro A: TMJ arthroscopic diagnosis and surgery; Clinical experience with 152 procedures over a 2½-year period. J Craniomandib Pract. In press.

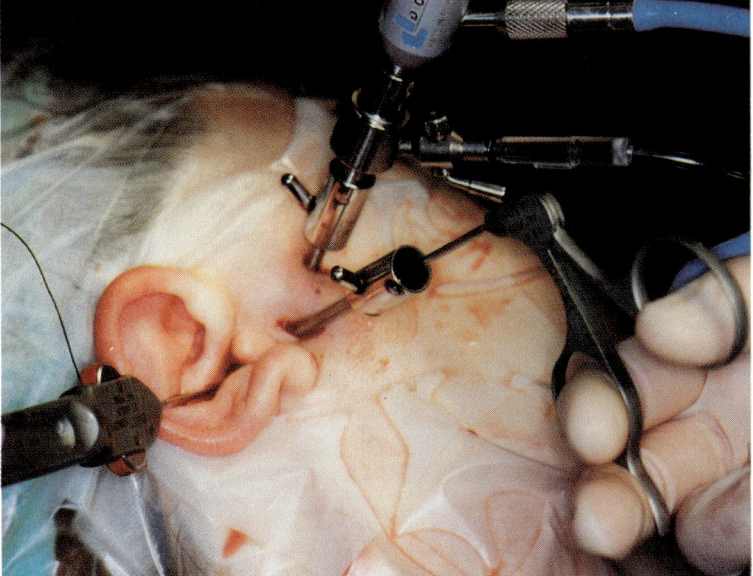

Figure 13–34. View of the right side of the face showing the use of the grasping forceps in the Shutt instrument suturing procedure. Note that the endaural cannula was removed to allow deeper placement of the Shutt instrument into the joint.

5. Tarro A: Arthroscopic diagnosis and surgery of the temporomandibular joint. J Oral Maxillofac Surg 46:282, 1988.
6. Israel H: Technique for placement of a discal traction suture during temporomandibular joint arthroscopy. J Oral Maxillofac Surg 47:311, 1989.
7. Ohnishi M: Arthroscopic surgery for hypermobility and recurrent mandibular dislocation. Oral Maxillofac Surg Clin North Am 1:00–00, 1989.

☐ F. Temporomandibular Joint Arthroscopy for Post-Arthrotomy Patients

DAVID C. HOFFMAN, D.D.S.

Arthroscopy of the temporomandibular joint (TMJ) has many diagnostic as well as therapeutic uses. One of the more complicated but rewarding applications is in the post-arthrotomy patient. We focus here on how arthroscopy allows the surgeon to evaluate problematic postoperative joints. The visualization of the soft tissue structures and integrity, the implant position and host response, the integrity of sutures and disc position are some of the benefits of the arthroscopic examination. Often, further patient care can be directed on the basis of arthroscopic findings.

Post-arthrotomy joint pathology can be addressed with an array of operative procedures. As a last resort, when further open surgery cannot be avoided, both the surgeon and the patient can benefit from the arthroscopic results in selecting the next surgical procedure. The post-arthrotomy patient may be categorized by previous procedures or by prevailing clinical symptoms. Indications for post-arthrotomy arthroscopy generally are based on patient evaluations, both subjective and objective.[1] In most situations, patients present with some component of postoperative problems. Typical previous procedures, problems, and symptoms are listed in Table 13–2.

Evaluation of these patients employs the usual protocols for any TMJ problem, including radiography, or other imaging modalities, history, and clinical examination, diagnostic blocks, and TMJ arthroscopy. Other adjunctive modalities are often needed as well. Because of the variety of TMJ surgical procedures, only the following generalizations can be made about the postoperative imaging techniques available, using either radiography or magnetic resonance imaging (MRI).[3–5]

1. Imaging of the post-arthrotomy joint often is difficult for two reasons. First, normal anatomic landmarks are often lost, making the views hard to interpret. Second, each imaging system favors either hard or soft tissue visualization, making no system complete. Traditionally radiography shows bony structures well, whereas MRI is best for disc or soft tissue. However, this difference is not always precise. Problems can arise with arthrography if there is scarring of the joint space that does not allow flow of the contrast material. Computed tomography (CT) scans are moderately effective in visualizing the soft tissues or the disc position but are best for viewing bone.

2. Hard tissue imaging is essentially unchanged in the post-arthrotomy patient, using either tomography or CT.

3. Demonstrations of alloplastic implants (Silastic or Proplast) or of autogenous grafts, (muscle, cartilage, or fascia) are significantly limited regarding position and integrity of the grafted material. Additionally, avascular necrosis associated with TMJ implants has been described by radiologists using T_2 MRI. When this is suspected, concomitant skeletal changes associated with the loss of vertical height or other supporting structures should be checked to confirm the diagnosis.

4. None of these techniques show true-to-life pathology of joint tissue surfaces (especially at the lower-power microscopic level used in arthroscopy).

Imaging, whether radiography or MRI, provides information that is at best difficult to evaluate as a means of directing a treatment of the problematic patient. All surgeons share the same concern about operating on a patient and being part of a never-ending plan that leads to a permanent or untreatable TMJ "cripple." Arthroscopic intervention has advantages that allow visualization of problematic joints and may also permit a more conservative approach than what may otherwise have be an open procedure. Although arthroscopy does not replace good imaging techniques, it certainly offers adjunctive real-life views of what would otherwise be a difficult joint to image.

In the following section, we look at specific operative procedures and discuss postoperative arthroscopic findings. Although there are a variety of findings and a host of arthroscopic procedures, some general rules will enhance arthroscopic technique.

When arthroscoping a previously opened or operated TMJ the following technical considerations are pertinent:

1. Postoperative TMJs have for the most part lost normal anatomy. Because of scarring and fibrosis of this space, normal anatomy must be re-established with judicious instrumentation or motorized equipment. The discs and the lateral joint capsules fibrose, often leaving no obvious joint space.[6, 7]

2. An outflow cannula should be inserted as soon as possible. This should be of larger

Table 13–2. INDICATIONS FOR TEMPOROMANDIBULAR JOINT ARTHROSCOPY FOR POST-ARTHROTOMY PATIENTS

Clinical Signs and Symptoms
1. Unprovoked pain in an operated joint
2. Pain on function in an operated joint
3. Decrease in range of motion in an operated joint
4. Hypermobility in a contralateral unoperated joint
5. Implant failure
6. Degenerating joint with concomitant changes in the skeletofacial form or occlusion
7. Return of clicking
8. Removal of a temporary implant spacer

Previous Surgical Procedures
1. Soft tissue disc repair; plication; tie-down
2. Discectomy with Silastic and implant or spacer
3. Discectomy with Proplast
4. Discectomy with autogenous graft
5. Total joint replacement

diameter if possible (e.g., Dyonics 2.9-mm cannula), which permits easy outflow and placement of instruments, if needed, as well as aggressive lavage to aid in visualization without excessive extravasation of fluid.

3. Shavers, suction punch, and forceps should be available. This equipment should be accompanied by the necessary skills of triangulation (Fig. 13–35).

4. In addition to the usual arthroscopic pathology, the surgeon should be familiar with the appearance of sutures, implants, and foreign-body or host response reactions (Fig. 13–36).

5. Knowledge of prior surgical techniques and procedures is mandatory.[8]

6. Understanding of TMJ anatomy is incumbent.[9]

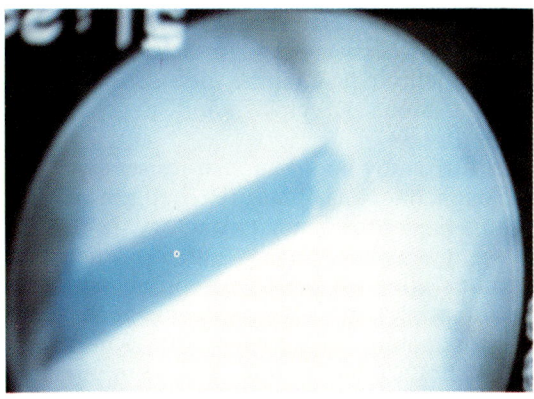

Figure 13–36. Blue PDS suture as seen through a 2.7-mm Dyonics arthroscope.

TMJ surgical procedures have been categorized using various classifications. In this discussion, they are divided into primary and secondary procedures. This distinction is based on whether this is a first or repeat TMJ surgical procedure. Under primary procedures, the most important and first distinction is the presence of the disc. The second concern in postsurgical evaluation is the type of implant placed. Although implants are constantly changing, the surgeon should have a historical perspective of previously used implants so that they may be identified.

The following list contains a group of common TMJ surgical procedures (not all are presently being used).

1. Full or partial posterior plication of disc[10]
2. Disc tie-down (Walker procedure)[11]
3. Discectomy with no implant[12]
4. Discectomy with no temporary spacer (Wilkes procedure)[8]
5. Discectomy with permanent Silastic spacers[13]
6. Proplast laminates or fossa implants[14]
7. Kent prostheses (fossa, condyle, or combined)[14, 15]
8. Other total joints (e.g., synthesis, Christianson)[8]
9. Silastic fossa implants
10. Autogenous grafts (e.g., concha cartilage, costochondral rib grafts, dermal grafts, fascia and temporalis muscle grafts)

Arthroscopy is not feasible in all of the procedures listed. To date, there have been no reports, published or otherwise reported, on arthroscopy of total joints, regarding total joint replacement systems. Arthroscopy of autogenous grafts also has not been reported but most likely has been attempted. This is technically difficult because of the lack of a definite joint space and the possibility of damage to the joint tissue.

ARTHROSCOPIC PRODECURES FOR POST-ARTHROTOMY DISC AND SOFT TISSUE SURGERIES

Patients who have had either a plication or a tie-down to correct an internal derangement may experience an array of postopera-

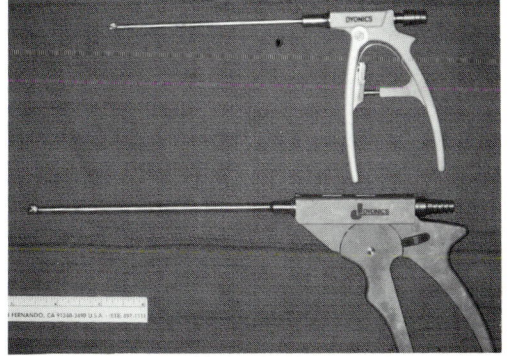

Figure 13–35. Examples of suction punches (2.7 mm and 3.4 mm) helpful in cleaning temporomandibular joints with extensive scarring.

tive problems. The simplest is a return of clicking, which can progress to a series of severe pathologic changes including perforations, fibrous ankylosis, and degenerative joint disease.

Arthroscopy can demonstrate several possible mechanisms of failure when these operations have proved unsatisfactory. In 1987, I presented a paper on this topic reporting five postoperative plications combined with tie-down procedures. To date, we have done approximately 15 postoperative soft tissue evaluations. The original data were presented at the Second International TMJ Arthroscopy Meeting in New York City. At that presentation, I recommended evaluating these on the basis of the following criteria[4,16]:

1. Synovium
2. Roofing
3. Integrity of sutures
4. Function
5. Adhesions

Synovium. This should be assessed in terms of vascularity, redundancy, integrity, fibrillation location, and growths.[16]

Roofing. Roofing is a term proposed by McCain to describe the extent of disc displacement. It can be measured by his technique of comparing the junction of the intermediate zone with the posterior retrodiscal tissue against the inferior and posterior slope of the eminence.[17]

Integrity of Sutures. Sutures can be visualized and should be evaluated for integrity, position, and the presence of the original knot. The suture line from a plication should be located; this will appear either intact or unravelled and either in or out of position. One should note tissue response above this suture line. A helpful hint during the arthroscopic procedure is to visualize through the arthroscope a similar suture not in the TMJ to identify clearly any suture material with regard to type or arthroscopic appearance.

Function. Function of the TMJ can be discerned by allowing the assistant to place the mandible in open, closed, and lateral positions and observing the TMJ. Arthroscopically, this procedure can elicit information about disposition, clicking, and any other intracapsular mechanical event.

Adhesions. The presence of adhesions is similar to that in other arthroscopic examinations. The adhesions may be relatively prolific or may be diffuse.

Case Histories

Case I

The patient is seen 18 months after a disc plication procedure and tie-down. The initial preoperative diagnosis was an anterior displaced disc with reduction; the clicking returned 18 months postoperatively with no other symptoms.

Arthroscopic Examination

Synovium: intact; no pathology
Roofing: 50% loss
Sutures: intact
Function: mobilized disc; good range of motion
Adhesions: none

The diagnosis was redisplacement of the disc, and the treatment plan was to repeat nonsurgical care on a p.r.n. basis.

Case II

A more symptomatic patient presented 12 months after a disc plication was performed during an open surgical procedure. The original diagnosis had been internal derangement with disc displacement.

Arthroscopic Examination

Synovium: synovitis, fibrillation and possible perforation
Roofing: 100% loss (complete disc displacement)
Sutures: unravelled and loose
Function: visualization of reducing disc
Adhesions: multiple

The diagnosis was a breakdown of the plication repair, with synovial tissue deterioration and scarring and possible perforation with displacement of the disc. Because there had been no immediate postoperative imaging of the disc, it was uncertain whether the displacement had actually been corrected, although clicking was absent for 12 months.

The treatment plan was to repeat basic care, including diet restrictions, TMJ rest, nonsteroidal anti-inflammatory medication, and appliance therapy. Arthroscopic surgery, which was not attempted at this time, might have been directed toward lysis of adhesions, stretching of the capsule and increasing mobility of the disc, and cleaning scar and deteriorating tissue; disc recapturing procedures were also a possibility.

Case III

This case was characterized by the most advanced pathology in the group reported on here. The patient underwent a disc plication that did well for 1 year; she reported that at this time she experienced a loud "pop" and severe pain in the TMJ. Postoperative arthroscopy was attempted by the primary surgeon, but there was no improvement. Arthroscopy may have failed owing to inability to enter the joint space, as described by the surgeon. Following this procedure, the patient experienced severe pain and restricted range of motion of the TMJ (opening limited to 10 mm).

A secondary procedure was performed, and a large perforation was visualized after removal of excessive scar tissue with a shaver. Once the perforation was identified, the margins were cleared with a suction punch and the disc was mobilized. Unfortunately, the lateral pole of the condyle was severely degenerated.

Arthroscopic Examination

Synovium: excessive fibrillation; synovitis
Roofing: 100% loss; anterior disc displacement
Sutures: not visualized
Function: restricted range of motion
Adhesions: multiple

The diagnosis was perforation and degenerative joint disease with disc displacement. The patient did well for 3 to 4 months but then had significant pain. The range of motion was increased, with more than 30 mm of opening and some translation. It was believed that if the patient could tolerate the pain, the return of function might allow for maturation of tissue and possibly have some "burnout" effect on the osteoarthritis. Unfortunately, the pain persisted and an open joint procedure was performed. Findings were consistent with those seen by arthroscopy, but the condylar head had deteriorated significantly (possibly from previous cortisone treatment).

SECONDARY SURGICAL PROCEDURES

Secondary surgical procedures often require removal of the disc. Although this can be done as a primary treatment for a severely perforated disc or for degenerative changes, it generally accompanies a secondary attempt. Removal of the disc, commonly known as a meniscectomy or discectomy, has received much attention in the literature over

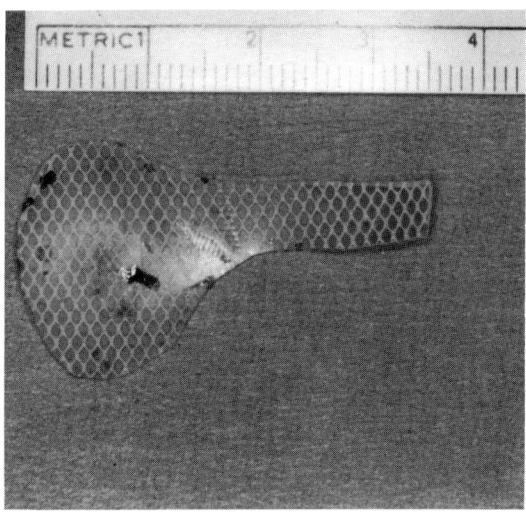

Figure 13–37. Gross photograph of a Silastic spacer showing wear in center and handle to remove under suture line.

the years. Discectomy, described by such surgeons as Dr. Silver and Dr. Wilkes, has been modified with the use of a Silastic spacer (Figs. 13–37, 13–38, and 13–39). A series of TMJ surgeries were done using the Silastic spacer for a period of 1 to 4 months and then removed. Arthroscopic biopsies and TMJ evaluations were reported in 1987 at the International Association of TMJ Arthroscopy Meeting. In this project, not all samples were problematic. However, the role of arthroscopy in evaluating the post-arthrotomy patient with regard to tissue reaction in the joint space was shown to have significance.

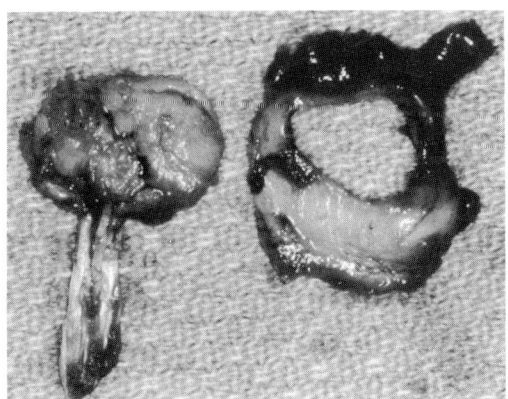

Figure 13–38. Gross photograph of tissue from disc that has broken down shows perforation and granulation tissue on the right. Sample on the left shows degenerative head of condyle with pterygoid muscle attached.

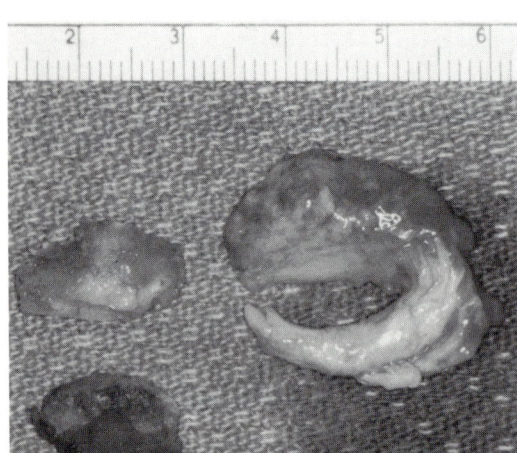

Figure 13-39. Gross photograph shows disc with perforation and adjacent fragments of tissue removed during the primary procedure of discectomy.

Arthroscopy has two major applications in post-discectomy TMJ procedures. First, the joint space can be evaluated to establish the extent and nature of the fibrous covering of the condyle. By inserting the arthroscope under the temporary spacer, the fibrous capsule can be evaluated. The range of response can vary from complete covering of the condylar head to a continuum of degenerative processes. A variety of findings can be seen, ranging from a tight fibrous response to irregular soft tissue covering small perforations and ultimately to large perforations with bony spicules extending through. Second, this tissue covering can be evaluated histologically when small samples are taken through the arthroscopic cannula as a direct biopsy, or using triangulation techniques. Arthroscopy makes this a relatively noninvasive procedure, and histologic samples can be taken from various regions in the TMJ.

The initial project done in 1987 evaluated ten post-discectomy patients. Samples of the ten TMJs evaluated showed a variety of responses. In some, the tissue forming the fibrous covering was tight and no portions of the condylar head could be visualized (Fig. 13-40). In other areas the condylar head could be seen, especially in areas consistent with markings on the Silastic spacer. The clinical ramifications of these findings ultimately could be directed toward postoperative care. Certainly, if the patient showed slow responsive changes in the fibrous capsule, continued unloading of the TMJ and TMJ rest could be two modalities of this type of treatment. In comparison, if a good fibrous covering was visualized, postoperative care could progress to the next stages of rehabilitation.

When the histologic samples of these TMJs were evaluated, a variety of responses were noted. Although the disc was not removed in its entirety, the majority of the fibrocartilage disc structure had been removed in all cases. The dissections for the discectomy involved removal of the disc from the retrodistal tissue up to the limits of the anterior band. In general, almost all traces of remaining tissue were removed, depending on their accessibility in the joint space. The fibrous capsule could be visualized (Fig 13-41). The nature of this fibrous capsule in these ten joints showed a variety of tissue types. The following list exemplifies the tissue responses seen histologically.

1. Typical fibrous tissue with strong connective tissue covering (Fig. 13-42 and 13-43)
2. Remnants of synovial tissue or regeneration of synovial tissue
3. Neovascularization of capsule with increased vascularity (Fig 13-44)
4. Irregular, fibrous connective tissue with fibrosis (Figs. 13-45 through 13-48)
5. Striated muscle tissue
6. Salivary or parotid gland tissue

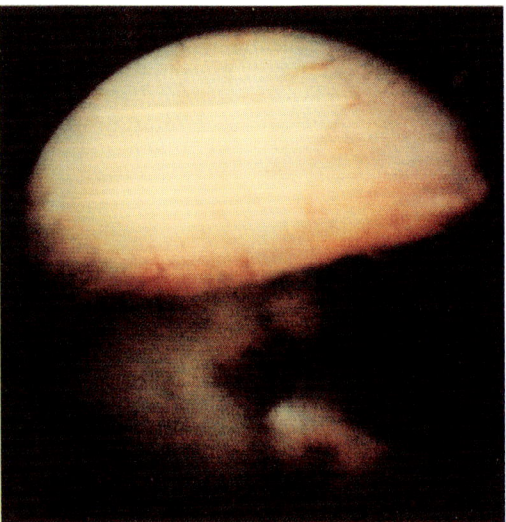

Figure 13-40. Arthroscopic view of synovium covering of temporomandibular joint following discectomy.

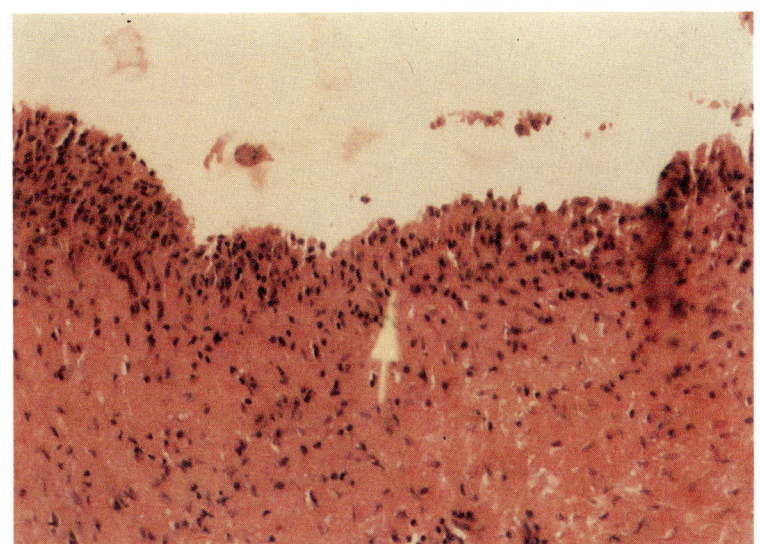

Figure 13–41. Tissue sample obtained following removal of Silastic spacer. Medium-power microphotograph shows synovial tissue with hyperplasia. Many hypertrophied cells *(arrow)* can be seen just beneath the surface.

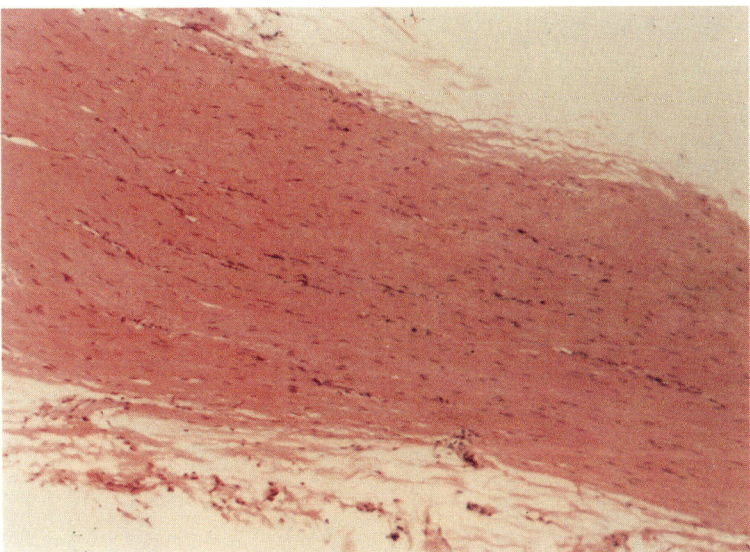

Figure 13–42. Tissue sample obtained following removal of Silastic spacer. Low-power microphotograph shows highly organized, dense fibrous tissue with low cellularity, partly lining the joint space.

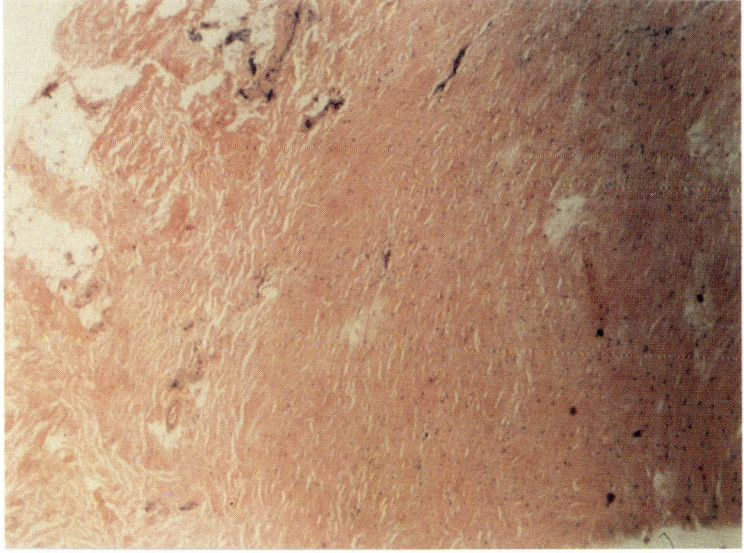

Figure 13–43. Tissue sample obtained following removal of Silastic spacer. Medium-power microphotograph shows low cellularity of dense fibrous tissue with hyalinization.

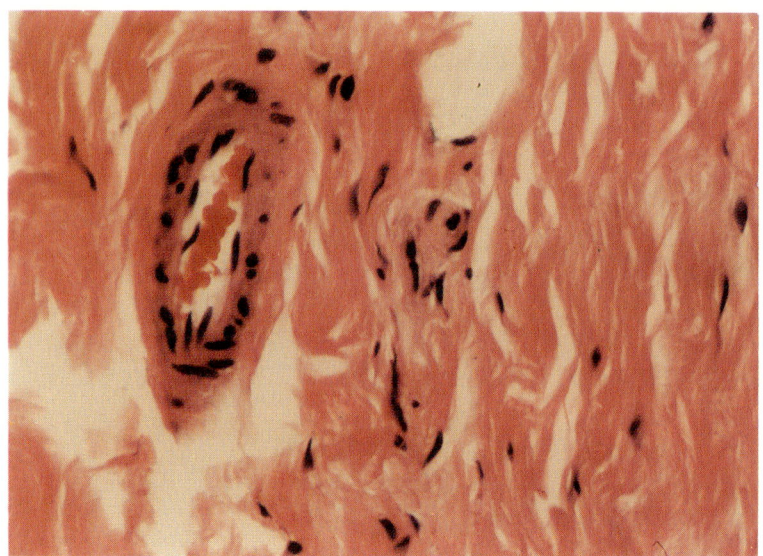

Figure 13–44. Vascularity of fibrous capsule following discectomy and removal of Silastic spacer. High-power microphotograph shows one of many small arteries against a background of dense fibrosis, with adjacent entrapped small nerve fibers.

Figure 13–45. Tissue sample obtained following removal of Silastic spacer. Low-power microphotograph shows papillary synovial fragments of dense fibrous tissue with focally increased intercellular matrix, having a chondroid appearance, and focally increased cellularity in the papillary fronds. Note the focus of dystrophic calcification (arrow).

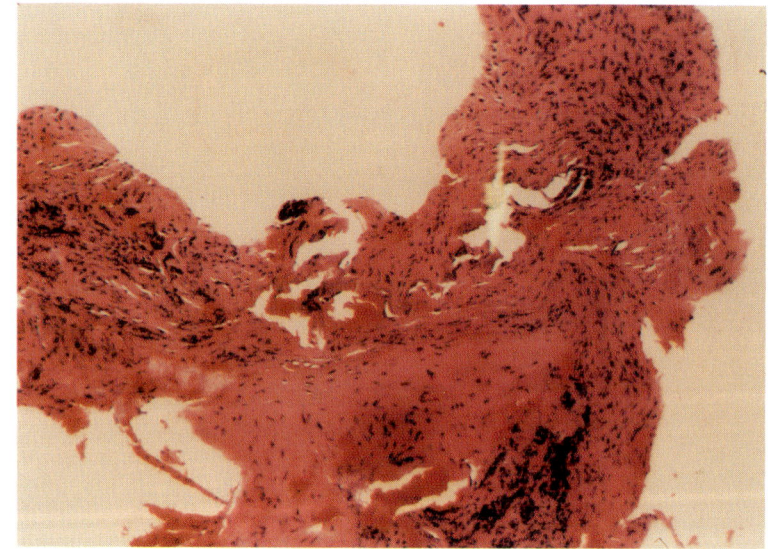

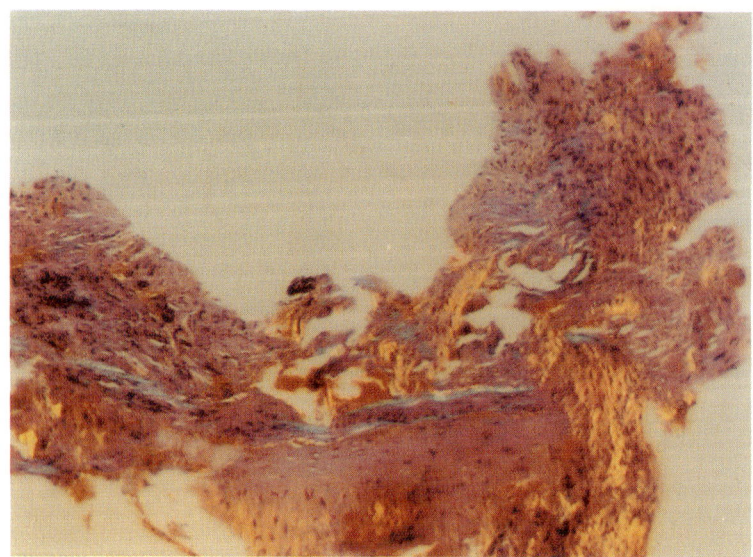

Figure 13–46. Low-power microphotograph from capsule following discectomy and removal of Silastic spacer. Examination under polarized light shows birefringent, yellow, dense, highly organized collagen in relatively acellular areas, as well as occasional wavy, large fragments of blue-white birefringent materials consistent with Silastic. There is little foreign-body reaction to Silastic, in contrast to that seen with Proplast (see Figs. 13–51 through 13–60).

F. Temporomandibular Joint Arthroscopy for Post-Arthrotomy Patients ■ 221

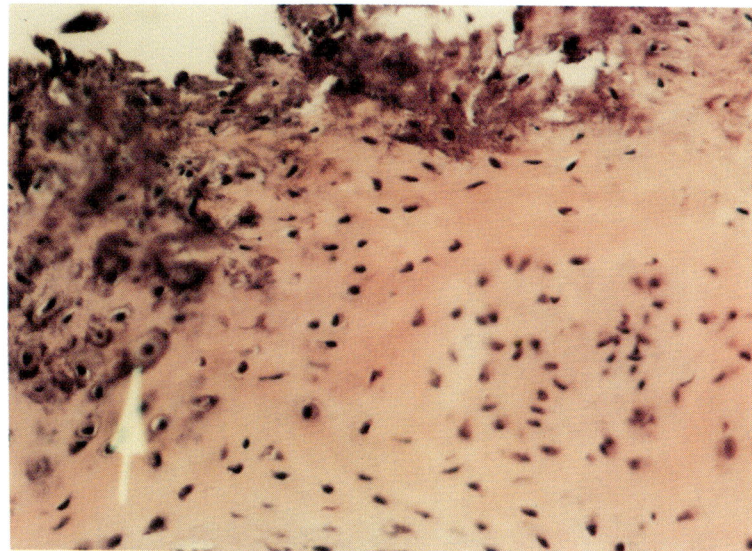

Figure 13–47. Tissue sample obtained following removal of Silastic spacer. High-powered microphotograph shows increased cellularity with many macrophages with increased intracellular matrix. There is dystrophic calcification *(arrow)* of the intercellular matrix in a loose filigree pattern surrounding stromal cells.

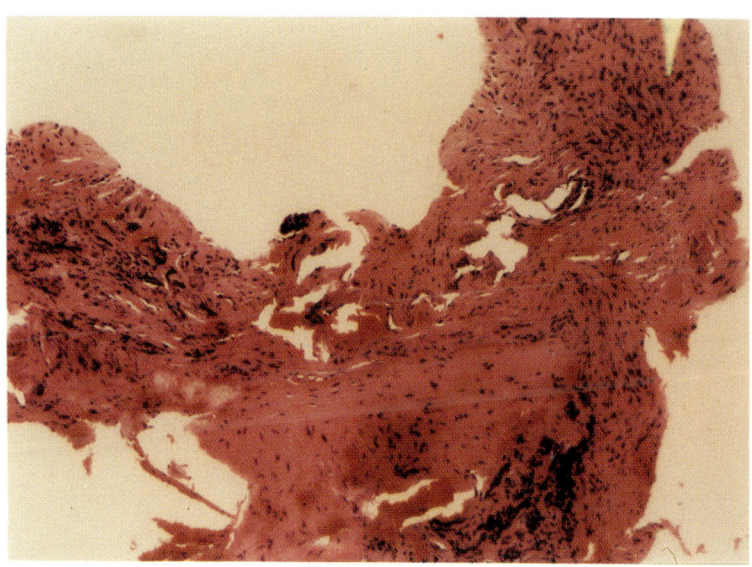

Figure 13–48. Tissue sample obtained following removal of Silastic spacer. Low-power microphotograph shows increased cellular areas of the fronds with macrophages, as seen in Figure 13–49.

7. Areas of calcification (Figs. 13–45, 13–47, and 13–49)
8. Fibrosis accompanying embedded Silastic in capsular samples (Fig 13–50)
9. Areas of cartilage formation (Fig. 13–47)
10. Foreign-body giant cell reaction

Although each sample contained only one or two of these findings, the variety of tissue responses indicated the multipotential cell types that can be found with this procedure. The clinical usefulness of this information became more relevant when samples showing calcification were visualized. In this instance, follow-up of a patient who showed early calcification revealed a bony ankylosis that had to be re-operated. One can conjecture whether a calcium-inhibiting agent such as etidronate disodium (Didronel) could have been used prophylactically.

Samples of the tissue responses are shown in the remaining histologic illustrations. Polarized light was useful when evaluating these samples to visualize Silastic embedded in the tissues.

When using the arthroscope to evaluate

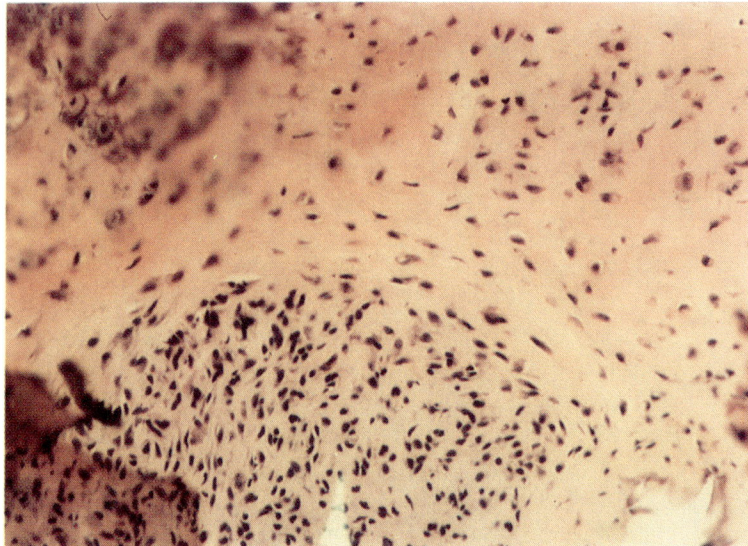

Figure 13–49. Tissue sample obtained following removal of Silastic spacer. Medium-power microphotograph shows fibrosis with increased extracellular matrix and cellular nodules of macrophages, with only occasional multinucleated giant cells and without recognizable foreign material.

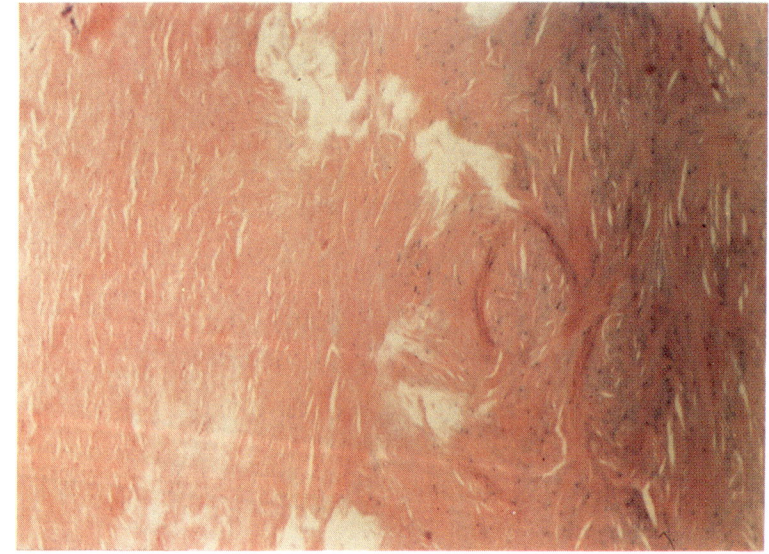

Figure 13–50. Tissue sample obtained following removal of Silastic spacer. Medium-power microphotograph shows dense fibrous tissue with hyalinization, low cellularity, and fibroplastic proliferation. The clear spaces contain faintly visible foreign material (Silastic) without foreign-body giant cell reaction.

post-discectomy joints, it is important to establish a correlation between clinical findings, radiographic findings, and histologic changes and the ultimate clinical course. This information can directly benefit postoperative care.

In conclusion, arthroscopy is a quick and simple method to assess the healing and repair following the use of a temporary spacer. Furthermore, arthroscopy may be beneficial from a research perspective in understanding the mechanism by which discectomy failure occurs. This may be due to continued degenerative breakdown of bone or fibrous tissue, to an irregular tissue-type growth that invades the capsule, or to the continued growth of adhesions.

When the diagnostic capabilities of this instrumentation are coupled with operative techniques, such as lysis of adhesions and lateral eminentia release, the result may be increased mobility in a postoperative course. Certainly, when a post-discectomy patient exhibits scarring down in the joint, arthroscopy may increase the range of motion in the TMJ. By stretching the limits of the capsule

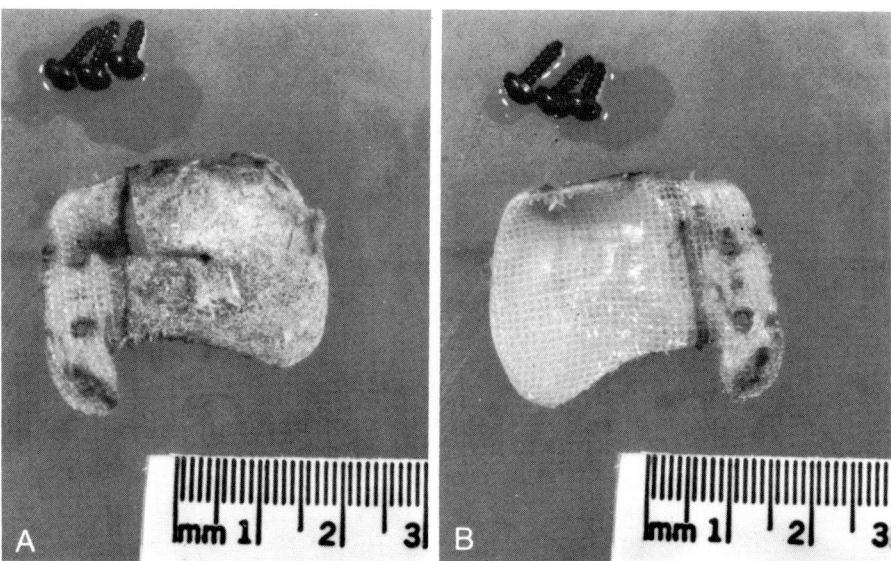

Figure 13–51. Kent Proplast laminate with reinforced Teflon used for fossa replacement. Superior *(A)* and inferior *(B)* surfaces are shown.

through either direct or indirect lysis and lavage, a greater interincisal opening can be obtained.

In the last major group of patients studied who had had TMJ arthrotomy, an alloplastic material had been implanted (Fig. 13–51). During the 1980s, the use of Proplast combination implants was popular. Unfortunately, this material caused a severe foreign-body reaction (Figs. 13–52 through 13–59). Arthroscopy made it possible to identify this reaction without resorting to arthrotomy of the TMJ.

When a patient who has had a Proplast implant placed in the TMJ develops clinical symptoms, the surgeon often experiences a dilemma. Further surgery may be a difficult decision for such a patient. Often, the patient has undergone multiple procedures, and another procedure is not necessarily in his or her best interest. However, assessment of the type of tissue reaction in the TMJ using routine imaging techniques is almost impossible in terms of visualizing a foreign-body giant cell response.

The patient with Proplast implants placed in the TMJ subsequently developed symptoms including radiographic evidence of loss of condylar height. In these patients, the arthroscopic appearance of a foreign-body reaction was dramatically and clearly visualized. Evaluation included comparison of gross specimens, arthroscopic samples, and histopathologic sections. It was apparent from the samples that Proplast elicits a specific type of foreign-body response and that arthroscopy visualizes this response predictably and consistently. On the head of the condyle, a "popcorn" lesion resembling a villonodular change could be seen. Microscopically this granulomatous tissue consistently showed embedded Proplast material with severe fibrosis and a foreign-body response. The arthroscopic appearance seen in

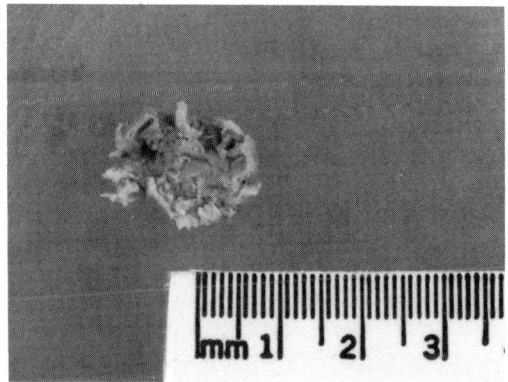

Figure 13–52. Tissue sample obtained from temporomandibular joint with Proplast implant. Gross photograph shows a single fragment of firm, fibrous tissue with many filiform extensions.

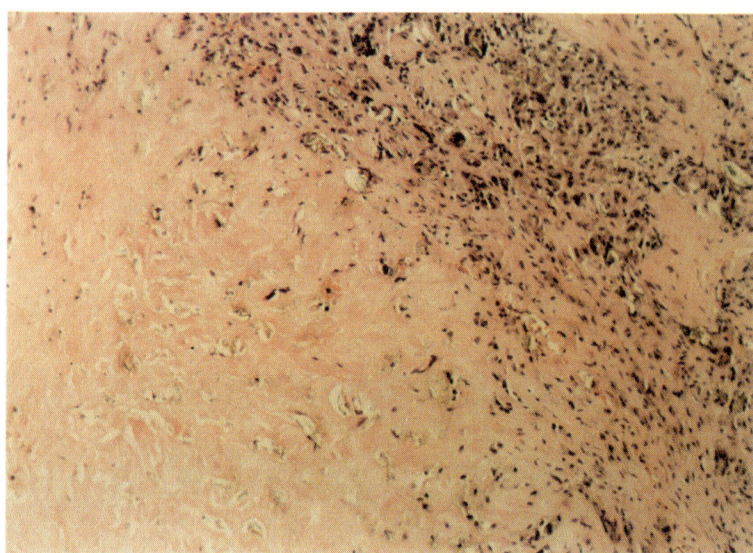

Figure 13–53. Tissue sample obtained following removal of Proplast spacer. Medium-power microphotograph shows fibrosis with hyalinized, relatively acellular, dense fibrous tissue with embedded minute, translucent fragments of foreign material (Proplast); on the opposite side of the field, there is a densely cellular infiltrate of macrophages with easily recognizable multinucleated foreign-body giant cells, some of which are around Proplast fragments.

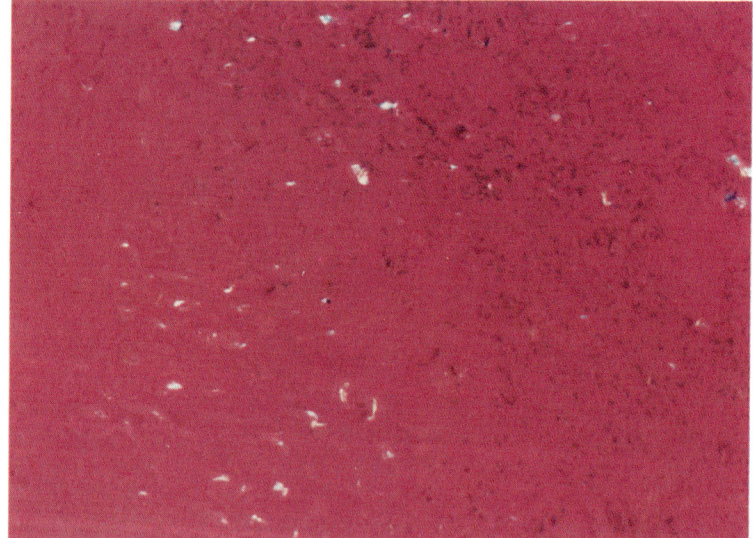

Figure 13–54. Tissue sample obtained following removal of Proplast spacer. Medium-power microphotograph (same field as Fig. 13–52) examined under polarized light shows birefringent, small, short, fibrous and often curved fragments (ranging in shape from round to oval) of Proplast in a relatively acellular area without adjacent macrophages, as well as in a hypercellular area with many surrounding macrophages.

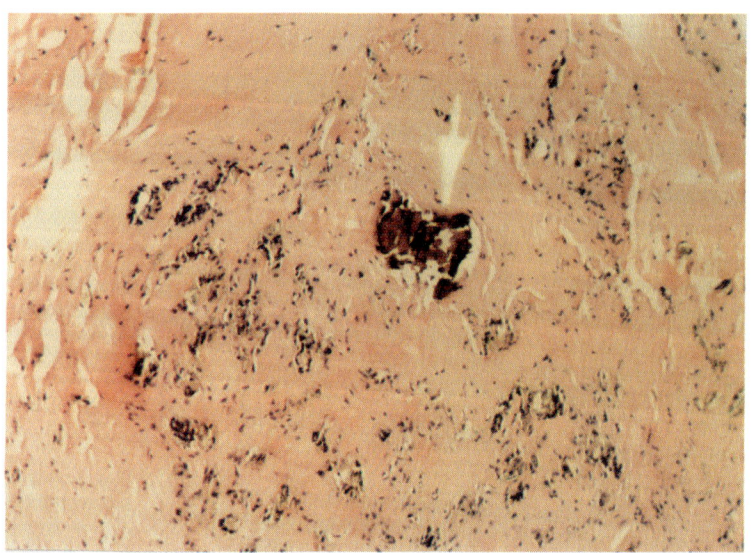

Figure 13–55. Tissue sample obtained following removal of Proplast spacer. Medium-power microphotograph shows hyalinized, dense, relatively acellular background of fibrosis with clusters of macrophages around colorless Proplast fragments. Note nodular focus *(arrow)* of dystrophic calcification, ossification, or embedded bone fragment.

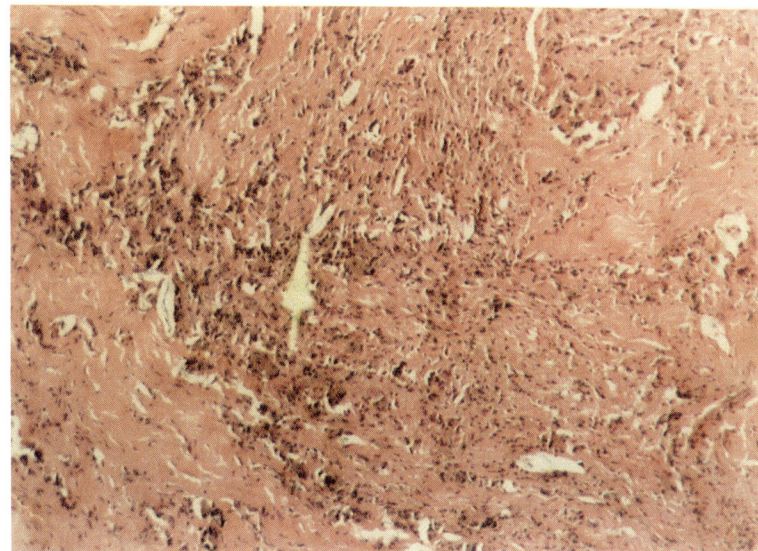

Figure 13–56. Tissue sample obtained following removal of Proplast spacer. Medium-power microphotograph shows fibrosis with dense, hyalinized collagen (embedded in which are irregular, elongated, colorless Proplast fragments) with adjacent cellular areas with many macrophages, some of which have formed multinucleated foreign-body giant cells (often at the edges of the Proplast fragments). Note the Proplast fragment *(arrow)* surrounded by foreign-body giant cells; Teflon fragments (not shown) are larger and more regular.

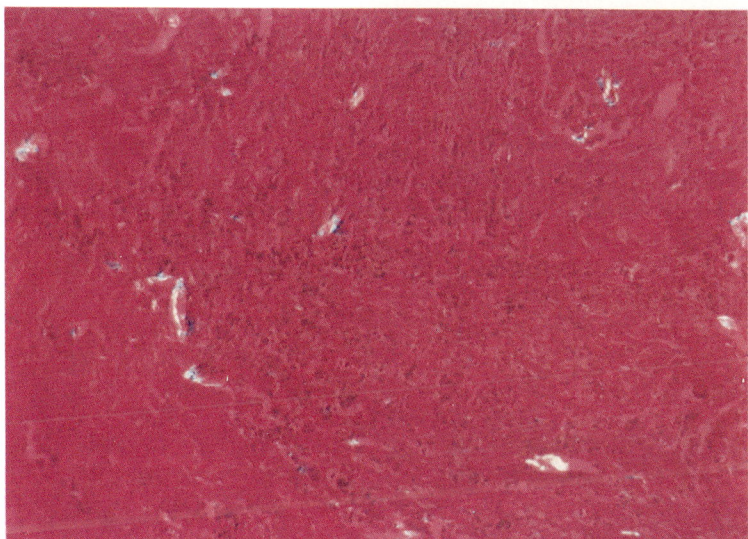

Figure 13–57. Tissue sample obtained following removal of Proplast spacer. Medium-power microphotograph (same field as Fig. 13–56) examined under polarized light shows minute, irregular, elongated, birefringent Proplast fragments; Teflon fragments (not shown) are more strongly birefringent.

Figure 13–58. Fibrous tissue sample removed from temporomandibular joint with Proplast implant. Gross photograph shows granulomatous reaction to Proplast foreign body. There are multiple fragments, ranging from firm to hard in consistency, of fibrous tissue, partly lining the joint space.

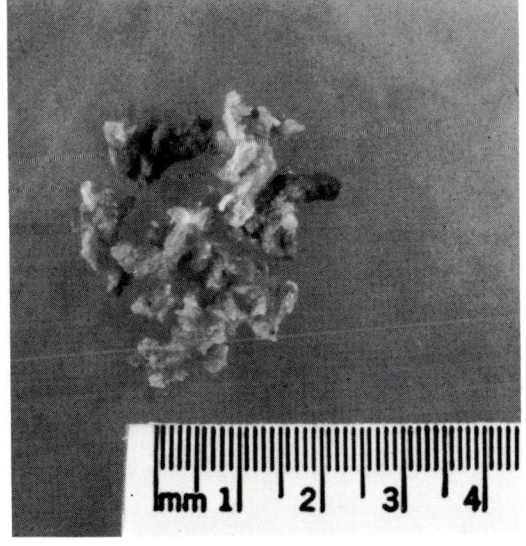

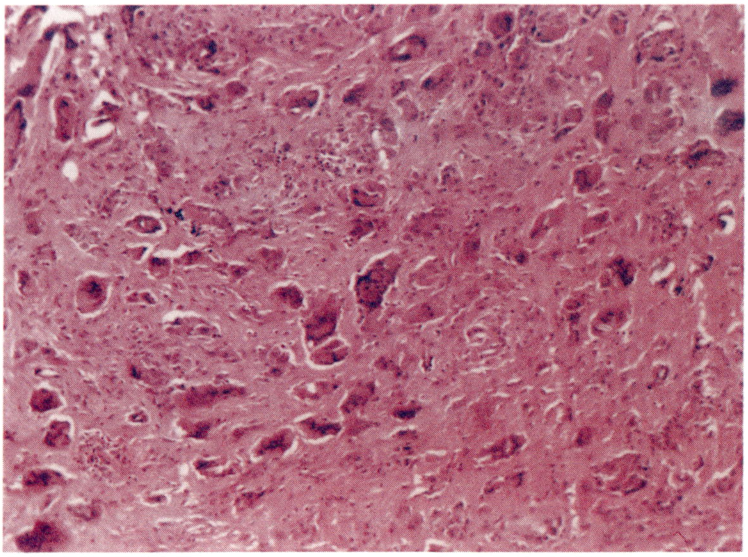

Figure 13–59. Tissue sample obtained following removal of Proplast spacer. Medium-power microphotograph shows granulomatous reaction with abundant multinucleated foreign-body giant cells against a background of hyalinized fibrous tissue with many macrophages. Proplast fragments can be seen in many of the giant cells.

Figure 13–60 is pathognomonic for this type of reaction.

It is interesting to note that the histologic responses of Silastic and Proplast are quite different. Silastic appears to cause predominantly bland fibrosis with a nodular fibrohistiocytic reaction around the material. There is little multinuclear foreign-body giant cell formation. Occasionally, there are some eosinophilic responses, but for the most part the walling of the Silastic fragments does not cause a granulomatous response (see Figs. 13–41 through 13–50).

The Proplast, however, does cause a predominantly granulomatous reaction showing typical foreign-body response with foreign-body multinuclear cells, increased fibrosis, and increased granulomatous mass that continues to grow and spread through the joint (see Figs. 13–42 through 13–55). The arthroscope can be used to clean out this material, as reported by Koslin[18] and others; however, it appears that the ultimate fate of these joints requires removal of the Proplast implant. In our clinical sample, all patients who have had a foreign-body response have had the Proplast implant removed and the joint debrided via arthrotomy.

Arthroscopic surgery can be beneficial to these patients in that further deterioration and foreign-body responses can be eliminated with the use of instrumentation and motorized equipment. Certainly, arthroscopy continues to limit the number of open joint procedures, which is a direct benefit to these patients.

CONCLUSIONS

Arthroscopy can be used to evaluate the post-arthrotomy patient who has undergone a simple soft tissue repair. In this instance, the benefits can be diagnostic as well as therapeutic. Release of adhesions and stretching of the joint capsule using arthroscopy can be of major benefit in increasing the range of motion. Although this may not necessarily limit the amount of pain a patient is experiencing, the resultant increase in joint function generally improves the ability of a joint to undergo normal repair.

Arthroscopy in more complicated TMJ surgical procedures is also beneficial. If the patient has had a meniscectomy with a Silastic spacer, the resultant fibrous capsule can be evaluated with the arthroscope at the time of removal. Familiarity with the previous open joint surgery is often a prerequisite for improving the use of this procedure.

In summary, arthroscopy often limits the need for and amount of subsequent joint procedures, and it may benefit the patient both diagnostically and therapeutically.[2, 19]

ACKNOWLEDGMENT:

The contribution of Steven L. Goldberg, M.D., to the preparation of this chapter is greatly appreciated.

F. Temporomandibular Joint Arthroscopy for Post-Arthrotomy Patients

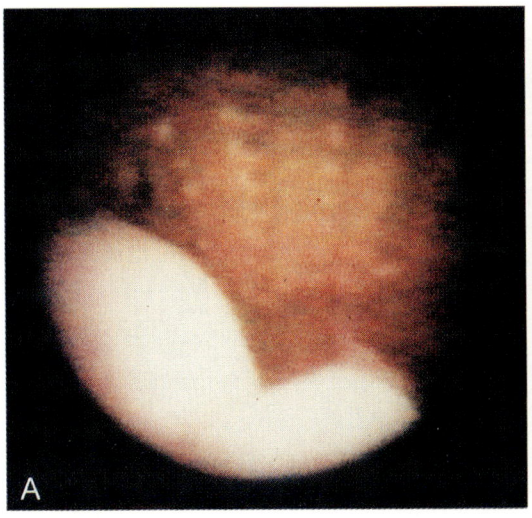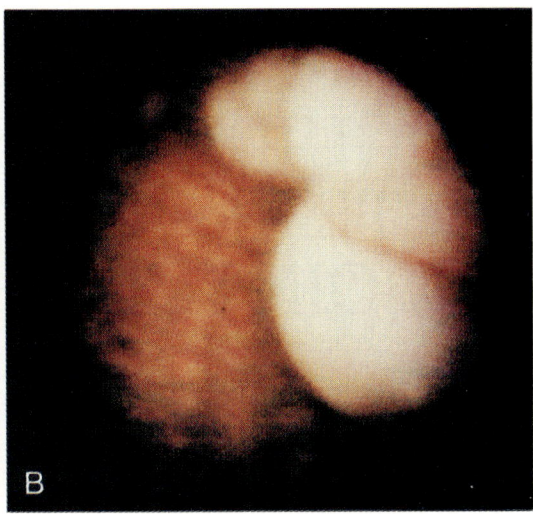

Figure 13–60. *A* and *B,* Arthroscopic photographs of Proplast implants in fossa and foreign-body lesions on the condyle. The granulatory tissue is pathognomonic of foreign-body reactions.

References

1. Schwartz LL: Pain associated with the TMJ. JADA 51:305, 1955.
2. Moses JJ, Poker ID: TMJ arthroscopic surgery: An analysis of 237 patients. J Oral Maxillofac Surg 47:790, 1989.
3. Merrill RG: Historical perspectives and comparison of temporomandibular joint surgery for internal disk derangements and arthropathy. J Craniomandib Pract 4:75, 1986.
4. Holmlund AB, Hellsing G: Arthroscopy of the temporomandibular joint: A comparison study of arthroscopic and tomographic findings. J Oral Maxillofac Surg 17:128, 1988.
5. Blaustein D, Heffez L: Diagnostic arthroscopy of the temporomandibular joint. Part II: Arthroscopic findings of arthrographically diagnosed disk displacements. Oral Surg 65:9, 1988.
6. McCain JP: Arthroscopy of the human temporomandibular joint. J Oral Maxillofac Surg 46:648, 1988.
7. Holmlund AB: Diagnostic accuracy of temporomandibular joint arthroscopy. A comparison of findings during arthroscopy and arthrotomy. Oral Maxillofac Clin North Am 1:79, 1989.
8. Braun T: Temporomandibular joint surgery. Parts I and II: Surgical treatment of internal derangement. Selected Readings Oral Maxillofac Surg 1:3, 1989.
9. Murakami K-I: Arthroscopic anatomy of the temporomandibular joint. Oral Maxillofac Clin North Am 1:69, 1989.
10. McCarty WL: Surgery for internal derangements of the temporomandibular joint. J Prosthet Dent 42:191, 1979.
11. Walker RV, Kalamichi S: A surgical technique for management of internal derangement of the temporomandibular joint. J Oral Maxillofac Surg 45:299, 1987.
12. Silver CM: Long-term results of meniscectomy of the temporomandibular joint. J Craniomandib Pract 3:46, 1984.
13. Davis PK, Jones SM: The complications of Silastic implants: Experience with 137 consecutive cases. Br J Plast Surg 24:405, 1971.
14. Kent JN, Dusek J, Smith P: Proplast-Teflon implants for treatment of TMJ degenerative disease. [Abstract] 61st Annual Meeting of the American Association of Oral and Maxillofacial Surgeons, 1978.
15. Temporomandibular joint condylar prosthesis: A ten year report. J Oral Maxillofac Surg 41:245, 1983.
16. Heffez L, Blaustein P: Diagnostic arthroscopy of the temporomandibular joint. Part I: Normal arthroscopic findings. Oral Surg 64:653, 1987.
17. McCain JP, de la Rua H, Le Blanc WG: Correlation of the clinical, radiographic and arthroscopic findings in internal derangements of the TMJ. J Oral Maxillofac Surg 47:913, 1989.
18. Koslin M: Second International TMJ Arthroscopic Surgery Symposium, December 1987, New York City.
19. Tarro AW: Arthroscopic treatment of anterior disc displacement: A preliminary report. J Oral Maxillofac Surg 47:347–348, 1989.

Suggested Further Reading

Bronstein SL: Diagnostic and operative arthroscopy. Historical perspectives and indications. Oral Maxillofac Clin North Am 1:59, 1989.

Dolwick MF, Aufdemorte TB, Cornelius JD: Histopathologic findings in TMJ internal derangements. [Abstract] J Dent Res 63:267, 1984.

White RD: Retrospective analysis of 100 consecutive surgical arthroscopies of the temporomandibular joint. J Oral Maxillofac Surg 47:1014–1021, 1989.

Chapter 14

GUIDELINES FOR TEMPOROMANDIBULAR JOINT ARTHROSCOPY

SIDNEY L. BRONSTEIN, D.D.S., M.SC.D., F.A.C.D.

An exceptionally significant event occurred in the summer of 1986 when the First International Symposium on Temporomandibular Joint Arthroscopy convened in New York City. This conference was assembled under the sponsorship of the Hospital for Joint Diseases Orthopaedic Institute and directed by Drs. Joseph McCain and Stuart Springer. Papers that were presented at that symposium dealt solely with the developing diagnostic and treatment modality of temporomandibular joint (TMJ) arthroscopy. Information pertinent to this subject was presented by oral and maxillofacial surgeons, orthopedic surgeons, and physical therapists.

A notable consequence of this symposium was the formation of the International Study Group (ISG) for the Advancement of TMJ Arthroscopy, involving clinical practitioners and research investigators from the United States, Asia, and Europe. From this group have come deliberations, debates, and decisions regarding arthroscopic education and training, hospital credentialing, continuing education, and general guidelines and principles for the practice of TMJ arthroscopy. The efforts of the ISG significantly encouraged development of the Position Statement on TMJ Arthroscopy by the American Association of Oral and Maxillofacial Surgeons (AAOMS) (Appendix A) and the formation of an ad hoc advisory committee of the AAOMS for clarification of criteria for health insurance coverage for this procedure.

Mastery of the techniques for TMJ arthroscopy requires extensive commitment. Oral and maxillofacial surgeons have been especially successful in developing skills for this procedure; because of their specialized surgical skills and their extensive knowledge of the anatomy, physiology, and pathology of this joint, they found themselves in the leadership role in utilizing this new technique. This proficiency follows successes in open joint surgery based on biologic principles of restoration of normal joint anatomy, muscle physiology, and masticatory function. Moreover, with the application of newer knowledge of synovial disease and fibrocartilage responses to injury, the surgery now involves less invasive maneuvers that promote faster healing and return of function.

Because of this rapid input of new information and the development of new techniques and instruments, the need for continuing education in TMJ arthroscopy has grown commensurately. Symposia, didactic courses, and laboratory workshops using cadavers are presented throughout the United States and are now convening in many foreign countries. Advanced workshops utilizing newer techniques of operative TMJ arthroscopy are offering training at a more skilled level of expertise for improved treatment of TMJ articular disease.

HOSPITAL CREDENTIALING

The clinical practice of TMJ arthroscopy requires that the patient be in a hospital atmosphere either as an inpatient or outpatient, under general anesthesia. This has affected hospital credentialing procedures in a major way, at least in larger hospitals. The ISG and the AAOMS have developed and presented position statements addressing hospital credentialing.

It has been suggested that the granting of initial clinical privileges require the following: (1) certification or eligibility for certification by the respective surgical boards and current privileges in open TMJ surgery (almost certainly in larger hospitals there will be surgeons not meeting this requirement who are already quite proficient in TMJ surgery); (2) documentation of significant experience in TMJ arthrotomy within the past 5 years, with a majority of these cases performed as an operating surgeon; (3) documentation of attendance at didactic and/or clinical continuing education courses on the subject of TMJ arthroscopy for 16 or more hours; (4) documentation of participation in a hands-on fresh cadaver technique workshop; and (5) satisfactory performance of at least three TMJ arthroscopic procedures, proctored by a surgeon holding full privileges in TMJ arthroscopy. In some areas, these proctors probably would not be available or there would be only a few arthroscopists upon whom this chore would fall; therefore, some modification of this requirement would be necessary.

In most hospitals, medical staff reappointment occurs biennially. Continuation of clinical privileges would require some form of documentation regarding maintenance of current expertise, knowledge, and advances in the practice of TMJ arthroscopy. Five arthroscopic cases per year plus proof of attendance at seminars, symposia, and/or cadaver workshops could satisfy this requirement.

Many modern oral and maxillofacial surgery residency programs now include TMJ arthroscopy as an integral, significant portion of their training. Those residents who have demonstrated competency in TMJ arthroscopic procedures during their training would also need to meet the requirements listed previously; however, information regarding proficiency could be provided and substantiated by the program director or by attending surgeons in the program who are experienced in TMJ arthroscopy. Compliance in this manner would necessarily exclude those specific requirements listed previously concerning case documentation, course attendance, and workshop participation.

CLINICAL PRACTICE

Anyone in whose practice arthroscopy plays a major role would do well to be familiar with the formal position paper prepared by the AAOMS (Appendix A). The information it contains is very useful to present both to referring doctors and to third-party providers to explain the application of arthroscopy in oral and maxillofacial surgical practice.

Diagnostic and surgical staging in the treatment of diseases of the TMJ, as devised by Dr. Clyde Wilkes, is very useful in the practice of TMJ arthroscopy. It is especially applicable to treatment planning and development of a prognostic sense for this procedure, and it also offers a means by which clinicians may discuss cases using the same reference criteria. This classification (Table 14–1) is divided into five stages: early, early intermediate, intermediate, late intermediate, and late. These stages using clinical, radiologic, and surgical criteria describe the onset and progression of internal derangement of the TMJ.

Another descriptive category, arthroscopy (developed by Dr. Ralph Merrill and the author), has been proposed to be considered under the same five stages. The criteria developed for this additional category attempt to follow the clinical symptoms and radiographic signs outlined by Wilkes, as well as the surgical findings. The arthroscopic criteria are presented in Table 14–2.

Generally a certain finite period of initial nonsurgical management is prescribed for TMJ arthropathies. If symptoms persist and arthroscopy is chosen as the next treatment phase, further patient care and presurgical preparation may include the continued use of a load-transferring or load-altering orthotic, use of indicated imaging techniques to further confirm or define the intracapsular structural status, and a detailed discussion with the patient concerning surgical outcome expectations and the importance of strict compliance post-arthroscopically with dietary restrictions and physical therapy. An informed consent for this procedure (Appendix B), thoroughly understood by the patient and his or her family, must be obtained.

Table 14–1. STAGING CRITERIA FOR INTERNAL DERANGEMENTS OF THE TEMPOROMANDIBULAR JOINT WITH RESPECT TO CLINICAL, RADIOLOGIC, AND SURGICAL FINDINGS*

Early Stage
Clinical: No significant mechanical symptoms, other than reciprocal clicking (early in opening movement, late in closing movement, and soft in intensity); no pain or limitation of motion
Radiologic: Slight forward displacement, good anatomic contour of disc, and normal tomograms
Surgical: Normal anatomic form, slight anterior displacement, and passive incoordination (clicking) demonstrable

Early/Intermediate Stage
Clinical: First few episodes of pain, occasional joint tenderness and related temporal headaches, beginning major mechanical problems, increase in intensity of clicking sounds, joint sounds later in opening movement, and beginning transient subluxations or joint catching and locking
Radiologic: Slight forward displacement, slight thickening of posterior edge or beginning anatomic deformity of disc, and normal tomograms
Surgical: Anterior displacement, early anatomic deformity (slight to mild thickening of posterior edge), and well-defined central articulating area

Intermediate Stage
Clinical: Multiple episodes of pain, joint tenderness, temporal headaches, major mechanical symptoms—transient catching, locking and sustained locking (closed locks), restriction of motion, and difficulty (pain) with function
Radiologic: Anterior displacement with significant anatomic deformity/prolapse of disc (moderate to marked thickening of posterior edge) and normal tomograms
Surgical: Marked anatomic deformity with displacement, variable adhesions (anterior, lateral, and posterior recesses), and no hard tissue changes

Intermediate/Late Stage
Clinical: Characterized by chronicity with variable and episodic pain, headaches, variable restriction of motion, and undulating course
Radiologic: Increase in severity over intermediate stage, abnormal tomograms, and early to moderate degenerative remodeling hard tissue changes
Surgical: Increase in severity over intermediate stage, hard tissue degenerative remodeling changes of both bearing surfaces, osteophytic projections, multiple adhesions (lateral, anterior, and posterior recesses), and *no perforation* of disc or attachment

Late Stage
Clinical: Characterized by crepitus on examination, scraping, grating, grinding symptoms, variable and episodic pain, chronic restriction of motion, and difficulty with function
Radiologic: Anterior displacement, *perforation* with simultaneous filling of upper and lower compartments, filling defects, gross anatomic deformity of disc and hard tissues, abnormal tomograms as described, and essentially degenerative arthritic changes
Surgical: Gross degenerative changes of disc and hard tissues, *perforation* of posterior attachments, erosions of bearing surfaces, and multiple adhesions equivalent to degenerative arthritis (sclerosis, flattening, anvil-shaped condyle, osteophytic projections, and subcortical cystic formation)

*Radiologic findings refer to arthrographic, magnetic resonance, and tomographic imaging where applicable.
(Reprinted with permission from Wilkes CH: Internal derangements of the temporomandibular joint. Arch Otolaryngol Head Neck Surg 115:470, 1989. Copyright 1989, American Medical Association.)

As mentioned earlier, arthroscopic procedures are performed in an operating room environment, outpatient or inpatient, using general anesthesia, with standard surgical aseptic technique and draping (Fig. 14–1). A suggested operating room set-up for the equipment and personnel is illustrated in Appendix C. Diagnostic arthroscopy may require only 20 to 30 minutes per side to complete, whereas a difficult, complicated operative case may require up to 2 hours per TMJ. However, the longer the TMJ is being manipulated arthroscopically, the more the tissues can become swollen with irrigating medium, the more they may become distorted, and the greater chance there is for iatrogenic tissue injury. The chances for extravasation of fluid into the surrounding tissues also increase.

Certain pitfalls are commonly encountered as one enters the early clinical practice of TMJ arthroscopy. These should be recognized and corrected. Instruments must be in the desired joint space; irrigation must be adequate, with freely flowing inflow and outflow; joint movement must be sufficient to allow development of space for the instrumentation; and a trained surgical team is necessary.

Table 14–2. STAGING CRITERIA FOR INTERNAL DERANGEMENTS OF TEMPOROMANDIBULAR JOINT WITH RESPECT TO ARTHROSCOPIC FINDINGS

Early Stage
Roofing, 80% (closed position) to 100% (open or protrusive positions); incipient bilaminar zone elongation; incipient loss of articular surface smoothness; normal synovium, vascularity, superior compartment recesses, and disc flexure (junction of discal eminence and superior lamina)

Early/Intermediate Stage
Roofing, 50% (closed position) to 100% (open or protrusive positions); bilaminar zone elongation with decreased disc flexure; early adhesive synovitis with beginning adhesion formation; slight lateroanterior capsular stretching and laxity

Intermediate Stage
Advanced bilaminar zone elongation with accordion-shaped redundancy and loss of disc flexure; prominent synovitis and adhesion formations; diminished lateral recess with capsular prolapse

Substage A
Roofing, 5% (closed position) to <15% (open or protrusive positions); chondromalacia, Grades I–II (softening, blistering, or furrowing)

Substage B:
No roofing (nonreducible disc displacement); pseudowall formation in anterior synovial pouch; chondromalacia, Grades II–III (blistering, furrowing, ulceration, fraying, fibrillation, surface rupture)

Intermediate/Late Stage
Increased severity of superior compartment pathology over intermediate stage disease; hyalinization of retrodiscal surface; chondromalacia, Grades III–IV (ulceration, fraying, fibrillation, surface rupture, cratering, bone exposure)

Late Stage
Prominent articular surface fibrillations; advanced synovitis and generalized adhesions; perforation; retrodiscal metaplasia; false capsule formation in anterior synovial pouch; chondromalacia, Grade IV (cratering, bone exposure)

Prognostication for operative arthroscopy is closely dependent on the severity of the disease. Good prognosis may be predicted when the disc morphology is essentially normal (Fig. 14–2). This is seen most often in the initial episode of acute painful hypomobility of short history. Chronic painful hypomobility or dysfunctional hypermobility in the early, early/intermediate, or intermediate stages carries a favorable prognosis if disc deformation seen by arthrography or MRI is minimal (Fig. 14–3).

Hypermobile joints are somewhat more difficult to treat, but if the disc can be well mobilized by lysis of adhesions and the translation of the condyle improved, the

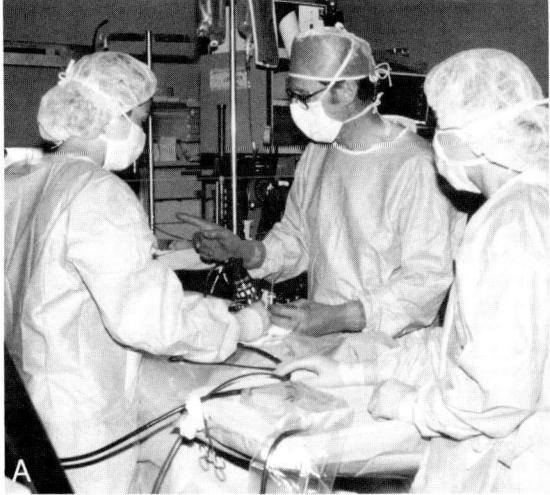 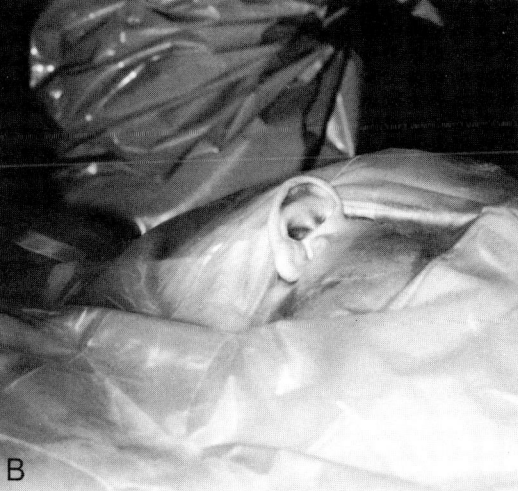

Figure 14–1. *A,* Operating room set-up showing positions of surgeon, assistant, and instrument nurse; *B,* sterile preparation and draping of right temporomandibular joint area.

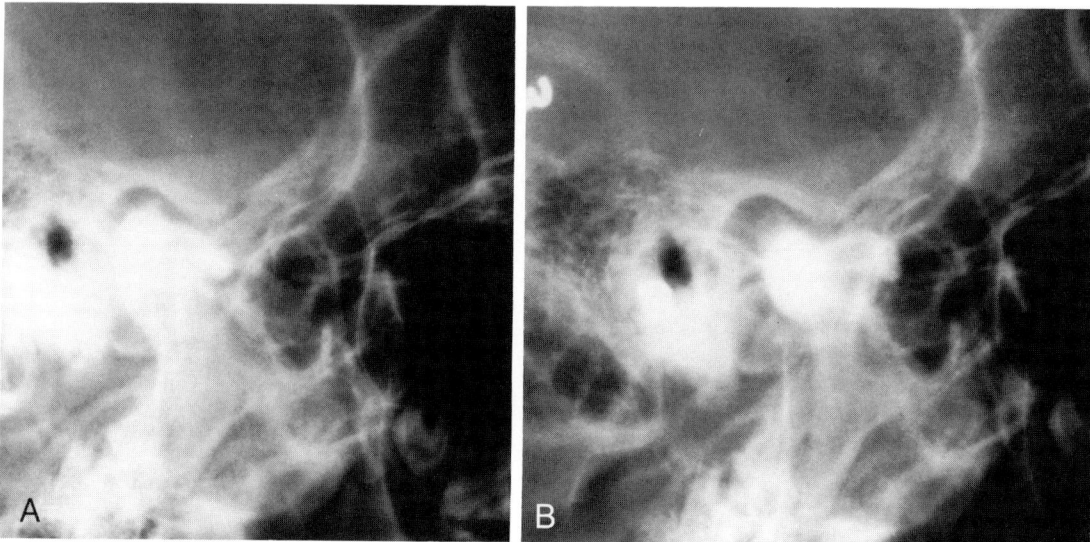

Figure 14–2. Arthrograms of reducible anteriorly displaced disc showing essentially normal disc morphology: *A*, closed position; *B*, maximal open position.

prognosis can be very good. The addition of sclerosing techniques has improved results in this situation.

Status postsurgical repair with minimal dysfunctional symptoms may also respond very favorably to operative arthroscopy. When disc deformation and degenerative joint disease are severe, a guarded prognosis must be entertained. Late/intermediate and late stage disease are examples of these situations (Fig. 14–4).

Documentation of surgical findings is extremely important so that the preoperative diagnosis can be confirmed, the surgical procedures can be displayed and studied at a later date, and the postsurgical status of the joint tissues can be recorded. Although the required operative report may adequately describe the conditions found, the procedures accomplished, and the postoperative status of the joint, videotapes, pictures from video printers and still photographs taken during surgery offer additional, striking, useful documentation and provide effective teaching material.

Planned progressive involvement in arthroscopy is the best training for a neophyte arthroscopist. Early cases should be diagnostic in nature or combined with arthrotomy. After reaching the joint capsule, time can be spent inserting the arthroscope through the capsule, familiarizing oneself with the arthroscopic anatomy, attempting triangulation, and then comparing the naked-eye view, after opening into the joint compartment, with the arthroscopic pictures. This method may then be applied through skin punctures, prior to actually opening into the TMJ, in order to experience the more realistic "feel" of entering the TMJ with an arthroscope.

Following thorough familiarization with the instrumentation as described, lysis and lavage of adhesions with a blunt trocar, through direct visualization, can be performed and perfected. This involves learning the triangulation technique, a rather difficult exercise in hand/eye coordination. As the next progression in the learning curve, visualized hand instrumentation can be accomplished with hooked or blunt probes, with blunt trocars, or with other instruments to achieve adhesiolysis, lavage, and disc reduction. Accompanying these procedures, injection of the posterior attachment and/or the oblique protuberance with sclerosing solution can be utilized to maintain the hypermobile disc in its reduced position, or intraligamental steroids may be indicated to treat severe synovitis of the retrodiscal tissues and generalized arthritis.

As a subsequent step, biopsy forceps can be introduced into the arthroscopic cannula, and tissue samples can be obtained for diagnosis and study. Cutting instruments such as knives or scissors may be used to lyse adhe-

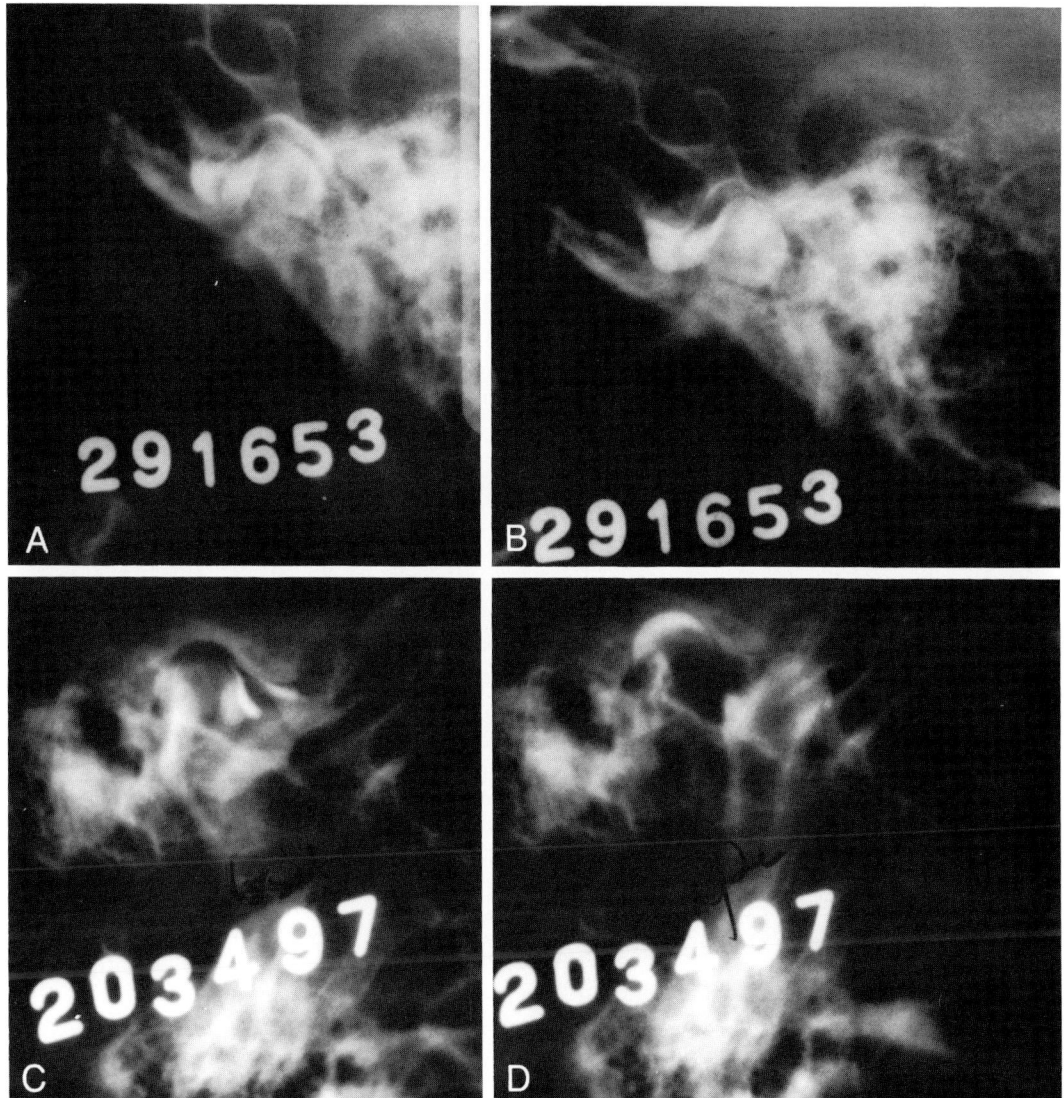

Figure 14–3. Arthrograms of chronic locking (*A*, closed; *B*, open) and of dysfunctional hypermobility (*C*, closed; *D*, open), showing minimal disc deformity.

sive pseudowalls in the anterior synovial pouch. The use of motorized instruments can then be easily mastered for lysis, lavage, and debridement of TMJs with chondromalacia or proliferative synovial problems.

Electrosurgical procedures for anterior release of the lateral pterygoid muscle, allowing disc reduction and subsequent cauterization of the posterior attachment, are very advanced arthroscopic procedures. Many simpler procedures must be mastered before these should be attempted, and additional cadaver workshops should be attended.

Performance review of patient care and treatment results is extremely important so that the value of this modality can be assessed and so that clinical progress can be correlated with the disease stage. Cases progressing after several months to arthrotomy must be studied, as these cases are considered failures of arthroscopy. Patient follow-up objectives should include the absence of preoperative clinical signs and symptoms, improvement in diet and ranges of motion, and decrease of pain and dysfunction.

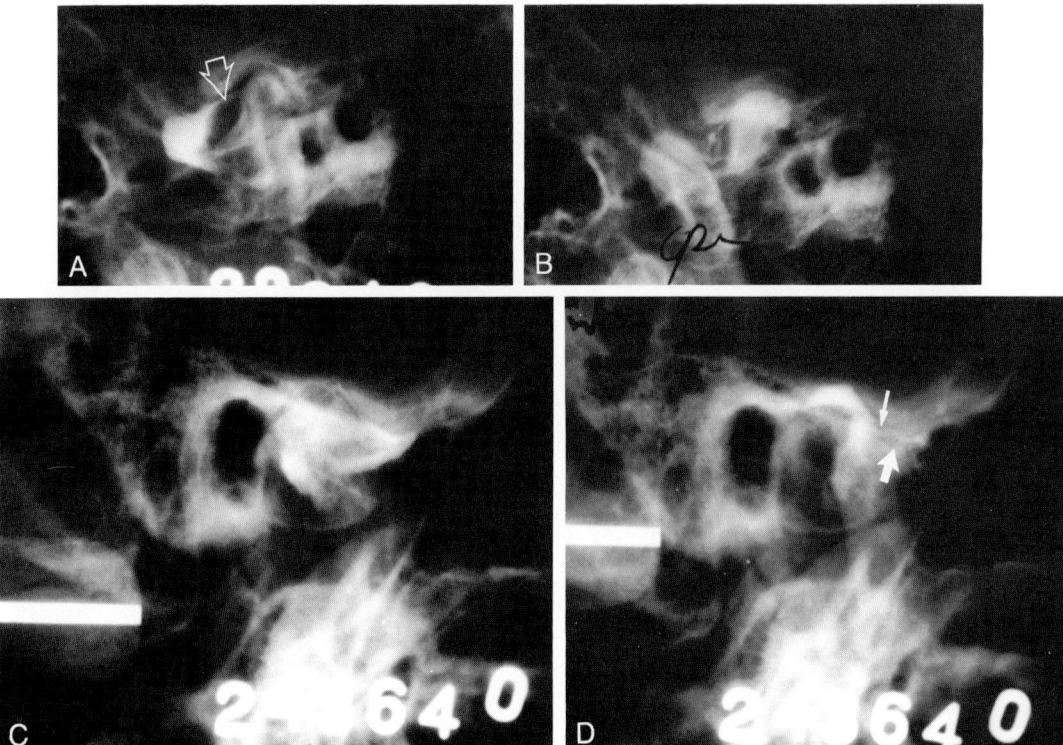

Figure 14–4. *A* and *B*, Arthrograms of anterior disc displacement with reduction (*A*, closed [arrow]; *B*, open) showing extreme thickening of the disc; *C* and *D*, arthrograms of degenerative joint disease with perforation (*C*, closed; *D*, open) showing thinning of the disc *(thin arrow)* and condylar bony changes *(wide arrow)*.

SUMMARY

TMJ arthroscopy occupies a very vital and valuable place in the armamentarium of treatment for TMJ disease. Although this is a new application of an existing technique, the dissemination of information to referring colleagues and to third-party payors must be accomplished so that patients can be better treated through their health insurance coverage. In addition, differentiation between an actual intra-articular joint problem with side effects of muscle involvement and the typical nonarticular myofascial pain dysfunction problem, which is not an arthropathy, needs to be established. Only by establishing these clinical entities as separate conditions can the surgical disease be well defined and claims presented to insurance companies for benefit. The supportive or nonsurgical segment of surgical treatment is then a portion of the surgical fee and should be determined for coverage in the same way that casting, orthotics, crutches, and so forth are components of other joint therapies.

Section IV
Arthroscopic Pathology of the Temporomandibular Joint

Chapter 15

SOFT TISSUE PATHOLOGY

A. Intracapsular Fibrosis of the Superior Compartment of the Temporomandibular Joint

Ronald M. Kaminishi, D.D.S.,
Christopher L. Davis, D.D.S., M.D.

Arthroscopic surgery has afforded new insights into temporomandibular joint (TMJ) pathology. In the past, diagnoses of TMJ dysfunction centered on the articular disc and myofascial dysfunction. With the ability to view the intracapsular environment in a more physiologic state, new vistas have opened in the study of TMJ pathophysiology. The arthroscope has provided a means of accomplishing microsurgical evaluation of tissues in a physiologic fluid medium. Up to this time we have viewed the "forest" from afar by many different means. This has resulted in a myriad of TMJ theories. Now we can "walk among the trees," and a more precise concept of what constitutes TMJ pathophysiology is evolving. The concept of recapturing, repositioning, replacing, substituting, or eliminating the articular disc may not be the ultimate goal in years to come.

It is said that perception is reality. When the TMJ is first viewed via an arthroscope, it is difficult to process the overwhelming amount of new information. The purpose of this chapter is to help process what we perceive so that we can expand our awareness of the reality.

Disc immobility is a common finding in TMJ disease. It has been shown that the disc may become immobilized in many different positions, ranging from within the fossa to beyond the eminence.[1] Such variations in position may be found in patients with normal range of motion as well as in those with bony ankylosis and nearly total immobility.[2]

The question arises: What factors are contributing to disc immobilization? One major factor is intracapsular fibrosis and fibro-osseous pathosis.

SIMPLE FIBROUS BANDS (Fig. 15–1)

The simplest of these bands are the fibrous adhesions. These range from lacy, spider web–like threads to thick fibrous bands. Histologically, they range from immature to very mature fibrous tissue. They most commonly connect the superior aspect to the inferior aspect of the joint compartment. Superiorly, they are attached via periosteum or articular cartilage to the bone of the fossa or eminence. Inferiorly, they may be attached to the retrodiscal tissue, disc, or "pseudodisc."

The term pseudodisc is used here to designate adaptive retrodiscal tissue. This may be seen in the normal position of the disc when the true disc is actually displaced anteriorly, medially, or laterally.

The superior aspect or roof of the upper compartment includes the fossa and the posterior slope, apex, and anterior slope of the eminence. In the lower compartment the superior aspect includes the inferior surface of the normal retrodiscal tissue, disc, or adaptive retrodiscal tissue (pseudodisc).

In the upper compartment the inferior aspect or floor includes the superior surface of the normal retrodiscal tissue, articular disc, or adaptive retrodiscal tissue. In the lower compartment the inferior aspect or floor is the superior aspect of the condyle. Most arthroscopic studies have been done in the upper compartment of the TMJ; therefore, our discussion will focus primarily on this area.

How do these bands develop? This can only be theorized from current knowledge. The bony components of the normal joint are covered with articular cartilage, thickest in the areas where articular forces are especially transmitted (e.g., the articular eminence and head of the condyle); the nonloading areas of the joint are lined with synovial tissue. We know that when there is abnormal joint function, such as micro- or macrotrauma, the synovium is easily injured. This very delicate tissue then rapidly undergoes a healing response. Of particular interest during this healing is the stage of fibrin formation by the underlying connective tissue.[3] This changes the surface of the synovium from a layer of synovial cells bathed in synovial fluid to a layer of fibrin; a "super-slippery" surface designed for minimal to zero friction becomes a "sticky" surface. This is most likely the etiology of the "suction cup" effect described by Sanders[4] as one of the findings in TMJ closed lock. The surfaces adhere together, the fibrin progresses to a more mature fibrous type of tissue, and intra-articular fibrosis occurs.

Other findings in the formation of intracapsular fibrosis are hematomas, subsynovial hyperemia, and ecchymosis, all of which are frequently identified in the TMJ. When these hematomas are investigated closely, the normal sequence of transition to fibrin and fibrous tissue within these structures may be found, sometimes to the point of observing immature fibrous bands separating as the arthroscope is manipulated in and around the mature hematomas.

FIBROSYNOVIAL BANDS (Fig. 15–2)

The fibrosynovial band has the same core as the simple fibrous band, except there is now a layer of synovial tissue covering the fibrous tissue. This appears to be a natural progression of the simple fibrous band. Histologic studies show the synovial cells at the

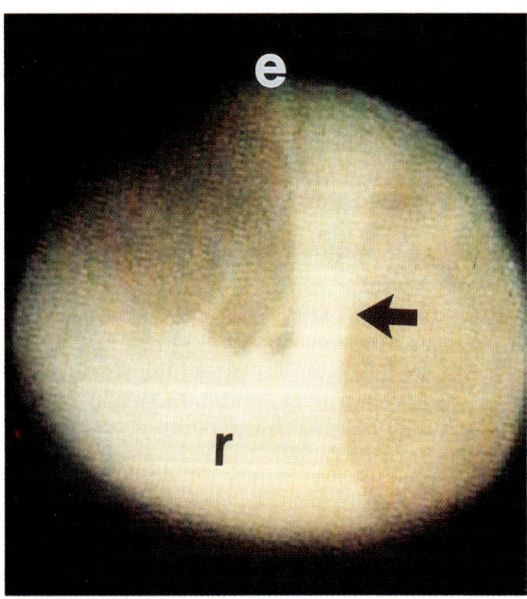

Figure 15–1. Simple fibrous band (arrow), left temporomandibular joint. e = eminence; r = retrodiscal tissue.

A. Intracapsular Fibrosis of the Superior Compartment of the Temporomandibular Joint ■ 237

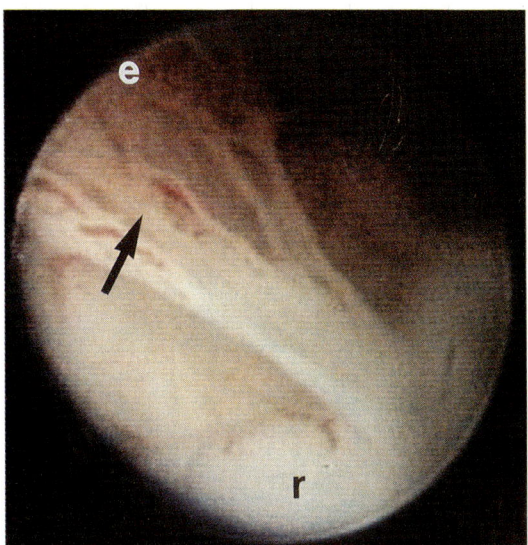

Figure 15–2. Fibrosynovial bands *(arrow)*, left temporomandibular joint. e = eminence; r = retrodiscal tissue.

capsule, one may observe distinct, thick bands of fibrous tissue within or protruding from the capsule. They usually are not parallel to the homogeneous fibers of the normal capsule, although this may occur.

When manipulated with a probe, these bands may be very rigid. In the presence of such fibrosis on the lateral capsule, the lateral paradiscal groove found along the inferior aspect is usually obliterated. The intracapsular details of such lesions can only be seen arthroscopically. Thickened or partially fibrosed capsules are commonly encountered during arthrotomy. Because they require transection to perform the arthrotomy, their clinical significance has not been well understood. Arthroscopically transecting or stretching these restrictive bands has helped improve joint immobility and reduce pain.

DISCO-OSSEOUS BANDS (Figs. 15–4 and 15–5)

This category consists of a fibrous band attached to medullary bone, whereas almost all the other types of fibrosis described are attached to the cortical bone via the periosteum. The disco-osseous band penetrates the cortex via an orifice in that layer. Each band appears to have its own individual orifice. When the band is transected and the orifice explored, it appears that the origin of the

base of these lesions proliferating and migrating across the fibrous tissues.[3] This indicates a more mature lesion, possibly indicative of a more chronic problem.

Occasionally one encounters an area of distinct fibrosis between the eminence and the junction of the bilaminar zone (normal retrodiscal tissue) and the disc or pseudodisc. If this is seen in the early stage of transition from fibrin to mature fibrous tissue, the tissue may be very friable or soft. As the arthroscope is positioned for close inspection, the tissue will spontaneously separate. Small areas of microhemorrhage can be seen and may cloud the field of vision. Sometimes the entire area of fibrosis can be resected by the arthroscopic examination alone. However, if the tissues have matured, the resection and surgical release may be very difficult and time-consuming. If the pathologic process has progressed to calcification or ossification, arthrotomy will be required.

CAPSULAR FIBROSIS (Fig. 15–3)

The normal capsule both medially and laterally is seen arthroscopically as a homogeneous series of vertical or oblique fibers and may be covered by a layer of synovial tissue. The synovium will contain varying degrees of small subsynovial vessels. In a pathologic

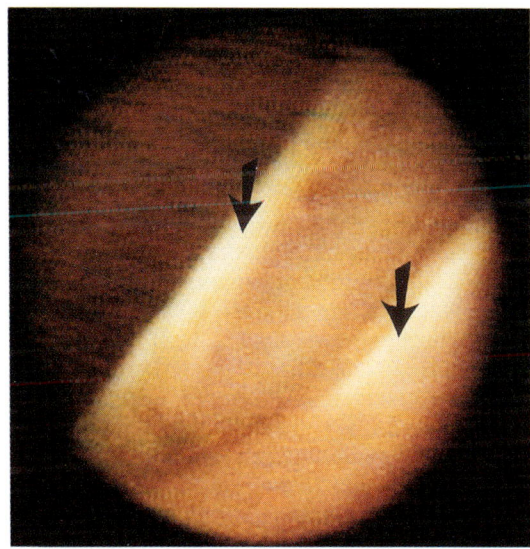

Figure 15–3. Capsular fibrosis *(arrows)*.

15 Soft Tissue Pathology

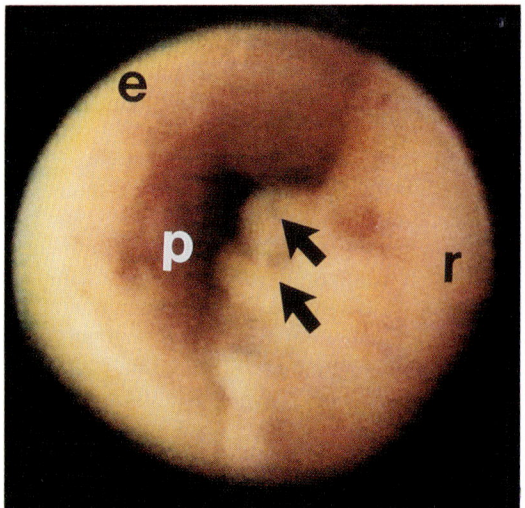

Figure 15–4. Disco-osseous band *(arrows)*. e = eminence; p = perforation; r = retrodiscal tissue.

learning curve of arthroscopic surgical orientation one can and will be fooled by these false walls. The pseudowalls will completely partition the enclosed portion of the joint space, giving the illusion of a short joint.

Partial Fibrous and Fibrosynovial Pseudowalls (Fig. 15–6)

As the name implies, these walls only partially traverse the medio-lateral dimension of

fibrosis is the medullary bone. This arthroscopic discovery may help to explain one of the etiologic factors in intracapsular pain: there are few pain fibers within the TMJ but many pain fibers in the bone.

These bands, which have been observed primarily penetrating the articular eminence, may vary in size. They may be singular or there may be many. Inferiorly, they have been observed attached to the adaptive bilaminar zone of an anteriorly displaced disc. Most were easily resected and consisted of delicate fibrous tissue.

PSEUDOWALLS

The term pseudowall is used to describe fibrous or fibrosynovial "walls" of tissue, partly or completely traversing the joint space from the medial to lateral capsule. These are usually attached superiorly to the anterior slope, apex, or posterior slope of the eminence. The majority are found along the anterior slope. Inferiorly, the wall is attached to the normal retrodiscal tissue, pseudodisc, or disc.

For reasons yet unknown, the superior joint space may be separated into one or more compartments via these pseudowalls. Pseudowalls are not normal anatomic findings but, in fact, are distinct pathologic entities; thus the description "false wall." During the

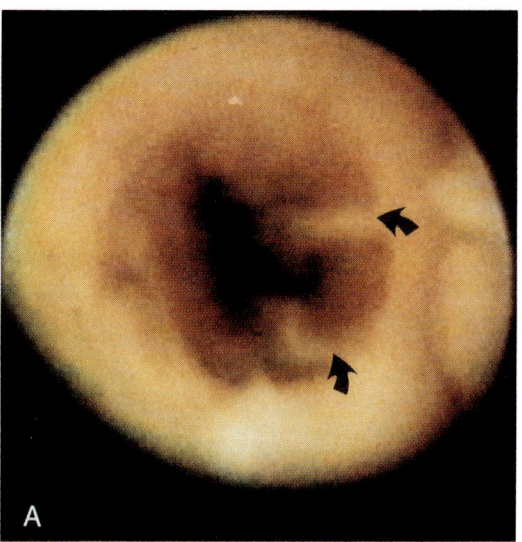

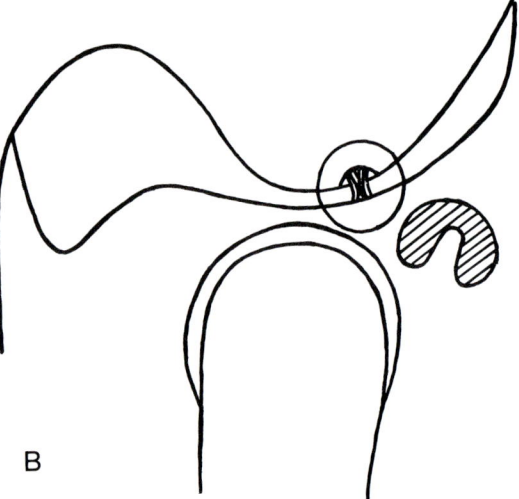

Figure 15–5. Osseous perforation in eminence region. *A*, Disco-osseous bands *(arrows)*; *B*, schematic showing location of bands in *A*.

A. Intracapsular Fibrosis of the Superior Compartment of the Temporomandibular Joint ■ 239

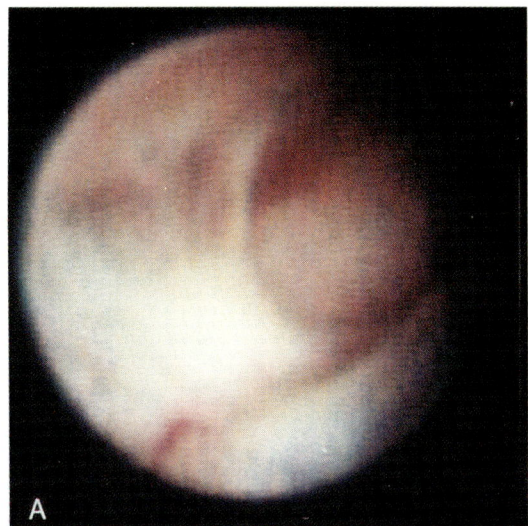

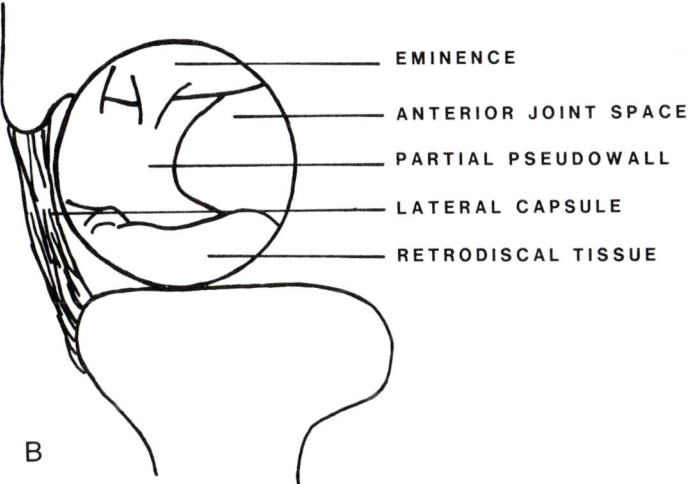

Figure 15–6. *A*, Partial fibrosynovial pseudowall in anterior pouch; *B*, Coronal schematic of pseudowall in *A*, viewed anteriorly.

the TMJ. They may start at either the medial or lateral capsule. They connect the superior aspect to the inferior aspect of the joint space. The medio-lateral dimension may vary, and the maturity of the fibrous tissue within the wall may not be homogeneous. As with the fibrous bands, there may be a covering of synovial tissue, with subsynovial vasculature traversing the fibrous tissue.

Intermittent Fibrous and Fibrosynovial Pseudowalls (Fig. 15–7)

This category of pseudowall is composed of columns of fibrous bands, usually wider than the simple fibrous bands. These intermittent columns alternate with an open space. Superiorly and inferiorly, these are attached as mentioned earlier. In some cases the columns are connected by sheets of synovial tissue. When viewed arthroscopically from a distance, one can see alternating white and dark bands; the white bands are the fibrous tissue columns, and the dark are the opening continuing into the anterior aspect of the joint space. One must remember that without the arthroscope light the joint will be dark. Only when one comes close to this structure can a thin sheet of synovium sometimes be seen connecting the columns. If the inspection is done too vigorously, the synovium is easily obliterated.

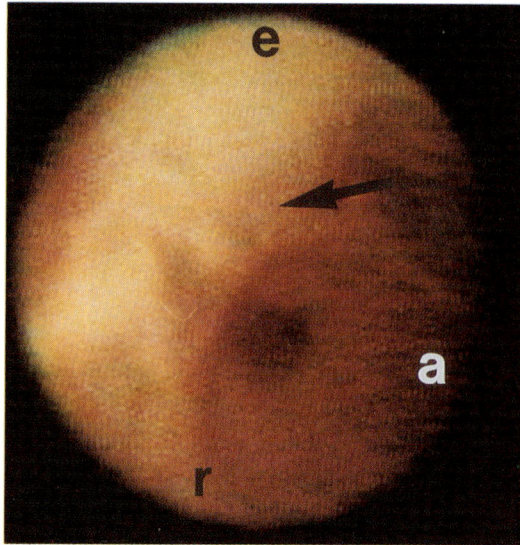

Figure 15-7. Intermittent pseudowall *(arrow)* with orientation similar to that in Figure 15-6B. e = eminence; r = retrodiscal tissue; a = anterior synovial pouch.

Total Fibrous and Fibrosynovial Pseudowalls (Fig. 15-8)

As the name implies, these are walls that totally separate the superior joint space into different compartments. Most commonly, a simple wall separating the anterior recess from the rest of the joint is found. This wall is usually attached to the anterior slope near the apex of the eminence. Inferiorly, it may be attached to displaced retrodiscal tissue in various stages of adaptation or to the disc itself. The fibrous wall is composed of disorganized fibrous tissue. The posterior surface of the wall usually appears smooth. From afar, the surface may appear as a homogeneous fibrous matrix apparently formed by parallel fibrous bands; however, on close inspection the fibrous tissue is seen to be haphazard in organization and thickness. There may be voids in the wall that appear as black spots. In reality, these are voids in the wall through which the anterior joint space can be seen. The anterior surface of these walls varies from tissue totally covered by coagulated blood and hematoma to a very rough, chaotic-appearing aggregation of fibrous tissue (Fig. 15-9). Except as a vertical partition, there usually does not appear to be any organized development of this side of the wall. When the walls are transected, a significant amount of hemorrhage usually occurs, demonstrating that vascular elements are present within this structure. There is also early biopsy evidence that peripheral neurologic structures are present within these pseudowalls—a finding that deserves further investigation.

The majority of these walls are covered on the posterior surface by a layer of synovium of varying thickness. The subsynovial vasculature and hyperemia also vary greatly. It can

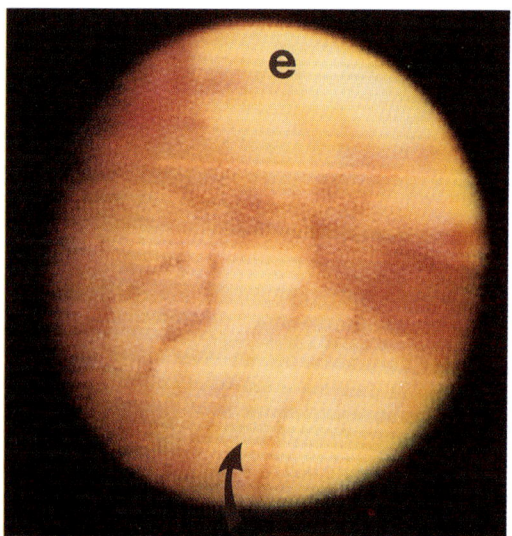

Figure 15-8. Total fibrosynovial pseudowall *(arrow)*, viewed anteriorly. See 1 in Figure 15-10B for orientation.

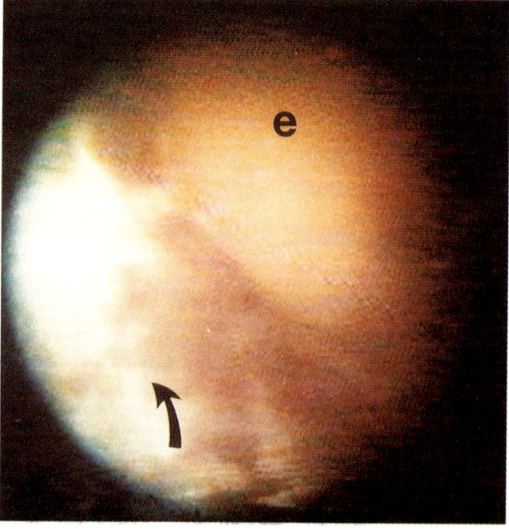

Figure 15-9. Total fibrosynovial pseudowall at posterior slope of eminence *(arrow)*, viewed anteriorly. e = eminence. See 2 in Figure 15-10B for orientation.

A. Intracapsular Fibrosis of the Superior Compartment of the Temporomandibular Joint ■ 241

be safely stated that the synovium usually has various degrees of inflammation present on these walls. The synovium appears to easily bridge voids or defects in the fibrous tissue. Thus, fibrosynovial pseudowalls usually present a homogeneous, uniform surface texture. Again, on close inspection darker areas underlying the synovial layer reveal the inconsistencies of the fibrous wall.

There have been no observations or reports of synovium covering the anterior aspect of any pseudowall.

More than one pseudowall can be present in the superior joint space. It is perplexing to see such a structure; it is most perplexing to see more than one. In one case, the posterior wall was found on the posterior slope of the eminence, attached inferiorly to the retrodiscal tissue; again, it totally traversed the joint from the medial to lateral capsule. The second wall was located at the anterior slope of the eminence, attached inferiorly to the adapting retrodiscal tissue of the anteriorly displaced disc. As with all total pseudowalls, it traversed the joint from the medial to lateral capsule. Thus, it could be seen that the superior joint space was separated into three distinct joint spaces (Fig. 15–10).

INTEROSSEOUS FIBROSIS (Fig. 15–11)

Chronic, severe TMJ disease may result in a large perforation or obliteration of the inter-

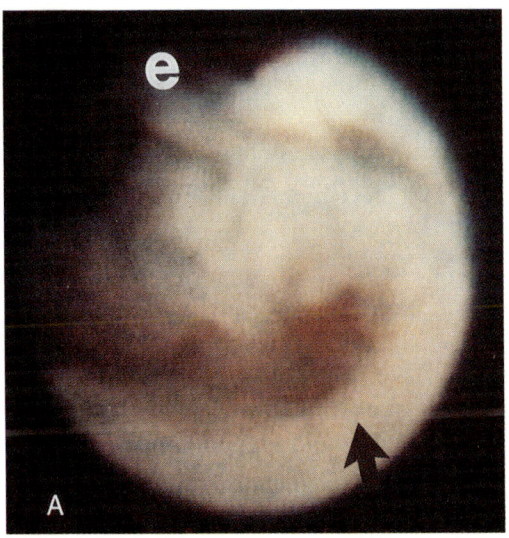

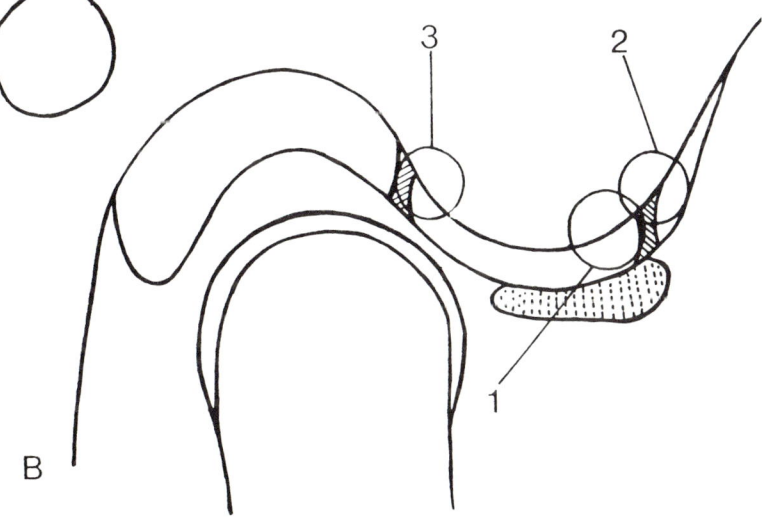

Figure 15–10. A, Second pseudowall in the same temporomandibular joint as in Figure 15–9 (arrow), viewed posteriorly. e = eminence. See 3 in B for orientation. B, Schematic showing orientation for Figures 15–8 (1), 15–9 (2), and 15–10A. (3).

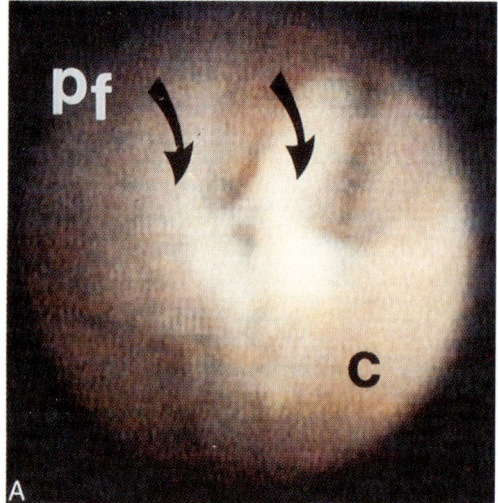

ankylosis. When clearly diagnosed prior to treatment arthroscopic procedures may be contraindicated. Occasionally, in closed-lock dysfunction of the TMJ, bony ankylosis is indistinguishable from intracepsular fibrosis. It may be possible to enter the posterior recess of the superior joint space.

In Figure 15–12 it appears that a fibrosynovial total pseudowall is present. However, in this instance, when attempts were made to transect the pseudowall, osseous elements were discovered. Incidentally, when an anterior portal was attempted, a distinct diagnosis of bony ankylosis was made. Because the arthroscopic pictures of the total fibrosynovial pseudowall and of bony ankylosis are virtually identical, it is speculated that there may be a correlation between the two.

SUMMARY

Fibrosis within the capsule of the TMJ has been seen for many years. This is recognized in both superior and inferior joint spaces. Now, with the aid of the arthroscope, we can definitively evaluate differences in this fibrosis. By selectively transecting, removing, and/or stretching various types of fibrosis we have observed significant therapeutic results. The challenge is to use this added information in the continuing search for the true pathophysiology of TMJ disease.

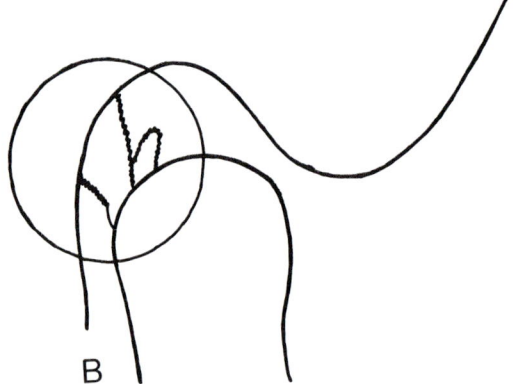

Figure 15–11. *A*, Interosseous fibrosis *(arrows)*. c = condyle, pf = posterior fossa. *B*, Schematic showing orientation of *A*.

articular disc. Perforations of this nature may expose greater than 75% of the articulating surface of the condyle to the superior joint space.

Interosseous fibrosis may occur between the osseous elements of the fossa or eminence and the condyle. These usually are thick, very mature fibrous elements. They are attached to the bone of the fossa, eminence, and condyle. Synovial coverings have not been observed in these types of lesions. Visualization of such pathosis under function shows how restrictive they are to translation of the condyle.

FIBRO-OSSEOUS AND OSSEOUS ADHESIONS (Fig. 15–12)

These findings are more realistically referred to as fibro-osseous ankylosis or bony

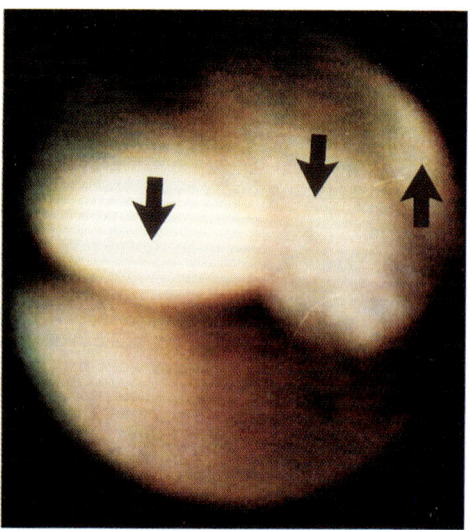

Figure 15–12. Nodules of bony ankylosis *(arrows)*, anterior view.

References

1. Davis CL, Kaminishi RM, Burnett K: TMJ arthroscopy and MR imaging. J Calif Dent Assn 16:52–66, 1988.
2. Kircos LT, Ortehdahl DA, Mark AS: Magnetic resonance imaging of the TMJ disc on asymptomatic volunteers. J Oral Maxillofac Surg 45:10, 1987.
3. Kao R, Lee C: Synovial lesions. [Lecture Presentation] Squaw Valley, CA: Craniomandibular Institute, 1989.
4. Sanders B, Buoncristiani R: Diagnostic and surgical arthroscopy of the TMJ: Clinical experience with 137 patients over 2 years. Craniomandib Disord Facial Oral Pain 1(3):202–213, 1987.

Suggested Reading

Dandy DJ: Arthroscopy of the Knee. London: Gower Medical Publishing, 1984.

Hohmann EL, Elde RP, Rysavy JA, et al: Innervation of periosteum and bone by sympathetic vasoactive intestinal peptide–containing nerve fibers. Science 232:4752, 1986.

Johnson L: Arthroscopic Surgery. St Louis: Mosby, 1986.

Merrill R (ed): Oral Maxillofac Surg Clin North Am 1:1, 1989.

Moses J, Sartoris D, Glass R, et al: The effect of arthroscopic surgery lysis and lavage of the superior joint space on TMJ disc position and mobility. J Oral Maxillofac Surg 47:674–678, 1989.

Ohnishi M: Arthroscopy of the temporomandibular joint. J Stomatol Soc Jap (Kokubyo Gakkir Zasshi) 42:207–213, 1975.

Sakada S, Maeda K: Characteristics of innervation and nerve ending in CAT mandibular periosteum. Bull Tokyo Med Dent Univ 8(2):77–84, 1967.

Tanaka S, Ito T: Histochemical demonstration of adrenergic fibers in the fascia, periosteum, and retinaculum. Clin Orthop 126:276–281, 1987.

B. Synovial Chondromatosis

MOHAN THOMAS, D.D.S., F.A.C.D., DANIEL BUCHBINDER, D.M.D.

Synovial chondromatosis is an uncommon, benign condition characterized by the formation of multiple small cartilaginous nodules in the synovial membrane via metaphasia within the subintimal connective tissue layer of the synovial membrane.[1–3] These nodules may detach from the synovial membrane and enter the joint compartment as free intra-articular loose bodies[2–4] or joint mice.[5] Loose bodies have been reported to occur in practically every joint. These bodies can become secondarily calcified or ossified, giving the classic radiographic appearance of "rice grain"–like globules. Calcification of the joint mice, and hence positive radiographic findings, is present in only 50% of cases.[5] Other radiographic signs include widening of the joint space, irregularity of the joint surface, and sclerosis of the glenoid fossa and mandibular condyle.[6]

A review of the literature indicates that the condition is usually monarticular and affects mostly the larger joints of the body, especially the knee, hip, ankle, and elbow. Rarely is the condition seen in the temporomandibular joint (TMJ). The first case of synovial chondromatosis of the TMJ was described by Axhausen in 1933.[7] Subsequently, only 45 cases have been reported in the English medical literature (Table 15–1).[1–39]

Synovial chondromatosis is thought to be the result of the metaplastic proliferation of embryonal mesenchymal rests in the subintimal layer of the synovium, thus leading to the formation of nodules that may be released into the joint space as loose bodies, may remain attached to the synovium, or may coalesce within the joint space forming a solid mass. The cartilaginous nodules can also become secondarily calcified or ossified.[5] It is postulated that the fibroblasts just beneath the surface membrane of the synovium can become metaplastic and deposit chondromucin. Once a cartilaginous focus has formed, the nodules grow by active proliferation of chondrocytes. As the villous folds of the synovial membrane containing the developing cartilaginous deposits enlarge, they become pedunculated, separate from their pedicles, and mobile bodies are present within the joint space.[5, 24] Although detached in the joint space, the joint mice are

Table 15–1. REPORTED CASES OF SYNOVIAL CHONDROMATOSIS OF THE TEMPOROMANDIBULAR JOINT

Axhausen, 1933[7]	Gaillard et al, 1981[17]
Trevor, 1952[38] *	Tagaki and Ishikawa, 1981[35]
Feist and Gibbons, 1960[16]	Brants and Kusen, 1982[14]
Schneider, 1960[30]	Morrish et al, 1984[25]
Inovay, 1962[20]	Blankestijn et al, 1985[1] ‡
Kusen, 1969[21]	Boccardi et al, 1985[12]
Schulte and Rhyne, 1969[31]	De Bont et al, 1985[13]
Silver et al, 1971[32]	Silver et al, 1986[33]
Ballard and Weiland, 1972[10]	Thompson et al, 1986[37]
Alling et al, 1973[9]	Casselman et al, 1987[2]
Tasanen et al, 1974[36]	Cannon, 1987[5]
Rosen et al, 1977[29]	Nokes et al, 1987[26]
Akhtar et al, 1978[8]	Hamilton et al, 1987[18]
Raibley, 1977[27]	Manco and Deluke, 1987[23]
Lomba et al, 1977[22]	Von Arx et al, 1988[39]
Noyek et al, 1977[6]	Forsell et al, 1988[3]
Ronald et al, 1978[28] †	
Blenkinsopp, 1978[11]	Hertzog and Mafee, 1990[19]
Miller et al, 1978[24]	Sun et al, 1990[34]
Fee et al, 1979[15]	

Superior numbers indicate reference source.
*Two cases reported.
†Four cases reported.
‡Three cases reported.

nourished by the synovial fluid and remain viable and continue to grow.[5, 39]

The pathogenesis of synovial chondromatosis remains unresolved. Several proposed possible etiologic factors in cases affecting the TMJ have been proposed and include (1) injury to the joint area (macrotrauma), (2) chronic low-grade trauma (microtrauma), (3) inflammation, (4) malocclusion, (5) subluxation, and (6) tension states.[3, 13, 28] Synovial chondromatosis of the larger joints affects men twice as often as it does women, usually in the fourth and fifth decades of life. However, when the TMJ is affected, the condition shows a great predilection for women, with a 4:1 female to male ratio.[17] The age range of those affected is from 18 to 75, with a mean of 47 years.[1] All reported cases have been monarticular, with the right TMJ affected in the majority of cases.

The diagnosis of TMJ synovial chondromatosis must be considered for patients complaining of slowly progressive preauricular swelling, pain, and crepitus in the region of the TMJ, and a limited range of motion of the joint. Other signs and symptoms include otalgia, malocclusion, stiffness of the joint, popping, deviation of the jaw on opening, and inability to open the mouth.[1] It is important to differentiate this process from neoplasms of the parotid gland, which can present with similar symptoms. In two cases reviewed, superficial parotidectomies were performed before the correct diagnosis was established.[8, 37, 39] Magnetic resonance imaging (MRI), computed tomography (CT) scans, and sialography may be used to rule out extracapsular spread, parotid involvement, and intracranial extension.[2, 19, 23, 26, 34, 37]

Extracapsular extension has been reported in only four cases.[8, 10, 35, 37] The first case of intracranial extension was reported by Nokes et al in 1987;[26] a second case of intracranial extension was reported by Sun and co-workers in 1990.[34] With the use of MRI and CT, they were able to see the extension of the mass into the middle cranial fossa and identified a clear tissue plane between the mass and the temporal lobe. CT may assist in confirming the intra-articular localization of the loose body opacities. Radiographic confirmation is sometimes difficult, especially with plain films, since there may be a varying degree of calcification of these nodules, making them "invisible" on the radiographs (Fig. 15–13). Plain film diagnosis depends on identification of variable numbers of cartilaginous lesions within the joint capsule.[6] Blankestijn and colleagues[1, 6] reported the particles to be calcified in only 16 of the 28 cases they reviewed. The presence of intra-articular calcification, on the other hand, is not pathognomonic of synovial chondromatosis. In fact, osteochondral fractures, avascular necrosis, osteochondritis dissecans, rheumatoid and tuberculous arthritis, and osteoarthritis (detached osteophytes) can all produce loose joint bodies or joint mice.[1, 2, 10, 11, 31, 32]

It is the multiplicity of the loose bodies that favors the diagnosis of synovial chondromatosis.[39] Conditions producing intra-articular bodies were summarized by Blenkinsopp in 1978 (Table 15–2).[11, 39] The presence of numerous loose bodies in the joint space strongly suggests the diagnosis of synovial chondromatosis. The loose bodies are usually white in color, firm or hard in consistency, and rice- or pearl-like in shape, with a smooth or sometimes lobulated surface.[13]

B. Synovial Chondromatosis ■ 245

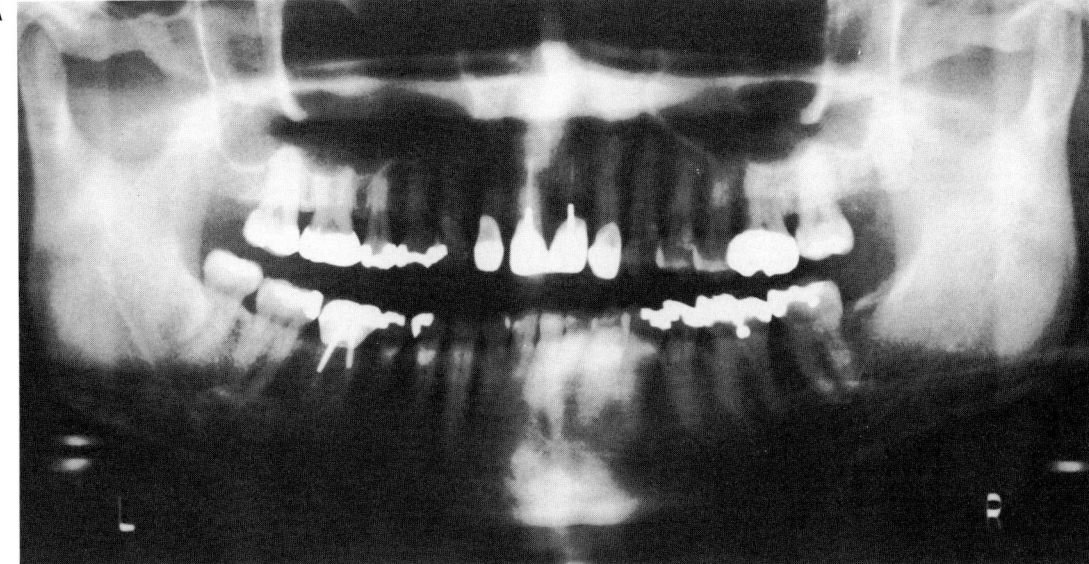

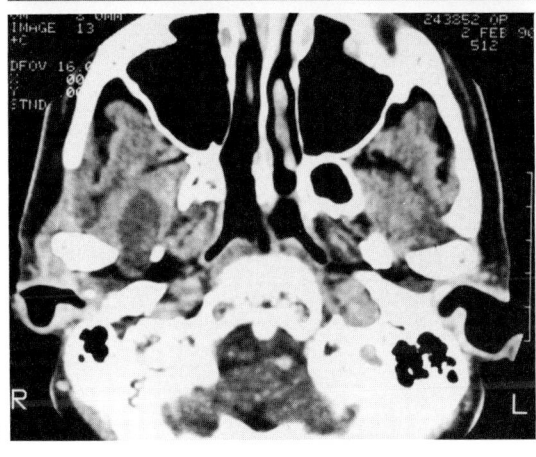

Figure 15–13. *A*, Orthopantomogram of patient with synovial chondromatosis of the right temporomandibular joint (TMJ). Note that there is no evidence of calcification within the joint space. *B*, Computed tomography scan of the right TMJ of the same patient, showing the presence of a "mass" in the joint space.

Casselman[2] summarized the diagnostic advantages of CT studies of synovial chondromatosis affecting the TMJ: (1) exact topographic localization of the opacities within the joint, (2) demonstration of the intrinsic features of the intra-articular bodies (i.e., sclerotic margins or less dense central areas), (3) detailed depiction of surrounding osteoarticular structures as well as their topographic relationships, and (4) the most sensitive detection of residual loose bodies in the postoperative joint.

Confirmation of the diagnosis can be attained only after histologic examination of the resected specimen. Although histopathologic examination usually reveals worrisome features such as nuclear pleomorphism and multinucleated cells in the area of chondroid tissue, the lesion is essentially benign in nature (Fig. 15–14).[3] There have been a few reports of malignant transformation of synovial chondromatosis to chondrosarcoma in the joints,[18] but in review of the literature no

Table 15–2. CONDITIONS PRODUCING INTRA-ARTICULAR BODIES

No. of Loose Bodies	Pathology
50–500	Synovial chondromatosis
1–10	Osteoarthritis
1–3	Osteochondritis dissecans
1–3	Intracapsular fractures
	Tuberculosis of pyogenic arthritis
	Rheumatoid arthritis
	Neurotropic arthritis

Based on Blenkinsopp PT: Loose bodies of the temporomandibular joint: Synovial chondromatosis or osteoarthritis. Br J Oral Surg 16:12–20, 1978.

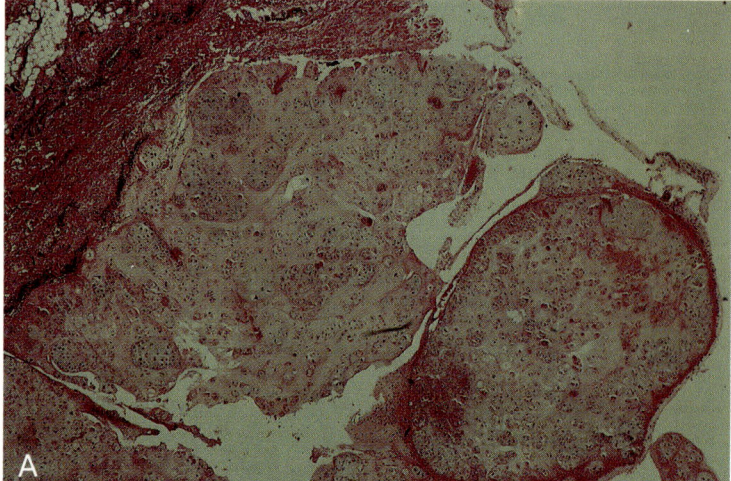
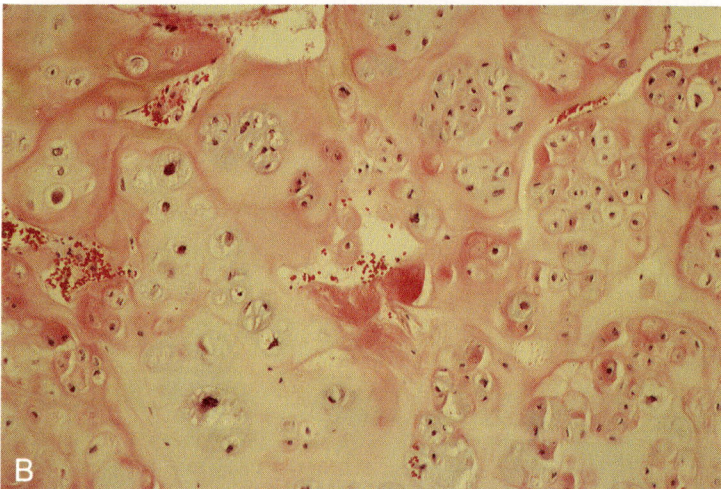

Figure 15–14. *A*, Low-power photomicrograph of a section of an H and E–stained surgical specimen from the patient in Figure 15–13, showing cartilaginous nodules containing mature chondrocytes incorporated in the synovial membrane. *B*, High-power photomicrograph of same case showing cloned chondrocytes with atypical and hyperchromatic nuclei.

cases of malignant transformation have been reported involving the TMJ.

The therapy of synovial chondromatosis described in the literature ranges from conservative surgical removal of loose bodies and lavage of the joint to removal of the nodules with a total synovectomy, meniscectomy, and even condylectomy to gain access to the medial synovial lining.[1, 6, 32, 34, 39] The most widely accepted treatment modality remains joint debridement with synovectomy. Most authors have advocated a preauricular approach to the joint. Arthroscopic debridement of the joint has also been performed successfully by one of the authors (M.T.) (Fig. 15–15). Once the joint mice have been removed the synovium should be carefully inspected and, if found to be diseased, removed.[2] Synovial removal should be as complete as possible to prevent recurrence of the lesion.[1, 3, 15, 34, 37, 39]

References

1. Blankestijn J, Panders A, Vermey A, Scherpbier AJ: Synovial chondromatosis of the temporomandibular joint. Report of three cases and a review of the literature. Cancer 55:479–485, 1985.
2. Casselman JW, Demeulemeister L, Bossuyt M, et al: CT findings in synovial chondromatosis of the temporomandibular joint. Comput Assist Tomogr 11(5):898–900, 1987.
3. Forsell K, Happonen R, Forsell H: Synovial chondromatosis of the temporomandibular joint. Report of a case and review of the literature. Int J Oral Maxillofac Surg 17:237–241, 1988.
4. Chandler E: Loose bodies. *In* O'Connor's Textbook of Arthroscopic Surgery. Philadelphia: JB Lippincott, 1984, pp 227–235.

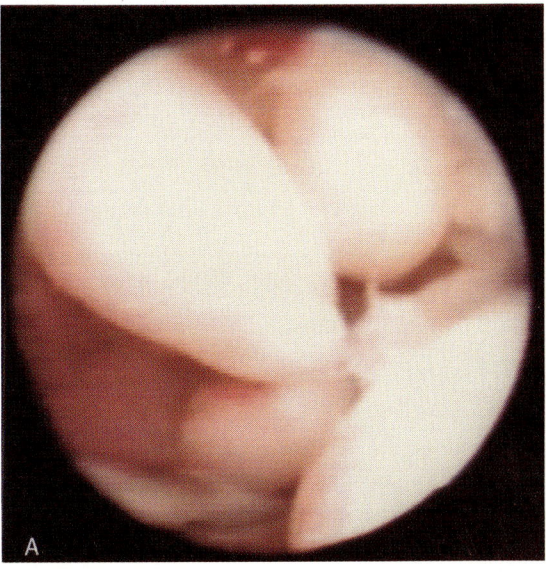 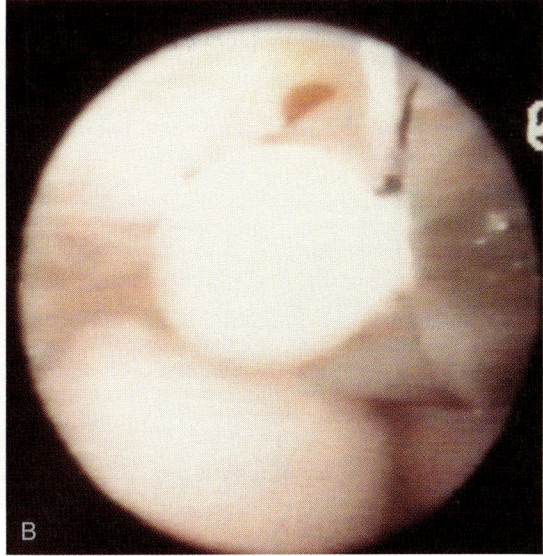

Figure 15–15. *A*, Arthroscopic view of free temporomandibular joint (TMJ) "mice." *B*, Debridement of TMJ using cup forceps under direct vision through a second portal placed more anteriorly. (Courtesy of Dr. Robert Schwartz.)

5. Cannon CR: Osteochondrosis of the temporomandibular joint presenting as an apparent parotid mass. Ann Otol Rhinol Laryngol 96:330–332, 1987.
6. Noyek AM, Holgate RC, Fireman SM, et al: The radiologic findings in synovial chondromatosis (chondrometaplasia) of the temporomandibular joint. J Otolaryngol [suppl] 6:45–48, 1977.
7. Axhausen G: Pathologie und Therapie des Kiefergelenkes. Fortschr Zahnheilk 9:171–186, 1933.
8. Akhtar M, Mahajan S, Koh E: Synovial chondromatosis of the temporomandibular joint. J Bone Joint Surg 59:266–267, 1977.
9. Alling C, Rawson D, Staats O, Middleton R: Synovial chondromatosis of the temporomandibular joint. Parts 1 and 2. J Oral Surg 31:604–606, 691–693, 1973.
10. Ballard R, Weiland LH: Synovial chondromatosis of the temporomandibular joint. Cancer 30:791–795, 1972.
11. Blenkinsopp PT: Loose bodies of the temporomandibular joint: Synovial chondromatosis or osteoarthritis. Br J Oral Surg 16:12–20, 1978.
12. Boccardi A, Gatti G, Cataldi A: Chondromatosi articulare temporo-mandibolare. Reperti tomografici e TC. Radiol Med (Torino) 71:73–75, 1985.
13. de Bont LGM, Blankestijn J, Panders A, Vermey A: Unilateral condylar hyperplasia combined with synovial chondromatosis of the temporomandibular joint. Report of a case. J Maxillofac Surg 13:32–36, 1985.
14. Brants JF, Kusen GJ: Synoviale chondromatosis van het kaakqenricht. Acta Stomatol Belg 79:37–44, 1982.
15. Fee WE, Windhorst P, Niggins R, Pang L: Synovial chondromatosis of the temporomandibular joint. Otolaryngol Head Neck Surg 87:741–748, 1979.
16. Feist J, Gibbons TG: Osteochondromatosis of the temporomandibular joint. Radiology 97:291–294, 1960.
17. Gaillard A, Delaire J, Jacquemarie D, Buzelin J: La chondromatose synoviale de l'articulation temporomandibulare. A propos d'un cas. Rev Stomatol Chir Maxillofac 82:105–108, 1981.
18. Hamilton A, Davis R, Hayes D, Mollam R: Chondrosarcoma developing in synovial chondromatosis. J Bone Joint Surg 69B:137–140, 1987.
19. Herzog S, Mafee M: Synovial chondromatosis of the TMJ: MRI and CT findings. Am J Neuroradiol 11:742–745, 1990.
20. Inovay J: A rare case of benign synovialoma of the mandibular joint. Oral Surg 15:775–780, 1962.
21. Kusen GJ: Chondromatosis: Report of a case. J Oral Surg 27:735–738, 1969.
22. Lomba JA, Cabanas R, Marrero I; Synovial chondrometaplasia of the temporomandibular joint: Report of a case. J Oral Surg 35:675–681, 1977.
23. Manco LG, Deluke DM: CT diagnosis of synovial chondromatosis of the temporomandibular joint. AJR 148:574–576, 1987.
24. Miller AS, Harwick RD, Daley DJ: Temporomandibular joint synovial chondromatosis: Report of a case. J Oral Surg 36:467–468, 1978.
25. Morrish RB, Hansen LS, Ware WH: Synovial chondromatosis of the temporomandibular joint. A case report. J Craniomandb Pract 2:65–70, 1984.
26. Nokes SR, King PS, Garcia R, et al: Temporomandibular joint chondromatosis with intracranial extension. MRI and CT contributions. AJR 148:1173–1174, 1987.
27. Raibley SO: Villonodular synovitis with synovial chondromatosis. J Oral Surg 44:279–284, 1979.
28. Ronald JB, Keller EE, Weiland LH: Synovial chondromatosis of the temporomandibular joint. J Oral Surg 36:13–19, 1978.
29. Rosen PS, Pritzker KPH, Greenbaum J, et al: Synovial chondromatosis affecting the temporomandibular joint. Case report and literature review. Arthritis Rheum 20:736–740, 1977.

30. Schneider G: Zur Chondromatose des Kiefergelenks. Dtsch Zahnarztl Z 2:1233–1241, 1960.
31. Schulte WC, Rhyne RR: Synovial chondromatosis of temporomandibular joint. Report of a case. J Oral Surg 28:906–913, 1969.
32. Silver CM, Simon SD, Litchman HM, Dyckman J: Synovial chondromatosis of the temporomandibular joint. J Bone Joint Surg 53A:777–780, 1971.
33. Silver CM, Motamed M, Moonan DE: Chondromatosis of the temporomandibular joint arising in the meniscus. J Oral Maxillofac Surg 44:70–73, 1986.
34. Sun S, Helmy E, Bays R: Synovial chondromatosis with intracranial extension. A case report. Oral Surg Oral Med Oral Pathol 70:5–9, 1990.
35. Takagi M, Ishikawa G: Simultaneous villonodular synovitis and synovial chondromatosis of the temporomandibular joint: Report of a case. J Oral Surg 39:694–701, 1981.
36. Tasanen A, Lamberg MA, Kotilainen R: Osteochondromatosis of the temporomandibular joint. Oral Surg 38:845–849, 1974.
37. Thompson K, Schwartz HC, Miles JW: Synovial chondromatosis of the temporomandibular joint presenting as a parotid mass: Possibility of confusion with benign mixed tumor. Oral Surg 62:377–380, 1986.
38. Trevor D: A case of synovial chondromatosis of the temporomandibular joint. Postgrad Med J 28:408–409, 1952.
39. Von Arx DP, Simpson MT, Batman P: Synovial chondromatosis of the temporomandibular joint. Br J Oral Maxillofac Surg 26:297–305, 1988.

■ Chapter 16

ARTICULAR PATHOLOGY: DISC DISPLACEMENT AND LATERAL IMPINGEMENT SYNDROME

JEFFREY J. MOSES, D.D.S.

The etiology of pain in the temporomandibular joint (TMJ) diagnosed with internal joint derangement (IJD) is unclear. Similarities of pain and limitation of motion between the impingement phenomenon of the shoulder and IJD of the TMJ have led me to believe that an impingement process is occurring in the TMJ between the lateral third of the condyle and the eminence. This belief is based on observations obtained from the arthroscopic endaural view, coronal magnetic resonance imaging (MRI), and anteroposterior protruded-position laminograms performed on patients who had failed nonsurgical efforts to correct TMJ dysfunction yet did not exhibit classic disc displacement.

This chapter presents the anatomy and pathophysiology of this phenomenon, its surgical management, and research results from preoperative and postoperative MRI scans studying disc position and mobility of operative arthroscopy.

ANATOMY AND PATHOPHYSIOLOGY

There are many theories regarding TMJ dysfunction; however, the following questions arise in almost every discussion: What are the causes of the pain, and why can one joint with disc displacement not hurt and another, perhaps with a less serious problem, be severely tender?

Part of the answer involves the histochemical characteristics of pain mediators within the joint fluid.[1] The direct and indirect results of inflammation on the capsule and associated musculature also play a role in pain symptoms.[2,3] Review of studies of similar joint pain and restricted mobility in the shoulder with acromial impingement syndrome show a striking resemblance to observations made on the TMJ (Fig. 16–1).[2-8] This has led to the investigation of the lateral TMJ articulation by tomographic examinations, MRI, and direct arthroscopic examination. It has become apparent that there is a process of pathology ranging from seemingly minor capsulitis with proliferative synovial changes to frank degenerative disease with disc/capsular impingements.

Disc displacement actually may occur late in the pathophysiology of internal joint derangement (Table 16–1). Early inflammatory changes, initiated by macrotrauma or microtrauma, may lead to a loss of the lubricating nature of the hyaluronic acid and chondroitin sulfate within the synovial fluid. Capsulitis itself, with the synovium proliferating in an attempt to repair or regenerate damaged intracapsular structures, combines with inflammation and leads to the production of hyaluronidase, which breaks down the hyaluronic acid within the TMJ. A loss of lubrication ensues, leading to increased surface "stickiness," resulting in capsular fibrosis and relative immobility of the TMJ, especially within the superior joint compartment, on attempted translatory movements of the mandible.

If allowed to mature, the adhesions may

250 ■ 16 Articular Pathology: Disc Displacement and Lateral Impingement Syndrome

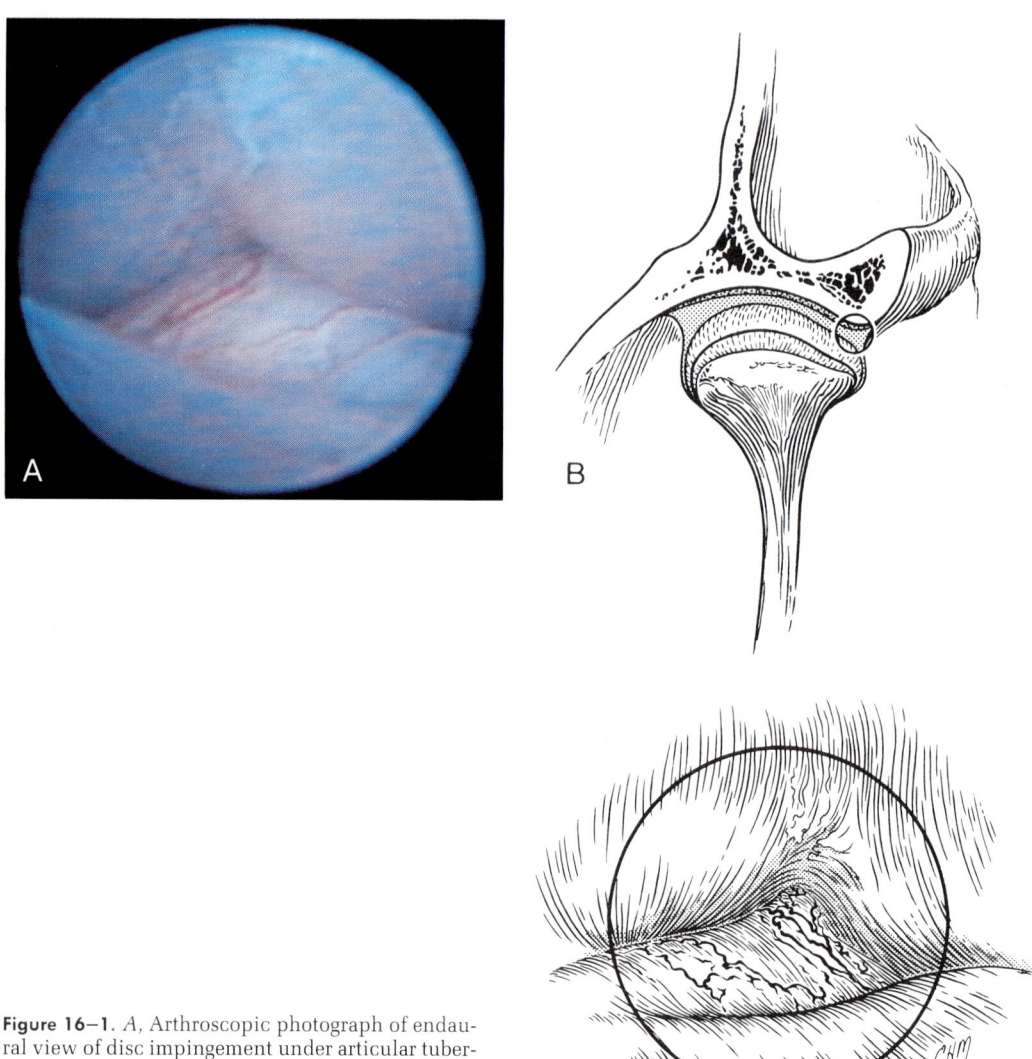

Figure 16–1. *A*, Arthroscopic photograph of endaural view of disc impingement under articular tubercle; *B*, drawing of location of endaural view seen in *A*; *C*, drawing of endaural photograph seen in *A*.

Table 16–1. PROGRESSIVE STAGES OF IMPINGEMENT LESIONS

Stage	Diagnosis	Clinical Course	Treatment
I: Inflammation	Acute capsulitis and synovitis	Reversible	NSAID, rest, physical therapy, orthotic splint, intracapsular irrigations and lavage
II: Fibrosis	Chronic adhesive capsulitis, proliferative synovitis, discal displacement or immobility, synovial plicae	Recurrent pain with activity	Arthroscopic lysis of adhesions, lateral eminencia release and capsular stretch, lavage, physical therapy, orthotic splint appliance (OSA)
III: Bony remodeling and attachment migration	Discal displacement or immobility, hyperplastic eminencia tubercle, degenerative joint disease	Progressive disability	Lateral eminencia release, capsular stretch, lateral eminencia osteoplasty, physical therapy, OSA

vascularize and become part of the restriction (Fig. 16–2). On attempted opening, lateral adhesive components can cause incoordination of disc/condyle/eminence dynamics. Strain is placed on the lateral disc attachments as the condyle is forced to begin translation from within the inferior joint compartment. The disc, while relatively immobile in its relationship to the articular eminence, may or may not be displaced at this time (Fig. 16–3).

Over a period of time, translation solely in the inferior joint compartment may cause a gradually increasing laxity of the lateral disc attachment, allowing the anatomic migration of the disc anteromedially. The patient also may experience a "closed lock," depending on the morphologic changes within the disc and its ability to form a mechanical obstruction (Fig. 16–4).

As the disc slowly migrates forward and medially, movement within the superior joint compartment generally remains minimal. The inferior joint compartment begins to act as the translatory compartment for the "wide-open" mouth position.

Anterior disc displacement traditionally has been diagnosed via arthrographic studies, and more recently with MRI. A sagittal view may reveal a well-placed disc; however, the MRI coronal view allows diagnosis of

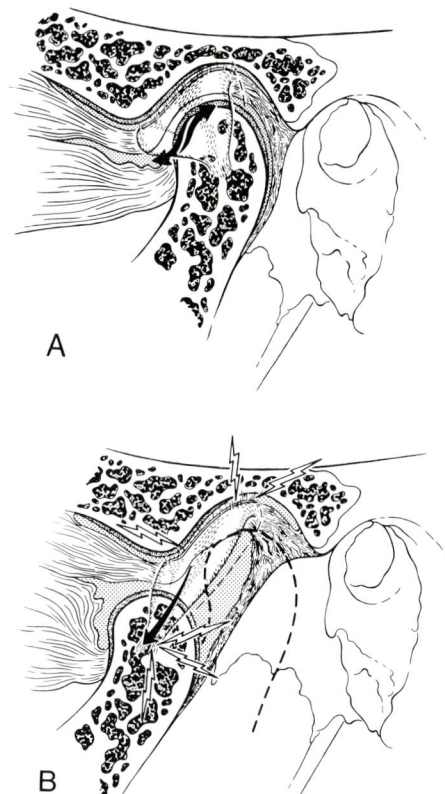

Figure 16–3. *A*, Drawing depicting relative disc immobility after maturation and vascularization of adhesions; translation is forced to occur in the lower compartment. Arrow indicates the location of the lateral discal attachment, which is strained and possibly painful. *B*, Eventually there is laxity of the lateral disc attachments and increased translatory movements in the lower joint compartment. Arrow indicates the location of the lateral discal attachment, which is strained and possibly painful.

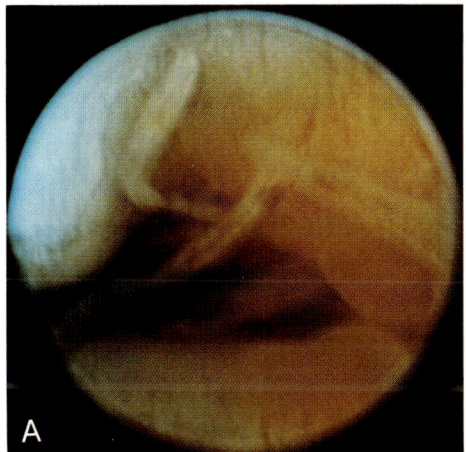

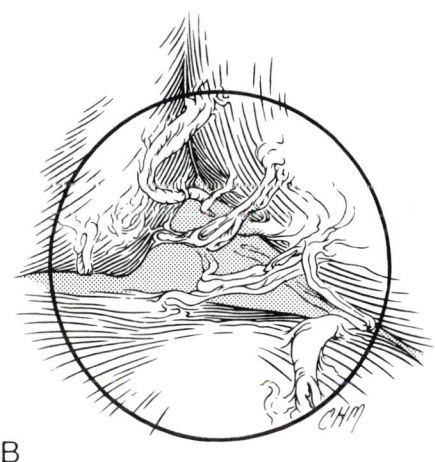

Figure 16–2. *A*, Arthroscopic photograph of endaural view of articular eminence, demonstrating inflamed synovial proliferative tissue and early adhesions; *B*, drawing of endaural view seen in *A*. Location of this tissue is the same as that seen in Figure 16–1*B*.

252 ■ 16 Articular Pathology: Disc Displacement and Lateral Impingement Syndrome

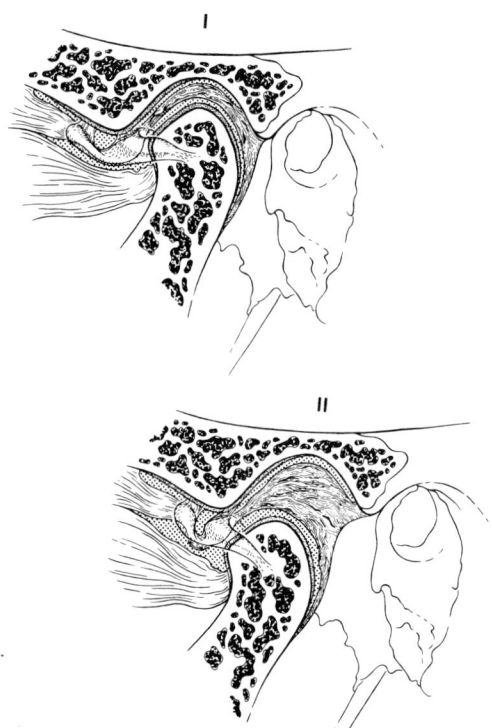

Figure 16–4. Disc migration (I) and changes in disc morphology (II) leading to "closed lock." Superior compartment adhesions restrict translatory movements.

medial or lateral disc displacement. MRI correlative studies on more than 100 arthroscopic confirmations of disc displacement have shown that discs that appeared in normal anatomic position on sagittal views were actually rotated on their condyles with medial displacement (Fig. 16–5).

Diagnosis of disc pathologies, based on two-dimensional studies, can be misleading. In some cases the posterior band almost becomes longitudinally placed anteroposteriorly along the lateral rim of the condyle. This may lead to a "bulging" out of the capsule on coronal MRI (Fig. 16–6). In other cases, images of a disc more medially displaced may have a "sucked-in" appearance of the lateral capsule on coronal MRI, which is termed lateral capsular prolapse (Fig. 16–7). Lateral capsular prolapse may play a role in the development of the lateral impingement phenomenon.

As disc displacement progresses anteromedially, the lateral attachment migrates forward as a result of the gradual and progressive pull of the condyle, which stretches it during attempted translation in the inferior joint space.[9, 10] The attachment carries with it the bone of the condylar lateral pole, developing the anterior "beaking" or "lipping" commonly seen in sagittal tomography (Fig. 16–8). "Beaking" represents an adaptation of condylar remodeling to forces placed on it, rather than a true osteophyte.

If the load is not redistributed,[11] areas of perforation can occur (Fig. 16–9), and further degenerative changes may develop along with adaptive remodeling of both hard and soft tissues. The concept of load distribution is a fundamental biomechanical principle that is crucial to the understanding of joint structure and function. The entire physiologic function of the joint and its associated structures is load distribution. Damage occurs when factors inhibit load distribution. Dysfunction occurs when metaplasia and adaptive remodeling cannot repair this damage by restructuring load distribution.

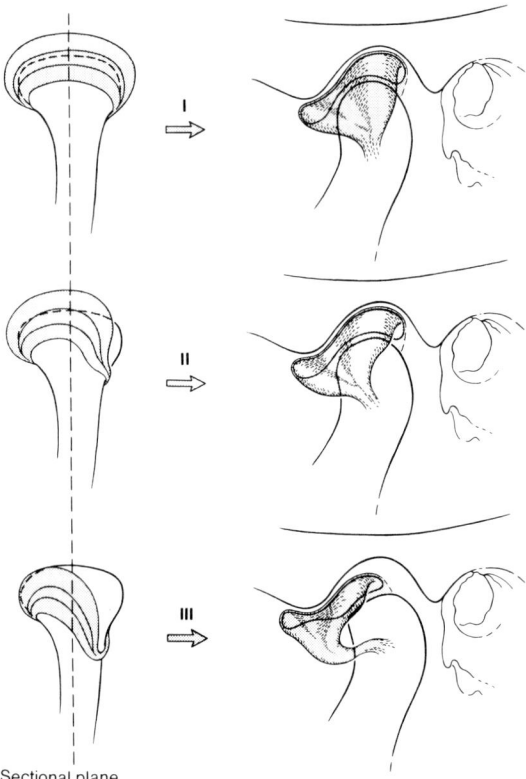

Sectional plane

Figure 16–5. Disc that appears to be well placed on sagittal imaging (I) actually may be rotated on the condyle with medial displacement (II) and in time may suffer increased laxity of the lateral collateral disc attachments (III).

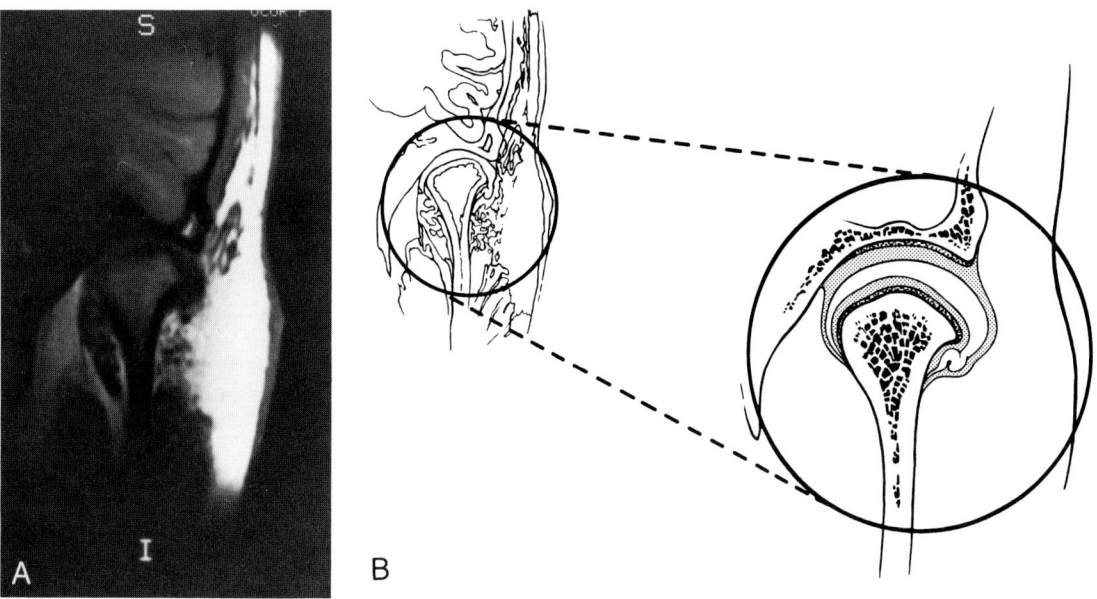

Figure 16–6. *A*, Magnetic resonance image, coronal view, of the temporomandibular joint, demonstrating lateral capsular bulge; *B*, sketch of the image shown in *A*.

A review of arthroscopic cases reveals that the majority of pathologic adhesions and restricted motion lie within the lateral third of the joint. The soft tissues of the capsule become fibrotic and constricted, with inactivity and/or inflammation restricting mandibular movement. From the endaural arthroscopic approach, viewing anteriorly along the lateral trough of the superior compartment, inflamed synovial proliferation and projection are seen (see Fig. 16–2), as well as adhesions binding the disc to the eminence and capsule, leading to restricted mobility and possibly pain.

In the advanced stage, areas of lateral condylar resorption, best seen in anteroposterior tomograms (Fig. 16–10), correlate with the hypertrophic articular tubercles (Fig. 16–11*A–C*) that impinge upon the lateral third of the disc. If the joint space has diminished

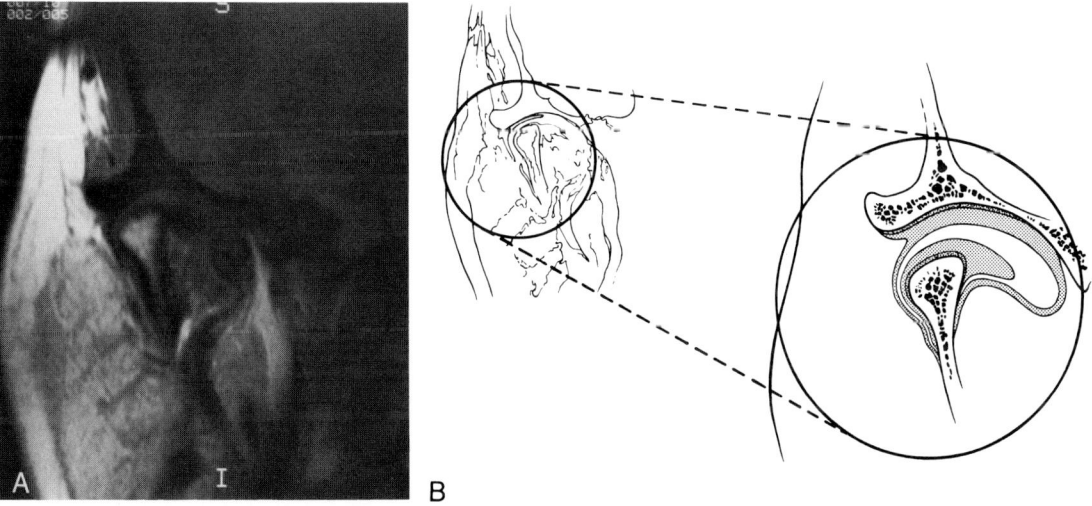

Figure 16–7. *A*, Magnetic resonance image, coronal view, demonstrating lateral capsular concavity and medial discal displacement; *B*, drawing of the image shown in *A*.

254 ■ 16 Articular Pathology: Disc Displacement and Lateral Impingement Syndrome

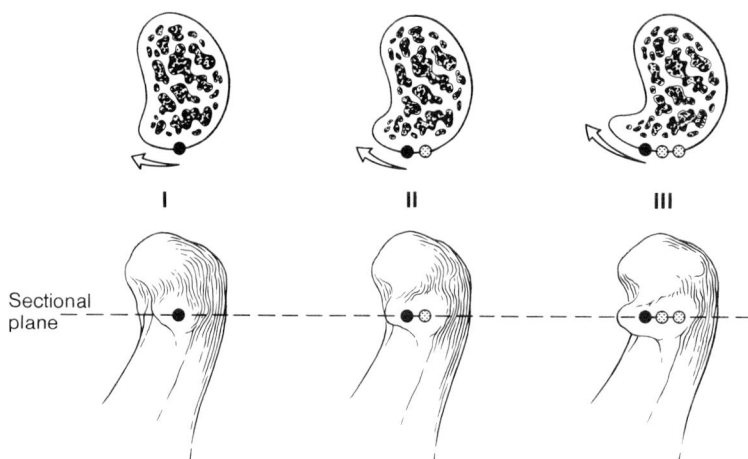

Figure 16–8. Drawing depicting progressive development of anterior "beaking" or "lipping" commonly seen on sagittal tomograms.

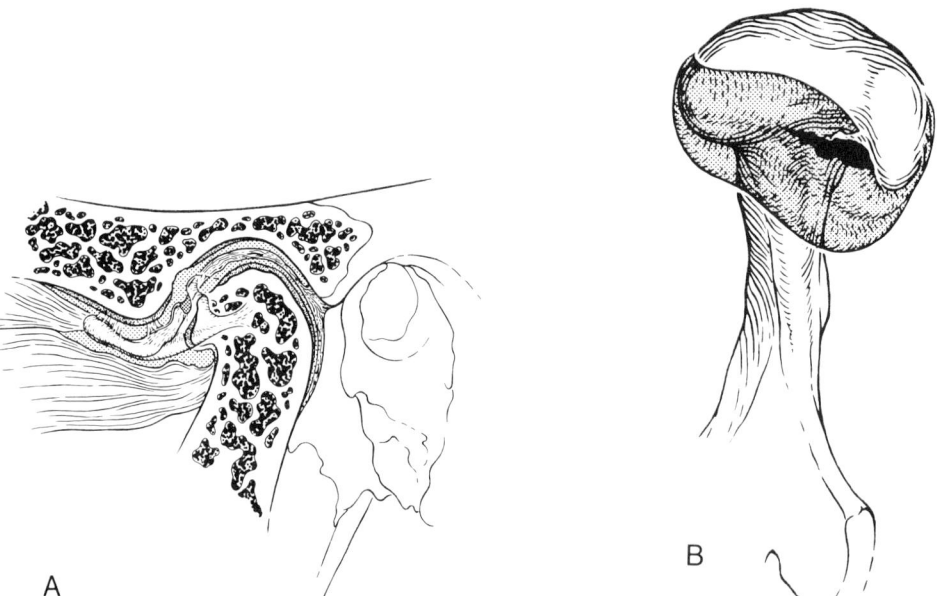

Figure 16–9. Further degeneration of hard and soft tissues in response to undistributed load. *A*, discal, lateral ligamental, and bony changes; *B*, disc perforation.

16 Articular Pathology: Disc Displacement and Lateral Impingement Syndrome ■ 255

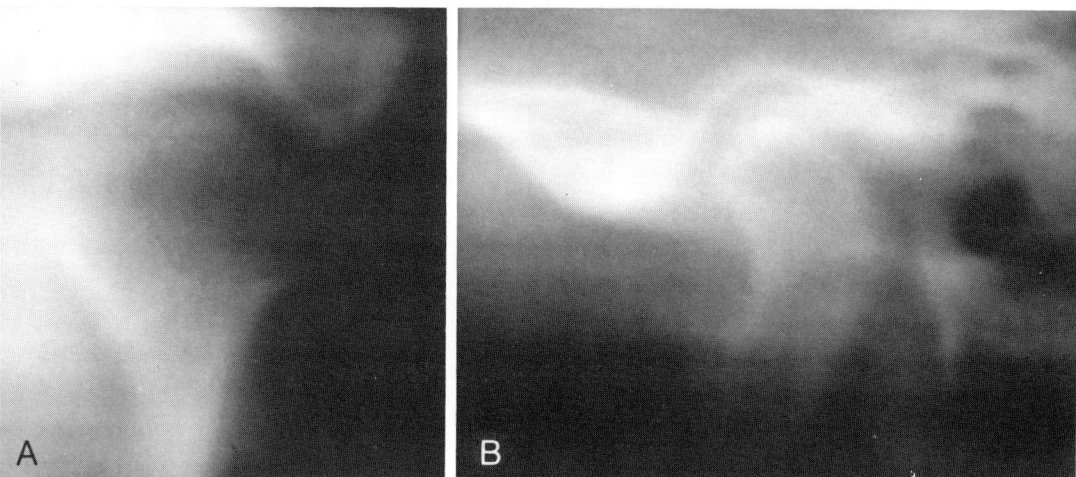

Figure 16–10. *A*, Coronal tomogram taken in slightly protruded position showing bony lateral impingement and prominent articular remodeling of lateral one-third of the condyle; *B*, sagittal tomogram of the same temporomandibular joint.

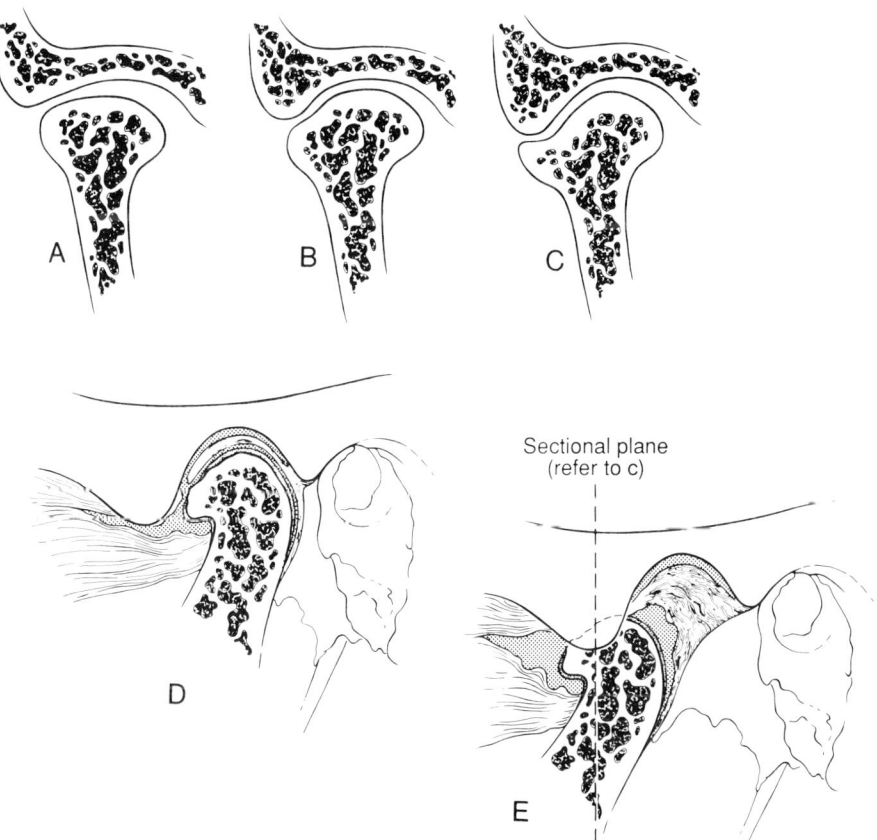

Figure 16–11. Drawings showing advanced stages of condylar remodeling and/or resorption. Areas of lateral condylar resorption correlate with hypertrophic articular tubercles *(A–C)* in response to disc displacement and loss of joint space.

with degenerative changes this becomes especially important, as the condyle will articulate more heavily in that lateral area on protrusive and opening movements (Fig. 16–11D and E). In my experience, disc perforation occurs most frequently in the lateral posterior bilaminar zone/disc junction correlating with this lateral impingement.

Pain itself is not a disease. "Pain merely halts the function to allow healing. The gradual increase in function allows the programming of mesenchymal cell differentiation."[12,13] The goals of treatment should include decreasing functional load and increasing the capacity of cells to accomplish articular remodeling.

Clinical studies utilizing the lateral eminence release (LER) and capsular stretch (CS) procedures, combined with routine arthroscopic lysis of adhesions and lavage (L/L), have relieved both pain and restricted mandibular mobility in over 92% of patients (Table 16–2).[14] Patients with lateral tubercle impingements on the disc seem to require

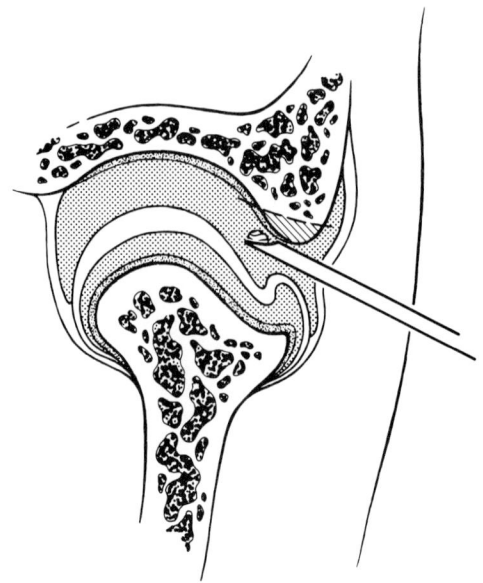

Figure 16–12. Drawing showing arthroscopic osteoplasty of hypertrophic articular tubercle.

additional eminoplasty, which gains joint space and relieves load concentration from that area (Fig. 16–12).

MRI analysis study revealed a consistent result of no change in disc position in the closed-mouth status, both before and after arthroscopic surgery, in 92 patients.[15] The study revealed an increase in mobility of the disc following arthroscopic release that was directly correlated with the clinical success of pain reduction and restoration of normal mandibular function.

The mobilization of tissues within and around the joint, combined with reduction of load concentrations, enhances mesenchymal cell reprogramming, allowing potential formation of pseudodisc articulations and condylar remodeling. Studies are in progress at the present time investigating whether condylar remodeling occurs long-term following arthroscopic procedures (Fig. 16–13).

Table 16–2. THE EFFECT OF TMJ ARTHROSCOPIC SURGICAL LYSIS AND LAVAGE OF SUPERIOR JOINT COMPARTMENT ADHESIONS ON DISC POSITION AND MOBILITY*

Preoperative Findings
100% (92 patients)
  had anteriorly displaced discs without reduction.
35% (32 patients)
  had radiologic evidence of degenerative joint disease.
15 joints
  had arthrographically demonstrated perforations.

Postoperative Findings
92% (85 patients)
  had persistent anteriorly displaced discs.
8% (7 patients)
  demonstrated reduced discs.
80% (73 patients)
  had joints that showed evidence of disc mobilization when compared to the preoperative examination.

Summary and Conclusions
1. Arthroscopic lysis and lavage of TMJ was effective in 92% of the cases.
2. Arthroscopic surgery of this type will not result in disc reduction.
3. Disc mobility rather than repositioning of the disc may play a significant part in the success of the treatment.

*Preoperatively, 100% of the patients included in this study had arthrograms and tomograms, and 85% had MRI scans; postoperatively, 100% of the patients had MRI scans to evaluate disc position and mobility.

References

1. Quinn J: Personal communication.
2. Ellman H: Arthroscopic subacromial decompression. Orthop Trans 9:48, 1985.
3. Neer CS II: Anterior acromioplasty for the chronic impingement syndrome in the shoulder: A preliminary report. J Bone Joint Surg 54A:41, 1972.
4. Hawkins RF, Kennedy JC: Impingement syndrome in athletes. Am J Sports Med 8:151, 1980.

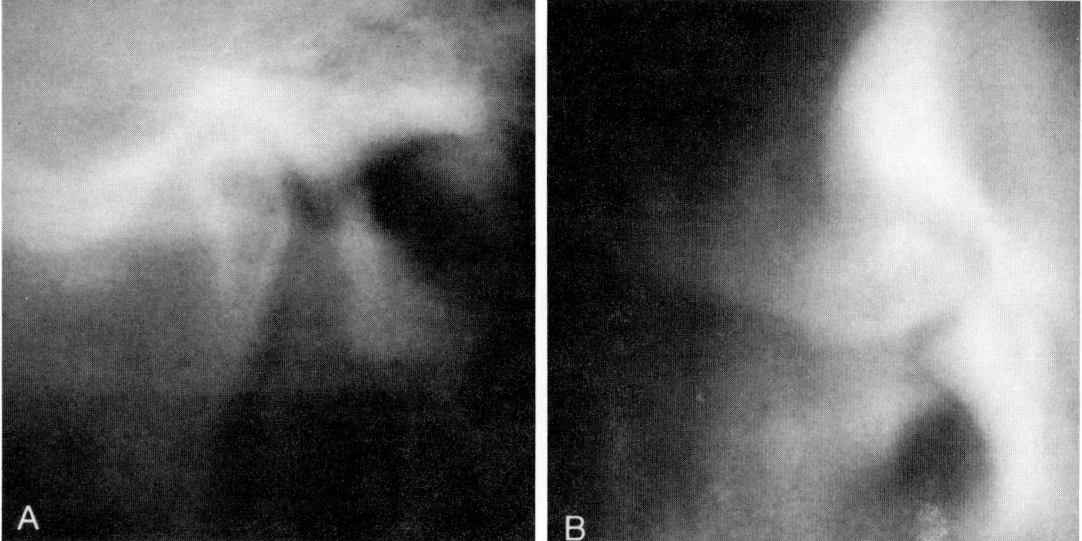

Figure 16-13. *A,* Preoperative sagittal tomogram of a temporomandibular joint (TMJ) with adhesions: *B,* 1-year postoperative sagittal tomogram of same TMJ showing adaptive remodeling following lysis of adhesions and joint lavage.

5. Neer CS II: Impingement lesions. Clin Orthop 173:70, 1983.
6. Pujadas GM: Coracoacromial ligament syndrome. J Bone Joint Surg 52A:136, 1979.
7. Post M, Cohen J: Impingement syndrome: A review of late state II and early state III lesions. Orthop Trans 9:48, 1985.
8. Raggio CL, Warren RF, Sculco T: Surgical treatment of impingement syndrome: 4-year follow-up. Orthop Trans 9:48, 1985.
9. Backwood HJJ: Arthritis of the mandibular joint. Br Dental J 115:317, 1963.
10. Juniper RP: The pathogenesis and investigation of TMJ dysfunction. Br J Oral Maxillofac Surg 25:105–112, 1987.
11. Tay David KL: The pathogenesis of disc displacement in the temporomandibular joint: A reassessment of the role of closed-locked positions. J Gnathol 6(1), 1987.
12. Moffett B: Instructional Course Lecture, Pacific Clinical Research Foundation, 1988.
13. Moffett BC, Johnson LC, McCabe JB, Askew HC: Articular remodeling in the adult human temporomandibular joint. Am J Anat 115:119–142, 1964.
14. Moses J, Poker I: TMJ arthroscopic surgery—an analysis of 237 patients. J Oral Maxillofac Surg 47:90–94, 1989.
15. Moses J, Poker I: Correlation studies of effects of TMJ arthroscopic surgical lysis of superior joint compartment adhesions and lavage. J Oral Maxillofac Surg 47: 674–678, 1989.
16. Eggleton D, Langton T: General Principles of TMJ Physical Therapy Management—Pre- and Postsurgical. San Diego, CA: UCSD School of Medicine, TMJ Management Symposium Booklet, 1988.
17. Eggleton D, Langton T: General Principles of TMJ Physical Therapeutics—Pre- and Post-surgical Considerations. San Diego, CA: UCSD Medical Center, Pacific Clinical Research Foundation Course Booklet, Advanced TMJ Arthroscopy, 1989.

Chapter 17

HARD TISSUE PATHOLOGY

A. Osteoarthrosis

*LAMBERT G. M. DE BONT, D.D.S., PH.D.,
BOUDEWIJN STEGENGA, D.D.S.,
and GEERT BOERING, D.D.S., PH.D.*

Osteoarthrosis is a noninflammatory disorder in which initial alterations of the articular cartilage, and possibly also of the synovial membrane and subchondral bone, cause a vicious cycle of cartilage breakdown accompanied by attempts to repair. When the degrading process exceeds the response of repair, the osteoarthrotic disorder progresses into clinically detectable stages.[1,2]

Osteoarthrosis of the temporomandibular joint (TMJ) frequently is associated with an internal derangement, because the gliding capacity of the articular disc is impaired by the degrading process, giving rise to disc displacement. In our opinion, in many cases disc displacement should be considered as an accompanying sign of early osteoarthrosis rather than its cause.[2,3]

Because osteoarthrosis is the most common TMJ affliction and the degenerative changes can be observed during arthroscopy, it makes sense to describe the degenerative changes in detail.

CHONDROMALACIA

Fibrocartilage is composed of chondrocytes and fibrocytes surrounded by a dense intercellular matrix of collagen fibrils and a ground substance that is composed predominantly of proteoglycan aggregates (see Chapter 4B). The collagen fibrils are organized in a three-dimensional network. The proteoglycan aggregates are entangled throughout the network of collagen fibrils. Proteoglycans are highly hydrophilic and expand easily by uptake of water from the synovial fluid through osmosis. The resulting internal hydrostatic pressure is resisted by the collagen network.[4]

In the early stages of osteoarthrosis, swelling of the articular cartilage resulting from an increased volume of the proteoglycan–water gel is observed. Because no element in the cartilage other than the collagen fiber network has tensile strength, the most acceptable explanation for the increased hydration is a decrease in the stiffness of the collagen network caused by fragmentation of the collagen fibrils.[4-6] This fragmentation also results in a progressive thinning of the articular cartilage.[7] Changes in the fibrous component of the matrix of articular cartilage, characterized by degenerative alterations of the collagen fibrils and destruction of their spatial arrangement, also have been demonstrated in osteoarthrotic cartilage of mandibular condyles.[8,9] Phenomena such as fibrillation (an increased roughness of the articular surface) and splitting (the presence of horizontal and vertical clefts) accompany disintegration of the collagen fiber network.[10]

The term *chondromalacia* is used rather loosely by the medical profession to describe a clinically distinctive post-traumatic softening of the articular cartilage of the patella in young persons. The anatomic lesions usually are microscopically indistinguishable from those of early osteoarthrosis, although subtle differences have been described. A focal softening associated with increased water content and swelling of cartilage is described as an early stage of chondromalacia. This presumably results from localized breakdown of collagen fibrils within the matrix.[11] Chondromalacia of the TMJ has been introduced as being essentially the same disease as chondromalacia of the patella, and four grades of chondromalacia are described.[10]

The various pathologic findings of TMJ osteoarthrosis have been described by Blackwood,[12] but he was doubtful whether some of the minor histologic changes found in his material represented true osteoarthrotic changes. He suggested that resorption of the subchondral bone and fibrosis of the adjacent bone marrow, which are indicative of osteoarthrosis, according to Bauer,[13] might be part of the normal remodeling process of the mandibular condyle. However, resorption of subchondral bone and fibrosis of marrow spaces frequently are accompanied by extensive horizontal splitting and clustering of chondrocytes, creating degenerative lesions underneath the unaffected articular zone. This complex phenomenon may be considered "chondromalacia" in slightly affected areas, but we agree with those who consider these phenomena to form part of a primary degenerative disease or osteoarthrosis.[11, 14] Chondromalacia is a clinical term applied to the degenerative process involving articular cartilage in osteoarthrotic joints. We support the suggestion of Bean and colleagues[15] that the definition of osteoarthrosis should be broadened to include the degenerative changes of the deeper zones of the articular cartilage and the subchondral bone that occur simultaneously with a microscopically intact articular surface. Therefore, we suggest that chondromalacia should be considered a clinical description to indicate the initial stage of osteoarthrosis rather than a new or separate disease entity.

OSTEOARTHROSIS

There are several hypotheses regarding the initial changes in osteoarthrosis. According to Freeman and Meachim,[7] fatigue failure due to repetitive overloading results in decreased collagen network stiffness, which leads to increased hydration of the proteoglycan–water gel.[7] Radin and co-workers[16] hypothesized that cartilage breakdown is induced by a reduction of the resilience of subchondral bone due to microfractures as a result of excessive loading. Consequently, in Radin's opinion the primary lesion in osteoarthrosis is to be expected in the subchondral bone.[17] Other theories are based on the concept of an intrinsically reduced adaptive capacity of the joint. Furthermore, a reduction of the quantity or an alteration in the quality of the synovial fluid likely impairs the nutritional support of the articular cartilage, possibly resulting in decreased quality and gradual loss of the cartilage matrix. Changes in synovial fluid production will also reduce its lubricating capacity and thus impair joint function.[2] It has been hypothesized that cartilage or synovial cell breakdown, resulting in the release of proteolytic or collagenolytic enzymes, induces enzymatic matrix degeneration.[18] Whatever the initial event will be, it may give rise to degenerative tissue breakdown (i.e., osteoarthrosis) (Fig. 17–1).

Initial cartilage degeneration (chondromalacia) may progress to more progressive pathologic changes[19] and clinical symptoms[20] in later stages. Collagen network disintegration and proteoglycan depletion cause

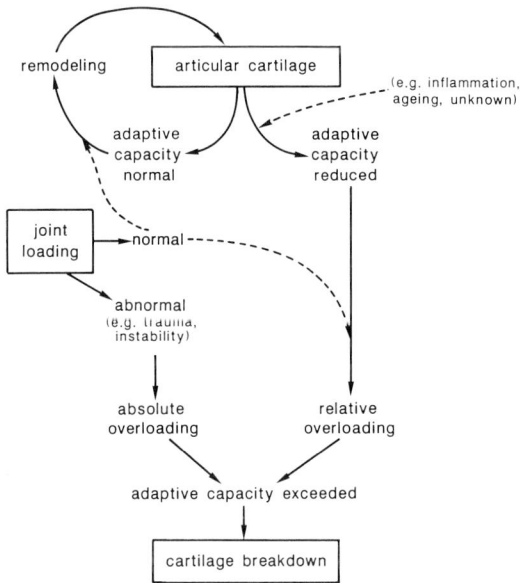

Figure 17–1. Relationship between the adaptive capacity of cartilage, joint loading, and the initiation of degenerative cartilage breakdown. (Reprinted with permission from Stegenga B, de Bont LGM, Boering G: Osteoarthrosis as the cause of craniomandibular pain and dysfunction: A unifying concept. J Oral Maxillofac Surg 47:249–256, 1989.)

a vicious cycle of cartilage breakdown (Fig. 17–2). In addition, increased friction may induce wear, leading to cartilage thinning. The major clinical symptoms in this stage include joint pain and stiffness of short duration, especially after periods of inactivity. Further cartilage destruction may eventually lead to focal bone denudation. Clinically, pain and tenderness on palpation, joint crackling and crepitus, and limitation of joint motion are the main symptoms.[20] Signs of sclerosis and osteolytic cysts may be detected radiographically.[19] Gradual enlargement of the area of bone exposure due to abrasive wear leads to regressive remodeling, resulting in flattening and loss of bone height. As part of this remodeling process, new bone and fibrous tissue may be formed at the periphery of the region of tissue destruction (peripheral remodeling), which may be radiographically detectable as osteophytic lipping.[19, 21]

The TMJ obeys the same biologic laws as do all other synovial joints and their associated musculoskeletal components. Throughout life, TMJ articular cartilage and the underlying bone display shifting equilibria between changes in form and function by tissue remodeling, just as do all other joints of the body (Figs. 17–3 and 17–4).[22] Increased or decreased functional stress affects the biologic properties of the cartilage tissue.[23] Increased loading may stimulate remodeling, involving increased synthesis of proteoglycans and collagen fibrils.[24]

Early alterations in TMJ osteoarthrosis are characterized by structural failure of articular cartilage focally due to loss of proteoglycans, increased water content, and a probably highly significant change in the arrangement and size of collagen fibrils.[8, 9] Initially, cartilage changes are subclinical, but they can set up a vicious cycle of cartilage breakdown (Fig. 17–5, Stage I). The repair process following or accompanying the cartilage breakdown may maintain the joint in a steady state, possibly for many years. In comparison, the degenerative process may exceed the reparative attempts because of aggravating environmental factors, resulting in progression of the osteoarthrosis process (vertical paths in Fig. 17–5) and clinically significant effects (Fig. 17–5, Stage II).[2] Although osteoarthrosis may develop without disc displacement (Fig. 17–5, Stage IIA), internal derangement appears to be highly correlated with TMJ osteoarthrosis (Fig. 17–5, Stage IIB). Both cartilage breakdown, which affects the sliding properties of the joint surfaces, and alterations of the synovial fluid, which give rise to increased friction and adhesive wear, impair disc movement. This may induce repetitive stretching of the disc attachments, which may gradually elongate to an extent that permits disc displacement. At first, the disc can be actively repositioned during movement (reducible disc displacement), but eventually this condition may progress to permanent disc displacement.

In the case of anterior disc displacement, the bilaminar zone becomes subjected to compressive loading. This may lead to an inflammatory response, causing pain and further maladaptive changes such as thinning, fatty degeneration, and perforation. However, adaptive changes in the bilaminar zone (decreased vascularity, decreased elastin content, presence of cartilage cells, and fibrosis of the anterior part of the bilaminar zone) also have been described.[25–27] In all stages of internal derangement, pain may be present owing to secondary synovitis[28] and irritation of disc attachments, capsule, and perhaps also superficial bone. Inflammatory mediators and enzymes produced by the

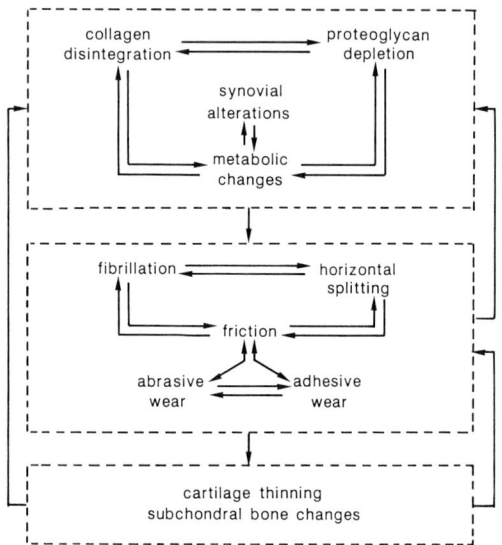

Figure 17–2. Vicious cycles of cartilage breakdown due to alterations in the functionally interdependent cartilage components and the synovial fluid. (Reprinted with permission from Stegenga B, de Bont LGM, Boering G: Osteoarthrosis as the cause of craniomandibular pain and dysfunction: A unifying concept. J Oral Maxillofac Surg 47:249–256, 1989.)

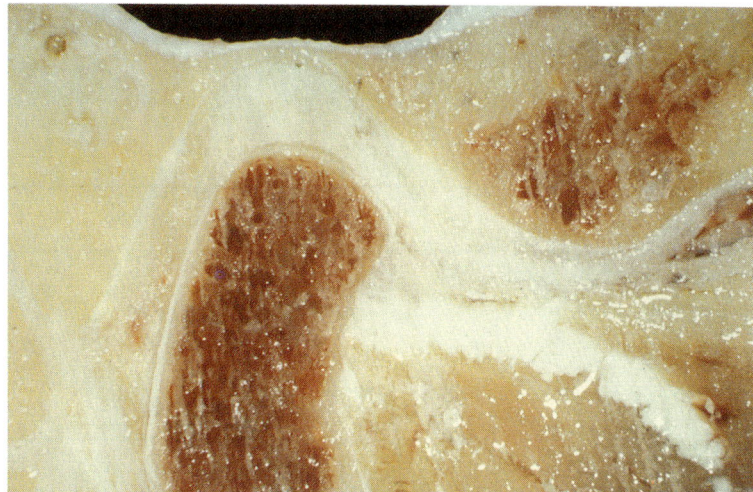

Figure 17–3. Autopsy specimen of a normal temporomandibular joint.

chondrocytes may stimulate the inflammatory process.[18]

Progressive cartilage breakdown eventually leads to denudation of the subchondral bone (Fig. 17–5, Stage III). Although radiographic signs may be present in previous stages, gross bony alterations are seen especially in this stage. They consist of the characteristic radiographic signs of osteoarthrosis such as sclerosis of the subchondral bone, osteophytic lipping, cyst formation, flattening of the condyle and eminence, and decreased height of the mandibular ramus.[21] Eventually, bony remodeling leads to the end stage of osteoarthrosis, described as "burned-out osteoarthrosis"[21] and as "internal rearrangement."[29] Most clinical signs and symptoms of the previous stages tend to subside; only crepitation may remain.

Characteristic histopathologic features of TMJ osteoarthrosis, including horizontal splitting, clustering of chondrocytes, bone marrow fibrosis, sclerosis, cyst formation, and reduction in TMJ size,[3] are shown in Figures 17–6 through 17–11. Disc displacement and changes in shape and size of the disc are considered to be part of the osteoarthrotic process.

ARTICULAR SURFACE CHARACTERISTICS

Articular surface characteristics have been studied by scanning electron microscopy

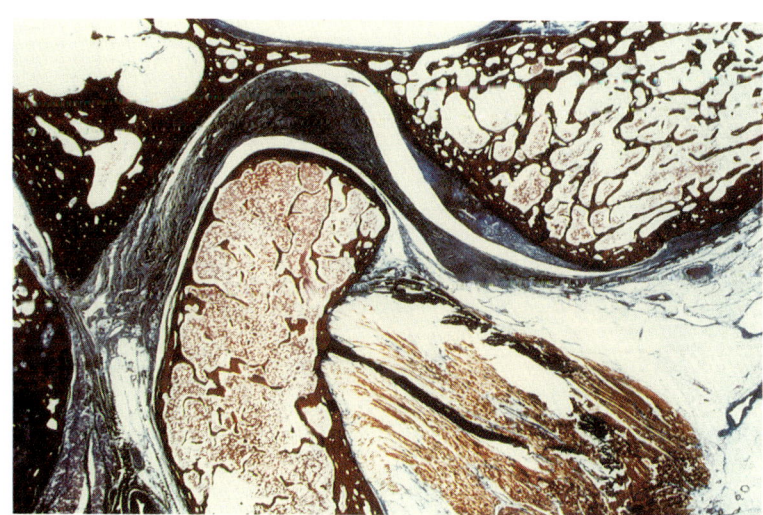

Figure 17–4. Midsagittal light microscopic survey section of the temporomandibular joint, shown in Figure 17–3. The articular cartilage covering of the mandibular condyle and the articular eminence as well as the cartilage of the articular disc are clearly observable. (Azan staining; magnification × 3.5.)

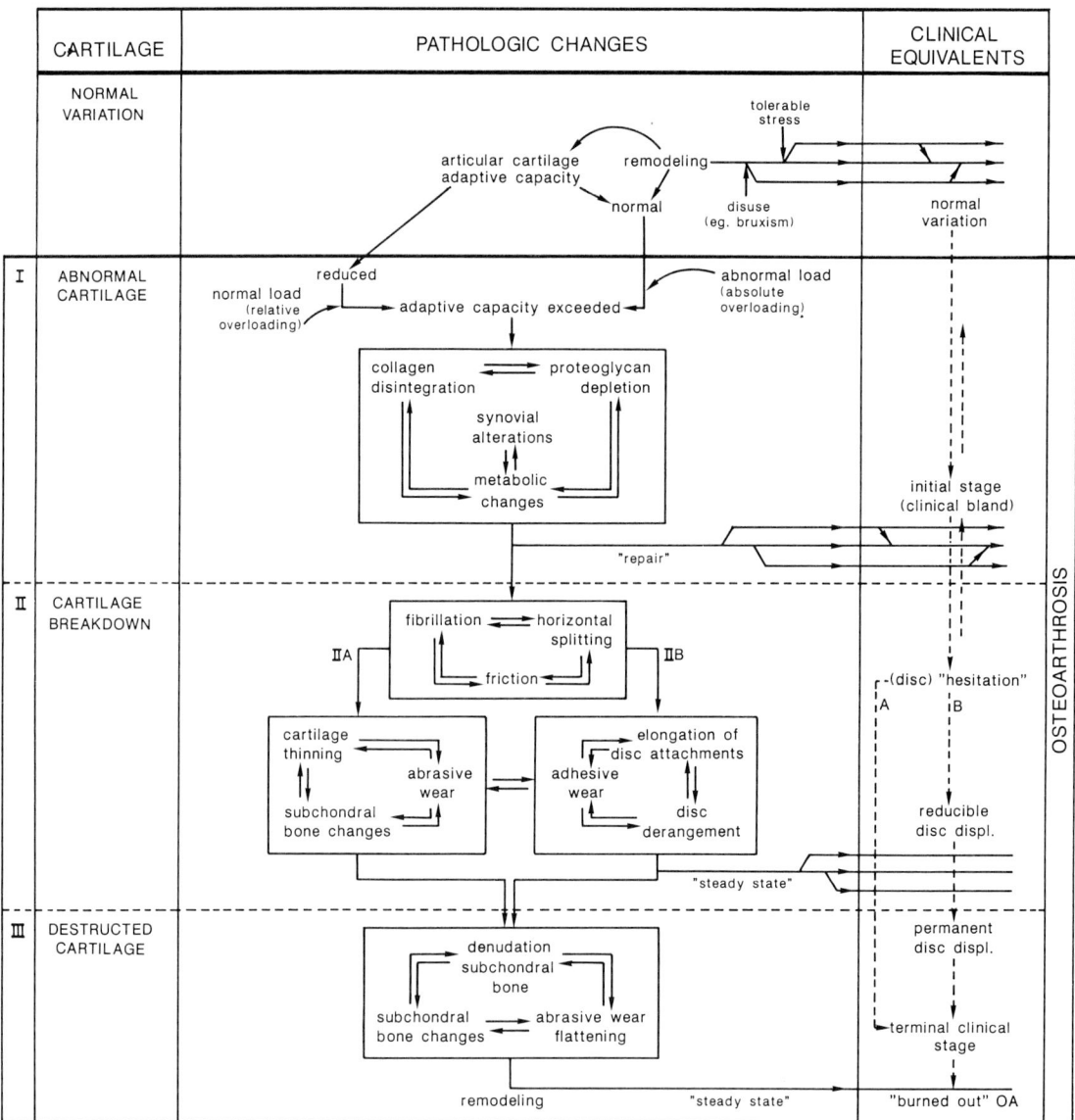

Figure 17–5. The temporomandibular joint osteoarthrosis concept. In the sequence from normal cartilage to destroyed cartilage, and from normal variation to osteoarthrosis, three stages are distinguished, corresponding to the accompanying clinical signs. OA = osteoarthrosis. (Reprinted with permission from Stegenga B, de Bont LGM, Boering G: Osteoarthrosis as the cause of craniomandibular pain and dysfunction: A unifying concept. J Oral Maxillofac Surg 47:249–256, 1989.)

A Osteoarthrosis ■ 263

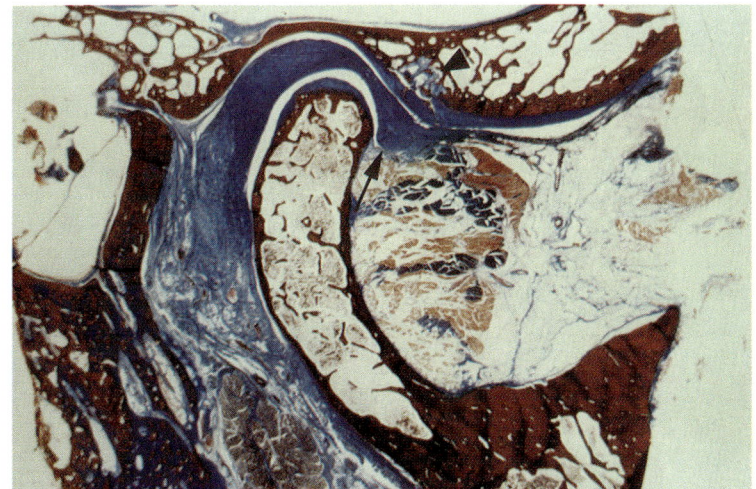

Figure 17–6. Midsagittal light microscopic survey section of a temporomandibular joint with a deformed disc. Note the shape of the anterior band *(arrow)* and the degenerative changes at the articular eminence *(arrowhead).* (Azan staining; magnification × 3.2.)

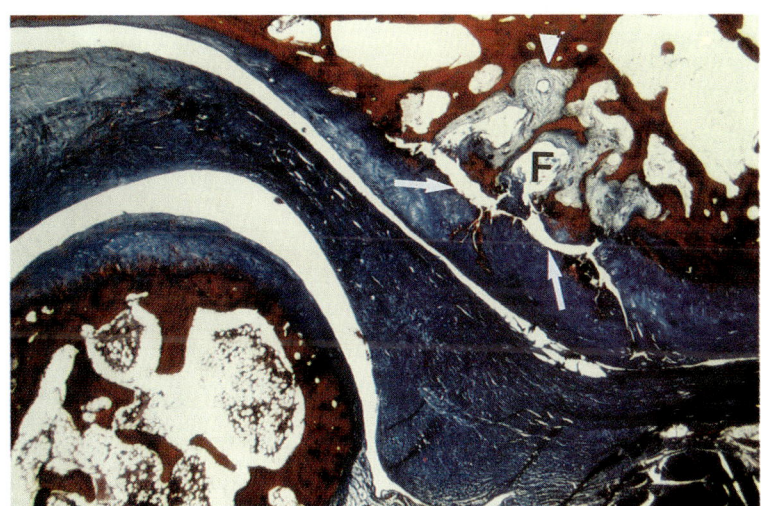

Figure 17–7. Detail of Figure 17–6, showing horizontal splitting of the articular cartilage *(arrows)* parallel to the articular surface and the subchondral bone and fibrosis (F) of the marrow spaces of the articular eminence. Note the cystlike fibrosis *(arrowhead).* The articular surfaces seem smooth and unaffected. (Azan staining; magnification × 14.)

Figure 17–8. Detail of Figure 17–7, showing the irregular border of the subchondral bone and the splitting articular cartilage. The articular cartilage shows fibrillation at the edge of the split *(arrows).* (Azan staining; magnification × 50.)

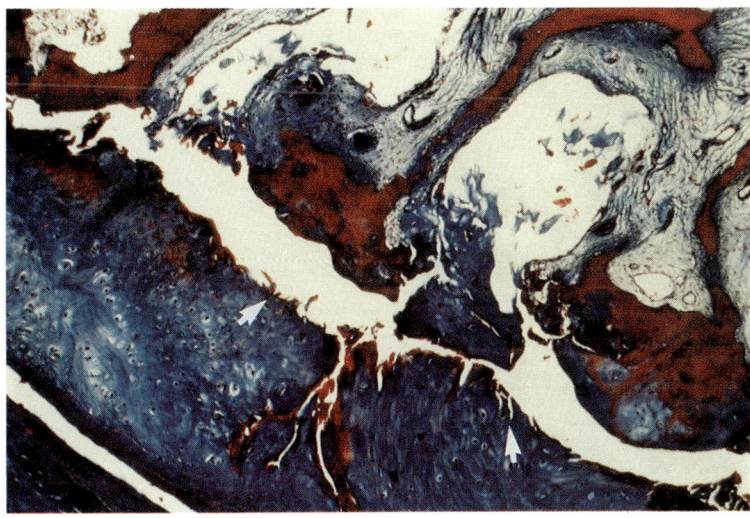

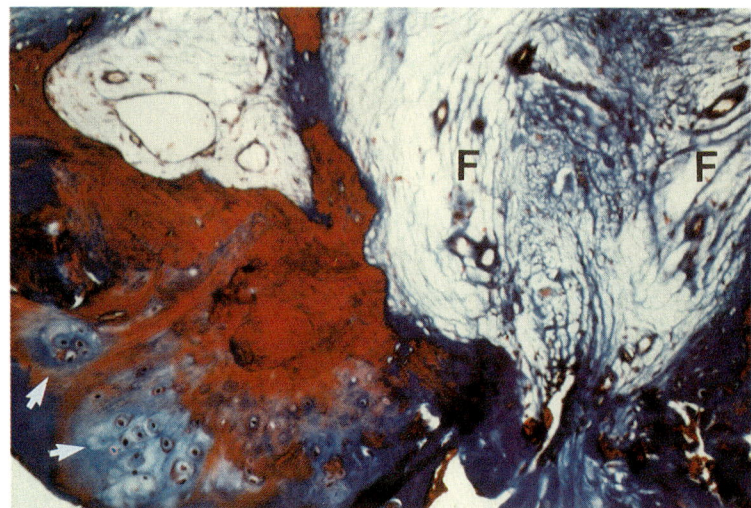

Figure 17–9. Detail of Figure 17–8, showing clustering of chondrocytes underneath the horizontal split *(arrows)* and fibrosis of the marrow spaces (F). (Azan staining; magnification × 125.)

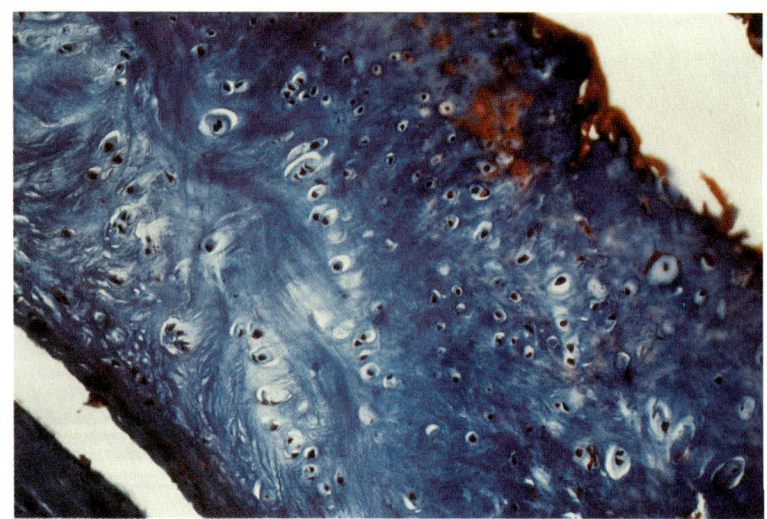

Figure 17–10. Detail of Figure 17–8, showing the articular cartilage above the split. No zonal differentiation is observable. Note the chondrocytes. (Azan staining; magnification × 125.)

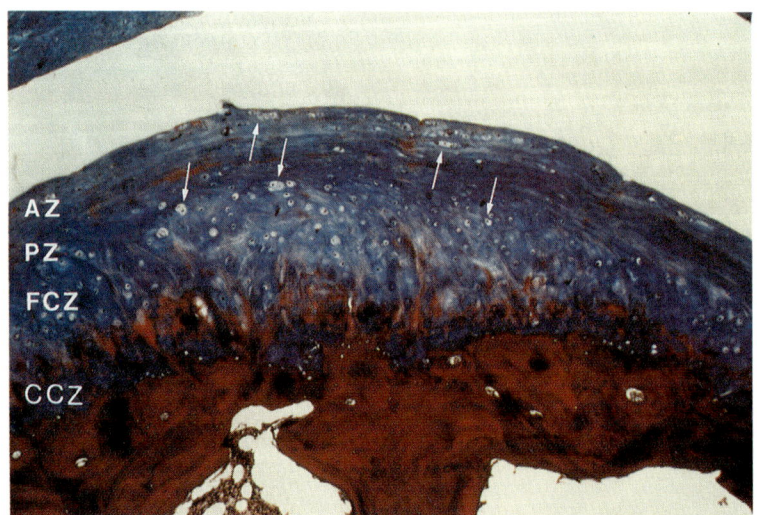

Figure 17–11. Detail of Figure 17–7, showing the summit of the mandibular condyle. Zonal differentiation is observable. Note the chondrocytes situated throughout the tissue *(arrows)*. AZ = articular zone; PZ = proliferative zone; FCZ = fibrocartilaginous zone; CCZ = calcified cartilage zone; SB = subchondral bone. (Azan staining; magnification × 50.)

(SEM) of the articular cartilage of TMJ autopsy specimens.[9, 30] After dissection, the mandibular condyles were routinely washed with a saline solution. SEM images of the articular surface of the mandibular condyle showed characteristic features of collagen fibrils organized in collagen fiber bundles (Figs. 17–12 and 17–13).

For experimental reasons, we changed the method of tissue processing several times during our SEM experiments; occasionally, the mandibular condyles were not washed after dissection. The SEM images of the articular surface of the unwashed condyles showed a smooth surface, like asphalt pavement (Figs. 17–14 and 17–15). The smooth material superimposed on the collagen network of the articular surface probably represents a thin layer consisting of ground substance of the articular cartilage or a layer of synovial fluid on the articular surface, fixed by the fixation fluid during tissue processing. The lamina splendens, as described by some light microscopists, basically has the same origin.[31]

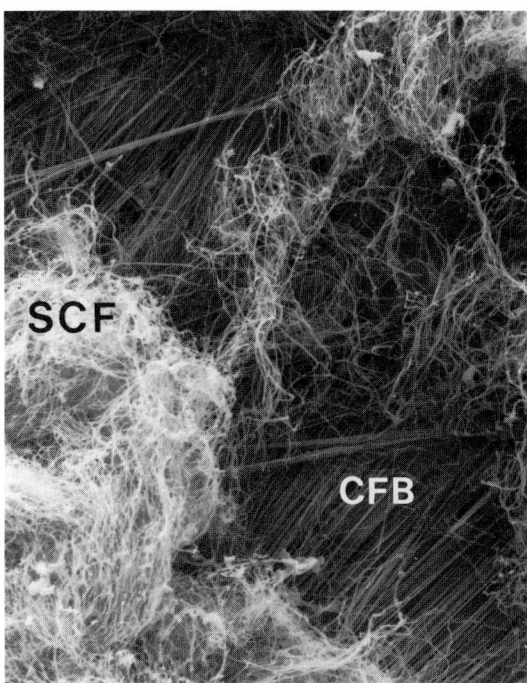

Figure 17–13. Detail of scanning electron microscopic image of the articular surface of the mandibular condyle, showing the individual fibrils in the collagen fiber bundles (CFB) and the small coiled fibrils (SCF) with a cotton-wool appearance. (Magnification × 1680.)

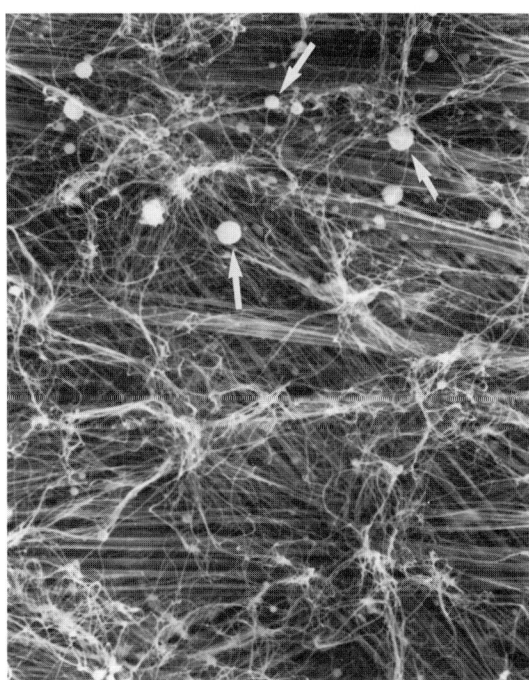

Figure 17–12. Scanning electron microscopic image of the articular surface of the mandibular condyle, showing the individual fibrils in the interwoven collagen fiber bundles. The small globules (arrows) represent free fatty acids, fixed by osmium tetroxide. (Magnification × 1060.)

DISCUSSION

Knowledge of TMJ morphology is necessary for understanding both its normal function and dysfunction. Processes like remodeling, aging, and osteoarthrosis affect joint morphology. Remodeling is a process of reversible biologic adaptation in which mechanical forces stimulate the cellular formation and resorption of articular tissue and bone and, therefore, changes the structure or morphology of the tissue concerned.[24, 32, 33] Progressive, regressive, and circumferential remodeling are the three distinguishable types of remodeling that occur in synovial joints.[32, 34, 35] Aging is a process of senescence-related events in the joint tissues that are associated with chronologic age, exclusive of and distinct from osteoarthrosis.[36] Osteoarthrosis, a primarily noninflammatory disorder of diarthrodial joints, is characterized by deterioration and abrasion of the articular cartilage and by a simultaneous remodeling process in the underlying bone.[37–39] Although the differences between remodeling, aging, and osteoarthrosis were

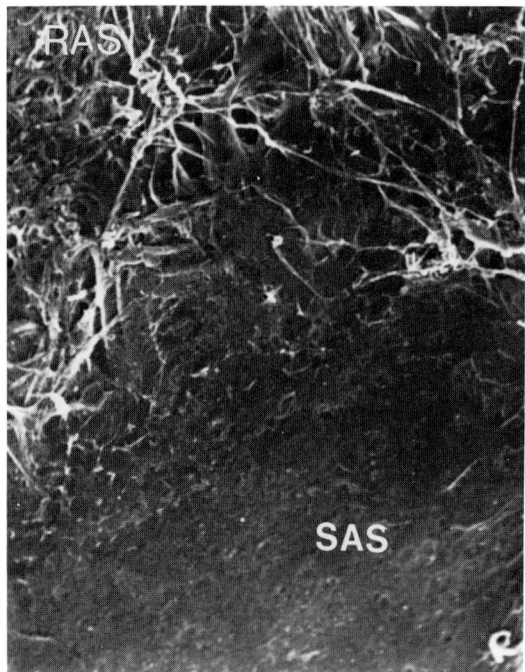

Figure 17–14. Scanning electron microscopic image of the articular surface of the mandibular condyle, showing a demarcation area between rough (RAS) and smooth (SAS) articular surfaces. The rough articular surface represents an area perhaps affected by mild fibrillation. The smooth surface probably represents a thin layer of ground substance or synovial fluid on the articular surface and resembles asphalt pavement. (Magnification × 52.)

means (e.g., arthroscopy, biopsy, histology), may progress to several characteristic stages,[2] although we should realize that in some cases the disease will remain subclinical. The natural course of internal derangement and osteoarthrosis has recently been described by Nickerson and Boering[44] and is presented in Figure 17–5. Osteoarthrosis of the TMJ is a self-limiting disorder. Not all cases will progress to the final stage; even if the final stage is reached, it "burns out" in 85 to 90% of all cases in 2 to 3 years.[21, 44]

Internal derangement of the TMJ, defined as displacement or a malrelation of the disc to the condyle and articular eminence, plays an important role in TMJ dysfunction.[3, 40, 45–50] Although the causal relationship between disc displacement and osteoarthrosis has not yet been proven, frequently it is assumed that internal derangement of the TMJ leads to osteoarthrosis,[49, 51–53] analogous to such a progession in, for example, the canine knee after experimental section of a cruciate ligament.[54] However, despite the

described by Moffett and colleagues[32] and Sokoloff,[36] it is nevertheless difficult to define the boundaries between age-related changes and osteoarthrosis on one hand, and between remodeling and osteoarthrosis on the other.[32, 34, 36] Because all of the adaptive mechanisms characteristic of remodeling play an active role in osteoarthrotic joints, as well as in aged joints, it is also difficult to distinguish histologically a joint that can be regarded as aged and a joint that has become pathologically affected.[24] We agree with Johnson's statement[34] that osteoarthrosis results from decompensated or unbalanced remodeling. However, as mentioned by Carlsson and co-workers,[39] there are no generally accepted histologic criteria for osteoarthrosis of the TMJ, despite the basic studies of Blackwood, Moffett, Steinhardt, and Toller.[14, 32, 35, 40–43]

Early cartilage degeneration, not radiographically detectable but obvious by other

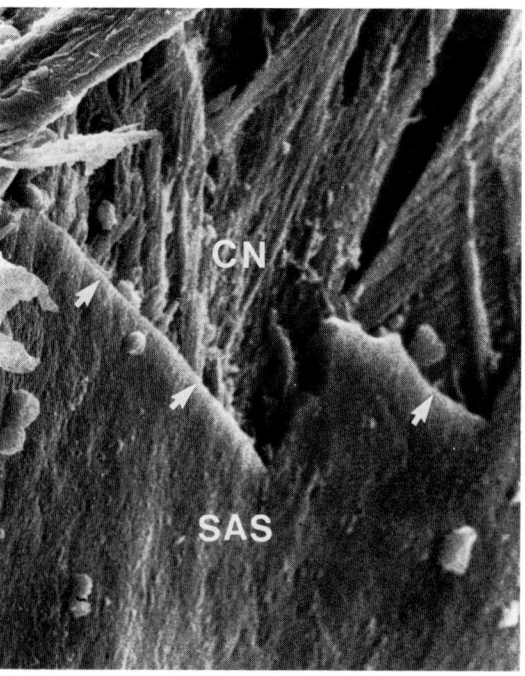

Figure 17–15. Scanning electron microscopic image of the articular surface of the mandibular condyle that was broken while it was deeply frozen in liquid nitrogen. The line of the break is clearly visible *(arrows)*; it demarcates the smooth articular surface (SAS), which resembles asphalt pavement, from the underlying collagen network (CN). (Magnification × 890.)

high correlation between disc displacement and osteoarthrosis, as found in histopathologic studies,[26, 35, 40, 45] internal derangement seems to be one of the accompanying signs of TMJ osteoarthrosis.[3]

The adaptive capacity of some joint structures to new environmental factors is not fully discussed in the literature. For example, the posterior attachment of the disc, which is positioned on top of the condyle when the disc is anteriorly displaced, may become more dense over a period of time while the tissue of this attachment is loaded during joint function. This adaptive capacity is probably one of the explanations for the good long-term prognosis of many closed-lock cases as described by Boering.[21, 44] The original loose connective tissue, containing many elastic fibers, seems to become more and more dense during its adaptation to loading.

Arthroscopy is a relatively recent development in oral and maxillofacial surgery and a most exciting area, not only for diagnostic and therapeutic procedures but also, certainly, for research. However, arthroscopy is restricted to inspection of the articular surfaces. This means that it has a restricted capacity to detect degenerative changes such as splitting of the articular cartilage and fibrosis of the bone marrow (see Figs. 17–7 through 17–11). These can only be detected microscopically and not by inspection of the joint surfaces during arthroscopy or during open joint surgery. The articular surfaces frequently seem unaffected, whereas the degenerative changes are clearly present in the deeper layers of the articular cartilage.[3]

Inspection of the articular surface by SEM reveals a network of interwoven collagen fiber bundles and, superposed on this network, small coiled fibrils with a cotton-wool appearance.[30] Perhaps this appearance is the result of fraying, a sign of wear at the articular surface. SEM of osteoarthrotic cartilage of the TMJ reveals signs of fatty degeneration and collagen network disintegration. Fatty degeneration, as emphasized by Ghadially,[31] is one of the remarkable phenomena in osteoarthrotic cartilage. However, healthy articular cartilage also shows lipid debris in the matrix as a result of cell necrosis.[31, 55, 56] It is reasonable to expect that the rate of formation and abundance of lipid debris in the matrix corresponds to the rate of development of osteoarthrosis, which is attended by high cell turnover. The free fatty acids, as shown by SEM (see Fig. 17–13), are the result of fatty degeneration, which produces this intramatrical lipidic debris. SEM of the articular cartilage surface reveals different pictures, depending on the manner of tissue processing and on the magnification that is used. In this respect, there is some resemblance between SEM and arthroscopy, because both look at surface structures and produce pictures with a certain magnification.

References

1. Stegenga B, de Bont LGM, Boering G: A proposed classification of temporomandibular disorders based on synovial joint pathology. J. Craniomandib Pract 7:107–118, 1989.
2. Stegenga B, de Bont LGM, Boering G: Osteoarthrosis as the cause of craniomandibular pain and dysfunction: A unifying concept. J Oral Maxillofac Surg 47:249–256, 1989.
3. de Bont LGM, Boering G, Liem RSB, et al: Osteoarthrosis and internal derangement of the temporomandibular joint. A light microscopic study. J Oral Maxillofac Surg 44:634–643, 1986.
4. Maroudas A: Physiochemical properties of articular cartilage. In Freeman MAR (ed): Adult Articular Cartilage, 2nd Ed. London: Pitman Medical, 1979, pp 215–290.
5. Maroudas A: Balance between swelling pressure and collagen tension in normal and degenerate cartilage. Nature 260:808–809, 1976.
6. Meachim G: Ways of cartilage breakdown in human and experimental osteoarthrosis. In Nuki G (ed): The Aetiopathogenesis of Osteoarthrosis. London, Pitman Medical, 1980, pp 16–28.
7. Freeman MAR, Meachim G: Ageing and degeneration. In Freeman MAR (ed): Adult Articular Cartilage, 2nd Ed. London, Pitman Medical, 1979, pp 487–540.
8. de Bont LGM, Liem RSB, Boering G: Ultrastructure of the articular cartilage of the mandibular condyle: ageing and degeneration. Oral Surg Oral Med Oral Pathol 60:631–641, 1985.
9. de Bont LGM, Boering G, Liem RSB, et al: Osteoarthritis of the temporomandibular joint: A light microscopic and scanning electron microscopic study of the articular cartilage of the mandibular condyle. J Oral Maxillofac Surg 43:481–488, 1985.
10. Quinn JH: Pathogenesis of TMJ chondromalacia and arthralgia. In Merrill RG (ed): Disorders of the TMJ I: Diagnosis and Arthroscopy. Oral Maxillofac Surg Clin North Am: 47–57, 1989.
11. Sokoloff L: Pathology and pathogenesis of osteoarthritis. In McCarty DJ (ed): Arthritis and Allied Conditions. A Textbook of Rheumatology, 9th Ed. Philadelphia, Lea and Febiger, 1979, pp 1135–1153.
12. Blackwood HJJ: Arthritis of the mandibular joint. Br Dent J 115:317–326, 1963.
13. Bauer WH: Osteo-arthritis deformans of the temporomandibular joint. Am J Pathol 17:129–140, 1941.
14. Toller PA: Temporomandibular arthropathy. Proc R Soc Med 67:153–159, 1974.

15. Bean LR, Omnell KA, Öberg T: Comparison between radiologic observations and macroscopic tissue changes in temporomandibular joints. Dentomaxillofac Radiol 6:90–106, 1977.
16. Radin EL, Paul IL, Rose RM: Osteoarthrosis as a final common pathway. In Nuki G (ed): The Aetiopathogenesis of Osteoarthrosis. London, Pitman Medical, 1980, pp 84–89.
17. Radin EL: Biomechanical considerations. In Moskowitz RW, Howell DS, Goldberg VM, et al (eds): Osteoarthritis, Diagnosis and Management. Philadelphia, WB Saunders, 1984, pp 93–107.
18. Fassbender HG: Significance of endogenous and exogenous mechanisms in the development of osteoarthritis. In Helminen HJ, Kiviranta I, Säämänen AM, et al (eds): Joint Loading. Bristol, Wright, 1987, pp 352–374.
19. Meachim G, Brooke G: The pathology of osteoarthrosis. In Moskowitz RW, Howell DS, Goldberg VM et al (eds): Osteoarthritis, Diagnosis and Management. Philadelphia, WB Saunders, 1984, pp 29–42.
20. Moskowitz RW: Osteoarthritis—symptoms and signs. In Moskowitz RW, Howell DS, Goldberg VM, et al (eds): Osteoarthritis, Diagnosis and Management. Philadelphia, WB Saunders, 1984, pp 149–154.
21. Boering G: Arthrosis Deformans van het Koakgewricht. Temporomandibular joint arthrosis: an analysis of 400 cases. Leiden, Stafleu & Tholen, 1966, pp 87–144.
22. Moffett BC: Classification and diagnosis of temporomandibular joint disturbances. In Solberg WK, Clark GT (eds): Temporomandibular Joint Problems. Biologic Diagnosis and Treatment. Chicago, Quintessence, 1980, pp 21–31.
23. Helminen HJ, Jurvelin J, Kiviranta I, et al: Joint loading effects on articular cartilage: a historical review. In Helminen HJ, Kiviranta I, Säämänen AM, et al (eds): Joint Loading. Bristol, Wright, 1987, pp 1–46.
24. Meikle MC: Remodeling. In Sarnat BG, Laskin DM (eds): The Temporomandibular Joint. A Biological Basis for Clinical Practice, 3rd ed. Springfield Ill, Thomas, 1979, pp 205–226.
25. Hall MB, Brown RW, Baughanan RA: Histological appearance of the bilaminar zone in internal derangement of the temporomandibular joint. Oral Surg Oral Med Oral Pathol 58:375–381, 1984.
26. Scapino RP: Histopathology associated with malposition of the human temporomandibular joint disc. Oral Surg Oral Med Oral Pathol 55:382–397, 1983.
27. Isberg A, Isacsson G: Hyperplastic soft tissue formation in the temporomandibular joint associated with internal derangement, a radiographic and histological study. Oral Surg Oral Med Oral Pathol 61:32–38, 1986.
28. Holmlund A, Hellsing G: Arthroscopy of the temporomandibular joint: Occurrence and location of osteoarthrosis and synovitis in a patient material. Int J Oral Maxillofac Surg 17:36–40, 1988.
29. Ogus H: The mandibular joint: Internal rearrangement. Br J Oral Maxillofac Surg, 25:218–226, 1987.
30. de Bont LGM, Boering G, Havinga P, et al: Spatial arrangement of collagen fibrils in the articular cartilage of the mandibular condyle: A light microscopic and scanning electron microscopic study. J Oral Maxillofac Surg 42:306–313, 1984.
31. Ghadially FN: Fine structures of synovial joints. A text and atlas of the ultrastructure of normal and pathological articular tissues. London, Butterworths, 1983, pp 20–102.
32. Moffet BC, Johnson LC, McCabe JB, et al: Articular remodeling in the adult human temporomandibular joint. Am J Anat 115:119–142, 1964.
33. Moffett BC: Definitions of temporomandibular joint derangements. In Moffett BC (ed): Diagnosis of Internal Derangements of the Temporomandibular Joint. Vol 1: Double-contrast Arthrography and Clinical Correlation. Seattle, Univ. of Washington, 1984.
34. Johnson LC: Joint remodeling as the basis for osteoarthritis. J Am Vet Med Assoc 141:1237–1241, 1962.
35. Blackwood HJJ: Cellular remodeling in articular tissue. J Dent Res 45:480–489, 1966.
36. Sokoloff L: The pathology of osteoarthrosis and the role of ageing. In Nuki G (ed): The Aetiopathogenesis of Osteoarthrosis. London, Pitman Medical, 1980, pp 1–15.
37. Sokoloff L: The Biology of Degenerative Joint Disease. Chicago, Chicago University Press, 1969, pp 1–12.
38. Kopp S, Carlsson GE, Hansson T, et al: Degenerative disease in the temporomandibular, metatarsophalangeal and sternoclavicular joints. An autopsy study. Acta Odontol Scand 34:23–32, 1976.
39. Carlsson GE, Kopp S, Öberg T: Arthritis and allied diseases of the temporomandibular joint. In Zarb GA, Carlsson GE (eds): Temporomandibular Joint Function and Dysfunction. Copenhagen, Munksgaard, 1979, pp 269–320.
40. Steinhardt G: Untersuchungen über die Beanspruchung der Kiefergelenke und ihre geweblichen Folgen. Deutsche Zahnheilkunde 91:1–78, 1934.
41. Blackwood HJJ: Pathology of the temporomandibular joint. J Am Dent Assoc 79:118–124, 1969.
42. Toller PA: Ultrastructure of the condylar articular surface in severe mandibular pain-dysfunction syndrome. Int J Oral Surg 6:297–312, 1977.
43. Toller PA, Wilcox JH: Ultrastructure of the articular surface of the condyle in temporomandibular arthropathy. Oral Surg Oral Med Oral Pathol 45:232–245, 1978.
44. Nickerson JW, Boering G: Natural course of osteoarthrosis as it relates to internal derangement of the temporomandibular joint. In Merrill RG (ed): Disorders of the TMJ I: Diagnosis and Arthroscopy. Oral Maxillofac Surg Clin North Am: 1:27–45, 1989.
45. Steinhardt G: Zur Pathologie und Therapie des Kiefergelenkknackens. Dtsch Z Chir; 241:531–552, 1933.
46. Farrar WB: Diagnosis and treatment of anterior dislocation of the articular disc. NY J Dent 41:348–351, 1971.
47. McCarty WL: Diagnosis and treatment of internal derangements of the articular disc and mandibular condyle. In Solberg WK, Clark GT (eds): Temporomandibular Joint Problems. Biologic Diagnosis and Treatment. Chicago, Quintessence, 1980, pp 145–164.
48. Katzberg RW, Dolwick MF, Helms CA, et al: Arthrotomography of the temporomandibular joint. AJR 134:995–1003, 1980.
49. Dolwick MF: The temporomandibular joint: normal and abnormal anatomy. In Helms CA, Katzberg RW, Dolwick MF (eds): Internal Derangements of the

50. Isberg-Holm AM, Westesson P-L: Movement of disc and condyle in temporomandibular joints with and without clicking. A high-speed cinematographic and dissection study on autopsy specimens. Acta Odontol Scand 40:167–179, 1982.
51. Weinberg LA: The etiology, diagnosis and treatment of TMJ dysfunction-pain syndrome: differential diagnosis. J Prosthet Dent 43:58–70, 1980.
52. Farrar WB, McCarty WL: A Clinical Outline of Temporomandibular Joint Diagnosis and Treatment, 7th Ed. Montgomery, Normandie Publications, 1982; pp 11–37.
53. Westesson P-L, Rohlin M: Internal derangement related to osteoarthrosis in temporomandibular joint autopsy specimens. Oral Surg Oral Med Oral Pathol 57:17–22, 1984.
54. Stockwell RA, Billingham MEJ, Muir H: Ultrastructural changes in articular cartilage after experimental section of the anterior cruciate ligament of the dog knee. J Anat 136:425–439, 1983.
55. Ghadially FN, Meachim G, Collins DH: Extra-cellular lipid in the matrix of human articular cartilage. Ann Rheum Dis 24:136–146, 1965.
56. Ghadially FN. Ultrastructural Pathology of the Cell and Matrix, 2nd Ed. London, Butterworths, 1982; pp 881–936.

B. Chondromalacia

MOHAN THOMAS, D.D.S., F.A.C.D., CHRISTOPHER LANE, D.D.S.

The term *chondromalacia*, meaning a softening of the articular cartilage, was originally coined by the orthopedic surgeon Konig in 1924, and has remained in the international literature ever since.[1,2] The term was applied initially to any anterior patellofemoral arthralgia. This clinical syndrome was then called chondromalacia patellae post-traumatica because it was used to define the status of the knee after trauma. Subsequently, several studies on cadavers described lesions of chondromalacia without any evidence of trauma and post-traumatica was eliminated from the terminology.[3,4] Although the condition described as chondromalacia usually refers to the patella, it can be used to describe this condition in any diarthrodial joint, including the temporomandibular joint (TMJ). Studies have shown that the chondromalacia affecting the patella is the same as the chondromalacia that affects the TMJ.

Chondromalacia is a clinical term applied to the degenerative process involving articular cartilage in osteoarthritic joints. This chapter discusses chondromalacia as it affects the TMJ, including its etiology, mechanism by which it causes pain, classification, and treatment modalities.

PATHOGENESIS

Softening changes in articular cartilage may be observed in the early stages of osteoarthritis, but transient, localized, post-traumatic, and precocious soft cartilage lesions also occur that are unrelated to arthritis or joint degeneration. These lesions have different etiologies and natural histories, but are all characterized by loss of articular cartilage turgor and eventual disruption of the lamina splendens.

The articular cartilage of the TMJ is composed of fibrocartilage, unlike the articular cartilage of the knee, which is composed of hyaline cartilage. The primary difference between fibrocartilage and hyaline cartilage is in the type of collagen and the number of chondrocytes. Hyaline cartilage contains Type II collagen, whereas fibrocartilage contains predominantly Type I collagen or a combination of Types I and II.[5] The proliferative zone of the TMJ fibrocartilage also contains some undifferentiated mesenchymal cells that have the potential for repairing the tissue.[6] Normal articular cartilage is an avascular, aneural, alymphatic, and hypocellular tissue; it is composed of a matrix and ground substance.[7]

The matrix is an aggregate of collagen fibers that have great tensile strength but cannot support compressive loading. The ground substance contains complex sugars (i.e., glycosaminoglycans), which are mucopolysaccharides composed of keratin sulfate and chondroitin sulfate. The sugars are extremely hydrophilic and imbibe water, which ultimately constitutes 70% of articular cartilage by volume.[8] This water content provides the turgor and shock-absorbing capacity of articular cartilage and maintains the tension on arcades of collagen fibers within the matrix.[8, 9] The combination of matrix and ground substance, which has been compared with concrete reinforced with steel wire mesh, is responsible for supporting the compressive loading of the joint.[8–10]

Compressive and shearing forces damage the most superficial chondrocytes, resulting in the release of cathepsin B and other collagenases such as metalloproteinase.[9] The collagenases act on the cartilage ground substance by splitting the proteoglycan chains and producing water loss.[11] After degradation of the proteoglycans, water is reabsorbed into the fibrillar mesh, causing a fragmentation of the collagen fibrils.[4] This fragmentation also results in a progressive thinning of the articular cartilage.[4, 12] The reabsorbed water produces a loss of cartilage resilience, resulting in softening of the cartilage and reduced ability to withstand compressive and shearing forces (Fig. 17–16).[4]

Changes in the fibrous component of the matrix of articular cartilage, characterized by degenerative alterations of the collagen fibrils and destruction of their spatial arrangement, have been demonstrated in osteoarthritic cartilage of the TMJ and patella.[2, 6, 13] Phenomena such as fibrillation (increased roughness of the articular surface) and splitting (the formation of horizontal and vertical clefts) accompany disintegration of the collagen fiber network. Zimny and Redler[14] believe that in chondromalacia, dedifferentiation of superficial chondrocytes to fibroblasts occurs, promoting fibrillation.[14] The ultimate degenerative progression leads to the exposure of subchondral bone. Denuded of articular cartilage, the subchondral bone becomes hyperostotic and eburnated in response to concentrated force loading.

ETIOLOGY

The etiology of chondromalacia is still not well understood. Several theories have been proposed, all of which have some scientific merit but are not conclusive in explaining all the nuances of the pathology. It is generally agreed that cartilage is an avascular, aneural, alymphatic tissue that, when injured, does not go through the phases of repair normally associated with vascularized tissue (i.e., necrosis, inflammation, and repair).

The presence of trauma is considered the primary event in the etiology of chondromalacia.[2, 4, 15] The joints are subjected to trauma (i.e., wear and tear) throughout our lives; thus, by a certain age, all individuals will have chondromalacia to some degree. The question is how much wear and tear the articular cartilage can handle while still maintaining the homeostatic integrity of the tissue. Other causative factors that affect the composition of the cartilage matrix or the metabolic activity of the supporting chondrocytes include unfavorable loading situations, hemarthrosis, sepsis, gout, malnutrition, and the mucopolysaccharidoses (e.g., sarcoidosis).[2]

Trauma as it relates to chondromalacia is divided into two categories: acute trauma and microtrauma. In acute trauma, there is a sudden, direct injury associated with high stress loading in a short time frame, leading to (1) the loss of a piece of cartilage from the surface of the condyle or (2) death of the chondrocytes over a section of the articular surface. These types of injuries are common in contact sports and automobile accidents and may be seen with whiplash-type injuries. Microtrauma is a repetitive process of damage to the articular surface. Examples of microtrauma affecting the TMJ include clenching and stress bruxism. The sequential pathogenesis of degenerative changes of articular cartilage terminating in chondromala-

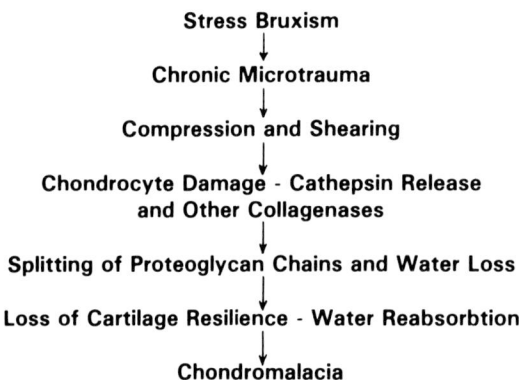

Figure 17–16. Sequential pathogenesis of the degenerative changes of articular cartilage. (Reprinted with permission from Quinn JH: Pathogenesis of temporomandibular joint chondromalacia and arthralgia. Oral Maxillofac Surg Clin North Am 1:47–57, 1989.)

cia is as follows: stress bruxism leading to chronic microtrauma, leading to compression and shearing of the most superficial chondrocytes.

The probable etiology of the arthralgia associated with chondromalacia is related to friction, compression, and impingement of degenerating articular cartilage and to synovitis.[2, 4, 16] Degeneration of collagen fibrils and fragmentation of the cartilage produce a roughened surface that increases friction as the articular disc translates anteriorly and posteriorly on the posterior slope and peak of the articular eminence.[4] As the surface of the fibrocartilaginous disc continues to break down, the amount of friction increases. Once the frictional shearing between the disc and the articular eminence begins to mobilize the fibrocartilage attached to the underlying subchondral bone, the abundant sensory nerve fibers in the subchondral bone are stimulated to produce pain. With further degeneration and breakdown, the articular cartilage loses the ability to withstand compression because of the loss of proteoglycan. Collagen fibrils in the articular cartilage have tensile strength that withstands shearing forces, but unless the proteoglycan component is sufficient, the cartilage cannot withstand compressive forces.[4, 6, 15, 17] Subsequently, compressive and shearing forces of the functioning joint can be brought to bear directly on the subchondral bone, causing irritation of the sensory nerve pain fibers in the bone.

PAIN

According to Quinn,[4] the principal cause of TMJ pain is probably impingement of fragments of degenerating cartilage hanging from the articular eminence, between the articular eminence and the disc. As the disc moves downward and forward on the posterior slope of the eminence, traction on the fibrillar degenerative cartilage fragments that are attached to the subchondral bone stimulates the sensory nerve pain receptors. Synovitis, or inflammation of the synovial membrane, is one of the earliest signs of degenerative arthritis resulting from microtrauma. Most workers believe that it is primarily caused by degenerative cartilage debris within the TMJ, which has been produced by microtrauma and collagenase activity. Synovitis eventually leads to the degeneration of the posterior slope, the peak of the articular eminence, and the disc.

Microscopic debris normally is absorbed and digested by the synovial membrane and macrophages.[4, 6, 13, 14, 18] When excessive amounts of particulate material are present, it is impossible for all of it to be ingested and removed by the synovial membrane. Chemical mediators of inflammation and pain from the arachidonic acid cascade are produced from the excess particulate material, resulting in synovitis. These mediators—bradykinin, prostaglandin E_2, leukotriene B_4, and thromboxane B_2—are believed to be present in the painful dysfunctional TMJ.[4, 17]

PROGRESSIVE STAGES

Chondromalacia of the TMJ is characterized by four discrete stages of progression that have been observed clinically using the arthroscope.[4] These are Stage I, softening; Stage II, furrowing; Stage III, ulceration and fibrillation; and Stage IV, crater formation and subchondral bone exposure (Table 17–1, Figs. 17–17 through 17–20). The same stages are seen arthroscopically by the orthopedic surgeon when observing chondromalacia of the patella.

As previously discussed, the precise series of events leading to overt cartilage lesions associated with chondromalacia are unknown. However, the lesions encountered in symptomatic joints do have an hypothesized natural history. Lesions can be initiated from the surface down or from the deeper basal cartilage layers up to the surface.

Surface degeneration occurs when the superficial proteoglycan content is decreased to the point where there is a significant reduction of the mechanical stiffness of the cartilage surface. Proteoglycans have been shown to be the key components of the extracellular matrix responsible for maintenance of mechanical integrity. As the superficial collagen fibers and matrix lose their mechanical stiffness, wear against the tissue continues. A process of fibrillation then ensues. This type of degradation leaves the cartilage vulnerable to increased wear and tear, resulting in focal shredding and further loss of the cartilage matrix. Lesions of this type eventually result in complete cartilage loss and eventual eburnation of the subchondral plate of bone (Stage IV chondromalacia). Although this

Table 17–1. ARTHROSCOPIC FINDINGS IN PROGRESSIVE CHONDROMALACIA OF THE TEMPOROMANDIBULAR JOINT (TMJ) AND KNEE

Stage	Finding	Cause
I	Softening	Digestion of the ground substance, proteoglycan, by collagenases from injured chondrocytes (see Fig. 17–16); clinically identified by palpation of the articular cartilage with an examining probe and determining its compressibility (both TMJ and patella).
II	Furrowing (TMJ) Blistering (patella)	Disruption of some of the deep-zone collagen fibrils at the calcified and noncalcified cartilage attachment and hydrated swelling of the proteoglycan-depleted areas among the fibrils in the TMJ (see Fig. 17–17); in the patella, rupture of fibrils is thought to occur at a more superficial level.
III	Ulceration and fibrillation	First, rupture of the deeper collagen fibrils from their calcified and noncalcified cartilage attachments; then disruption of the parallel fibrils of the articular surface (see Fig. 17–18). This produces fibrillar strands of degenerating cartilage hanging from the posterior slope and peak of the articular eminence that are seen suspended in the Ringer's lactate used to inflate the superior joint space of the TMJ for arthroscopic examination. The same degenerative changes are obvious in the articular cartilage of the patella.
IV	Crater formation; subchondral bone exposure	Further rupture of the deep fibrils and a progressive breakdown of the superficial and intermediate cartilage fibrils, with ultimate exposure of the subchondral bone in both the TMJ and patella (see Fig. 17–19).

Reprinted with permission from Quinn JH: Pathogenesis of temporomandibular joint chondromalacia and arthralgia. Oral Maxillofac Surg Clin North Am 1:47–57, 1989.

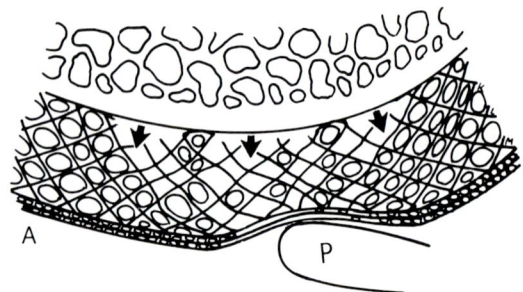

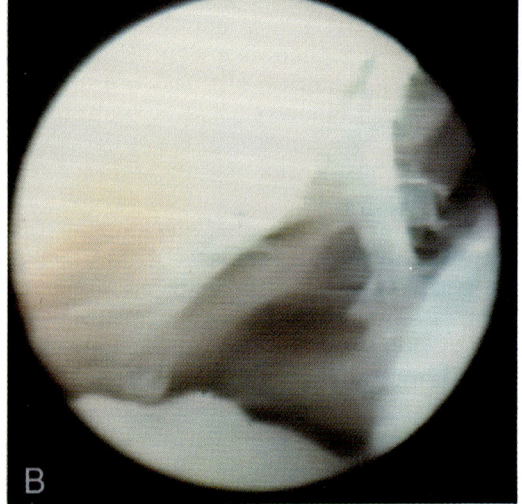

Figure 17–17. *A*, Stage I chondromalacia: Softening of articular cartilage. Degradation and loss of proteoglycan by lysosomal chondrocyte enzymes are indicated diagrammatically by missing circles within the fibril meshwork in the temporomandibular joint. p = examining probe. *B*, Arthroscopic view of palpation with probe of temporal compartment, showing softening of articular cartilage. (*A*, reprinted with permission from Quinn JH: Pathogenesis of temporomandibular joint chondromalacia and arthralgia. Oral Maxillofac Surg Clin North Am 1:47–57, 1989; *B*, courtesy of Dr. Robert Schwartz.)

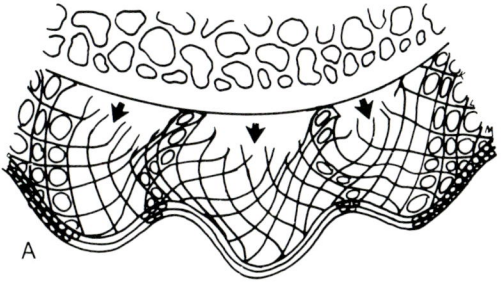

TREATMENT

The treatment of chondromalacia depends on the stage of degeneration present. Studies show that articular cartilage that is superficially damaged will not regenerate to its full thickness and frequently does not heal completely.[4, 12] Surface chondrocytes do not re-

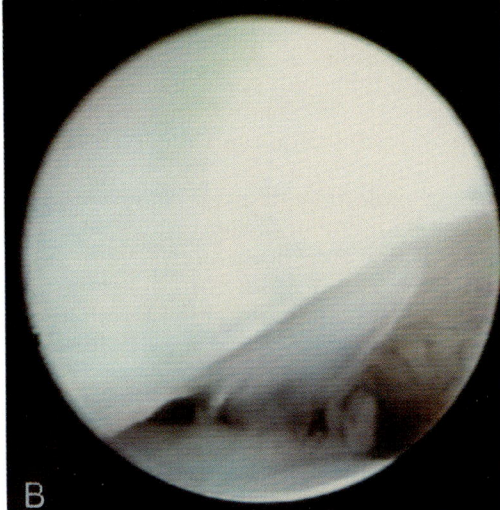

Figure 17–18. *A*, Stage II chondromalacia: Rupture of deep fibrils. Initial rupture of intermittent fibrils occurs by compression and shearing forces after loss of proteoglyans in the deeper layers of the temporomandibular joint articular cartilage. *B*, Arthroscopic photograph showing "furrowing" of the temporomandibular joint cartilage on the posterior slope of the articular eminence secondary to rupture of deep fibrils.

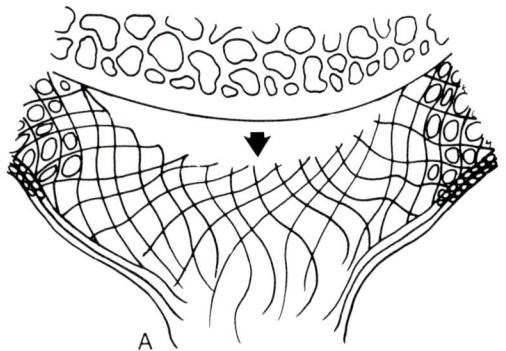

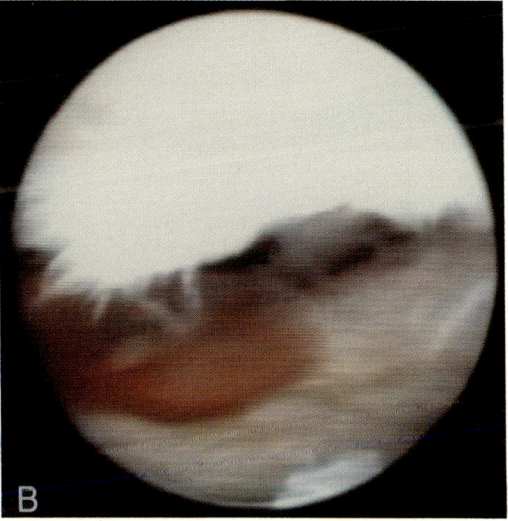

Figure 17–19. *A*, Stage III chondromalacia: Rupture of parallel fibrils of the articular zone. Fibrillar degeneration of cartilage is secondary to rupture of the parallel fibrils of the articular zone with preceding rupture of deeper zone fibrils. *B*, Arthroscopic view showing fibrillar degeneration of cartilage on the posterior slope of the articular cartilage. (*A*, reprinted with permission from Quinn JH: Pathogenesis of temporomandibular joint chondromalacia and arthralgia. Oral Maxillofac Surg Clin North Am 1:47–57, 1989.; *B*, courtesy of Dr. Robert Schwartz.) (Reprinted with permission from Quinn JH: Pathogenesis of temporomandibular joint chondromalacia and arthralgia. Oral Maxillofac Surg Clin North Am 1:47–57, 1989; *B*, courtesy of Dr. Robert Schwartz.)

type of lesion will not heal, further degeneration can be allayed by correction of this biomechanical instability.

Basal degeneration is visualized arthroscopically by the presence of "blisters." The affected articular cartilage is subject to high stress in a region where such levels are not normally encountered. This type of overloading results in delamination of the basal collagen network from the calcified deepest zone of cartilage. The end result is a large blister that rises above the surrounding contiguous cartilage. The blister void space is filled by interstitial water, which adds to the lack of mechanical integrity. The final result of both fibrillation and basal degeneration associated with chondromalacia is the eventual destruction and loss of cartilage matrix.[3, 19, 20]

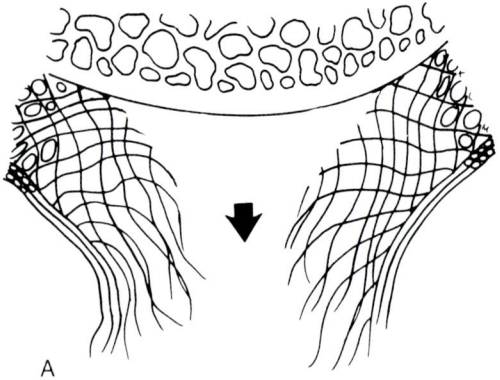

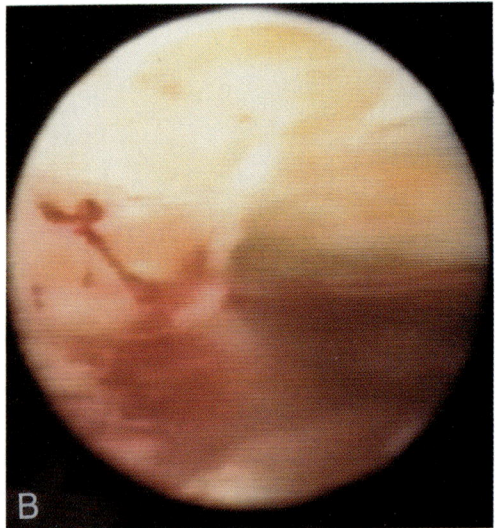

Figure 17-20. *A*, Stage IV chondromalacia: Advanced fibrillar degeneration of full thickness of the articular cartilage with subchondral bone exposure. *B*, Arthroscopic photograph of fibrillar degeneration of articular cartilage with bone exposure. (*A*, reprinted with permission from Quinn JH: Pathogenesis of temporomandibular joint chondromalacia and arthralgia. Oral Maxillofac Surg Clin North Am 1:47–57, 1989; *B*, courtesy of Dr. Robert Schwartz.)

suction punch forceps and/or motorized minishavers. Post-traumatic chondromalacia has been found to respond favorably to arthroscopic shaving.[21] This treatment is believed to be justified because degenerating fibrils break down into particulate debris, producing mediators of inflammation and pain. Shahriaree[16] also states that the removal of degenerating fibrillar cartilage too close to the bone may actually further expose the bone. Therefore, the defects should not be deepened beyond what is necessary to create a reasonably smooth contour and to decrease surface friction. This cartilage has no significant potential for healing in the superficial zones, yet protection against deep ulceration and pitting is provided by smoothing the gross irregularities of articular surfaces.

The treatment for Stage IV chondromalacia with exposed bone is abrasion arthroplasty to remove the surface down to bleeding bone, which encourages granulation tissue to form and possibly cover the bone with fibrocartilage.[2, 12, 16]

The treatment for acute synovitis with moderate to advanced hyperemia is to inject betamethasone directly into the subintimal tissue of the synovial membrane, perferably under arthroscopic control.

Regardless of the cause of chondromalacia in any specific patient, the treatment objective and aggravating forces are the same. Efforts should be directed toward maintaining

generate themselves because they derive their nutrition from the synovial fluid. Full-thickness cartilage degeneration down to subchondral bone heals because of the ability of the bone, with its abundant blood supply, to produce new tissue.[12] According to Shahriaree,[2, 16] when sufficient fibrillar degeneration is obvious on arthroscopic examination, as seen in Stages III and IV chondromalacia, one should use a motorized shaver unit to remove carefully the majority of the degenerating hanging strands of fibrillar cartilage (Fig. 17–21). These cartilaginous loose bodies act as abrasives and are best removed by

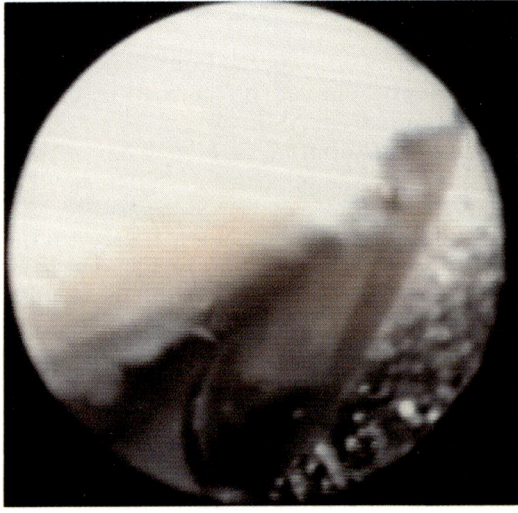

Figure 17-21. Use of motorized shaver in the management of chondromalacia.

adequate nutrition for the chondrocytes and avoiding shear forces and excessive loading of affected areas of the joint surface.

SUMMARY

Arthroscopy provides a low-morbidity approach to the management of pathologic manifestations of chondromalacia. Inflammatory responses are reduced by the removal of actual or potential particulate matter, bone fragments, metabolites, and degradative enzymes. The reduction of these enzymes helps to protect and preserve the integrity of collagen fibers within the matrix. By smoothing and abrading irregular surfaces, tissue patching can be induced to replace destroyed articular cartilage. Via arthroscopic spongilization of the subchondral plate, stabilization of blistered articular cartilage can sometimes be accomplished. This results in clot formation, providing an adherent mesh between bone and cartilage. Through arthroscopic intervention and early joint mobilization, the morbidity associated with surgical treatment of chondromalacia is greatly reduced. Because arthroscopic surgical techniques obviate major capsular incisions, postoperative functional inhibition and the inflammatory changes resulting from copious hemarthrosis associated with arthrotomy are minimized.[22] Finally, with the advent of TMJ arthroscopic diagnosis and surgery, it is possible to prevent the ultimate advanced degeneration of the articular cartilage and resulting bone loss of advanced osteoarthritis.[4]

References

1. Konig F: Mikroskopische Beobachtungen am Knorpelgewebe mit Ultraviolettem Licht. Verh D Phys Ges Z Wurzburg (Sitzungsberichte 10–15) 49:160, 1924.
2. Shahriaree H (ed): O'Connor's Textbook of Arthroscopic Surgery. Philadelphia: Lippincott, 1984, p 266.
3. Owre AA: Chondromalacia patellae. Acta Chir Scand [Suppl 41] 77:9, 1936.
4. Quinn JH: Pathogenesis of TMJ chondromalacia and arthralgia. Oral Maxillofac Surg Clin North Am 1:47–57, 1989.
5. Miller EJ: Biochemical characteristics and biological significance of the genetically distinct collagens. Mol Cell Biochem 13:165, 1976.
6. Bentley G, Dowd G: Current concepts of etiology in treatment of chondromalacia patellae. Clin Orthop Rel Res 189:209, 1984.
7. de Bont LGM: Temporomandibular joint: Articular cartilage structure and function. [Thesis] Groningen, The Netherlands: University of Groningen, 1985.
8. Mankin HJ: The articular cartilage: A review. American Association of Orthopaedic Surgeons Instructional Course Lectures 19:204, 1970.
9. Meachin G, Stockwell RA: The matrix. In Freeman MAR (ed): Adult Articular Cartilage, 2nd Ed. London: Pitman Medical, 1979, pp 1–67.
10. Mankin HJ: Reaction of articular cartilage to injury in osteoarthritis. N Engl J Med 291:1285, 1974.
11. Harris ED: Role of collagenases in joint destruction. In Sokoloff L (ed): The Joints and Synovial Fluid, Vol 1. New York: Academic Press, 1978, p 243.
12. Friedman MJ, Galick GS, Brna JA, et al: Chondromalacia of the knee: A comparison between those treated with and without intra-articular shaving. [Abstract] Arthroscopy 8(2):131, 1987.
13. de Bont LGM: Osteoarthritis and internal derangement of the TMJ: A light microscopic study. J Oral Maxillofac Surg 44:634, 1986.
14. Zimny ML, Redler J: An ultrastructural study of patella chondromalacia in humans. J Bone Joint Surg 5A:179, 1969.
15. Outerbridge RE: The etiology of chondromalacia patellae. J Bone Joint Surg 43B:752, 1961.
16. Shahriaree H: Chondromalacia. Contemp Orthop 2(5):27, 1985.
17. Egg D: Concentrations of prostaglandins D-2, E-2, F-2α, 6 Keto F-1α and thromboxane B-2 in synovial fluids from patients with inflammatory joint disorders in osteoarthritis. Z Rheumatol 43:89, 1984.
18. Hasselbacher P: Structure of the synovial membrane. Clin Rheum Dis 7:57, 1981.
19. Aleman O: Chondromalacia post-traumatica patellae. Acta Chir Scand 63:194, 1928.
20. Hirsch C: A contribution to the pathogenesis of chondromalacia of the patella: Physical, histologic and chemical study. Acta Chir Scand [Suppl] 90:83, 1944.
21. Ogilvie-Harris DJ, Jackson RW: The arthroscopic treatment of chondromalacia patellae. J Bone Joint Surg 66B:660, 1984.
22. Whipple TL: Osteoarthritis and chondromalacia. In Parisien S (ed): Textbook of Arthroscopic Surgery. New York: McGraw-Hill, 1989, pp. 135–145.
23. Meyers ER, Mow VC: Biomechanics of cartilage and its response to biomechanical stimuli. In Hall S (ed): Cartilage, Vol 1. New York: Academic Press, 1983, pp 313–341.

Chapter 18

CONNECTIVE TISSUE PATHOLOGY: ARTHRITIDES

A. Rheumatoid Arthritis

ANDERS HOLMLUND, D.D.S., PH.D.

Rheumatoid arthritis (RA) is a systemic, chronic inflammatory disease. The incidence is about 1% in the Western World, with a predominance for women.[1] The onset is usually in the third or fourth decade of life but the disease may occur at any age, from childhood to late adulthood. The joints of the extremities are predominantly affected, in most cases with a symmetric pattern. The disease course may be variable, ranging from mild to severe and destructive, causing invalidism. Because there is no definite cure, management is necessary over a long period of time, often involving prolonged medical, surgical, and physical therapy. The reported incidence of TMJ involvement varies widely, from 2% to 86%,[2] reflecting the fact that there is a lack of definite clinical and radiographic criteria for RA of the TMJ.[3,4] Investigations involving more accurate diagnostic methods such as arthroscopy will probably elucidate this matter.

PATHOGENESIS

The cause of RA is unknown. It is thought that an unknown agent, possibly a virus, stimulates the formation of antibodies that, for some reason, act as new antigens. These antigens give rise to formation of anti-idiotype antibodies that, in their turn, will be phagocytosed by leukocytes. The leukocytes then release lysosomal enzymes and possibly other products as well. Cell-mediated immunity also seems to be involved in the disease process.

RA is basically a synovial disease, and although cartilage and bone are frequently involved, this is a consequence of the destructive process that takes place in the synovium. The early signs are edema, accumulation of chronic inflammatory cells, and increased vascularity. The synovial lining undergoes hyperplasia that spreads over the articular surfaces and isolates the cartilage from its nutritional synovial fluid. The disease may then produce destruction of cartilage and subchondral bone and fibrosis of the soft tissues. The joint may be fused by fibrous tissue or bone, causing marked impairment of joint mobility.

DIAGNOSIS

Clinical Findings

New detailed diagnostic criteria have recently been proposed by the American Rheumatism Association.[5] Clinical findings in RA of the TMJ largely follow those of other synovial joints. However, it has been difficult to differentiate RA from other joint affections such as osteoarthrosis because clinical signs and symptoms often coincide.[3,4] Symmetric involvement of the TMJ and changes in occlusion of the teeth causing a progressive bite opening may indicate a rheumatoid affection.[6] Abnormal bite opening often occurs late in the disease, when destruction of cartilage and subchondral bone has appeared. Early-phase TMJ rheumatoid arthritis may therefore be extremely difficult to diagnose on clinical grounds only.

Radiographic Findings

Radiographic examination has long been the basis for the diagnosis of osteoarthrosis and RA. Refined techniques such as corrected sagittal tomography and computed tomography (CT) have shown high diagnostic accuracy in detecting hard tissue changes. Nevertheless, proposed radiographic features of TMJ RA are not specific[3, 7] and, with the possible exception of erosions, give no information about the degree of cartilage destruction.

Arthroscopic Findings

Comprehensive evaluation during the last decade[8-11] has gained the general acceptance of arthroscopy as an important diagnostic tool. Furthermore, arthroscopic and histologic features of synovial inflammation have been highly correlated.[12, 13] A study performed on the TMJ indicated high diagnostic accuracy of arthroscopy in regard to osteoarthrosis and synovitis.[14] Early diagnosis and treatment of RA of the TMJ is necessary in order to avoid such complications as progressive open bite and ankylosis. Arthroscopic examination may therefore be of utmost importance.

The arthroscopic picture may vary widely, depending on how early or late in the disease process the examination is performed and whether disease-modifying therapeutic agents have been given.[13] Variation may be considerable within a single TMJ, and all stages of macroscopic inflammation, and even areas with normal appearance, may be present within the same joint.[12] Recent studies[7, 15] indicate that the arthroscopic findings in RA of the TMJ are similar to those for other synovial joints.

The following arthroscopic features can be identified:

1. Synovium: increased vascularity (Fig. 18–1), capillary hyperemia (Fig. 18–2), granulation formation (Fig. 18–3), villus formation (Fig. 18–4), effusion (Fig. 18–5), and fibrosis (Fig. 18–6)
2. Cartilage: fibrillation (Fig. 18–7), lesions of cartilage and subchondral bone (Fig. 18–8), and bone exposure and eburnation (Fig. 18–9).

Early features of synovial involvement may be increased vascularity and capillary hyperemia; the more severe the disease, the

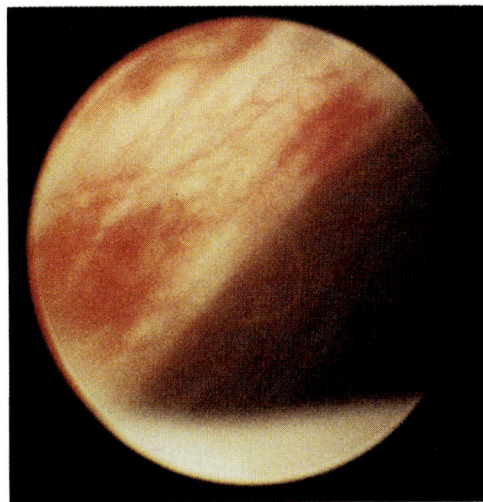

Figure 18–1. Right temporomandibular joint (TMJ), superior compartment: Increased vascularity of the medial capsule of the TMJ in early-phase rheumatoid arthritis.

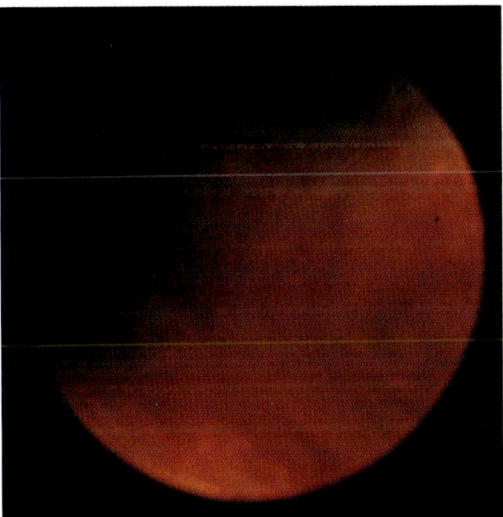

Figure 18–2. Left temporomandibular joint, superior compartment: Close-up view of the posterior disc attachment, displaying capillary hyperemia.

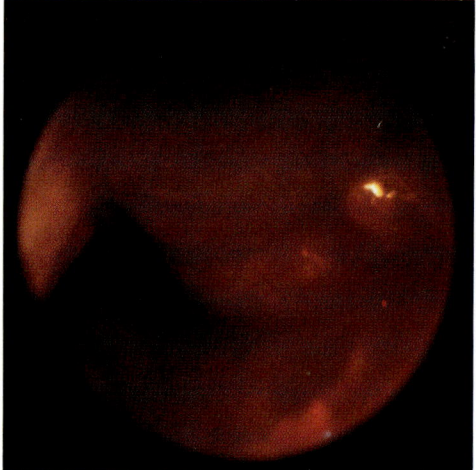

Figure 18-3. Right temporomandibular joint, superior compartment: Hyperplasia and granulation tissue formation of the posterior disc attachment.

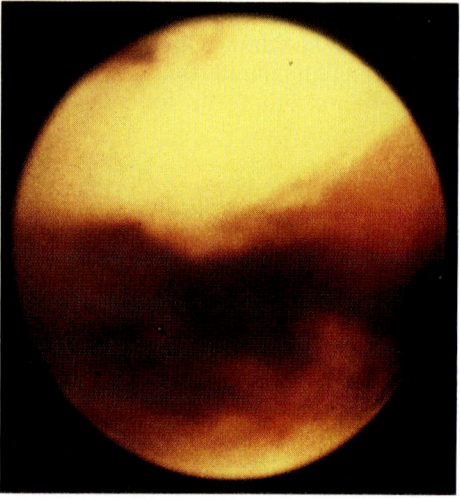

Figure 18-5. Right temporomandibular joint, superior compartment: Effusion and chronic inflammation with debris in the joint cavity.

more features will be found. The same is true of the cartilage, in which findings may vary from early superficial changes, such as localized areas with fibrillation, to lesions and exposure of subchondral bone. Marked fibrosis or even ankylosis may occur. Arthroscopic examination is then often impossible.

Synovial Biopsy

Obtaining synovial biopsy during arthroscopy is usually a quick and uncomplicated procedure. Sampling of biopsy material may be performed under direct vision or using a so-called semi-blind or indirect technique. (Techniques for biopsy procedures are described elsewhere in this text.) It is important to use a well-designed forceps in order to avoid damage caused by compression of the synovial sample. A specimen with a diameter of 1 to 3 mm is sufficient for histologic examination. Histologic features indicating RA include proliferation of the synovial lin-

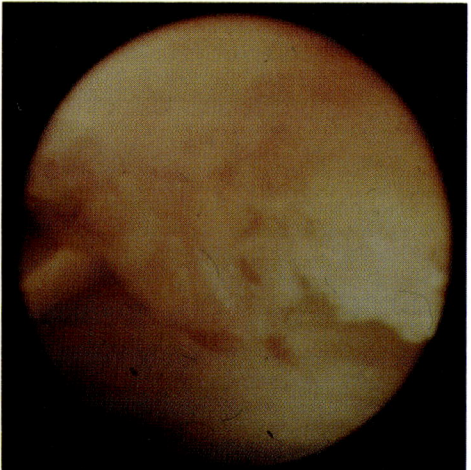

Figure 18-4. Left temporomandibular joint, superior compartment: Small villi with hyperemic tops.

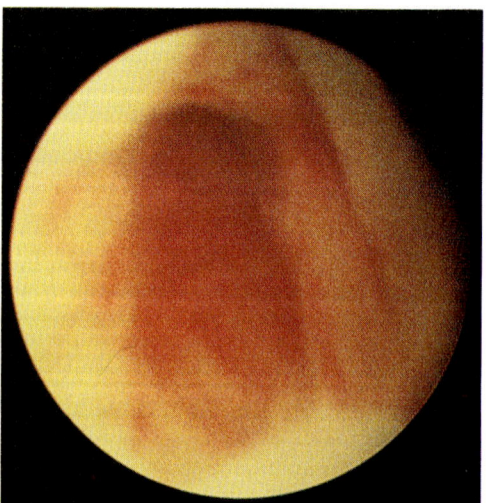

Figure 18-6. Right temporomandibular joint, superior compartment: Fibrosis (adhesions) and capillary hyperemia of the posterior part of the joint.

A. Rheumatoid Arthritis 279

Figure 18–7. Left temporomandibular joint, superior compartment: Early changes of the cartilage (fibrillation). The disc below is unaffected.

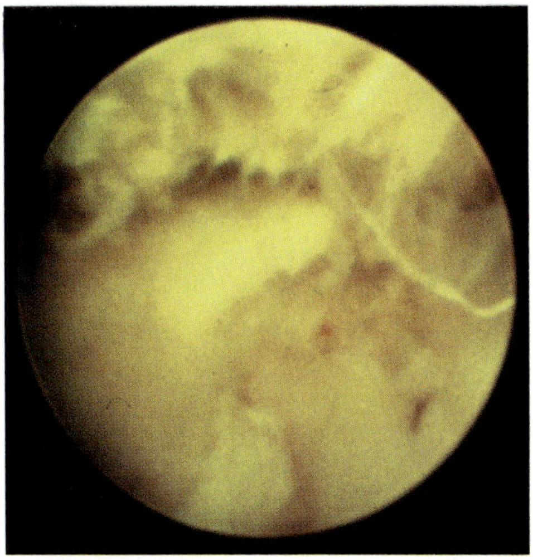

Figure 18–9. Left temporomandibular joint, superior compartment: A small lesion of subchondral bone surrounded by eburnated bone. The disc below shows pronounced fibrillation.

ing, infiltration of lymphocytes and plasma cells, increased vascularity, and fibrosis.

TREATMENT

Rheumatoid arthritis is a systemic disease and thus initially the patient should be given systemic therapy. Systemic medication is beyond the scope of this chapter; however, proper knowledge of current concepts of medication and concomitant side effects must be emphasized. Local treatment of the different joints and physical therapy of the muscle groups involved often are necessary. A team approach involving physicians, orthopedic surgeons, and physical therapists, therefore, seems most appropriate.

The treatment for RA of the TMJ follows the same general guidelines, although stomatognathic physiologists, dentists, and oral and maxillofacial surgeons will replace the orthopedic surgeons. Nonsurgical management must not be overlooked, and strategies for such treatment have been proposed.

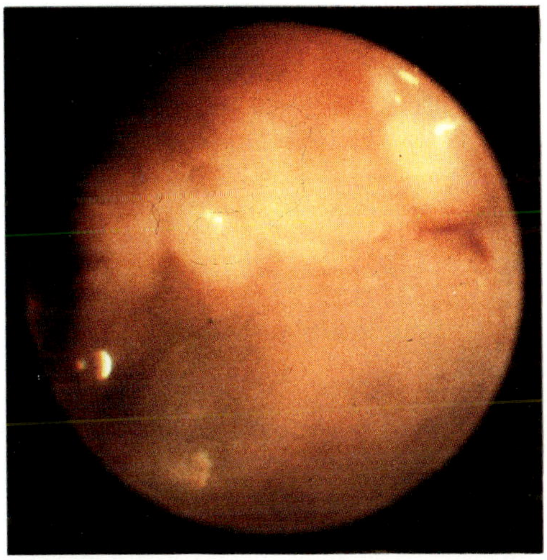

Arthroscopy

The importance of early treatment of RA, including local treatment, has been mentioned previously. At present arthroscopy seems to be the only method that provides possibilities for such treatment based on a proper diagnosis. The following procedures may be performed.

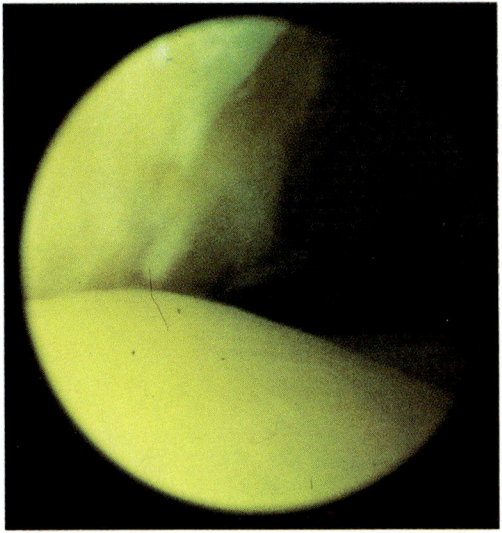

Figure 18–8. Right temporomandibular joint, superior compartment: Close-up view of the central part of the glenoid fossa showing remodeling and lesions of cartilage and subchondral bone.

Lavage

Thorough irrigation of the joint with isotonic saline solution has been effective in alleviating symptoms in rheumatoid disease of both the knee joint[16] and the TMJ.[17] A possible explanation for the relief of symptoms is that debris and other inflammatory products are removed. Irrigation with diluted sodium hyaluronate has been advocated as an alternative.[18]

Intra-articular Injections

Intra-articular injections of corticosteroids have proved efficacious.[19, 20] There is, however, ambiguity regarding the local side effects on the joint cartilage.[21, 22] Kopp and colleagues[23] have reported a study of the long-term effects of intra-articular injections of sodium hyaluronate and corticosteroids on chronic TMJ arthritis. No side effects have been reported with sodium hyaluronate and it may, therefore, be preferable to steroids. Technically, injection of sodium hyaluronate is a simple procedure and may be performed simultaneously with the arthroscopic examination. In cases with only minor areas of synovial inflammation, sometimes found in early-phase RA, subsynovial injections of small volumes of corticosteroids may be a suitable alternative procedure. These injections are performed during direct arthroscopic observation.

Synovial Resection and Lysis

Hypertrophic synovium or granulation tissues often are found in joints with advanced RA, proceeding over the cartilage and isolating the cartilage from its nutrition. Destruction of cartilage follows. The removal of such granulation tissue may arrest or even cure the disease. Synovectomies are best performed with so-called shavers (Fig. 18–10). This procedure demands considerable technical skill and must always be performed under direct vision. Bleeding often obscures the visibility, and the procedure perhaps should be limited to cases with well-defined lesions.

Fibrosis and adhesions frequently are found in RA joints, eliciting impairment of joint mobility. Knives, scissors, or shavers may be used in order to cut or remove these bands under direct arthroscopic observation.

Open Surgery

Arthroscopic surgery of the knee has reduced considerably the frequency of postop-

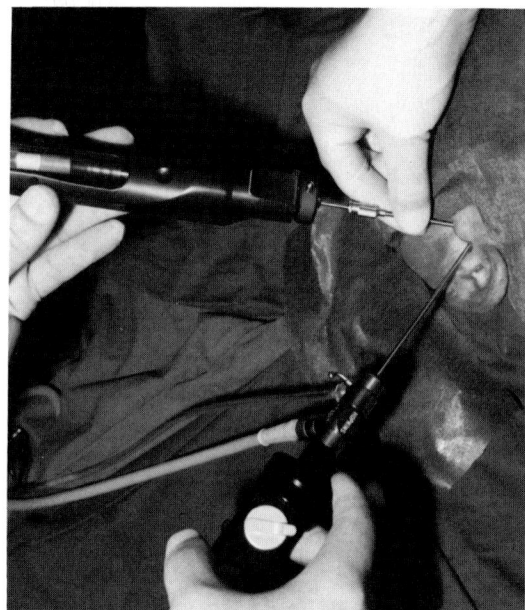

Figure 18–10. Synovial resection in the left temporomandibular joint using a minishaver by triangulation technique.

erative complications. Furthermore, postoperative hospital and sick leave periods have been reduced. However, it is important to understand that there are limitations. In certain cases of RA of the TMJ, it is inappropriate or even contraindicated to investigate or treat by means of arthroscopy. Examples are cases with marked impairment of joint mobility due to fibrous or bony ankylosis. These cases are more safely and better managed by open surgery. Joints exhibiting pronounced granulation or villus formation are also best treated by open surgical procedures.

SUMMARY

The diagnosis of RA of the TMJ has been difficult, mainly because of lack of specific clinical and radiographic criteria. Arthroscopy provides accurate information regarding intra-articular conditions and supplies possibilities for early local treatment. The procedures described may arrest the disease, give long-term relief of symptoms, and thereby improve the quality of life for many of these patients. Arthroscopy also provides a considerable potential for basic research work and evaluation of different therapeutic procedures.

References

1. Rubin E, Farber JL: Pathology. Philadelphia: JB Lippincott, 1988, p 1375.
2. Carlsson GE, Kopp S, Oberg T: Arthritis and allied diseases of the temporomandibular joint. In Zarb GA, Carlsson GE (eds): Temporomandibular Joint: Function and Dysfunction. St Louis: CV Mosby, 1979, pp 293–320.
3. Ogus H: Rheumatoid arthritis of the temporomandibular joint. Br J Oral Surg 12:275–284, 1975.
4. Tegelberg A, Kopp S: Clinical findings in the stomatognathic system for individuals with rheumatoid arthritis and osteoarthritis. Acta Odont Scand 45:65–75, 1987.
5. Arnett FC, Edworth SM, Bloch DS, et al: The 1987 revised American Rheumatism Association criteria for classification of rheumatoid arthritis. Arthr Rheum 31:315–324, 1988.
6. Zarb GA: Non-surgical treatment of rheumatoid and degenerative arthritis of the TMJ. In President's Conference on the Examination, Diagnosis, and Management of Temporomandibular Joint Disorders. Chicago: JADA, 1982, pp 133–136.
7. Holmlund A, Hellsing G: Arthroscopy of the temporomandibular joint: A comparative study of arthroscopic and tomographic findings. Int J Oral Maxillofac Surg 17:128–133, 1988.
8. Eikelaar HR: Arthroscopy of the knee. [Dissertation]. Groningen: Rijksuniversiteit Groningen, Royal United Printers Hoitsema BV, 1975.
9. Eriksson E, Lindvall N, Sebik A, Silfverskiold I: A comparison between arthroscopy and arthrography of the knee. Acta Orthop Scand 52:126, 1981.
10. Gillquist J, Hagberg G: Findings at arthroscopy and arthrography in knee injuries. Acta Orthop Scand 49:398–402, 1978.
11. Johnson L: Diagnostic and Surgical Arthroscopy: Knee and Other Joints. St Louis: CV Mosby, 1981, pp 373–375.
12. Lindblad S, Hedfors E: Intra-articular variation in synovitis. Local macroscopic and microscopic signs of inflammatory activity are significantly correlated. Arthr Rheum 28:977–986, 1985.
13. Rooney M, Condell D, Quinlan W, et al: Analysis of the histologic variation of synovitis in rheumatoid arthritis. Arthr Rheum 31:956–963, 1988.
14. Holmlund A: Diagnostic accuracy of temporomandibular joint arthroscopy. Oral Maxillofac Surg Clin North Am 1:1, 1989.
15. Holmlund A, Hellsing G: Arthroscopy of the temporomandibular joint. Occurrence and location of osteoarthrosis and synovitis in patient material. Int J Oral Maxillofac Surg 17:36–40, 1988.
16. Jayson MIV, Dison AStI: Arthroscopy of the knee in rheumatoid disease. Ann Rheum Dis 27:503–511, 1968.
17. Holmlund A, Hellsing G, Wredmark T: Arthroscopy of the temporomandibular joint: A clinical study. Int J Oral Maxillofac Surg 15:715–721, 1986.
18. Weiss L: Basic structure of diarthrodial joints. In Parisien JS (ed): Arthroscopic Surgery. New York: McGraw-Hill, 1988, pp 12–13.
19. Kopp S, Wenneberg B: Effects of occlusal treatment and intra-articular injections on temporomandibular joint pain and dysfunction. Acta Odont Scand 39:87–96, 1981.
20. Wenneberg B, Kopp S: Short-term effect of intra-articular injections of a corticosteroid on temporomandibular joint pain and dysfunction. Swed Dent J 2:189–196, 1978.
21. Balch RW, Gison JMC, El-Ghobarey AF, et al: Repeated corticosteroid injections into the knee joint. Rheumatol Rehab 16:137–140, 1977.
22. Saxne T, Heinegard D, Wollheim FA: Proteoglycans in synovial fluid: The effect of intra-articular corticosteroid injections. Br J Rheum 24:221, 1985.
23. Kopp S, Carlsson GE, Haraldsson T, Wenneberg B: Long-term effect of intra-articular injections of sodium hyaluronate and corticosteroids on temporomandibular joint arthritis. J Oral Maxillofac Surg 45:929–935, 1987

B. Systemic Inflammatory Arthritides with Temporomandibular Joint Involvement

HARRY SHEN, M.D., MOHAN THOMAS, D.D.S., F.A.C.D.

RHEUMATOID ARTHRITIS

Rheumatoid arthritis (RA) is estimated to occur in approximately 3% of adults in the United States with a female-to-male ratio of about 2.5 to 1.[1] Patients with RA have a chronic, symmetric, erosive polyarthritis that characteristically involves the proximal interphalangeal (PIP) and metacarpophalangeal joints of the hands. The PIP and metacarpophalangeal joints of the feet are similarly affected. The disease can affect large joints, such as the hips, or small joints, such as the cricoarytenoids. Unlike osteoarthritis, in RA the distal interphalangeal joints typically are spared. The reported incidence of temporomandibular joint (TMJ) involvement has varied widely, from 2% to 86%, reflecting the fact that there is a lack of definite clinical criteria for RA of the TMJ.[2-4] Between 55% and 70% of patients have jaw symptoms at some time during their illness.[5-8]

RA is primarily a synovial disease, although cartilage and bone frequently are involved. This is usually a consequence of the destructive process that occurs in synovium. The early signs are edema of the synovial lining with infiltration of chronic inflammatory cells and increased vascularity. The hyperplastic synovial lining invariably spreads over the articular surface, thereby isolating the cartilage from its nutritional synovial fluid. It is not unusual to find joint impairment in end-stage disease due to fibrosis or bony ankylosis.

Clinically, it may be difficult to diagnose RA in the TMJ; however, as the disease progresses and if there is symmetric involvement in the TMJ, changes in the occlusion of teeth and a progressive open bite may occur. The radiographic features of RA are not specific, although erosions of the condylar head or other active leading surfaces may be observed using various radiologic techniques. Radiographic studies revealed alterations in about 78% of the joints examined.

The arthroscopic findings in RA depend on the stage of the disease process. In synovium one or all of the following signs may be present: increased vascularity, capillary hyperemia, granulation formation, villus formation, effusion, and fibrosis. Cartilage may exhibit one or all of the following: fibrillation, lesions of cartilage and subchondral bone, and bony exposure with eburnation. Synovial biopsies obtained during arthroscopic procedures may show proliferation of the synovial lining and infiltration of lymphocytes and plasma cells with increased vascularity and fibrosis.[9]

Many patients with TMJ involvement have cervical involvement that may lead to instability at the C1-C2 level with the attendant risk of subluxation and cord compression.[10] It is important to obtain radiographs of the cervical spine as part of any preoperative evaluation of a patient with RA. Patients with more severe disease often have rheumatoid nodules, characteristically found over the olecranon bursa. Some of these patients develop systemic features, including vasculitis, pulmonary involvement, scleromalacia perforans, and Felty's syndrome. A significant percentage of patients have secondary Sjögren's syndrome.

One of the laboratory hallmarks of RA is the presence of positive rheumatoid factor (RF). These are usually IgM antibodies directed against the Fc portion of IgG immunoglobulins. In a small percentage of patients, the IgM RF is negative, and it is possible to demonstrate IgA RF or the so-called "hidden" IgG RF. RF is not specific for RA, because it can be found in other autoimmune illnesses such as Sjögren's syndrome and systemic lupus erythematosus as well as in patients who have chronic infections, such as subacute endocarditis. Although the precise etiology of RA is unknown, there is clearly a genetic component to the disease, because the human leukocyte antigen HLA-DR4 phenotype is strongly associated with the presence of clinical RA.

Since RA is a disease that involves multiple joints as well as other organs, it should be treated systemically as well as locally. Nonsurgical treatment for RA of the TMJ should include the use of an orthotic and physical therapy. Arthroscopic surgical treatment of rheumatoid arthritis may include lavage and perhaps injection of diluted sodium hyaluronate, which may relieve symptoms.[11] Intra-articular injection of corticosteroids, particularly synovial injections under arthroscopic control, have proved to be therapeutically effective.[12, 13] Operative arthroscopic management of rheumatoid arthritis may include debridement of the proliferative tissue within the joint via a partial or subtotal synovectomy, employing a wide variety of instrumentation including suction forceps and motorized shavers. For further information on RA and its manifestations, arthroscopic management, and treatment, see Section A of this chapter.

SYSTEMIC LUPUS ERYTHEMATOSUS

Systemic lupus erythematosus (SLE) is a chronic inflammatory disease with a plethora of evidence indicating immune dysfunction. Its etiology is unknown; however, genetic, hormonal, and environmental factors are all known to play a role. The prevalence of SLE ranges from 4 to 250 cases per 100,000, with a female-to-male ratio of 10 to 1. The strongest HLA association is with the HLA-DR3 allele; an association with HLA-DR2 has also been made. Musculoskeletal features include arthralgias and arthritis as well as tenosynovitis. The arthropathy may mimic that of RA; however, the deformities are usually reducible. Involvement of the TMJ is unusual but has been reported.[14–16] Osteonecrosis most often affects the hips but may affect other joints and is seen in both the untreated and steroid-treated patient. Other clinical manifestations include alopecia, mucocutaneous lesions, cardiac involvement, pulmonary parenchymal disease, serositis, central and peripheral nervous system involvement, renal disease, and hematologic abnormalities. Among the last are the anemia of chronic disease and autoimmune hemolytic anemia.

Coagulation abnormalities include thrombocytopenia and the presence of antibodies called lupus anticoagulants, which are paradoxically named, since clincially they are associated with thromboembolic and not hemorrhagic events. Other laboratory findings include antinuclear antibodies and antibodies to double-stranded DNA, which is one of the hallmarks of the disease. The presence of high titers of anti-DNA antibodies is often accompanied by low levels of complement and clinically active disease. Anti-Sm antibodies, which are found in about one fourth to one third of patients, are highly specific for SLE.

Lupus erythematosus is a systemic disease and should be managed with systemic therapy (steroids and/or cytotoxic drugs) together with local treatment of the TMJ if it is involved. Management and treatment when the TMJ is involved can be effected through a combination of nonsurgical and surgical modalities. Nonsurgical modalities include fabrication and use of an orthotic and physical rehabilitation, along with change of dietary habits to include soft foods. Patients with thrombotic events may be treated with anticoagulants, which of course should be discontinued, if possible, prior to any surgical procedure. It is very important to have a complete evaluation of the patient's status and, in particular, a hematologic work-up prior to any operation.

The patient group that has been treated at the Hospital for Joint Diseases Orthopaedic Institute, New York, has responded fairly well to nonsurgical therapy along with an alteration of dietary intake. Clinically these patients often present with pain specific to the joint area, along with limited interincisal opening registering between 10 and 20 mm.

Arthroscopic features of the disease process in synovium includes one or all of the following: synovial proliferation showing increased vascularity and capillary hyperemia, villus formation, effusion, and fibrosis. In cartilage, one or more of the following may be seen: fibrillation, lesions of cartilage and the subchondral bone, and perhaps areas of bony exposure with eburnation (Figs. 18-11 through 18-14 and 18-17). Arthroscopic treatment includes one or both of the following procedures: (1) simple lysis with lavage and (2) joint debridement via partial or subtotal synovial resection with the use of suction punch or motorized mini-shavers (Figs. 18-15 through 18-17).

MIXED CONNECTIVE TISSUE DISEASE

Mixed connective tissue disease is characterized by the presence of features typical of two or more well-defined connective tissue disorders. For example, a patient may present with physical and laboratory findings consistent with SLE and subsequently develop an erosive, deforming arthritis with high RF titers consistent with a diagnosis of RA. Most of these patients have extremely high titers to the autoantibodies known as extractable nuclear antigen (ENA).

SJÖGREN'S SYNDROME

Patients with Sjögren's syndrome typically are middle-aged women who have complaints of dry eyes (keratoconjunctivitis sicca) and dry mouth (xerostomia). Primary Sjögren's syndrome usually appears as the sicca complex together with arthralgias and/or nondeforming arthritis. Sjögren's syndrome is a generalized disorder of the exocrine glands. Other manifestations include renal tubular acidosis and central or peripheral nervous system involvement.

Complications of Sjögren's syndrome include benign and malignant lymphoproliferation, which often arises in the salivary glands. Serologically, patients have high titers of rheumatoid factor, a positive antinuclear antibody (ANA) assay, and often anti-Ro (SSA) or anti-La (SSB) antibodies. Secondary Sjögren's syndrome includes not only the sicca symptoms but also an associated autoimmune disease, most commonly RA, followed by SLE and less frequently by scleroderma, polymyositis, or polyarteritis nodosa. Parotid and submandibular gland enlargement is often noted (Fig. 18-18). Bi-

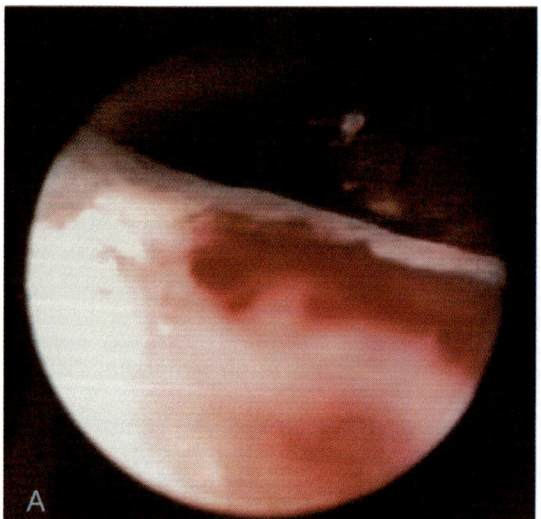
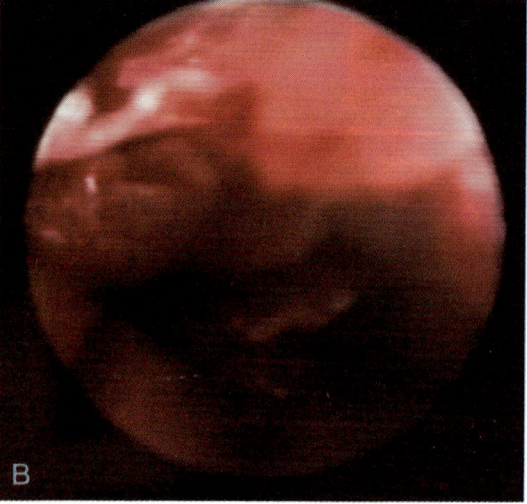

Figure 18-11. Arthroscopic views of the right temporomandibular joint in a patient with systemic lupus erythematosus: *A*, increased vascularity and hyperemia in the retrodiscal tissue; B, synovial proliferation, granulation formation, and hyperemia.

B. Systemic Inflammatory Arthritides with Temporomandibular Joint Involvement

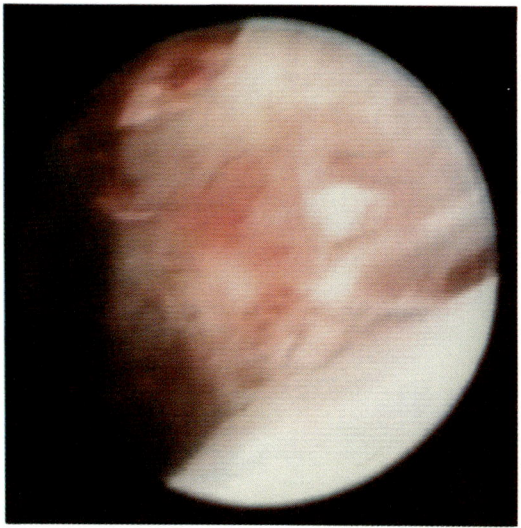

Figure 18–12. Arthroscopic view of the right temporomandibular joint in a patient with systemic lupus erythematosus, showing synovial proliferation and increased vascularity in the anterior pouch.

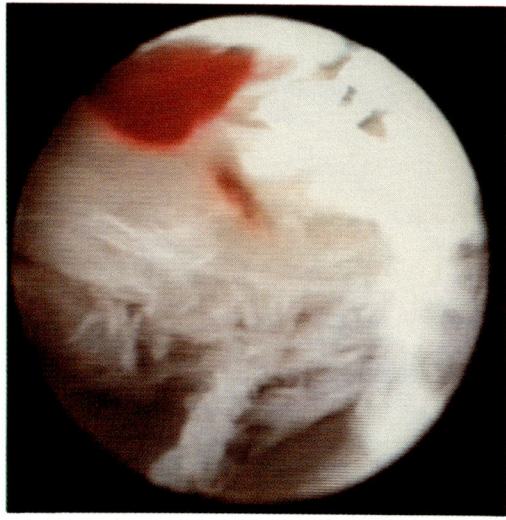

Figure 18–14. Arthroscopic view of the anterior pouch in a patient with systemic lupus erythematosus, showing villus formation and synovial hyperplasia in the right temporomandibular joint.

opsy of the minor salivary glands of patients with Sjögren's syndrome reveals an intense lymphocytic infiltrate destroying the acinar tissue. The focal sialoadenitis is scored according to the criteria of Chisholm and Mason.[17] Immunophenotyping of tissue from patients with Sjögren's syndrome reveals that a majority of the cells are CD4-positive T cells. The diagnosis can be further substantiated by a positive Schirmer test or positive rose bengal staining of the cornea. Only about 50% of patients who present with dry eyes or dry mouth will have an autoimmune illness. Other diagnostic possibilities include senile atrophy, use of medications such as tricyclic antidepressants, and local glandular disorders such as parotid tumors or infection.

SCLERODERMA

Scleroderma is an uncommon disease of unknown etiology, characterized by thickening and fibrosis of the skin and internal organ involvement including the heart, lungs, and gastrointestinal tract. Patients usually have Raynaud's phenomenon. The involvement of the skin of the face causes a characteristic drawn and pinched appearance (Figs. 18–19 and 18–20). Involvement of the mandible has been reported.[18] Laboratory findings include a positive ANA assay, usually in a speckled pattern. A less common but more specific finding is a nucleolar pattern on the ANA test. Patients may present with markedly reduced interincisal opening secondary to fibrosis or bony ankylosis. Surgical management including arthroscopy may not provide much improvement owing to the involve-

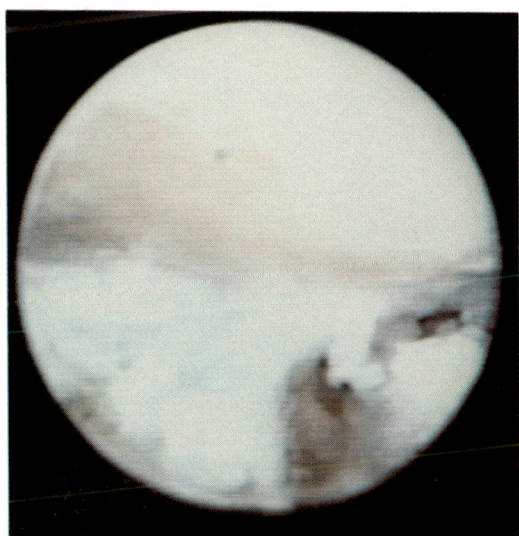

Figure 18–13. Arthroscopic view of the anterior pouch of the right temporomandibular joint in a patient with systemic lupus erythematosus, showing increased fibrosis and synovial proliferation.

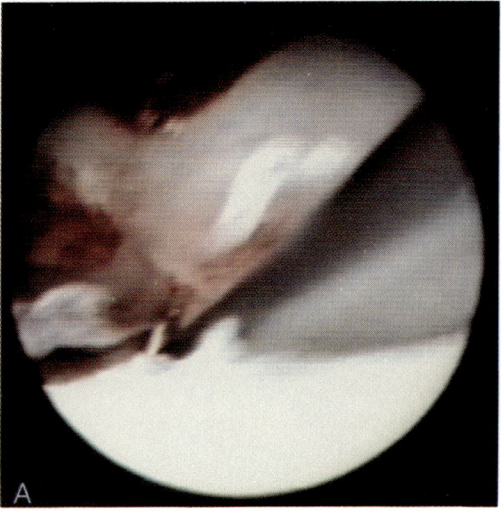 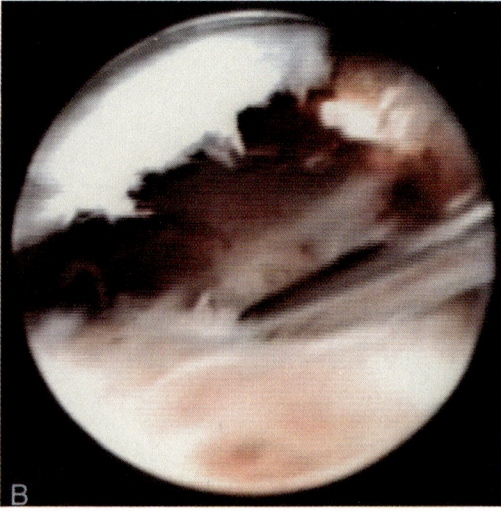

Figure 18–15. *A* and *B*, Arthroscopic photographs showing lysis and lavage with a blunt probe in the right temporomandibular joint of a patient with systemic lupus erythematosus.

ment of the overlying skin, which may lead to superficial breakdown and further scarring. Prognosis in the case of surgery is unpredictable and the long-term outcome is unknown.

POLYMYOSITIS AND DERMATOMYOSITIS

Polymyositis and dermatomyositis are inflammatory diseases of the muscles and differ clinically in that a patient with dermatomyositis has a characteristic skin rash. The dermatologic manifestations include a violaceous discoloration around the eyes (heliotrope rash) and dry scaly lesions over the metacarpophalangeal joints (Gottron's papules). The onset of illness is usually gradual, with evidence of weakness greater in the proximal muscles than in the distal. In older patients, especially those with dermatomyositis, there is an increased frequency of ma-

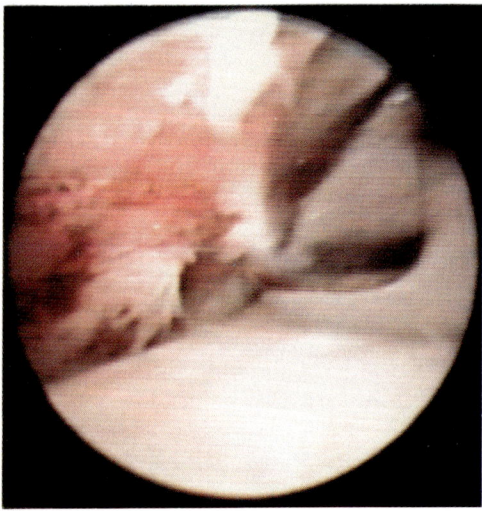

Figure 18–16. Arthroscopic photographs showing debridement with suction forceps in the right temporomandibular joint in a patient with systemic lupus erythematosus.

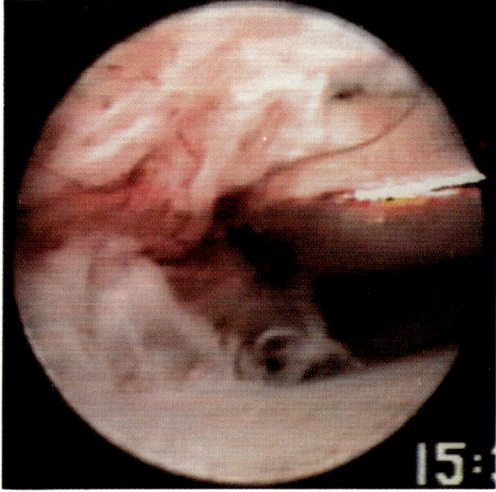

Figure 18–17. Arthroscopic view of the right temporomandibular joint in a patient with systemic lupus erythematosus, showing villus formation and the use of a motorized shaver for joint debridement and synovial resection.

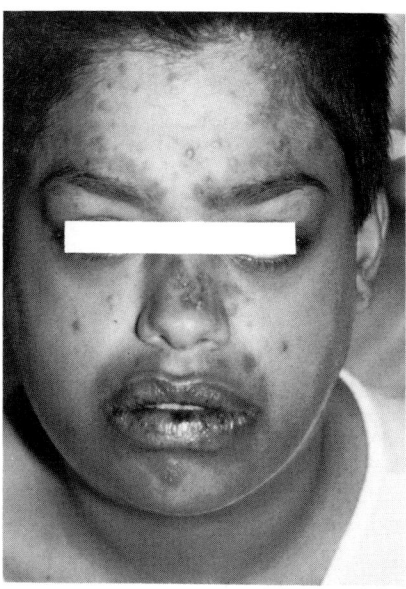

Figure 18–18. Parotid enlargement and rash in a patient with systemic lupus erythematosus and secondary Sjögren's syndrome.

lignancies; therefore it is important to search for an underlying neoplasm. Patients usually are ANA-positive and have elevated muscle enzymes, CPK, and aldolase. Electrodiagnostic studies show characteristic myopathic changes, and a muscle biopsy sample classically shows an inflammatory myositis.

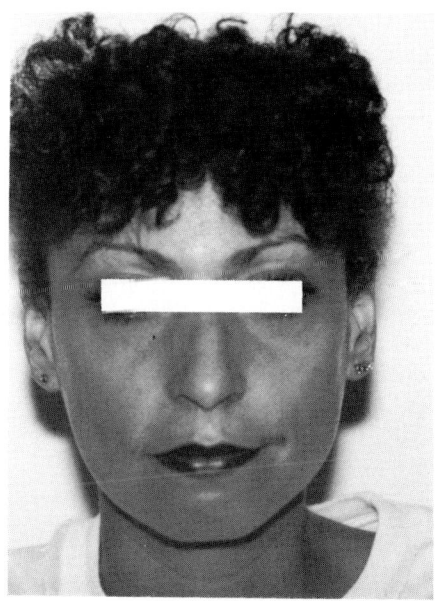

Figure 18–19. Drawn tight facies in a patient with scleroderma.

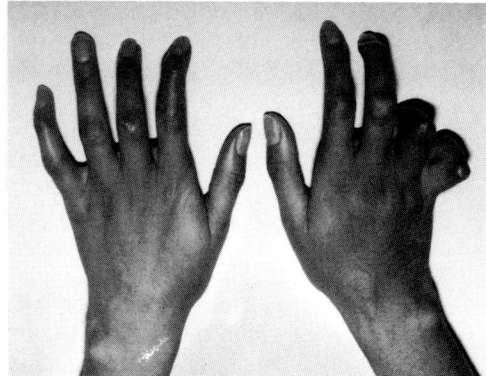

Figure 18–20. Hand contractures, tight atrophic skin, and healed ulcerations in the same patient shown in Figure 18–19.

TEMPORAL ARTERITIS

Temporal arteritis (giant cell arteritis) is a disease of older people; almost all reported cases occur in patients over the age of 50. The patient may complain of aching and stiffness in the shoulder girdle, neck, or hip girdle. Patients may complain of headache, fever, visual symptoms, scalp tenderness, pain in the teeth (particularly the maxillary), jaw or tongue claudication, and a sore throat. Patients may become blind; rarely, gangrene of the tongue or extremity occurs. A diagnostic temporal artery biopsy should be done as soon as possible and, when appropriate, corticosteroid therapy should be instituted. There usually is a markedly elevated sedimentation rate, but there are no other serologic abnormalities.

POLYMYALGIA RHEUMATICA

Temporal arteritis and polymyalgia rheumatica appear to be associated conditions; however, the exact relationship between the two is unknown. In polymyalgia rheumatica, no evidence for vasculitis can be demonstrated and the clinical course is milder. These patients usually respond dramatically to treatment with low doses (less than 10 mg per day) of prednisone.

TAKAYASU'S ARTERITIS

Takayasu's arteritis is an uncommon illness that usually involves the aorta or its major branches. It occurs primarily in children and young women. Pathologically there is a granulomatous arteritis of the involved vessels. In early disease, especially with carotid involvement, the symptoms may include fatigue, myalgia, and a low-grade temperature and may be indistinguishable from the symptoms of temporal arteritis. Later, in the pulseless phase of the illness, vascular insufficiency may develop; if it involves the head, atrophy of the skin of the face, with loss of hair or teeth, may develop. The other forms of vasculitis, such as polyarteritis nodosa, usually can be clinically differentiated from temporal arteritis.

ANKYLOSING SPONDYLITIS

Ankylosing spondylitis (AS) traditionally has been thought to affect young males primarily; however, more recent evidence suggests that the prevalence of AS is similar in males and females. Males are, however, more severely affected. The spondyloarthropathies may affect 1% of the population. AS is strongly associated with the presence of the genetic marker HLA-B27. Patients usually present with sacroiliitis, and during the course of their illness, about one third of patients will have asymmetric oligoarthritis that typically involves the lower extremity. Inflammation of the ligaments or tendons (enthesopathy) is common. TMJ involvement has been reported in about 10% of patients.[19] Relatively few patients develop the completely rigid "bamboo" spine. Extra-articular involvement may include constitutional features, eye disease, pulmonary disease (including pulmonary fibrosis as well as a rigid chest wall), and cardiovascular disease, which may encompass aortitis and conduction defects. Patients with AS or one of the other spondyloarthropathies are prone to develop heterotopic bone formation. Use of a diphosphonate or indomethacin to prevent extra-articular ossification may be indicated if a surgical procedure is performed. Prognosis is guarded.

PSORIATIC ARTHRITIS

Psoriatic arthritis is present in approximately 5% of patients with psoriasis. Clinically, patients most often have an asymmetric oligoarticular arthritis involving the distal and proximal interphalangeal joints of the hands and feet (Fig. 18–21). Other large joints may be involved. Patterns of presentation include arthritis mutilans, in which there is osteolysis of the involved distal digits, and spinal involvement with sacroiliitis and syndesmophyte formation. Destructive changes in the TMJ may be seen on radiographic studies.[20, 21] The diagnosis can be made with assurance when the patient presents with the typical pattern of joint involvement together with the skin lesions of psoriasis or the typical changes of psoriatic nail disease. Rarely, the patient may present with the arthritic changes without any skin disease. Often there is a strong family history of psoriasis. The most common genetic marker is HLA-Cw6, although other alleles such as B13, B17, B38, and B39 have been implicated. HLA-B27 is found in a majority of patients who have spondylitis. Psoriatic patients are uncommonly rheumatoid factor–positive. In psoriatic arthritis, the arthroscopic findings and surgical treatment are similar to those of RA.

REITER'S SYNDROME

Reiter's syndrome is an asymmetric, seronegative arthritis that usually involves the lower extremities and is accompanied by urethritis/cervicitis, dysentery, inflammatory eye disease, or mucocutaneous diseases such as circinate balanitis, oral ulcers, and keratoderma. The skin lesions may be indistinguishable from those of psoriasis. Often there is a history of an antecedent enteric illness such as *Shigella, Salmonella,* or *Yersinia* infection or venereal infection such as *Chlamydia.* Patients are sometimes mistakenly thought to have a sexually transmitted disease such as gonorrhea. In whites, about 80% of patients are HLA-B27–positive. Patients may present with erosive arthritis of the TMJ.[22] TMJ involvement may include a decrease in interincisal opening secondary to bony ankylosis (deposition of calcium).

GOUT AND PSEUDOGOUT

The crystal-associated forms of arthritis include gout and pseudogout.

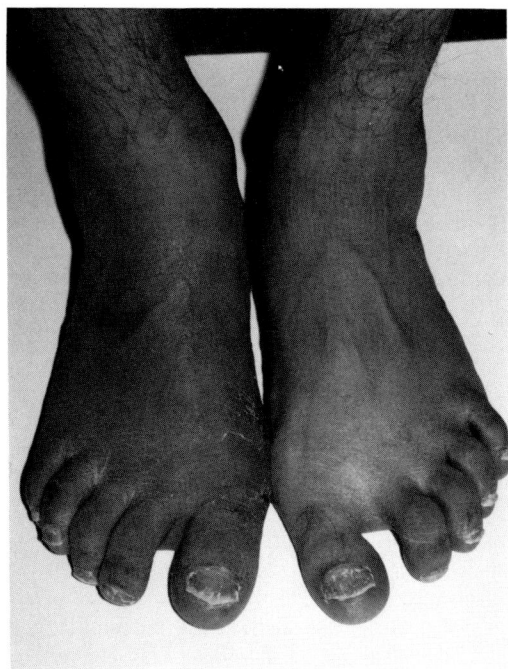

Figure 18–21. Deforming arthritis of the feet in a patient with psoriatic arthritis.

Gout

Gout is a disorder of purine metabolism characterized by an elevation of the serum urate level and the deposition of urate crystals in the intra-articular space. Gout may appear as acute, subacute, and chronic attacks of synovitis that occasionally may mimic RA or osteoarthritis. Attacks of gout classically affect the big toe (podagra), and attacks affecting the TMJ are rare (Fig. 18–22).[23] Acute attacks of gout must be distinguished from acute cellulitis. Renal involvement may take the form of parenchymal disease or kidney stones. Tophi, which are soft-tissue crystalline urate deposits, are usually found in patients with long-standing disease. Tophi commonly form over extensor surfaces, such as the olecranon bursa, but may form elsewhere, such as on the helix of the ear. Factors that may contribute to the gouty state include mutations in the enzymatic pathways of purine metabolism (e.g., hypoxanthine-guanine phosphoribosyltransferase deficiency), treatment with diuretics, and chronic lead poisoning. The laboratory hallmark of gout is the demonstration of negatively birefringent (yellow) intracellular needle-shaped urate crystals in the synovial fluid. The white blood cell count may be extremely elevated, and the possibility of a pyogenic infection must be ruled out by microscopy and culture.

Pseudogout

Pseudogout is indistinguishable clinically from gout. However, the crystals are composed of calcium pyrophosphate dihydrate (CPPD) that appear as weakly positive birefringent rhomboidal shapes.[24–26] CPPD deposition disease is clearly associated with a variety of metabolic disorders such as hyperparathyroidism, hemochromatosis, hypophosphatasia, and hypomagnesemia. A variable association has been found with conditions such as osteoarthritis, aging, hypermobility syndromes, hypothyroidism, and amyloidosis. The finding of CPPD crystals or chondrocalcinosis on radiographs should lead one to consider one of the aforementioned metabolic disorders.

BEHÇET'S SYNDROME

Behçet's syndrome originally was described as the clinical triad of recurrent aphthous ulcers of the mouth, genital ulcerations, and uveitis. It is now recognized that the syndrome encompasses synovitis, vasculitis, phlebitis, and meningoencephalitis. The arthritis usually involves the knees and ankles. It is a rare disease, the etiology of which is unknown.

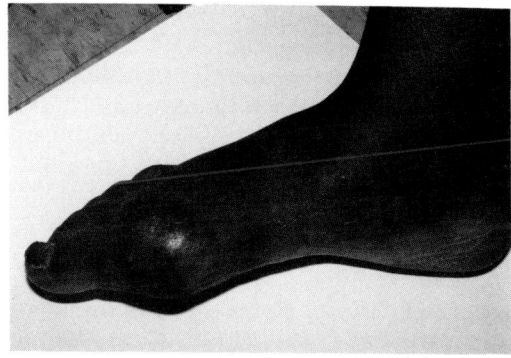

Figure 18–22. Acute gouty arthritis of the first metatarsophalangeal joint (podagra).

LYME DISEASE

Lyme disease is caused by the spirochete *Borrelia burgdorferi* and is transmitted by *Ixodes dammini* or related ticks. In the initial stage of the illness, there is a characteristic erythematous spreading skin rash (erythema chronicum migrans). From 30% to 40% of patients fail to recall any tick bites. Patients may develop arthritis or neurologic or cardiac problems. In the early phases of the disease, joint pains tend to be transient and migratory and are accompanied by enthesopathic symptoms. In the late, chronic phase, the arthritis is a persistent oligoarticular synovitis, with the most common joint involved being the knee. TMJ involvement has been reported.[27]

Lyme disease may mimic other inflammatory arthritides, and in some of the early case reports, patients were originally thought to have juvenile rheumatoid arthritis. *B. burgdorferi* is not usually cultured from these patients. The ELISA assay currently in common use to detect antibodies to the spirochete is highly sensitive, but it has been difficult to eliminate false-positive reactions. False-negative reactions can occur, as it takes 2 to 3 weeks for seroconversion to take place. Western blots are available to help distinguish false-positive test results. Patients with abnormal autoantibody production such as SLE have a high incidence of false-positive Lyme test findings.

RHEUMATOLOGIC MANIFESTATIONS OF THE ACQUIRED IMMUNODEFICIENCY SYNDROME (AIDS)

The AIDS epidemic has continued to grow, and more than a million people in the United States have been infected with the human immunodeficiency virus (HIV).[28] The manifestations of HIV disease include opportunistic infections, neoplasms, and neurologic, ocular, dermatologic, gastrointestinal, pulmonary, and renal diseases. This brief review focuses on the rheumatologic manifestations of HIV infection.

The most common type of rheumatic clinical presentation is Reiter's syndrome or reactive arthritis.[29, 30] Patients have severe, persistent oligoarticular arthritis of the lower extremities and often have extra-articular features such as urethritis, conjunctivitis, keratoderma blenorrhagicum, circinate balanitis, and painless oral ulcers. The symptoms may occur before there are overt signs of clinical immunodeficiency. HLA-B27 has been found in many of the white patients who have been studied. Other patients may present with arthritis, enthesopathy, and skin lesions that appear to be clinically identical to those in patients with psoriatic arthritis (Fig. 18–23).[31] A persistent, generalized lymphadenopathy has been described in patients with AIDS-related complex and is associated with the sicca syndrome.[32] Patients have positive Schirmer test results, positive rose bengal staining, and a positive salivary gland biopsy findings. The demographics are identical to those of HIV infection, in contrast to the situation in primary Sjögren's syndrome. Patients are rarely positive for rheumatoid factor, ANA, SSA, or SSB. HLA typing of affected individuals reveals that most patients are HLA-DR5 positive, which, again, is unlike the association seen in primary Sjögren's syndrome.

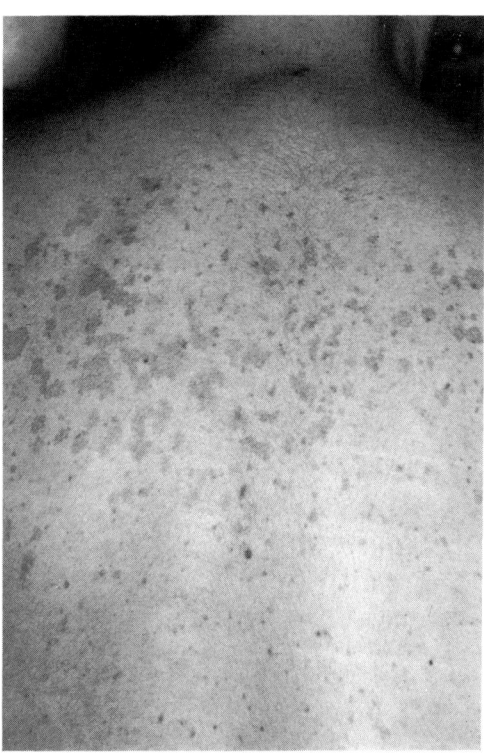

Figure 18–23. Psoriaform lesions in a patient with HIV/Reiter's syndrome. Similar skin lesions can be seen in patients with psoriatic arthritis, or non–HIV Reiter's syndrome.

JUVENILE RHEUMATOID ARTHRITIS

The inflammatory arthritides that begin in childhood are known collectively as juvenile rheumatoid arthritis (JRA) and undoubtedly represent diseases with different etiologies. By definition, patients with JRA become ill before the age of 16 years. About 25% of patients with JRA have involvement of the TMJ (Fig. 18–24).[33]

The classic systemic inflammatory arthritis of childhood is Still's disease, which on rare occasions begins in the third or fourth decade. The presentation includes fever of unknown origin; a morbilliform, erythematous, transient macular skin rash; lymphadenopathy; hepatosplenomegaly; serositis; and arthritis. TMJ involvement is relatively common in children. Inflammation of the joint may lead to ankylosis, and the chronic illness may cause a disturbance in growth centers that leads to micrognathia.[34–38] Serologic test results such as rheumatoid factor (RF) and ANA are usually negative. Still's disease is a diagnosis of exclusion, and other inflammatory arthritides as well as nonrheumatic illnesses such as infection (e.g., osteomyelitis) or tumor (especially leukemia) must be ruled out.

One subtype of JRA primarily affects very young girls and consists of an oligoarthritis affecting primarily the large joints of the lower extremity. Chronic uveitis, which is associated with this disorder, may progress to blindness if untreated. These children usually test ANA-positive and RF-negative.

Other types of JRA are notable more for the typical onset of disease at adolescence than for any remarkable clinical features. Children, most often girls, who are affected will have a chronic, symmetric, erosive polyarthritis that is RF-positive. The disease may progress to a deforming arthritis that is indistinguishable from classic RA in adults. Adolescent boys who have back pain and sacroileitis are clinically indistinguishable from adults who have ankylosing spondylitis. SLE frequently presents in older teen-age girls.

SUMMARY

A rheumatologic work-up is essential, particularly if the clinical presentation suggests systemic involvement, for the successful management of TMJ disorders. Surgical procedures should be complemented with systemic medications when appropriate, along with physical rehabilitation in order to maximize therapeutic effects.

[For further information please refer to Tables 18–1 and 18–2.]

References

1. Utsinger PD, Zvaifler NJ, Ehrlich GE (eds): Rheumatoid Arthritis. Etiology, Diagnosis, Management. Philadelphia: JB Lippincott, 1985, pp 139–140.
2. Carlsson GE, Kopp S, Oberg T: Arthritis and allied diseases of the temporomandibular joint. In Zarb GA, Carlsson, GE (eds): Temporomandibular Joint Function and Dysfunction. St. Louis: CV Mosby, 1979, pp 293–320.
3. Ogus H: Rheumatoid arthritis of the temporomandibular joint. Br J Oral Surg 12:275–284, 1975.
4. Tegelberg A, Kopp S: Clinical findings in the stomatognathic system for individuals with rheumatoid arthritis and osteoarthritis. Acta Odont Scand 45:65–75, 1987.
5. Ericson S, Lundberg M: Alterations in the temporomandibular joint at various stages of rheumatoid arthritis. Acta Rheum Scand 13:257, 1967.
6. Marbach JJ, Spiera H: Rheumatoid arthritis of the temporomandibular joints. Ann Rheum Dis 26:538, 1967.
7. Chalmers IM, Blair GS: Rheumatoid arthritis of the temporomandibular joint: A clinical and radiological study using circular tomography. Q J Med 42:369, 1973.
8. Akerman S, Kopp S, Nilner M, et al: Relationship between clinical and radiologic findings of the temporomandibular joint in rheumatoid arthritis. Oral Surg Oral Med Oral Pathol 66(6):639–643, 1988.
9. Rooney M, Condell D, Quinlan W, et al: Analysis of the histologic variation of synovitis in rheumatoid arthritis. Arthr Rheum 31:956–963, 1988.
10. Redlund-Johnell I: Severe rheumatoid arthritis of

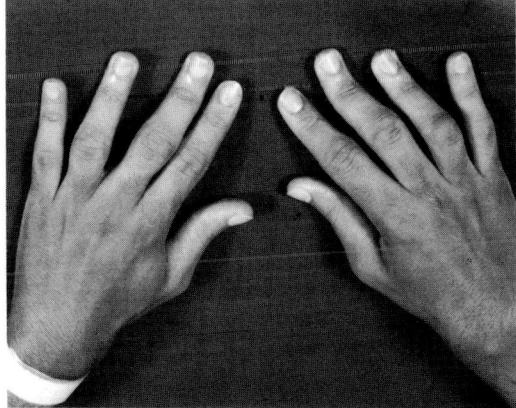

Figure 18–24. Deforming arthritis of the hands of a patient with juvenile rheumatoid arthritis.

Table 18-1. INFLAMMATORY ARTHRITIS: SOME COMMON CLINICAL MANIFESTATIONS

Disease	Joint Involvement			Skin Changes		
	Symmetry	Pattern	Deformity	Enthesopathy	Rash	Nodules
RA	Yes	Poly	Yes	No	No	Yes
OA	No	Var	No	No	No	No
AS	No	SI/spine	No	No	No	No
Reiter's syndrome	No	Oligo, lower	Var	Yes	Yes	No
Psoriatic arthritis	No	Oligo	Var	Yes	Yes	No
Gout; pseudogout	No	Oligo, lower	Var	No	No	Yes
SLE	No	Var	No	No	Yes	No
Sjögren's syndrome	No	Var	No	No	No	No
MCTD	No	Var	Var	No	Yes	No
Scleroderma	No	Overlying skin	Yes	No	Yes	No

RA = rheumatoid arthritis; OA = osteoarthritis; AS = ankylosing spondylitis; SLE = systemic lupus erythematosus; MCTD = mixed connective tissue disease; poly = polyarticular; var = variable; SI = sacroiliacl; oligo = oligoarticular.

Table 18-2. INFLAMMATORY ARTHRITIS: SOME COMMON LABORATORY FINDINGS

Disease	Laboratory Test				
	RF	ANA	Anti-DNA	SSA/SSB	HLA
RA	+++	−	−	−	DR4
OA	−	−	−	−	−
AS	−	−	−	−	B27
Reiter's syndrome	−	−	−	−	B27
Psoriatic arthritis	−	−	−	−	Cw6, B13, B16, B17, B27, B38
Gout; pseudogout	−	−	−	−	−
SLE	+	+++	+++	+	DR3, DR2
Sjögren's syndrome	++++	++	−	++	B8, DR3
MCTD	−	++	−	−	−
Scleroderma	−	++	−	−	A9, DR5

RF = rheumatoid factor; ANA = antinuclear antibodies; Anti-DNA = anti-deoxyribonucleic acid antibody; SSA/SSB = anti-Ro/anti-La antibodies; HLA = human leukocyte antigen; RA = rheumatoid arthritis; OA = osteoarthritis; AS = ankylosing spondylitis; SLE = systemic lupus erythematosus; MCTD = mixed connective tissue disease.

the temporomandibular joints and its coincidence with severe rheumatoid arthritis of the cervical spine. Scand J Rheumatol 16(5):347–353, 1987.
11. Weiss L: Basic structures of di-arthrodial joints. In Parisien JS (ed): Arthroscopic Surgery. New York: McGraw-Hill, pp 12–13, 1988.
12. Kopp S, Wennberg B: Effects of occlusal treatment and intra-articular injections on temporomandibular joint pain and dysfunction. Acta Odont Scand 39:87–96, 1981.
13. Wennberg B, Kopp S: Short-term effect of interarticular injections of corticosteroids on temporomandibular joint pain and dysfunction. Swed Dent J 2:189–196, 1978.
14. Liebling MR Gold RH: Erosions of the temporomandibular joint in systemic lupus erythematosus. Arthr Rheum 24:948, 1981.
15. Gerbracht D, Shapiro L: Temporomandibular joint erosions in systemic lupus erythematosus. [Letter]. Arthr Rheum 25:597, 1982.
16. Jonsson R, Lindvall A-M, Nyberg G: Temporomandibular joint involvement in systemic lupus erythematosus. Arthr Rheum 26:1506–1510, 1983.
17. Chisholm DM, Mason DK: Labial salivary gland biopsy in Sjögren's syndrome. J Clin Pathol 21:656–660, 1968.
18. Osial TA, Avakian A, Sassouni V, et al: Resorption of the mandibular condyles and coracoid processes in progressive systemic sclerosis (scleroderma). Arthr Rheum 24:729, 1981.
19. Davidson C, Wojtulewski JA, Bacon PA, et al: Temporomandibular joint disease in ankylosing spondylitis. Ann Rheum Dis 34:87, 1975.
20. Kudryk WH, Baker GL, Percy JS: Ankylosis of the temporomandibular joints from psoriatic arthritis. J Otolaryngol 14:336, 1985.
21. Kononen M: Clinical signs of craniomandibular disorders in patients with psoriatic arthritis. Scand J Dent Res 95(4):340–346, 1987.
22. Bomalaski JS, Jimenez SA: Erosive arthritis of the temporomandibular joint in Reiter's syndrome. J Rheumatol 11(3):400–402, 1984.

23. Gross BD, Williams RB, DiCosimo CJ, Williams SV: Gout and pseudogout of the temporomandibular joint. Oral Surg Oral Med Oral Pathol 63(5):551–554, 1987.
24. Ling D, Murphy WA, Kyriakos M: Tophaceous pseudogout. Radiology 138:162, 1982.
25. Pritzker KPH, Phillips H, Luk SC, et al: Pseudotumor of temporomandibular joint: destructive calcium pyrophosphate hydrate arthropathy. J Rheumatol 3:70, 1976.
26. Hutton CW, Doherty M, Dieppe PA: Acute pseudogout of the temporomandibular joint: A report of three cases and review of the literature. Br J Rheumatol 26(1):51–52, 1987.
27. Harris RJ: Lyme disease involving the temporomandibular joint. J Oral Maxillofac Surg 46:78–79, 1988.
28. AIDS and human immunodeficiency virus infection in the United States: 1988 update. MMWR 38:Suppl S4:1–38, 1989.
29. Winchester R, Bernstein DH, Fischer HD, et al: The co-occurrence of Reiter's syndrome and acquired immunodeficiency. Ann Intern Med 106:19–26, 1987.
30. Brancato L, Itescu S, Skovron ML, et al: Aspects of the spectrum, prevalence and disease susceptibility determinants of Reiter's syndrome and related disorders associated with HIV infection. Rheumatol Int 9:137–141, 1989.
31. Duvic M, Johnson TM, Rapini RP, et al: Acquired immunodeficiency syndrome–associated psoriasis and Reiter's syndrome. Arch Dermatol 123:1622–1632, 1987.
32. Itescu S, Brancato L, Buxbaum J, et al: Sjögren's syndrome associated with HIV infection. [Abstract]. Arthr Rheum 31(Suppl 2):S35, 1988.
33. Guyuron B: Facial deformity of juvenile rheumatoid arthritis. Plast Reconstr Surg 81(6):948–951, 1988.
34. Martis CS, Karakasis DT: Ankylosis of the temporomandibular joint caused by Still's disease. Oral Surg 35:462, 1973.
35. Larheim TA, Dale K, Tveito L: Radiographic abnormalities of the temporomandibular joint in children with juvenile rheumatoid arthritis. Acta Radiol 22:277, 1981.
36. Larheim TA, Haanaes HR, Dale K: Radiographic temporomandibular joint abnormality in adults with micrognathia and juvenile rheumatoid arthritis. Acta Radiol 22:495, 1981.
37. Sairanen E: On the etiology of growth disturbance of the mandible in juvenile rheumatoid arthritis. Acta Rheum Scand 16:136, 1970.
38. Larheim TA, Haanaes HR, Ruud AF: Mandibular growth, temporomandibular joint changes and dental occlusion in juvenile rheumatoid arthritis: A 17-year follow-up study. Scand J Rheumatol 10:225, 1981.

Section V

Postoperative Management

Chapter 19

POST-ARTHROSCOPIC PHYSICAL REHABILITATION OF THE TEMPOROMANDIBULAR JOINT

THOMAS M. EGGLETON, M.S., P.T.,
DENNIS P. LANGTON, B.S., P.T.

To paraphrase Dr. James S. Grisolia, the head and face are the focus of much human activity. The head is crowded with complex structures, reflecting its many functions. The neck contains many delicate structures needed for support and precise orienting of the head as well as those needed for all communication between the brain and body.[1] It follows that rehabilitation of the postoperative temporomandibular joint (TMJ) can be accomplished only by establishing a sound basis of knowledge of joint structure and function. Awareness and understanding of the mechanical and physiologic functions of the TMJ and surrounding structures, which directly or indirectly affect the pathology for which surgery is indicated, are also necessary.

This chapter presents an overview of specific rehabilitation techniques necessary for post-arthroscopic surgery of the TMJ. Emphasis is placed on evaluation and understanding of the primary and secondary surrounding structures.

PRESURGICAL EVALUATION

Given the axiom that TMJ dysfunction is a multfaceted problem, it is essential that a comprehensive physical assessment of the TMJ is done both intrinsically and extrinsically prior to surgery. A presurgical evaluation is critical not only for a full understanding of the pathology as it exists prior to the surgery but also to provide a standard of comparison for evaluating the patient postoperatively. The evaluation should include all functional and biomechanical aspects of the overall dysfunction.

History

Emphasis should be placed on ascertaining from the patient's life style any factor that may contribute functionally, anatomically, physiologically, or psychologically to his or her TMJ disorder.

Posture

Current research literature and clinical data indicate a direct relationship of posture to TMJ dysfunction.[2, 3] The effects of forward head posture include a change of tongue rest position; loss of vertical rest dimension of the mandible; change in habitual closure pattern of the mandible, leading to an open mouth breathing pattern; and, probably most significant, a change in the functional opening cycle of the mandible to precipitance of early translation.

Palpation

Palpation is a three-dimensional process, and understanding of anatomy on a three-dimensional basis[4] is both essential and required. Identification takes place by exclusion, whereby one must always picture the muscles, ligaments, and other structures that are localized above and next to each other in a specific topographic region. Examination includes identification of hyperactive and hypoactive muscular areas, hypertrophic muscles, and the location of trigger or tender points.[5, 6] Specific muscles for consideration include the temporalis, masseter, sternocleidomastoid, scalenus complex, supra- and infrahyoid muscles, and the prevertebrals, with particular relationship to the suboccipitals, medial pterygoids, splenius capitis, trapezius, and levator scapulae. Consideration should also be given to muscles of the anterior and posterior shoulder girdle.

Neuromuscular Examination

Testing can be on a general basis, designed to eliminate, as much as possible, neurologic disorders that may contribute to the symptomatology. Nerve roots cannot be specifically isolated for extrinsic testing; therefore, reflex, sensation, and muscle testing is performed on the dermatome and myotome areas. Specific muscle testing, along with palpation, assists in identifying physical trauma that may have occurred in the muscle itself. In the TMJ, muscles typically occur over a one-joint rather than a two-joint structure, such as is seen in the long head of the biceps. As a result, microtrauma occurs rather than actual rupture of the muscle.[7]

Auscultation

It is important to note not only the joint sounds themselves, but where they occur in the opening cycle. Auscultation should be done during movement in all directions. Although auscultation can be valuable, it must also be viewed critically, as there are several possible known patahologic reasons for joint sounds.[8] A Dopplergram may be useful in evaluating joint sounds.

Functional Mechanics of the Temporomandibular Joint

In the presurgical evaluation, the examiner needs to ascertain the current functional mechanics of the TMJ as well as the current mechanical state of the stomatognathic system and its relationship to the opening cycle. Therefore, such things as lip closure, lip position during swallowing, the swallowing pattern itself, rest position of the tongue, appearance of tongue thrust, and the respiratory pattern are included in a full functional examination.

In examining the dynamics of the opening and closing movements, several questions need to be answered:

1. On opening does the mandible deviate to one side?
2. Does the mandible deviate to one side and then return to the midline upon a click?
3. Does the mandible deviate to one side, then return to midline upon clicking, and then deviate to the opposite side?
4. Does this pattern repeat itself upon closure?
5. Does the pattern hold true for laterotrusion and protrusion?[9, 10]

With palpation over the lateral condyle, the examiner may note the rotation/translation relationships during the opening and closing cycle pre- and postoperatively.[9–11]

Spinal Evaluation

In establishing the overall effect of the structures extrinsic to the TMJ, testing of the segmental mobility of the cervical spine is important. Each individual cervical segment is tested in forward bending, backward bending, side bending, and rotation. This enhances the examiner's understanding of the roles of postural craniocervical relationships and neuromuscular factors on the craniomandibular system.

Typical problems identified in the presurgical evaluation, related to physical rehabilitation, include altered mandibular dynamics, mandibular hyper- versus hypomobility, muscle contraction pain, tongue thrust, tongue weakness, improper rest position of the tongue, improper rest position of the mandible, abnormal posture, spinal hypo- versus hypermobility, altered respiratory patterns, and headaches.

Specific presurgical problems related to the temporomandibular joint include the following:

1. Altered mandibular mechanics.
2. Presence or absence of capsular adhesions.
3. Altered proprioception presurgically caused by muscular and ligamentous tightness or imbalance.
4. Vascular changes such as ischemia of the condyle and proliferation of vessels in the posterior compartment and around the disc itself.[12,13]
5. Histologic changes in articular surfaces, including sclerosis, with progression to degenerative joint disease.
6. Loss of strength.
7. Loss of endurance.
8. Altered histology of the joint capsule and musculature including synovial hyperplasia and capsulitis,[14] muscle hypertrophy with increased number of sarcomeres, and stimulation of the release of potassium, histamine, serotonin, prostaglandins, and substance P.[15]

PREOPERATIVE REHABILITATION PROGRAM

A clear preoperative picture of the structure and function of the craniomandibular and vertebral system can be achieved from the initial evaluation. The goal of presurgical physical therapy is to enhance the surgical result and minimize any surgical trauma. Specific objectives include (1) diminishing presurgical pain; (2) relaxation of masticatory, precervical, and paracervical musculature; (3) expanding joint spaces; and (4) instructing in self-directed basic preoperative and immediate postoperative exercises that can be done until the rehabilitation process continues in the postoperative phase. These exercises emphasizes enhancing opening, using a rotational basis, and normalization of the translatoric movement within the TMJ to maintain disc mobility and prevent the occurrence of adhesions.

The goal of the preoperative rehabilitation program is not merely restoration of normal joint mobility following surgical procedures; such a program should also include planning the best way to increase motion, restore normal muscle length, and condition the entire craniomandibular and vertebral system for a satisfactory long-term result.

ROLE OF THE PHYSICAL THERAPIST IN EDUCATION

It is well understood and accepted in business circles that a person who has a good level of understanding of a problem is a much better participant in its solution. The same holds true in the field of health care. A patient who has an understanding of his or her pathology is more willing and participates more fully in the rehabilitation process.

In the area of patient education, the physical therapist can be of great assistance to the surgeon in helping the patient understand the surgical procedure and its goals and how the muscles and joints function in relationship to one another. Extrinsic factors such as standing and sitting posture, body mechanics, work activities, and activities of daily living affect the rehabilitation outcome and are reviewed with the patient by the physical therapist.

POSTOPERATIVE EVALUATION

A postoperative evaluation using the same presurgical criteria described previously will give the clinician a standard for comparison of the postsurgical result from a functional point of view. Immediate attention must be paid to the metabolic and neuromuscular effects of the actual trauma brought about by the surgical procedure. Range of motion and arthrokinematic evaluations should be limited to active ranges only, as there may be considerable muscle guarding, edema, and other postsurgical responses. If an extensive preoperative picture has been established, the postoperative evaluation can be completed with minimal repetition of motions, lessening the traumatic response to surgery.

POSTOPERATIVE REHABILITATION

Postoperative physical therapy must begin as soon as possible for three reasons. First, arthroscopic procedures require actual penetration of the joint capsule and superficial tissues. Surgical invasion of any joint yields metabolic and neuromuscular responses that may begin a healing phase that creates adhesions of various tissue layers to one another. Second, arthroscopy of the TMJ is often performed for the purpose of locating and releasing intrajoint adhesions of the capsule that have the properties necessary to begin new collagen bonding within a 48-hour period.[16] Third, the body responds to arthroscopic surgery of the TMJ in the same manner as it does to any other invasive procedure. The fact that a joint was involved yields additional response mechanisms, both metabolic and neuromuscular.[15, 17] We recommend that rehabilitation begins on the day of surgery or at least within 24 hours.

Immediate Considerations

Consideration during the first 24 hours should center on the following:

1. Immediate postoperative effusion.[18, 19]
2. Possible formation of hematoma due to the trauma of joint access.[20]
3. Alteration of the joint surface due to capsular trauma and procedures performed within the joint, such as sharp dissection of adhesions.
4. Changes in proprioceptive response due to the actual trauma to the joint capsule and physical alteration of joint surfaces.[15, 29]
5. Perceived pain.
6. Muscle guarding directly from stretch manipulation during the operative procedure and indirectly from perceived pain from the operative site.

Postoperative Goals and Treatment

Postoperative goals are best divided into immediate, short-term, and long-term categories. Immediate goals during the first 24 hours have been discussed previously. Included in this category is the immediate mobility of the TMJ, with emphasis on protective translation to maintain the surgical result and prevent adhesion formation.

Treatment Modalities (Table 19–1)

Contrast Applications of Heat and Cold. Heat and cold should be applied using a maximum of 8-minute intervals for each and ending with cold to maintain a constant vasoconstrictive effect to minimize edema.[21, 22]

Electrical Stimulation. High-voltage stimulation at pulse rates from 1 to 4, at proper intensity, creates a minimal visible contraction (Fig. 19–1)[21, 22] This acts as a mechanical pump to reduce effusion materials. Interferential current at various beat frequencies can be effective for edema, pain, and autonomic stimulation. Transcutaneous electrical nerve stimulation (TENS) has been shown to be beneficial in tissue healing, particularly bone.

Soft Tissue Rehabilitation Techniques. These techniques should be used on the muscles of the cervical and craniomandibular regions. Postsurgical muscle trismus is commonly noted, with trigger points and tender areas. These may be treated with muscle energy and soft tissue mobilization techniques (Fig. 19–2). We have found that there is soft tissue trauma to the upper cervical areas due to positioning of the patient's head during the operative procedure.

Joint Mobilization. Mobilization of the TMJ for vertical distraction is done to en-

Table 19-1. PATHOLOGIES AND MODALITIES THAT MAY BE USED IN THE PHYSICAL THERAPY MANAGEMENT OF PATIENTS WITH TEMPOROMANDIBULAR JOINT DISORDERS

Condition	Stage	Possible Treatment Modalities	Goals
Musculoskeletal (includes referred pain)	Acute	Cryotherapy, ultrasound, soft tissue massage, direct and indirect trigger point techniques, muscle energy techniques, proprioceptive neuromuscular facilitation, TENS. Iontophoresis and phonophoresis may also be helpful. The patient may be taught self–trigger point massage, spray and stretch techniques, home cryotherapy, and exercises.	Decrease pain, spasm, and inflammation and increase ROM; prevent adhesion formation.
	Subacute	Cryotherapy/moist heat (depending on the type of tissue), ultrasound, soft tissue massage and/or mobilization, direct and/or indirect trigger point techniques, proprioceptive neuromuscular facilitation, HVGS, therapeutic exercises. Conclude with cryotherapy; may include BFT. Home program continues; may add BFT.	Decrease inflammation, spasm, and fibrosis; increase tissue extensibility.
	Chronic	Cryotherapy/moist heat, ultrasound, HVGS, STM, PNF, postural exercise, iontophoresis, phonophoresis; frictioning, BFT. Conclude with cryotherapy, home exercises, self-stretching, and BFT.	Decrease spasm, fibrosis, adhesions, and inflammation.
Hypomobility (closed locked condition with or without reduction of displaced disc)	Acute*	Cryotherapy/ultrasound, indirect trigger point techniques, muscle energy techniques, PNF, therapeutic exercises, mobilization techniques, disc reseating (recapture) techniques; MHP and HVGS point stimulation to relax muscles. Home program may include cryotherapy, exercise, TENS, self-mobilization.	Decrease inflammation, spasm, and pain; soft tissue relaxation, disc relocation.
	Subacute*	Cryotherapy/MHP, ultrasound, STM, muscle energy techniques, trigger point techniques, HVGS, spray and stretch techniques, mobilization, disc reseating techniques, therapeutic exercise. Increase home exercise program to include mechanical changes with opening and self-mobilization.	Decrease spasm and inflammation; soft tissue relaxation with increased extensibility of fibrous capsule; disc relocation.
	Chronic*	Cryotherapy/MHP, ultrasound, STM, muscle energy techniques, trigger point techniques, HVGS, mobilization, therapeutic exercise, spray and stretch techniques. Home program emphasizes active	Increased extensibility of the fibrous joint capsule; destruction of adhesions.

Table 19-1. PATHOLOGIES AND MODALITIES THAT MAY BE USED IN THE PHYSICAL THERAPY MANAGEMENT OF PATIENTS WITH TEMPOROMANDIBULAR JOINT DISORDERS Continued

Condition	Stage	Possible Treatment Modalities	Goals
		mobility and normalization of joint mechanics.	
Hypermobility		Treatment modalities are the same as those for hypomobility. Mobilization techniques for both spine and TMJ should reflect areas of normalization of joint integrity and movement.	Decrease extensibility of certain tissues; decrease pain, spasm, etc.; prevent change to hypomobility.
Musculotendinous (cuff lesions, partial tears of joint capsule)	Acute	Cryotherapy, HVGS, indirect muscle relaxation techniques, iontophoresis, phonophoresis. Home stabilization and exercise program.	Decrease inflammation and pain; maintain muscle integrity.
	Subacute	Cryotherapy/MHP, HVGS, ultrasound, muscle relaxation techniques, iontophoresis, therapeutic stabilization exercise, mobilization. Continued home program with addition of self-mobilization.	Decrease inflammation, spasm, and pain; decrease protective responses; maintain muscle ROM.
	Chronic (progresses to adhesive capsulitis)	Cryotherapy/MHP, HVGS, ultrasound, muscle relaxation, mobilization, therapeutic exercises. Home program emphasizes ROM and self-mobilization.	Achieve normal joint integrity; destruction of adhesions.
Surgical repair	Acute	Cryotherapy with MHP for edema, HVGS, TENS, STM, muscle relaxation techniques, mobilization (depending of type of surgical repair).	Prevention of adhesions, edema, and pain; muscle relaxation techniques; maintain joint mechanics.
	Subacute	Cryotherapy/MHP, HVGS, ultrasound, STM, muscle relaxation techniques, mobilization, therapeutic exercise. Home program to maintain joint mechanics and prevent deformation.	Maintain joint integrity and mobility; normalized joint mechanics.
Adhesive capsulitis		Cryotherapy/MHP, HVGS, ultrasound, muscle relaxation techniques, mobilization, therapeutic exercise, TENS. Home program emphasizes maintained joint ROM and integrity as well as prevention of redeformation; self mobilization, stretching exercises, ADL training.	Achieve normal joint integrity; decrease pain, spasm, and protective muscle response; destruction of adhesions.
Postsurgical trismus	Acute	Cryotherapy/MHP, muscle relaxation techniques, mobilization, relaxation exercises, iontophoresis, phonophoresis.	Stimulate muscle relaxation; prevent edema and spasm; reduce pain; maintain joint integrity.
	Subacute	Cryotherapy, muscle relaxation techniques, mobilization, therapeutic exercises. Home program.	Reduce pain, edema, and spasm; normalize joint integrity and mechanics.

Table continued on following page

Table 19–1. PATHOLOGIES AND MODALITIES THAT MAY BE USED IN THE PHYSICAL THERAPY MANAGEMENT OF PATIENTS WITH TEMPOROMANDIBULAR JOINT DISORDERS Continued

Condition	Stage	Possible Treatment Modalities	Goals
Arthritis	Acute	Cryotherapy/MHP, iontophoresis, phonophoresis, mobilization, muscle relaxation. Home program maximizes muscle relaxation and minimizes joint pressure.	Decrease inflammation and pain; maintain joint function. Maximize joint space.
	Subacute	Cryotherapy/MHP, iontophoresis, phonophoresis, ultrasound, muscle relaxation, mobilization; home program to reduce joint friction and maintain ROM and flexibility.	Decrease pain, edema, and spasm; maintain joint integrity and mobility.
	Chronic		Reduction of pain, edema, and spasm; maintain joint integrity; retard progression of condition.

*Stages may change from chronic to subacute or from subacute to chronic, etc., in regard to joint integrity. Treatment should be altered as joint and muscle status changes.
Mobilization may refer to mobilization of vertebral, cranial, or temporomandibular joints. ROM = range of motion; TENS = transcutaneous electrical nerve stimulation; HVGS = High-voltage galvanic stimulation; BFT = Biofeedback techniques; STM = Soft tissue mobilization; PNF = proprioceptive neuromuscular facilitation; MHP = moist heat pack; TMJ = temporomandibular joint; ADL = activities of daily living.

courage synovial fluid production and lateral and protected translatoric joint capsule mobility (Fig. 19–3). Protective protrusive movements require anterior translation of the mandible from a long axis to distracted position with or without the presence of a postoperative orthotic. Mobilization of the vertebral system is based both on pre- and postoperative objective findings. Preoperative findings include specific segmental mobility limitations noted in the vertebral system, which may contribute to the surgical pathology. An example would be a restricted forward bending of vertebra of C1 or C7, as is often seen in forward head postures. Postoperative findings include limitations or changes in functional mobility that take place as acute trauma during the operative procedure, due to positioning and transportation of the patient while under anesthesia.

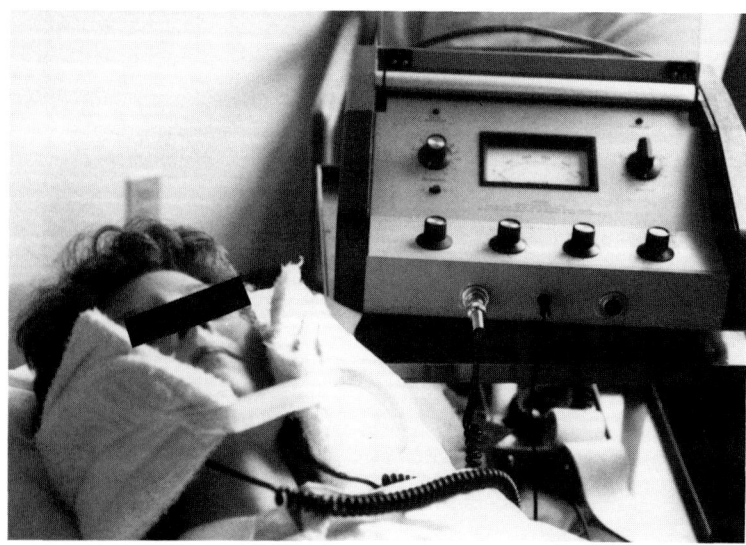

Figure 19–1. Immediate postoperative application of high voltage electrical stimulation.

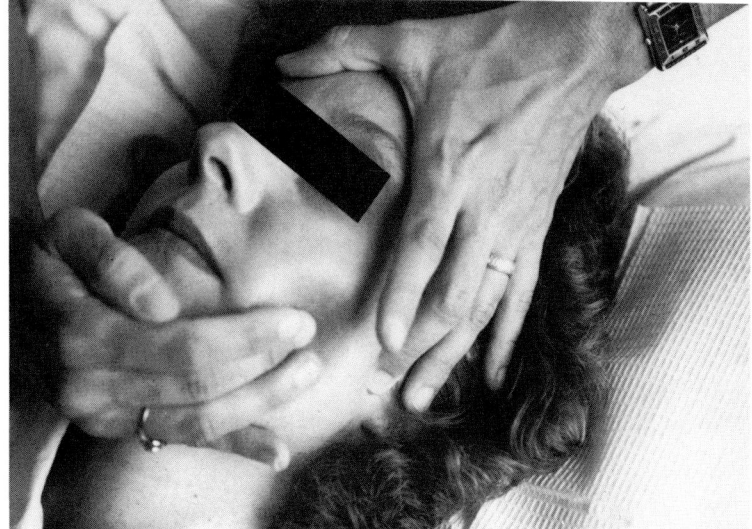

Figure 19-2. Indirect technique of strain/counterstrain for postoperative masseter pain.

Therapeutic Exercises. These exercises assist the patient in reducing muscle guarding as well as maintaining disc mobility. Postoperative magnetic resonance image studies indicate that the movement of the disc is more important than its relative position. Postoperative exercises include the following:

1. Placing the tongue against the roof of the mouth in the posterior one-third of the palate and then opening and closing the mouth in 1-second intervals with the tongue in that position.
2. Placing two tongue blades in the mouth across the lateral incisors and moving the mandible separately in protrusive, right laterotrusive, and then left laterotrusive movements (Fig. 19-4). (*Note:* retrusive movements have been intentionally omitted, as experience has shown that they serve no useful function.) Laterotrusive movements may be performed easily using a cotton roll between the incisors (Fig. 19-5). Again, these lateral movements should be done in one direction at a time.
3. Resistive opening exercises to facilitate inhibition of the mandibular closing muscles (Fig. 19-6). Exercises to relax the other muscles of the craniomandibular and vertebral system should also be begun immediately.

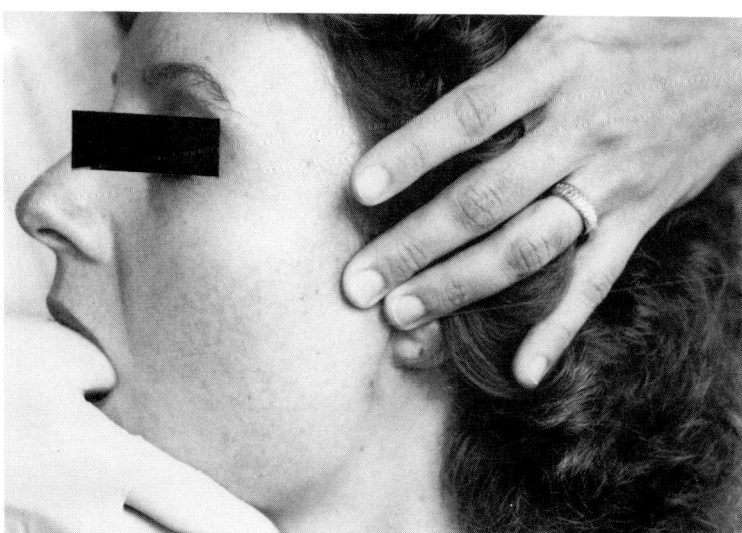

Figure 19-3. Intraoral joint mobilization for protective translatoric glide.

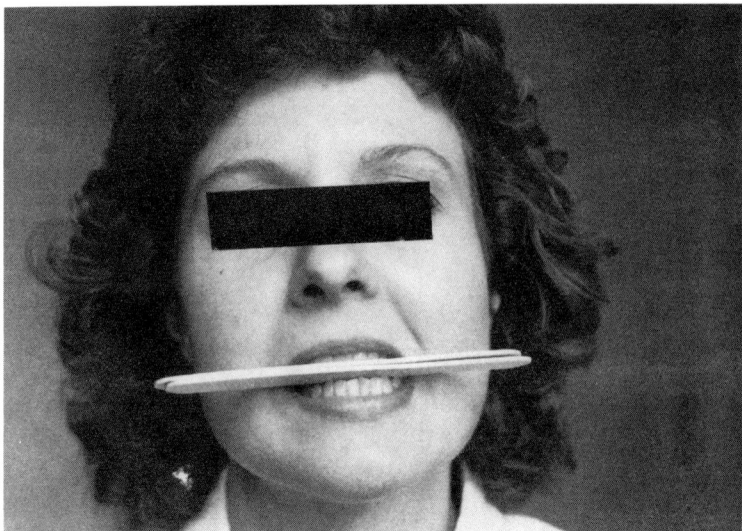

Figure 19–4. Home exercise to maintain protected laterotrusion.

Home Program. The modalities and exercises performed in the immediate postoperative phase, as previously described, should be modified so that they can be repeated easily at home. Establishment of and compliance with a home program regimen are absolute requirements for the long-term success of the surgical and therapeutic process. To assist in compliance, home exercise programs should be brief, easy to do in the required number of repetitions, and require a minimum of disruption of daily activities. Modalities should include short application of cold, using plastic bags of ice or frozen vegetables, and/or short applications of heat, using a moist compress. Home use of a TENS unit may also be useful for promoting tissue healing, particularly bone tissue, as well as for pain control.

Short-Term Goals

Short-term goals include therapy following the resolution of the immediate postoperative effusion, trauma, and edema and continuing for 21 to 30 days postoperatively. The therapist should concentrate on working with the patient on tongue and joint proprio-

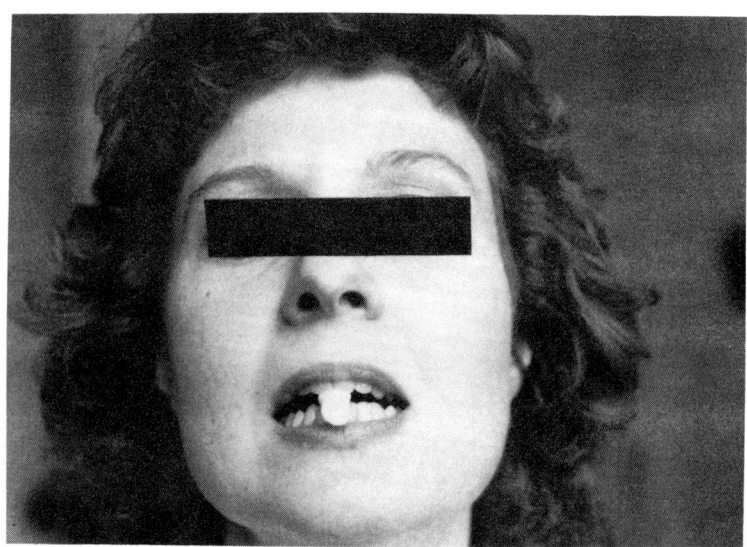

Figure 19–5. Home exercise using cotton roll for protected laterotrusion and proprioceptive training.

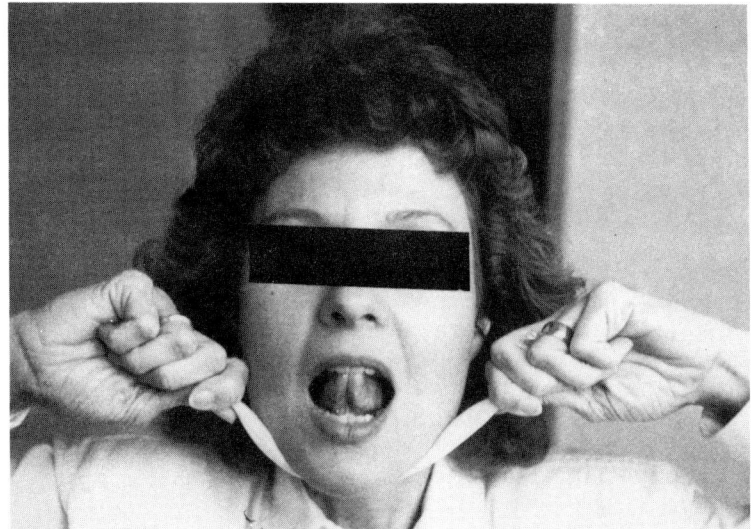

Figure 19–6. Home exercise for resisted opening with emphasis on rotational cycle.

ception to normalize movement into the newly gained range in all directions.[9, 22] Emphasis should be placed on the resting posture of the head and neck.[2]

In the absence of edema, the practitioner may use cold packs for 15 minutes to increase synovial viscosity and to improve lubrication and protection within the joint, or continuous moist hot packs may be applied for periods of less than 15 minutes to decrease collagen bonding.

The therapist may also use pulsed or continuous ultrasound as a mechanical deep-heating agent as well as for its other properties. It should be noted, however, that recent studies on aseptic necrosis in the mandibular condyle suggest caution in repeated use of ultrasound.[20]

Functional electrical stimulation may be utilized to stabilize hypermobility, prevent atrophy, and for ligamentous strengthening (Fig. 19–7).

Joint mobilization of the TMJs bilaterally emphasizes a normal rotation–translation relationship during all phases of opening. The goal is to maintain disc mobility.

Therapeutic exercises should also emphasize bilateral muscle function in all phases of

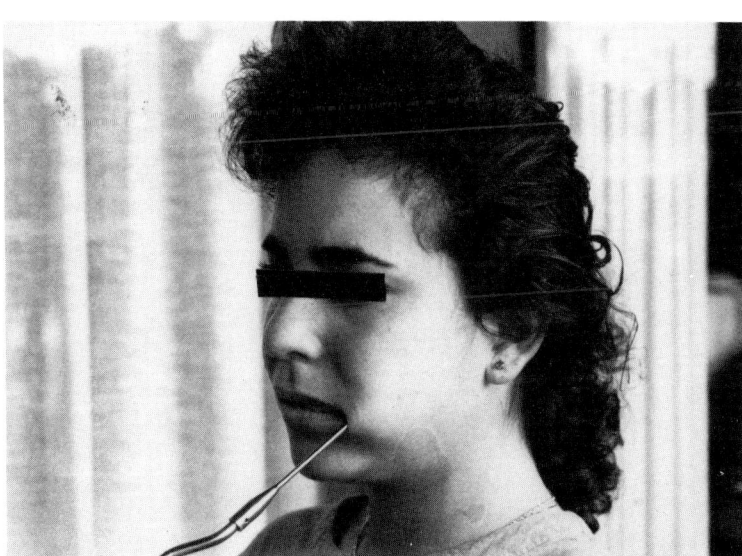

Figure 19–7. Intraoral electrical stimulation for masseter and medial pterygoid muscles.

opening. The goal is to attain symmetry, with both joints working in harmony. This is of particular significance in dealing with unilateral cases in which there is hypomobility on the operative side and hypermobility on the contralateral side.

Long-Term Goals

Long-term goals, following the initial 21- to 30-day period, center around maintaining the functional result of the surgery. In addition, extrinsic factors affecting the TMJ must be minimized. Vertebral posture and function that may adversely affect the TMJ require management. Goals should also address the modification or removal of any orthotic devices placed at the time of or prior to surgery and the inclusion of any future orthodontic and/or orthognathic considerations.

At this point, no additional physical therapy modalities are recommended, except to manage any acute exacerbations that may occur. Patients should be on a complete home rehabilitation program and should require only periodic follow-up for monitoring of movement and function as well as any fine-tuning of exercise programs. The sequence of visits is dependent on the degree of patient progress with considerations given to future treatment.

SUMMARY

A brief overview has been presented of the physical rehabilitation process for patients who undergo TMJ arthroscopy. Although further study of the specifics is indicated, the information supplied here will provide the practitioner with an understanding of general treatment goals. A thorough presurgical evaluation cannot be overemphasized, as it is the basis for knowledgeable postoperative treatment. Strong emphasis also has been placed on utilization of the physical therapist with specialized training and experience in dealing with patients with craniomandibular problems.

References

1. Grisolia JS: Course Materials, 1981.
2. Ayub E, et al: Head posture: A case study of the effects on the rest position of the mandible. J Orthop Sports Phys Therapy 5(4):179–183, 1984.
3. Clark GT: Craniocervical dysfunction levels in a patient sample from a temporomandibular joint clinic. JADA 115:231–236, 1987.
4. Dvorak J: General principles of palpation. In Manual Medicine. Manual Medicine Diagnostics. New York: Georg Thieme Verlag, 1984.
5. Travell JG: Myofascial Pain and Dysfunction. Baltimore: Williams & Wilkins, 1983.
6. Jones LH: Strain and Counterstrain. American Academy of Osteopathy, Colorado Springs, Colorado, 1981.
7. Soderberg GL: Muscle mechanics and pathomechanics. Phys Ther 63(2):216–220, 1983.
8. Moffett B: Anatomy and physiology of the temporomandibular joint and mechanics of growth and remodeling of the temporomandibular joint. Lecture syllabus: The Anteriorly Displaced Disc: How it Becomes Displaced and How it is Treated. Clinical Research Foundation, University of Washington. September, 1988.
9. Rocabado M: Temporomandibular Joint Disc Pathology. Tacoma, WA: Rocabado Institute, 1983.
10. Bourbon BM: Anatomy and biomechanics of the TMJ. In Krau SL (ed): TMJ Disorders: Management of the Craniomandibular Complex. New York: Churchill Livingstone, 1988.
11. Merlini L, et al: The relationship between condylar rotation and anterior translation in healthy and clicking temporomandibular joints. Schweiz Monatsschr Zahnmed 98:1181–2000, 1988.
12. Tanaka T: Advanced dissection of the temporomandibular joint. An instructional overview. Pacific Clinical Research Foundation, San Diego, California, 1988.
13. Isacsson G, et al: Internal derangement of the temporomandibular joint: Radiographic and histologic changes associated with severe pain. J Oral Maxillofac Surg 44:771–778, 1986.
14. Moses JJ: Personal communication.
15. Grieve GP: Modern Manual Therapy of the Vertebral Column. New York: Churchill Livingstone, 1982, pp. 206–249.
16. Johnson CL: Physical therapists as scar modifiers. Phys Ther 64(9):1381–1387, 1984.
17. Van Der Meulen JCH: Present state of knowledge on processes of healing in collagen structures. Int J Sports Med 3:4–8, 1982.
18. Moses JJ: Arthroscopy of the Temporomandibular Joint. Instructional Video, Stryker Corp.
19. Fryman VM: Basic Cranial Course Syllabus. College of Osteopathic Medicine of the Pacific, Pomona, California, 1987.
20. Schwartz RD: The role of synovium and articular cartilage. In Proceedings of Third International Conference in TMJ Arthroscopy. Hospital for Joint Diseases, New York, June 23–24, 1989.
21. Manheimer JS: Therapeutic modalities. In Kraus SL (ed): TMJ Disorders: Management of the Craniomandibular Complex. New York: Churchill Livingstone, 1988.
22. Rocabado M: Physical therapy for the postsurgical patient. J Craniomandib Disord Fac Oral Pain 3:75–82, 1989.

Chapter 20

PHARMACOLOGIC MANAGEMENT FOLLOWING ARTHROSCOPY

*RICHARD H. HAUG, D.D.S.,
MOHAN THOMAS, D.D.S., F.A.C.D*

The pharmacologic management of patients with temporomandibular joint (TMJ) disorders includes primary and secondary medications. The first line of therapy includes local anesthetics, analgesics, anti-inflammatory agents, anxiolytics, and antidepressants. The second line includes antipsychotics, antimigraines, anticonvulsants, muscle relaxants, and placebos. The pharmacologic therapy of rheumatic joint disorders includes narcotic and non-narcotic analgesics, anti-inflammatory agents, psychotherapeutic drugs, and medications such as gold, immunosuppressive agents, and antimalarials, which work by unknown mechanisms. The primary goals of the treatment of patients with joint disorders include control of pain, reduction of swelling, and relief of stiffness. Included in the overall management of this group of patients is control of anxiety and depression; this enhances the patient's well-being and may alter the perception of pain. The postoperative pharmacologic management of the arthroscopic surgical patient shares the same goals and concerns.

PHASES OF PHARMACOLOGIC THERAPY

The aims and considerations of pharmacologic therapy can be divided into immediate perioperative, short-term postoperative, and long-term postoperative.

The immediate postoperative phase begins in the operating room and ends with the hospital discharge of the patient. Pharmacologic therapy during this period includes those medicaments that may be delivered through the arthroscope and that may provide both short-term and long-term benefits. Local anesthesia may be introduced through the arthroscope or periarticularly to provide immediate postoperative pain relief. Glucocorticoids may be administered as one-time injections to provide an anti-inflammatory effect. Sodium hyaluronate may be introduced intra-articularly to enhance the viscoelasticity of the synovium.

The short-term postoperative phase begins at hospital discharge and continues for approximately 6 to 8 weeks after the surgical procedure. Concerns during this period include (1) control of postoperative pain so that physical therapy may be initiated and (2) the reduction of swelling, stiffness, and inflammation of the joints. Nonsteroidal, salicylate, and nonsalicylate anti-inflammatory agents are useful in the reduction of these signs and symptoms.

The long-term postoperative phase begins 6 to 8 weeks postsurgically. If pain persists after this period, serious consideration should be given to reconsidering the preoperative diagnosis, ruling out co-existing disease, and searching for pain of a nonarticular origin. Semisynthetic narcotic combinations and nonsteroidal anti-inflammatory agents are useful. Mood elevators and anti-anxiety drugs have been shown to be effective.

Immediate Postoperative Phase

Local Anesthesia

At the termination of the arthroscopic procedure, attention should be directed toward control of the surgically induced pain. A long-acting local anesthetic introduced through the arthroscope or by periarticular infiltration will be effective until enteral analgesics may be absorbed. Bupivacaine 0.25% is effective for this purpose; the duration of the anesthesia may last up to 7 hours, with prolonged analgesic effects. Bupivacaine is a local amide anesthetic that is metabolized in the liver and excreted through the kidneys. It is well tolerated by the tissues. The only absolute contraindication to its use is patient hypersensitivity. If an infiltration is used, paralysis of the facial nerve should be considered.

Glucocorticoids

A number of glucocorticoids are effective as anti-inflammatory agents when administered arthroscopically (Table 20–1). Although the dosages and concentrations may differ for individual drugs, the therapeutic effects are similar. At the macroscopic level, one-time intra-articular injections are effective in reducing local warmth, erythema, swelling, tenderness, and stiffness. Microscopically, edema, fibrin deposition, capillary dilatation, leukopedesis, and phagocytic activity are reduced. The pharmacologic effect is primarily local, but some mild systemic effects may be realized.

Glucocorticoids are available as synthetic and naturally occurring adrenocortical steroids. The relative anti-inflammatory efficacy differs with each drug (see Table 20–1). Metabolism occurs via the liver, with excretion in the urine or bile. One-time dosages will not render the patient adrenal-compromised or evoke any of the symptoms of Cushing's disease. The only contraindications are in patients with known hypersensitivity or systemic fungal infections.

Sodium Hyaluronate

Sodium hyaluronate is a high-molecular-weight polymer composed of disaccharide units and glucuronate. It is well tolerated by the body and has been used extensively for ophthalmologic surgery. A 1.0% solution may be injected intra-articularly to improve the viscoelastic properties of the joint and synovium postoperatively. Presently there are no known contraindications. Reports of side effects and adverse reactions have been insignificant.

Immediate Postsurgical Phase

Combination Semisynthetic Narcotic Analgesics

Combination semisynthetic narcotic analgesics are effective for various degrees of pain during the first few days postoperatively (Table 20–2). The chemical composition varies in this group of drugs; however, the semisynthetic narcotic component has effects similar to morphine, and the salicylate

Table 20–1. COMMONLY USED ANTI-INFLAMMATORY GLUCOCORTICOIDS FOR INTRA-ARTICULAR INJECTION

Generic Name (Trade Name)	Concentration (Dosage)	Relative Potency (1–30)	Contraindications
Triamcinolone diacetate (Aristocort)	40 mg/ml (5–40 mg)	5	Systemic fungal infections
Triamcinolone acetonide (Kenalog 10)	10 mg/ml (2.5–5 mg)	5	Systemic fungal infections
Betamethasone (Celestone)	3.0 mg/ml (1.5–3.0 mg)	30	Systemic fungal infections
Cortisone (Cortone)	25 mg/ml (25 mg)	1	Systemic fungal infections Hypersensitivity
Dexamethasone (Decadron)	4.0 mg/ml (0.8–1 mg)	25	Systemic fungal infections Hypersensitivity
Methylprednisolone (Depo-Medrol)	40 mg/ml (4–10 mg)	5	Systemic fungal infections Hypersensitivity
Prednisolone (Hydeltrasol)	20 mg/ml (5–20 mg)	4	Systemic fungal infections Hypersensitivity
Hydrocortisone (Hydrocortone)	25 mg/ml (10–25 mg)	1	Systemic fungal infections Hypersensitivity

Table 20-2. COMMONLY USED ANALGESICS

Generic Name (Trade Name)	Dosage and Administration	Drug Class	Effects	Principal Side Effects	Contraindications
Oxycodone 4.88 mg plus aspirin 325 mg (Percodan)	one tab po q4h; prn	Combination semisynthetic narcotic and salicylate analgesic	Relief of moderate to moderately severe pain	Drug dependence, vertigo, sedation, nausea	Hypersensitivity
Oxycodone 5.0 mg plus acetaminophen (Tylox 500 mg; Percocet 325 mg)	one tab po q4h; prn	Combination semisynthetic narcotic and nonsalicylate analgesic	Relief of moderate to moderately severe pain	Drug dependence, vertigo, sedation, nausea	Hypersensitivity
Dihydrocodeine 16 mg plus aspirin 326.4 mg plus caffeine 30 mg (Synalgos DC)	one tab po q4h; prn	Combination semisynthetic narcotic and salicylate analgesic	Relief of moderate to moderately severe pain	Vertigo, sedation, nausea	Hypersensitivity
Hydrocodone 50 mg plus acetaminophen 500 mg (Vicodin)	one tab po q4h; prn	Combination semisynthetic narcotic and nonsalicylate analgesic	Relief of moderate to moderately severe pain	Drug dependence, vertigo, sedation, nausea	Hypersensitivity
Tylenol 325 mg plus codeine 30 mg (Tylenol #3; Phenaphen #3)	one or two tabs po q4h prn	Combination opium alkaloid and non-opiate, non-salicylate analgesic	Relief of mild to moderately severe pain	Drug dependence, vertigo, sedation, nausea	Hypersensitivity
Acetaminophen 325 mg, 500 mg (Tylenol; Datril)	one or two tabs po q4h prn	Nonopiate, nonsalicylate analgesic	Relief of mild pain; anti-inflammatory, antipyretic	Hepatotoxicity after 10 days	Hypersensitivity
Aspirin 325 mg, 500 mg (Bayer; Bufferin; Anacin)	one or two tabs po q4h prn	Non-narcotic analgesic	Relief of mild pain; anti-inflammatory, antipyretic	Gastrointestinal irritation, interference with platelet aggregation	Hypersensitivity; drug-induced asthma, nasal polyps, urticaria; chickenpox, flu

or nonsalicylate analgesic can provide anti-inflammatory effects. These medicaments provide significant analgesia, sedation, and anti-inflammatory actions during the early postoperative period to allow the initiation of physical therapy. The only absolute contraindication is patient hypersensitivity. Drug dependence is a major concern. Vertigo, sedation, and nausea are significant side effects. These drugs are metabolized in the liver and excreted in the kidneys.

Non-Narcotic Analgesics

Non-narcotic analgesics that are useful in the control of mild pain in the postoperative phase are aspirin and acetaminophen (see Table 20-2).

The salicylates eliminate mild pain, reduce fever, and are effective anti-inflammatory agents. These drugs act peripherally. Metabolism occurs via the liver, with excretion by the kidneys. The only contraindication is hypersensitivity. With long-term use, gastrointestinal upset may occur, and platelet aggregation will be inhibited. Aspirin should be avoided by patients with gout, ulcers, and the syndrome of asthma, nasal polyps, urticaria, and angioedema.

Acetaminophen is an effective mild analgesic and antipyretic. It acts peripherally, is metabolized by the liver, and is eliminated by the kidneys. This medication does not produce the same gastrointestinal side effects of aspirin, nor does it inhibit platelet aggregation. Long-term use may result in hepatic toxicity; therefore, administration should be discontinued after 10 days.

Table 20-3. COMMONLY USED NONSTEROIDAL ANTI-INFLAMMATORY AGENTS

Generic Name (Trade name)	Dosage	Elimination	Effects	Principal Side Effects	Contraindications
Flurbiprofen (Ansaid)	50–100 mg po qid	Metabolized and excreted in urine within 24 hours	Anti-inflammatory, analgesic, antipyretic	GI upset, perforating ulcer, headache, coagulopathy	Hypersensitivity, drug-induced asthma
Sulindac (Clinoril)	200 mg po bid	Hepatic metabolism; renal excretion	Anti-inflammatory, analgesic, antipyretic	GI upset, dizziness, rash	Hypersensitivity, drug-induced asthma
Diflunisal (Dolobid)	500 mg po tid	Hepatic metabolism; renal excretion	Anti-inflammatory, analgesic, antipyretic,	Nausea, GI upset, rash, headache	Hypersensitivity, drug-induced asthma, rash
Piroxicam (Feldene)	20 mg po qid	Hepatic metabolism; excreted in urine and feces	Anti-inflammatory, analgesic, antipyretic	Nausea, GI upset, anemia	Hypersensitivity, drug-induced asthma, nasal polyps, angioedema
Indomethacin (Indocin)	25–50 mg po bid	Hepatic metabolism; excreted in urine and bile	Anti-inflammatory, analgesic, antipyretic	Nausea, GI upset, headache, dizziness	Hypersensitivity, drug-induced asthma, urticaria
Meclofenamate (Meclomen)	50 mg po qid	Hepatic metabolism; excreted in urine and feces	Anti-inflammatory, analgesic, antipyretic	Diarrhea, vomiting, GI upset, flatulence; enhances effect of anticoagulants	Hypersensitivity, drug-induced asthma, rhinitis, urticaria
Fenoprofen (Nalfon)	200–300 mg po tid	Hepatic metabolism; renal excretion in 24 hours	Anti-inflammatory, analgesic, antipyretic, anti-arthritic	GI upset, nausea, vomiting, constipation, dizziness, pruritus, palpitations, nervousness	Hypersensitivity, impaired renal function, drug-induced asthma, rhinitis, urticaria
Naproxen (Naprosyn)	250–500 mg po bid	Hepatic metabolism; renal excretion	Anti-inflammatory, analgesic, antipyretic	GI upset, headache, dizziness, pruritus, tinnitus, edema	Use of Anaprox, hypersensitivity, drug-induced asthma, nasal polyps, rhinitis
Ketoprofen (Orudis)	50–100 mg po bid	Renal excretion	Anti-inflammatory, analgesic, antipyretic	GI upset, nausea, diarrhea, flatulence, headache, edema	Hypersensitivity, drug-induced asthma, urticaria
Tolmetin (Tolectin)	400 mg po tid	Hepatic metabolism; renal excretion	Anti-inflammatory, analgesic, antipyretic	Nausea, GI upset, diarrhea, flatulence, headache, hypertension, edema, dizziness	Hypersensitivity
Diclofenac (Voltaren)	50–75 mg po bid	Hepatic metabolism; urinary and biliary excretion	Anti-inflammatory, analgesic, antipyretic	Abdominal cramps, constipation, nausea, diarrhea, headache, edema	Hypersensitivity, drug-induced asthma, urticaria
Ibuprofen (Motrin, Advil, Rufen, Medipren, Nuprin)	400–800 mg po qid	Hepatic metabolism; renal excretion	Anti-inflammatory, analgesic, antipyretic	Nausea, GI upset, dizziness	Hypersensitivity, drug-induced asthma, nasal polyps, angioedema
Ketorolac tromethamine (Toradol)	15–30 mg IM q6h	Partial hepatic metabolism; excreted in urine and feces	Anti-inflammatory, analgesic, antipyretic	GI ulceration, GI upset, nausea, drowsiness	Hypersensitivity, drug-induced asthma, nasal polyps, angioedema

GI = gastrointestinal.

Nonsteroidal Anti-Inflammatory Agents

Numerous nonsteroidal anti-inflammatory drugs (NSAIDs) are marketed (Table 20-3). These drugs may be used by the post-arthroscopic surgical patient for 6 to 8 weeks to reduce stiffness, swelling, and tenderness, so that normal function can be initiated. NSAIDs inhibit the production of mediators of the inflammatory response, including polypeptides of the kinin system, prostaglandins, lysosomal enzymes, and lymphokines. Dosages may vary, but the pharmacologic effects are similar. NSAIDs are metabolized by the liver and are eliminated in the urine or bile. Gastrointestinal disturbances are the most common side effects. Occasional skin rashes, headache, and vertigo have been reported. These drugs should be avoided by patients with the syndrome of asthma, nasal polyps, urticaria, and angioedema.

Toradol is a new NSAIDs. Although given IM, pharmacodynamics are similar to enteral NSAIDs. It is an effective analgesic and anti-inflammatory agent. IM injections are required. It should not be given with enteral NSAIDs.

Long-Term Postoperative Phase

If pain persists for more than 8 weeks following arthroscopic surgery, serious consideration should be given to reconsidering the diagnosis, co-existing disease, advanced disease, and pain of nonarticular origin. If the TMJ pathoses most amenable to arthroscopic surgical therapy have been addressed, then further investigation and management are in order. Myofascial pain and dysfunction, headaches, pains of vascular etiology, neuralgia, myalgia, pain of psychogenic origin, and pain that may be exacerbated by depression should be identified. The management of these disorders is beyond the scope of this text.
GM

SUMMARY

The pharmacologic management of the postoperative arthroscopic surgical patient should be first directed at operative pain. This may be controlled with a long-acting local anesthetic followed by an enteral combination semisynthetic narcotic analgesic. Control of short-term pain to allow the initiation of movement and physical therapy may be provided by narcotic analgesics, non-narcotic analgesics, and nonsteroidal anti-inflammatory agents. Improvement in function by enhanced viscoelastic properties of the synovium may be provided by administration of sodium hyaluronate. Intra-articular glucocorticoids and enteral NSAIDs may provide control of swelling, tenderness, redness, and stiffness during the postoperative course to allow function and effective physical therapy. Pain refractory to arthroscopic surgery may need to be addressed by additional surgery or therapy directed at nonarticular etiologies.

Suggested Further Reading

Barnhart ER: Physicians' Desk Reference. Medical Economics, 1990.

Hart FD: Rheumatic disorders. In Avery G (ed): Pharmacologic Therapeutics. WB Saunders, 1980.

Gregg JM: Pharmacological management of myofascial pain dysfunction. In Laskin DM, Greenfield W, Gale E, et al (eds): *The President's Conference on the Examination, Diagnosis, and Management of TMJ Disorders*. Chicago: American Dental Association, 1982, pp. 167–173.

Gregg JM, Rugh JD: Pharmacological therapy. In Mohl ND, Zarb GA, Carlsson GE, Rugh JD (eds): *A Textbook of Occlusion*. Chicago: Quintessence, 1988, pp. 351–356.

Kalkwarf KL, Hinrichs JE, Shaw DH: Management of the dental patient receiving corticosteroid medications. Oral Surg, Oral Med, Oral Pathol 54:396–400, 1982.

Travis RH, Sayers G: Adrenocorticotropic hormone, adrenocortical steroids, and their synthetic analogs. In Goodman LS, Gilman A (eds): *The Pharmacological Basis of Therapeutics*. New York: Macmillan, 1965, pp. 1608–1648.

Chapter 21

COMPLICATIONS OF TEMPOROMANDIBULAR JOINT ARTHROSCOPY

JEFFREY B. CARTER, M.D., D.M.D.

Temporomandibular joint (TMJ) arthroscopy and arthroscopic surgery have had very rapid growth since the initial description by Ohnishi in 1975.[1] Early investigations by Hellsing and colleagues[2] in 1984 confirmed that arthroscopy was a beneficial diagnostic procedure. Cadaver studies by Holmlund and Hellsing[3] further standardized the approach to maximize exposure and limit morbidity. After investigating additional cadavers, Westesson and co-workers[4] confirmed the relative safety of the technique.

The prospect of replicating the benefits of arthrotomy with a less invasive procedure ignited enthusiasm for clinical application of the new technology. From initial experiences with diagnosis and lysis and lavage, isolated incidents of surgical misadventures were documented in the maxillofacial literature. Intraoperative bleeding was first described by Goss and Bosanquet.[5] Transient peripheral facial nerve weakness was recorded by Holmlund and colleagues.[6] These complications were similar to those attributed to arthrotomy.

As experience with arthroscopy expanded, a spectrum of potentially catastrophic complications, which had not been previously associated with TMJ arthrotomy, emerged in the literature. McCain[7] reported one incident of a middle cranial fossa perforation and cerebrospinal fluid leak. Sanders[8] described one case of otitis media with resultant hearing loss. Van Sickels and co-workers[9] subsequently reported a case of middle ear damage and ossicular disruption. These outcomes directed a new focus toward a more comprehensive and systematic compilation of the complications encountered during the first generation of arthroscopic procedures.

CLASSIFICATION

In an attempt to analyze statistically the incidence and severity of complications from TMJ arthroscopy, Carter and Testa[10] in 1987 performed the first multicenter retrospective study. Their research reviewed 2225 cases of arthroscopy, composed mainly of diagnostic procedures and lysis and lavage. The study showed a global complication rate of 10%. The limitations of the study were its retrospective design and its reliance on the surgeon's recall to document complications. Nevertheless, when compared with the orthopedic literature, TMJ arthroscopy poses a significantly higher risk of infection. In a prospective study conducted by Small,[11] the overall complication rate for arthroscopy of the knee and other joints was 1.68%.

Despite the limitations of the study by Carter and Testa, several important conclusions were drawn. First, the great majority of complications were perioperative. Most were short-term problems that resolved in the immediate postoperative period, without long-term sequelae. Second, several catastrophic outcomes were reported that previously had not been seen with TMJ arthrotomy. These required immediate attention and intensified further research efforts and technical refinement. A classification scheme was proposed by Carter and Schwaber[12] to identify complications with an adverse outcome secondary to a specific etiology. Figure 21-1 outlines this classification scheme.

ANESTHETIC COMPLICATIONS

Ambulatory Surgery

The technique of TMJ arthroscopy is most often performed using general anesthesia. A nasoendotracheal tube is used so that manipulation of the mandible remains unobstructed. The majority of first-generation arthroscopic procedures can be accomplished skillfully with a reliably short operative time. As a result, most TMJ arthroscopy is performed on an ambulatory basis. This represents a significant shift from arthrotomy, for which hospitalization is usually required. Large clinical studies of TMJ arthroscopy by both Indresano[13] and White[14] support the fact that the procedure can be performed on an outpatient basis without complication.

Upper Airway Obstruction

From their early cadaver studies, Holmlund and Hellsing[3] discovered that arthroscopic techniques may puncture the medial capsule of the TMJ. During the procedure, a significant amount of irrigant can be flushed through the small volume of the joint space. During lavage, this fluid is irrigated under intense pressure. An improperly placed outflow cannula or excessive pressure on the inflow irrigant may perforate the medial wall, allowing the fluid to infiltrate the medial masticatory space. The irrigant may further extravasate into the lateral pharyngeal space and distort the airway. In a series of 100 joints, White[14] described two cases that required prolonged intubation in the recovery room because of this problem. Neither of these cases required overnight hospitalization.

McCain's study of joint anatomy[15] revealed that the average TMJ was 25 mm from the skin and the medial wall was 50 mm from the skin. These depths should be heeded while inserting the trocar and before initiating lavage. Additional factors that can lead to fluid extravasation include longer operative times, difficult triangulation procedures, and the development of more complex second-generation surgical procedures. Regardless of the procedure or operative time, surgeons should thoroughly examine the oropharynx

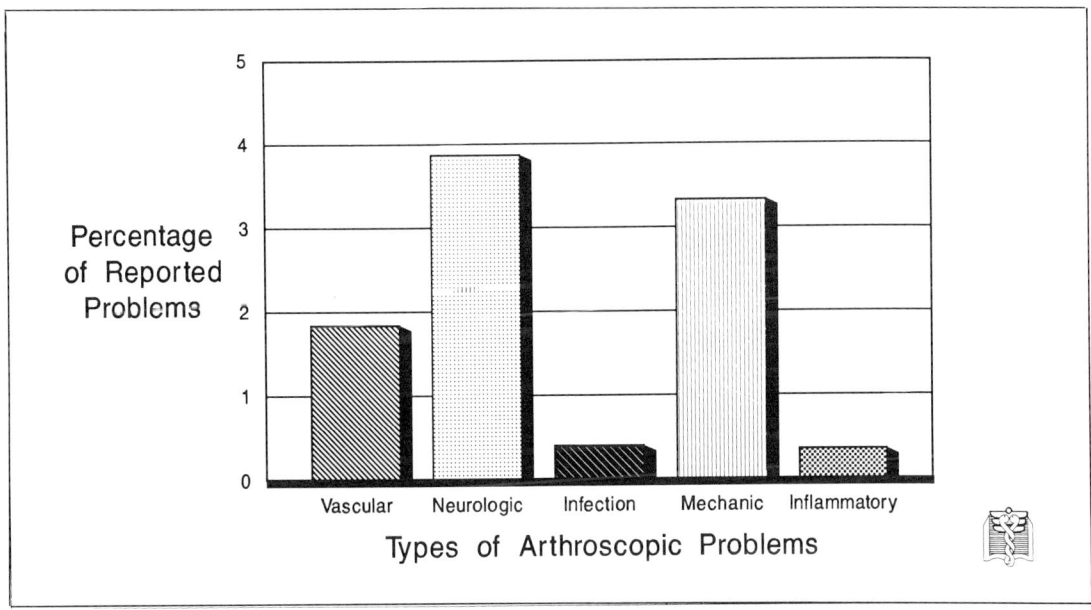

Figure 21-1. Complications of temporomandibular joint arthroscopy (N = 2225). (Reprinted with permission from Carter JB, Testa L: Complications of TMJ arthroscopy: A review of 2225 cases. J Oral Maxillofac Surg 46:M14–M15, 1988.)

prior to extubation to verify that the airway is clear of any distortion.

Arrhythmias

During TMJ arthroscopy, an adjunctive, vasoconstricting local anesthetic is used to distend the joint and promote hemostasis during the visual inspection. The vascular nature of the posterior synovial pouch and other nearby structures increases the risk of rapid absorption of the anesthetic, which can cause cardiac arrhythmia. Jones and Horn[16] reported one case of a patient who developed premature ventricular contractions with bigeminy after introduction of a 1:200,000 solution of epinephrine; the arrhythmia quickly resolved without treatment. Persistent ventricular irritability may require the introduction of intravenous lidocaine.

Manipulation of the mandible is critical to ensure complete inspection of the superior joint space. Sanders[8] was the earliest surgeon to recommend a first assistant for this task. Other surgeons prefer to use jaw distraction devices, which decrease the risk of contamination of the operative field. Either method of forced mandibular manipulation may result in inadvertent massage of the carotid body and may lead to an unsuspected bradycardia. Sinus bradycardia should be readily reversible by decreasing the manual manipulation over the carotid sinus. If it continues, atropine is indicated.

INFECTION

Incidence

Reports of postoperative infections following TMJ arthroscopy have been rare. In the retrospective study by Carter and Testa[10] in 1987, the overall rate of infection was less than 1%. Based on Small's data in 1988,[11] this rate is similar to that reported in the orthopedic literature.

Arthroscopic procedures may be contraindicated when infection is present in structures adjacent to the pathway of the endoscope. Nevertheless, in 1984 Murakami and co-workers[17] reported the successful use of arthroscopy to diagnose suppurative arthritis in the TMJ. In addition, they believed that lysis and lavage had a therapeutic benefit.

They reported no adverse postoperative complications from disseminated infection or regional cellulitis.

In 1986, Sanders[8] described one case of otitis media as a postoperative sequela subsequent to arthroscopy. In a retrospective study of arthroscopic surgery on 897 patients, Greene and Van Sickels[18] reported one incident of external otitis following lysis and lavage. Indresano[13] also reported one incident of external otitis that resolved without long-term consequences.

As surgeons move from the first-generation arthroscopic procedures to more complex and time-consuming maneuvers, theoretically the risk of infection increases. Tarro[19] published the results of 40 arthroscopic procedures consisting of an anterior release and the placement of a posterior suture. Of these, 14 joints also underwent electrocautery of the posterior ligament to aid in retention of the repositioned disc. Despite the complexity of these procedures, he reported only one postoperative infection. No organism was identified. The patient responded to a 5-day course of cephalexin 500 mg three times daily.

Prophylactic Antibiotics

The data of Small[11] in the orthopedic literature implicated *Staphylococcus aureus*, *S. epidermidis*, and *Streptococcus* spp. as the bacteria positively identified in the few cases of postoperative infection. An exhaustive review of the literature on TMJ arthroscopy found no reported cases of infection in which a causative organism was named. Surgeons have approached this problem empirically and have resorted to a wide variety of prophylactic regimens. Goss and Bosanquet[5] initially recommended the administration of one million units of intravenous penicillin as a bolus dose. Tarro[20] favored the use of 1 g of cefazolin as an intravenous bolus post-induction. In a larger clinical series by Moses and Poker,[21] the use of 1 g of cephalexin preoperatively was advocated, followed by oral cephalexin 500 mg every 6 hours for 5 days. White[14] recommended the use of a cephalosporin intravenously as well 4 days postoperatively. Both studies reported no significant infections.

At times when external otitis has occurred, adverse outcomes have not been reported.

Most workers state that the infection resolved spontaneously. White[14] suggested the routine use of corticosteroid ear drops for 5 days to alleviate inflammation within the canal.

In summary, the literature supports the use of prophylactic antibiotics; as with orthopedic experience, a cephalosporin is favored over penicillin. There is no documented difference in the infection rate with blast prophylaxis alone compared with blast prophylaxis followed by several days of oral antibiotics. Prescription of postoperative antibiotics is not warranted in most cases.

Preparation of the Surgical Site

TMJ arthroscopy is performed under sterile conditions. The preauricular area is isolated. When necessary, hair is shaved. The site is scrubbed for 10 minutes, and the ear canal is prepared with a sterile swab. White[14] documented one incident of an iatrogenic puncture of the tympanic membrane during this procedure. This complication is preventable by previous insertion of petroleum jelly–soaked gauze into the ear canal.

Instrument Preparation

The handling of delicate electronic video equipment is a new challenge for the oral and maxillofacial surgical scrub nurse. Conventional sterilization techniques of autoclaving at 270°F for 3 minutes suffice for hand instruments, trocars, and probes. Arthroscopes, video cameras, and power shavers and cords may be sterilized with ethylene oxide gas. In the orthopedic literature, Johnson[22] alternatively recommends the use of 2% glutaraldehyde sodium (Cidex) for a 30-minute soak. This technique is helpful in ambulatory suites in which multiple arthroscopies are scheduled in succession.

NEUROLOGIC INJURIES

Unlike arthroscopy performed on other joints, TMJ procedures are conducted in an area of great anatomic complexity. The arborizing pattern of the motor and sensory nerves creates a web that surrounds the structure (Fig. 21–2). Neurologic injuries are the most common complications reported in the larger retrospective studies by Greene

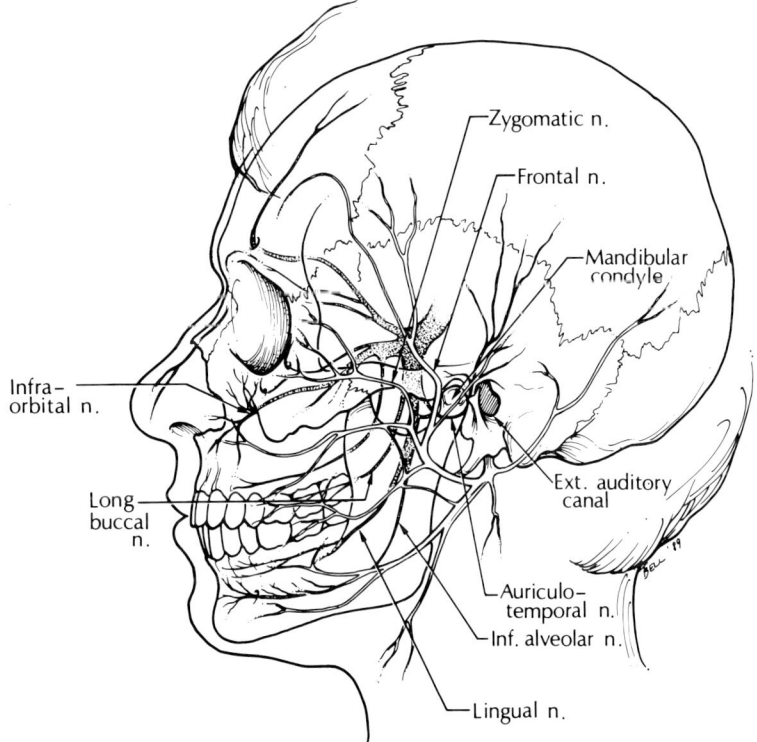

Figure 21–2. Neuroanatomy of the temporomandibular joint. (Reprinted with permission from Carter JB, Schwaber MK: Temporomandibular joint arthroscopy: Complications and their management. Oral Maxillofac Surg Clin North Am 1:185–199, 1989.)

and Van Sickels[18] and by Carter and Testa.[10]

Central Nervous System

The roof of the glenoid fossa is characterized by a thin, bony lamina that forms the floor of the middle cranial fossa. This structure is at risk for perforation by the misguided passage of an arthroscope or trocar. McCain[7] reported an incident in which an accessory instrument punctured the fossa and dura, resulting in a cerebrospinal fluid (CSF) leak. A neurosurgeon was immediately consulted, and the reconstructive arthroplasty was able to be completed as planned. A postoperative computerized tomography (CT) scan showed no damage to the cerebral cortex. In the review by Carter and Testa[10] of 2225 cases, this was the only documented case.

If the middle cranial fossa is punctured, management of the CSF leak should be supportive. A pressure dressing should be applied, and the patient should be hospitalized with the head elevated. In most cases, the dura seals and the leak spontaneously ceases. Persistent CSF leaks are an indication for neurosurgical intervention. A subarachnoid drain may be inserted, and the patient should have a CT scan (with bone windows) to evaluate the portal of entry. Surgical repair of such a defect rarely should be necessary.

Experience with newer imaging techniques on patients who have had previous arthroplasties and implants has revealed patterns of altered bony morphology in the glenoid fossa. Schellhas and colleagues[23] encountered some destruction of the roof of the fossa by an enlarging granuloma in patients who previously received a Teflon-Proplast implant (Vitek, Inc., Houston, TX). Because of the distorted anatomy, these patients are considered at high risk for probable CSF perforation. Application of arthroscopic techniques may be contraindicated in these patients.

Peripheral Nerve Injuries

Cranial nerves V and VII course very close to the capsule of the TMJ. The position of the auriculotemporal nerve makes it particularly vulnerable to injury. This has been well established from prior experience with open arthrotomy. Because of the risk of perioperative fluid extravasation, the potential for injury to this nerve may occur more readily during arthroscopic procedures. Motor weakness of cranial nerve VII appears to be less problematic with arthroscopy than with arthrotomy. However, because of cosmetic and ophthalmologic considerations, these risks must be defined by the surgeon.

Cranial Nerve V Injuries

Infraorbital Nerve. The infraorbital nerve exits at the infraorbital foramen and is the terminal branch of the second division of the trigeminal nerve (see Fig. 2–2). To date, the literature has not reported any incidence of injury to this nerve in an open TMJ procedure. However, when surgeons are first becoming acquainted with arthroscopy or when they are performing a second-generation technique, operative times may be prolonged and fluid extravasation is more likely to occur. If the infraorbital region is invaded, transient hypoesthesia may result. This usually resolves 2 to 3 hours postoperatively, although White[14] reported one case that took 3 days. No long-term morbidity has been associated with this problem.

Lingual Nerve. Prolonged anesthesia of the tongue in the postoperative period is usually secondary to technique. Inadvertent puncture of the medial capsular structures will cause medial extravasation of fluid into the pterygomandibular space. Hydrostatic pressure on the lingual nerve will result in a transient hypoesthesia. It is important during the postoperative examination to differentiate this type of neurologic injury from a complaint of numbness only in the tip of the tongue. Aggressive manipulation of the mandible by the surgical assistant may trap the tongue between the incisors. This type of injury usually resolves within a few days and requires only usual care.

Inferior Alveolar Nerve. The mechanism of injury to the inferior alveolar nerve can be either hydrostatic or mechanical. When fluid extravasation involves the lingual nerve, the inferior alveolar nerve is also involved. This common perioperative problem usually resolves before discharge from an ambulatory care facility.

Mechanical injury to the inferior alveolar nerve has been reported by Heffez and Blaustein.[24] Utilizing the technique described by Tarro,[20] a towel clamp is placed at the angle of the mandible in a percutaneous fashion. It was speculated that the jaws of the clamp perforated the lateral cortex of the mandible, resulting in a compression injury. Direct mechanical compression has a much poorer prognosis for recovery. To avoid this problem, Sanders[8] recommends that transoral manipulation be performed by a skilled first assistant. This technique accomplishes better movement with much less morbidity. Mandibular manipulation devices are now being introduced that offer greater distraction for intra-articular procedures. Their effectiveness at this point is uncertain.

Auriculotemporal Nerve. Because of its close proximity to the lateral capsule, the most frequently noted complication of TMJ arthroscopy is postoperative hypoesthesia of the auriculotemporal nerve.[12] Common mechanisms of injury include severance, contusion, and hydrostatic pressure. Rupture of the adjacent posterior capsular veins also is common and can result in a local hematoma. Because of the direct mechanical injury and hydrostatic pressure on this nerve, the duration of recovery is typically greater than with other nerve V injuries. Occasional complaints of dysesthesia have been reported. However, most patients have spontaneous resolution of sensory nerve dysfunction within 6 months.

Cranial Nerve VII Injuries

The temporozygomatic branch of the facial nerve is the most common nerve VII injury reported. Various techniques to reduce this risk have been reported in the literature. The inferolateral approach described by Murakami and Ono[25] in 1986 was designed to enter the TMJ away from this motor nerve. Based on cadaver dissections, Westesson and co-workers[4] suggested that a stepwise increase in the diameter of the trocar would gradually displace the nerve rather than sever it. Additional cadaver studies by Kurita and Bronstein[26] supported this view. McCain[27] developed a vector technique that utilizes preoperative measurements to predict the location of cranial nerve VII and to plan joint entry away from it.

Nevertheless, reports of injury to this nerve have remained frequent. The incidence was reported as 4% in the review by Carter and Testa[10] and 0.56% in the study by Greene and Van Sickels[18] (Table 21–1). Most of these cases were peripheral nerve VII injuries that resolved within 6 months. This is consistent with the case report by Indresano[13] of a temporozygomatic paresis that spontaneously resolved in the same amount of time. Applebaum and colleagues[28] reported the only documented case of a complete facial nerve paralysis. This patient had previously undergone open surgery and, therefore, represented a high risk for arthroscopy.

The management of a persistent temporozygomatic injury is directed toward supportive care to prevent corneal desiccation and abrasion. Taping of the eyelid at night and the use of artificial tears are beneficial supplements. In the unusual case of total paralysis, oculoplastic consultation for a lateral tarsorrhaphy should be considered.

As second-generation procedures and techniques develop, greater access to the anterior pouch will be required. The potential risk for injury to this nerve may increase over time.

Table 21–1. COMPLICATIONS OF TMJ ARTHROSCOPY*

Complications	No.	% of Total Treated
Sensory nerve injury	7	0.78
Facial nerve injury	5	0.56
Auditory canal perforation	4	0.45
Edema/extravasation of fluid	4	0.45
Bleeding resulting in ligation of an artery	1	0.11
External otitis	1	0.11
Total	22	2.5

* Based on 897 patients.
Reprinted with permission from Greene MW, Van Sickels JE: Survey of TMJ arthroscopy in oral and maxillofacial surgery residency programs. J Oral Maxillofac Surg 47:574–576, 1989.

VASCULAR INJURIES

Regional Anatomy

Compared with other joints, the neurovascular structures around the TMJ are very condensed. The blood supply to the head and neck is characterized by intricate collateral circulation. Therefore, although surgery in this region increases the potential for bleeding, the likelihood of a major vascular injury, with resultant loss of distal vitality, is much more remote than would be expected from arthroscopic procedures of extremity joints. The vascular structures that are the most vulnerable to TMJ arthroscopy are the terminal branches of the external carotid system and the tributaries of the superficial temporal vein (Fig. 21–3).

Arterial Complications

During operative arthroscopy, the TMJ is subject to numerous punctures. Locating the superficial temporal artery by palpation prior to joint distention may help to avoid unintentional penetration of the vessel. If the superficial temporal artery is pierced, a rapid, high-pressure bleeding point typically results. This can usually be controlled by direct digital pressure. A consequential hematoma sometimes forms, which may force termination of the arthroscopic procedure if the other anatomic landmarks are obscured from view. The literature suggests that significant arterial bleeding necessitating arthrotomy is rare. Greene and Van Sickels[18] reported only one episode that required ligation. Such profuse bleeding is a most unusual occurrence.

A delayed arterial complication was reported by Moses and Topper.[29] The patient had undergone TMJ arthroscopy and, postoperatively, complained of a preauricular "whishing" sound. An arteriogram confirmed the presence of an arteriovenous fistula. This postoperative vascular complication necessitated a secondary surgical procedure to ligate the fistula.

A second case of an arteriovenous fistula, in the postoperative period, was described by Preisler and associates.[30] This fistula was treated initially with interventional radiolo-

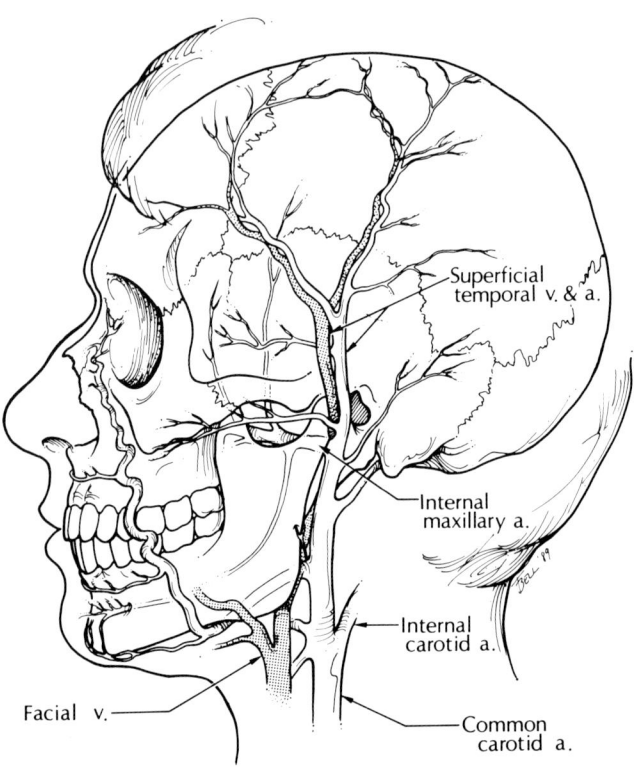

Figure 21–3. Vascular anatomy of the temporomandibular joint. (Reprinted with permission from Carter JB, Schwaber MK: Temporomandibular joint arthroscopy: Complications and their management. Oral Maxillofac Surg Clin North Am 1:185–199, 1989.)

gy. Successful embolization decreased this high-flow arteriovenous fistula but was followed by an ipsilateral slight-to-low frequency, sensineural hearing loss. Subsequent surgery resected the lesion, which was later histologically confirmed as arteriovenous fistula. No further complications were reported.

Venous Bleeding

In their experiences with open arthrotomy, maxillofacial surgeons have encountered the density and variability of venous structures around the TMJ. The two posterior capsular veins are nonpalpable, and their exact location cannot be ascertained prior to joint puncture. This problem, combined with the possible engorgement of the posterior portion of the deep temporal vein, represents the major bleeding hazard. Carter and Testa[10] found that the likelihood of a venous injury is much greater than is that of an arterial puncture. Of the 41 cases complicated by bleeding, 34% were arterial and 46% were venous. No adverse outcomes of venous bleeding have been reported. Hematoma formation has led to termination of the procedure but has not necessitated arthrotomy.

Intra-articular Bleeding

In first-generation TMJ arthroscopies, the likelihood of intra-articular bleeding is low. With the introduction of power shavers for synovectomy, anterior release procedures using electrocautery, and suturing techniques, the likelihood of intra-articular bleeding increases tremendously. Small[11] cited hemarthrosis as the most frequent complication of orthopedic arthroscopy. This is considered a significant problem if secondary aspiration of the joint is required. To date, there have been no reported cases of a postoperative hemarthrosis of the TMJ that required secondary aspiration. Techniques used to decrease the chances of intra-articular bleeding include the introduction of hypotensive anesthesia and the injection of local vasoconstrictors. There is no substitute for excellent visualization during the use of electrocautery or power instrumentation to prevent or control an intra-articular bleeding episode.

INSTRUMENT FAILURE

The advent of TMJ arthroscopy quickly spawned successive generations of newly manufactured instruments to meet the growing needs and demands of maxillofacial surgeons. In most cases, the new products are merely smaller-scaled versions of existing orthopedic technology to fit the anatomic constraints of the TMJ. These instruments are more delicate than their larger prototypes and in many cases are more fragile. Instrument breakage has occurred as a result of metallurgic defects. Even with optimal instrumentation, application of excessive force during a procedure may exceed the tolerances dictated by the size limitations. In cases in which grasping forceps cannot be used, a magnetic probe is very helpful in retrieving a metal fragment from the joint. This "golden retriever" will often prevent the need for arthrotomy.

At times when the proper instrument was not available, surgeons have improvised with other products of similar size. Literature on this type of resultant instrument breakage is anecdotal. Carter and Testa[10] described two cases of fragmentation of the distal tip of an angiocatheter that had been substituted for an evacuation cannula. This flexible, disposable device, used in lieu of the recommended metal instrument, was unable to withstand the multiple punctures required during the arthroscopic procedure (Fig. 21–4). The distal tip became a loose body within the joint. In one case reported, the tip was retrieved by grasping forceps, and an open procedure was avoided; in the other case, arthrotomy was required. The same outcome also has been documented more recently by White.[14] Each case involved recovering the plastic tip of an angiocatheter. Had the recommended specialty products been employed, this complication could have been prevented.

As the use of cutting instruments and other hinge-type hand instruments multiplies, the potential for instrument breakage will grow. The use of nonmetallic instruments is strongly discouraged. If instrument failure occurs, orthopedic practice recommends reporting the incident according to the criteria outlined in Table 21–2. Prior to surgery, patients should be informed of the possible need for an open joint procedure in the event of an irretrievable instrument.

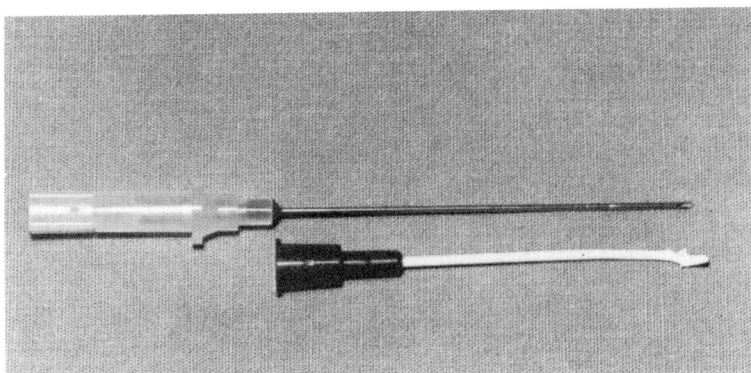

Figure 21-4. The flexible angiocath is subject to perforation and fracture after repeated insertion of a sharp stylet. (Reprinted with permission from Carter JB, Schwaber MK: Temporomandibular joint arthroscopy: Complications and their management. Oral Maxillofac Surg Clin North Am 1:185-199, 1989.)

Table 21-2. CRITICAL INFORMATION IN INSTRUMENT BREAKAGE

1. The procedure
2. The age of the instrument (years)
3. Part of the instrument that failed
4. Hinge pin location (intra- versus extra-articular)
5. Arthrotomy required (yes or no)
6. Metallurgic testing done (yes or no)
7. Manufacturer of instrument

OTOLOGIC INJURIES

In the spectrum of new complications that have evolved from the blind puncture technique, otologic complications have been reported. The close proximity of the posterior synovial pouch to the ear canal underlies most of these new developments.

In 1986, Sanders[8] described a single case of otitis media as the only complication in a large series of cases. He reported a slight hearing impairment, but no other details were mentioned. In 1987, Van Sickels and colleagues[9] reported one case in which they inadvertently slid a blunt trocar posteromedially through the ear canal and entered the middle ear space. This resulted in a perforation of the tympanic membrane and a slight dislocation of the malleus. A 50-dB conductive loss was noted postoperatively. Within 3 months, the ossicular chain appeared normal and the tympanic membrane was again intact. Air conduction thresholds improved significantly, but the patient was left with a residual 15-dB conductive loss.

In 1988, Applebaum and co-workers[28] reported three cases of enduring otologic impairment. Two patients developed a severe to profound sensorineural hearing loss, and the third had hearing loss with a large conductive component. Two of these patients had previously undergone open arthrotomy and thus had distorted anatomic structures and landmarks. The authors postulated that the sensorineural loss may have been secondary to damage of the oval or round window when the increased pressure of irrigation solution entered the middle ear.

Such alarming case reports instigated further audiologic investigation of patients choosing arthroscopic procedures. In 1989, Jones and Horn[16] compared the preoperative and postoperative audiograms of 14 patients who underwent arthroscopy. Regardless of the manipulation performed, no significant threshold shifts or changes in middle ear pressure were noted. Figure 21-5 shows the test results of one patient before and after surgery. Although this patient had a postoperative contusion on the anterior wall of the cartilaginous external auditory canal, no changes were noted from the preoperative audiogram. However, transient alteration in the resonating frequency of the ear canal as a result of the contusion was not investigated.

McCain and colleagues,[31] in a similar study, reported the results of preoperative and postoperative audiometry on 29 patients (44 joints). Two patients demonstrated a transient 10-dB hearing loss on the first postoperative day that was believed to be secondary to postsurgical edema. An additional patient showed a 15-dB shift in the lower frequencies and a transient 50-dB decline in the higher frequencies. The reason for this phenomenon was unclear, and it was not stated whether this change was conductive or sensorineural. All thresholds returned to normal within 2 months. No patients in the study showed any permanent change in hearing. These studies indicate that TMJ arthroscopy can be performed safely, without a high risk of permanent hearing loss, when safe techniques are practiced.

Management of Otologic Problems

Laceration of the External Auditory Canal

In Carter and Testa's retrospective study[10] of 2225 patients, three cases of external auditory canal perforation were reported. Greene and Van Sickels,[18] in their survey of 897 patients, enumerated four additional instances. The site of perforation is usually between the tragus and the bony portion of the canal. If a laceration occurs, bleeding should be controlled with bipolar cautery. Postoperatively, the canal should be treated with antibiotic/hydrocortisone ear drops for one to two weeks. If granulation tissue develops, bipolar cautery or silver nitrate should be used for treatment. There is little morbidity associated with perforations of the canal.

Tympanic Membrane Perforation

Perforation of the tympanic membrane is usually secondary to medial passage of the arthroscope. The tympanic membrane may also be damaged by vigorous canal preparation.[14] If perforation occurs in the anterior or inferior section of the membrane, spontaneous healing usually occurs without residual conductive loss. Injuries to the posterior aspect of the eardrum may result in ossicular damage and a more significant hearing impairment. Perforations of the posterior aspect, or large perforations in excess of 30% of the surface area, should be evaluated and managed by an otolaryngologist. Patients complaining of acute, profound postoperative hearing loss or vertigo should be referred immediately.

External Otitis and Otitis Media

Patient preparation for TMJ arthroscopy begins by cleaning the ear canal. If residual moisture remains in the canal, a localized proliferation of bacteria may occur and result in an inflammatory response. At the end of the procedure, the ear canal should be inspected and dried and the tympanic membrane should be visualized. If external otitis develops, the canal should be cleansed and an antibiotic hydrocortisone suspension ear drop should be instilled. In cases of severe inflammation, analgesics may be required. Although otitis media has been documented

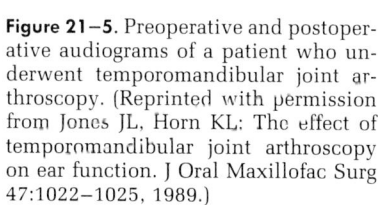

Figure 21–5. Preoperative and postoperative audiograms of a patient who underwent temporomandibular joint arthroscopy. (Reprinted with permission from Jones JL, Horn KL: The effect of temporomandibular joint arthroscopy on ear function. J Oral Maxillofac Surg 47:1022–1025, 1989.)

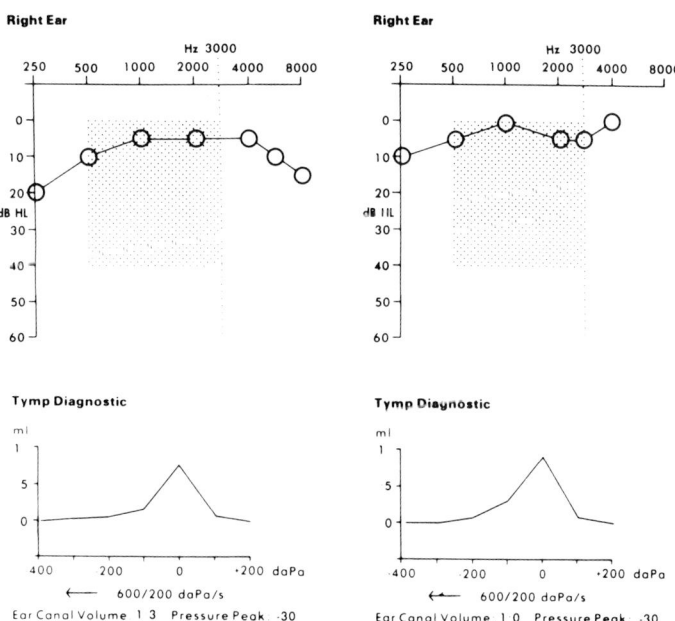

only once in conjunction with TMJ arthroscopy,[8] its appearance should alert the physician to prescribe systemic antibiotics. Amoxicillin 500 mg taken three times daily for 7 days is the usual treatment protocol. If effusion is persistent, more aggressive intervention may be required and the patient should be referred to an otolaryngologist.

INFLAMMATORY COMPLICATIONS

Postoperative Capsulitis

The term postoperative capsulitis is used to describe tenderness to palpation over the lateral capsule of the TMJ. This is a routine finding after violation of the skin and capsular structures by arthroscopic instruments. Persistent postoperative capsulitis has been an infrequent complication. Carter and Testa[10] reported only eight complaints of prolonged capsular tenderness following lysis and lavage. The details from this multicenter study were not sufficient to document whether these patients had undergone intraarticular steroid injections as part of their treatment. However, the reporting surgeons noted that the pain was managed medically with nonsteroidal anti-inflammatory medications and did not predispose these patients to a second operation.

Cutaneous Thermal Injury

As arthroscopists have advanced to the second generation of surgical procedures of the TMJ, the use of electrocautery and lasers has been frequently discussed in the literature. Although laser techniques remain in the investigational arena, cautery has been promoted for anterior release operations. When using cautery, it is essential to be cognizant of the position of the electrode tip relative to the insertion cannula. Contact between the activated electrode and the cannula can cause arcing of the current and result in a circumferential cutaneous injury. Figure 21–6 shows evidence of one of these rare wounds. After 18 months, a flat, pigmented unsightly scar remained that ultimately required scar revision. These complications are readily preventable with good visualization of the cautery tip and good hand–eye coordination.

Subcutaneous Fat Atrophy

The phenomenon of subcutaneous fat atrophy following TMJ arthroscopy was recently reviewed by Goldberg and colleagues.[32] A case was presented in which 10% triamcinolone acetonide was introduced into the superior joint space. A month after surgery, a preauricular depression was noted and pre-

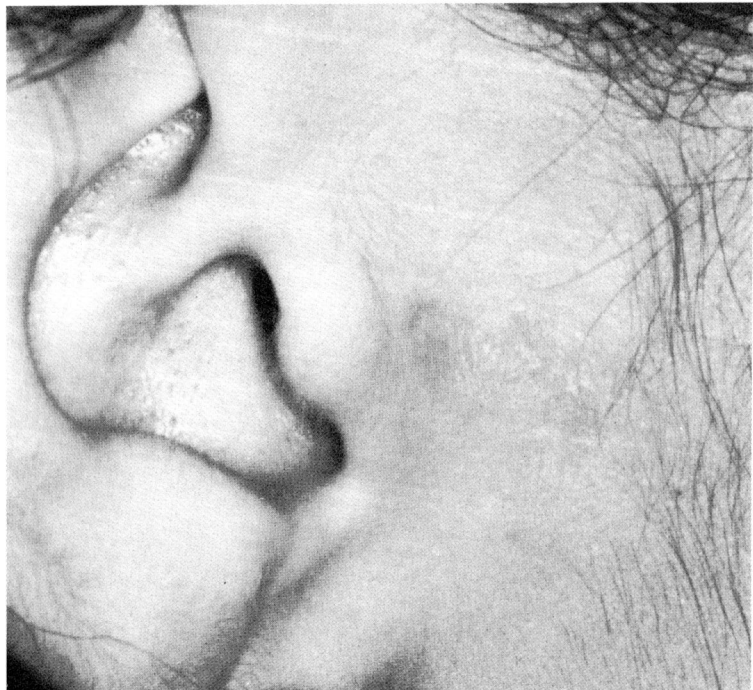

Figure 21–6. A cautery burn shown 18 months postoperatively. (Reprinted with permission from Carter JB, Schwaber MK: Temporomandibular joint arthroscopy: Complications and their management. Oral Maxillofac Surg Clin North Am 1:185–199, 1989.)

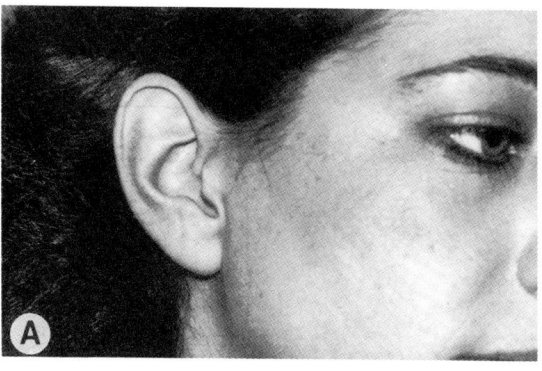 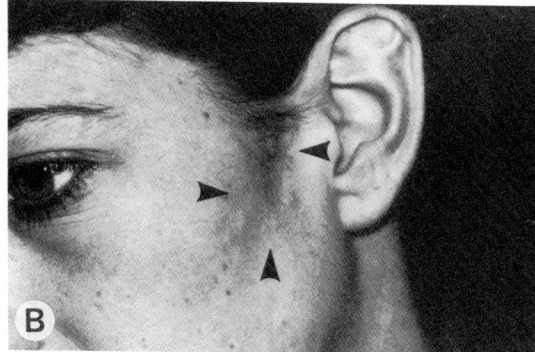

Figure 21-7. Clinical appearance of a patient 1 month following arthroscopic surgery. *A*, Normal right side; *B*, left side shows preauricular subcutaneous atrophy. (Reprinted with permission from Goldberg JS, Julian JB, Dachille R: Local subcutaneous atrophy following arthroscopy of the TMJ. J Oral Maxillofac Surg 44:614-617, 1986.)

sumed to be secondary to fat atrophy (Fig. 21-7). This contour defect took 6 months to resolve. The authors presented this as an unusual complication that occurred only once in 123 joints. They suggest the following considerations to minimize the problems of fat atrophy after TMJ arthroscopy:

1. Limit the site of insoluble steroids to deep injections.
2. Use the lowest effective concentration.
3. Avoid drug escape from deeper to superficial planes.
4. Be aware that this phenomenon is most often observed in pre-menopausal women.

SUMMARY

After 15 years of clinical experience with TMJ arthroscopy, a spectrum of complications has emerged. Although the majority are minor perioperative inconveniences, a few catastrophic problems have surfaced. When appropriate, informed consent should include a discussion of possible facial paralysis, altered sensory function, and hearing loss. The more unlikely problems of glenoid fossa puncture, bleeding, and instrument breakage should be discussed routinely.

References

1. Ohnishi M: [Arthroscopy of the temporomandibular joint] (author's trans.). Kokubyo Gakkai Zasshi 42:207-213, 1975.
2. Hellsing G, Holmlund A, Nordenram A, et al: Arthroscopy of the temporomandibular joint: Examination of 2 patients with suspected disk derangement. Int J Oral Surg 13:69-74, 1984.
3. Holmlund A, Hellsing G: Arthroscopy of the temporomandibular joint: An autopsy study. Int J Oral Surg 14:169-175, 1985.
4. Westesson P, Eriksson L, Liedberg J: The risk of damage to facial nerve, superficial temporal vessels, disk, and articular surfaces during arthroscopic examination of the temporomandibular joint. Oral Surg 62:124-127, 1986.
5. Goss AN, Bosanquet AG: Temporomandibular joint arthroscopy. J Oral Maxillofac Surg 44:614-617, 1986.
6. Holmlund A, Hellsing G, Wredmark T: Arthroscopy of the temporomandibular joint: A clinical study. Int J Oral Maxillofac Surg 15:715-721, 1986.
7. McCain JP: Arthroscopy of the human temporomandibular joint. J Oral Maxillofac Surg 46:648-655, 1988.
8. Sanders B: Arthroscopic surgery of the temporomandibular joint: Treatment of internal derangement with persistent closed lock. Oral Surg 62:361-372, 1986.
9. Van Sickels JE, Nishioka GJ, Hegewald MD, et al: Middle ear injury resulting from temporomandibular joint arthroscopy. J Oral Maxillofac Surg 45:962-965, 1987.
10. Carter JB, Testa L: Complications of TMJ arthroscopy: a review of 2,225 cases: Review of the 1988 Annual Scientific Sessions abstracts. J Oral Maxillofac Surg 46:M14-M15, 1988.
11. Small NC: Complications in arthroscopic surgery performed by experienced arthroscopists. J Arthroscopic Rel Surg 4:215-221, 1988.
12. Carter JB, Schwaber MK: Temporomandibular joint arthroscopy: complications and their management. Oral Maxillofac Surg Clin North Am 1(1):185-199, 1989.
13. Indresano AT: Arthroscopic surgery of the temporomandibular joint: Report of 64 patients with long-term follow-up. J Oral Maxillofac Surg 47:439-441, 1989.
14. White RD: Retrospective analysis of 100 consecutive surgical arthroscopies of the temporomandibular joint. J Oral Maxillofac Surg 47:1014-1021, 1989.
15. McCain JP: Complications of TMJ arthroscopy (letter). J Oral Maxillofac Surg 46:256, 1988.
16. Jones JL, Horn KL: The effect of temporomandibular joint arthroscopy on ear function. J Oral Maxillofac Surg 47:1022-1025, 1989.
17. Murakami K, Matsumoto K, Iizuka T: Suppurative arthritis of the temporomandibular joint: Report of a

case with special reference to arthroscopic observations. J Maxillofac Surg 12:41–45, 1984.
18. Greene MW, Van Sickels JE: Survey of TMJ arthroscopy in oral and maxillofacial surgery residency programs. J Oral Maxillofac Surg 47:574–576, 1989.
19. Tarro AW: Arthroscopic treatment of anterior disc displacement: A preliminary report. J Oral Maxillofac Surg 47:353–358, 1989.
20. Tarro AW: Arthroscopic diagnosis and surgery of the temporomandibular joint. J Oral Maxillofac Surg 46:282–289, 1988.
21. Moses JJ, Poker ID: TMJ arthroscopic surgery: An analysis of 237 patients. J Oral Maxillofac Surg 47:790–794, 1989.
22. Johnson L: Two per cent glutaraldehyde: A disinfectant in arthroscopy and arthroscopic surgery. J Bone Joint Surg 64A:237–239, 1982.
23. Schellhas KP, Wilkes CH, Deeb ME, et al: Permanent Proplast temporomandibular joint implants: MR imaging of destructive complications. AJR 151:731–735, 1988.
24. Heffez L, Blaustein D: Diagnostic arthroscopy of the temporomandibular joint. I: Normal arthroscopic findings. Oral Surg 64:653–670, 1987.
25. Murakami K, Ono T: Temporomandibular joint arthroscopy by infero-lateral approach. Int J Oral Maxillofac Surg 15:410–417, 1986.
26. Kurita K, Bronstein SL, Westesson P, et al: Arthroscopic diagnosis of perforation and adhesions of the temporomandibular joint: Correlation with postmortem morphology. Oral Surg Oral Med Oral Pathol 68:130–134, 1989.
27. McCain JP: An Illustrated Guide to Temporomandibular Joint Arthroscopy. Andover: Dyonics Corporation, 1987.
28. Applebaum EL, Berg LF, Kumar A, et al: Otologic complications following temporomandibular joint arthroscopy. Ann Otol Rhinol Laryngol 97:675–679, 1988.
29. Moses JJ, Topper DL: Arteriovenous fistula: An unusual complication associated with arthroscopic temporomandibular joint surgery. J Oral Maxillofac Surg 48:1220–1222, 1990.
30. Preisler SA, Koorbusch GF, Olson RAJ: An acquired arteriovenous fistula secondary to temporomandibular joint arthroscopy: report of a case. J Oral Maxillofac Surg 49:187–190, 1991.
31. McCain JP, Goldberg HM, de la Rua H: Preoperative and postoperative audiologic measurements in patients undergoing arthroscopy of the TMJ. J Oral Maxillofac Surg 47:1026–1027, 1989.
32. Goldberg JS, Julian JB, Dachille R: Local subcutaneous atrophy following arthroscopy of the TMJ. J Oral Maxillofac Surg 47:986–987, 1989.

Chapter 22

FUTURE DIRECTIONS IN TEMPOROMANDIBULAR JOINT ARTHROSCOPY

A. The Future

MOHAN THOMAS, D.D.S., F.A.C.D.,
CHRISTOPHER LANE, D.D.S.

Rapid technologic advances in temporomandibular joint (TMJ) arthroscopic surgical procedures have taken place over the last decade. Although these advances in technology are noteworthy, perhaps their widespread clinical application may be premature because of inadequate evaluation of long-term clinical trials. Furthermore, implementation of technical advances in surgical practice without long-term studies seems to indicate that they have a greater value than the existing techniques. The time to test the value and efficacy of these advances is perhaps before they are incorporated into daily medical and surgical practice.

The future of TMJ arthroscopy rests in the hands of researchers studying the pathophysiology of the TMJ and in those pursuing the advances in surgical techniques. Current topics of interest include the synovial apparatus and the production of synovial fluid, articular cartilage in both normal and diseased states, and autologous cartilage analogs. Surgical advances, including arthroscopic biopsy, laser-assisted arthroscopy, and the role of viscosurgery in arthroscopy, are presented in Chapters 13C, 22B, and 22C, respectively.

SYNOVIAL APPARATUS AND FLUID

The TMJ is a true diarthrodial joint that is lined by a synovial membrane containing 0.1 to 0.2 ml of synovial fluid, a dialysate of plasma.[1-3] We know that the components of connective tissue that line joints are cells (chondrocytes, fibroblasts, osteoblasts, endothelial cells, and synovial cells), fibers (collagen, reticular, and elastic), and ground substance (complex polysaccharides called glycosaminoglycans, predominantly hyaluronic acid).

Normally, the synovial membrane is impermeable to high molecular weight blood proteins resulting in a concentration of low molecular weight proteins in synovial fluid as compared with plasma.[4-6] However, in diseased states, the analysis of synovial fluid from the TMJ has revealed a different picture.[5,7] Elevated protein levels in synovial fluid are noted in inflammatory conditions, which reflect an increased permeability of the synovial membrane to plasma proteins[7-9] as well as to inflammatory cells.[1] Normal synovial fluid contains high concentrations of hyaluronic acid, which is highly viscous and plays an important role in joint lubrication.[4,6,9] Diseased states may bring about a reduction in the amount of hyaluronic acid. High levels of keratin sulfate have been reported in synovial fluid analyses of osteoarthritic joints.[10] Prostaglandin E_2 and leukotriene B_4 have been identified in the synovial fluid of painful dysfunctional TM joints.[11] Further work is being carried out in the quantitative and qualitative analysis of synovial fluid and suggests the possibility of synovial fluid sampling at the time of arthroscopy.

ARTICULAR CARTILAGE

The concept of healing articular cartilage lesions with allograft materials began over a century ago.[12-16] Research has shown that articular cartilage has a limited capacity for healing following traumatic insult or in reversing degenerative joint disease. The principal reason for this observation is that the tissue is unique in lacking both vascular supply and innervation.[17,18] Two possible mechanisms to initiate cartilaginous repair are (1) replication of chondrocytes in the regions adjacent to the defect (intrinsic repair) and (2) metaplasia of chondrocytes from connective tissue stem cells within the joint capsule from the synovium and subchondral bone (extrinsic repair).[17,18] Cartilage healing utilizing viable chondrocytes as a graft material has had mixed results. Preliminary studies as reported by Grande and associates[16] have resulted in a model for healing articular cartilage in the New Zealand white rabbit.[19,20] Their technique utilizes chondrocytes that have been cultured in vitro prior to subsequent autotransplantation. This is a model for intrinsic cartilage healing because the defect that is made does not violate the subchondral plate.

AUTOLOGOUS CARTILAGE ANALOG

The introduction of a novel technique for the repair of intra-articular condylar and discal cartilage has been studied by Thomas and Grande.[19] The results of this pilot study indicate that cartilaginous connective tissue can be harvested efficiently from the TMJ and that connective tissue cells can then be used to construct an in vitro tissue analog for repair of the articular disc. Investigators, including the author (MT), are currently in the process of implementing this technique for the repair of articular cartilage in the New Zealand white rabbit TMJ. However continued animal research is needed prior to human trials (see color plate).[16,19,21]

The development of an in vitro cartilaginous tissue derived from the cells of the subject's own disc would allow repair of the diseased tissue with an immunologically and histologically compatible tissue, eliminating rejection, allergic reaction, and second surgical site morbidity. The method described is a pilot study based on an animal model. The ultimate goal would be to harvest fibrocartilage shavings of the articular disc during diagnostic arthroscopy. These shavings would then be processed and cultured to provide an autologous cartilage analog for subsequent autotransplantation to repair defects or lesions of the temporomandibular disc.

After successful cartilage analog development, its functional ability depends on securing the graft intra-articularly. Analogs have been successfully attached by means of suturing[22] and adhesives. Currently two commercially available adhesives are capable of securing chondrocyte allografts intra-articularly. The two materials are fibrin glue (Tissucol, Tisseel; by Immuno, A.G., Vienna, Austria) and mussel adhesive protein (MAP;

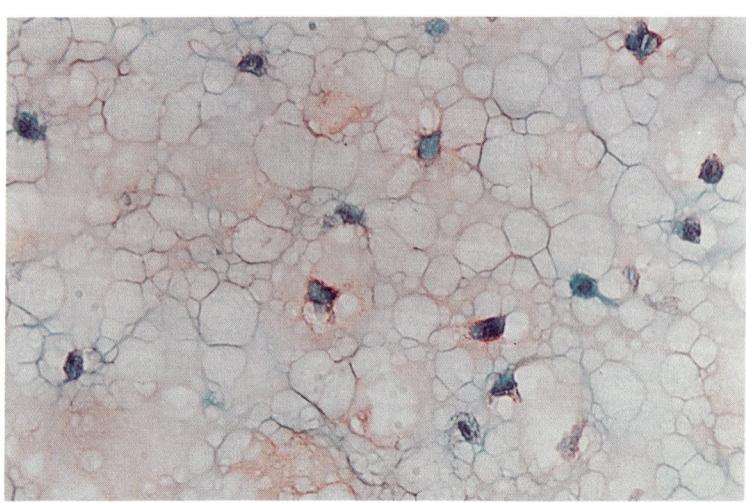

Histologic specimen of tissue analog stained with safranin O and fast green showing chondrocytes in the matrix (200×).

by Biopolymers, Farmington, CT). The results of the series that evaluated MAP as a material for the adhesion of chondrocyte allografts were significantly better than those for fibrin glue; however, more research and clinical trials are necessary prior to its widespread use.[23]

Kurita and colleagues[22] have studied the use of 8–0 polyglycolic acid sutures (Dexon, Cyanamid of Great Britain Ltd., Gosport Hampshire, Great Britain) versus fibrin glue. They have found no appreciable macroscopic or histologic difference between condyles in which fibrin sealant or sutures were applied for fixation of the articular soft tissue cover.

ARTHROSCOPY

Arthroscopically assisted suturing for traction and repositioning of the articular disc has been reported by Israel and Tarro (see Chapter 13E).

Another technical advance has been the use of lasers in TMJ arthroscopy. Bradrick and associates have studied the morphologic and histologic changes in the canine TMJ tissues following arthroscopically guided laser exposure.[25] The study of lasers through the arthroscope in TMJ surgery has proved to be most promising. Cutting, coagulating, debriding, and contact cutting have all been studied as have the effects of exposure of low level neodymium:yttrium aluminum garnet (Nd:YAG) laser energy on articular cartilage (see Chapter 22B).[24,25]

Laser Arthroscopy

The Nd:YAG laser emits light at 1064 nanometers in the non-visible spectrum. Through a low power He-Ne sighting beam, the Nd:YAG laser beam appears red. This beam has been shown to have no effects on the articular cartilage. Another laser that has been used in TMJ arthroscopy is the KTP:532 contact laser, which emits light in the visible spectrum at 532 nanometers. A sighting beam is not required with this laser because its beam is in the visible spectrum and is green. It may prove to be safer in the TMJ, because its contact is less, thus less penetration of the tissue occurs compared with the Nd:YAG laser. The KTP:532 has been utilized through the arthroscope for anterior release and posterior cauterization procedures.

VISCOSURGERY

Viscosurgery is the application of viscoelastic substances to protect tissues and facilitate their manipulation. Viscoelastic substances have been safely utilized by many ophthalmologists for vitreous humor exchange. The use of the fluid Healon (Pharmacia Ophthalmics Inc., Pasadena, CA), a viscoelastic preparation of sodium hyaluronate, in arthroscopy has been reported. Weiss has found Healon fluid to be safe and effective as a standard irrigating fluid because it provides better visualization and protects joint tissues. This fluid may also actually reduce iatrogenic damage (see Chapter 22C).

CONTINUOUS PASSIVE MOTION

Advances in the area of continuous passive motion (CPM) devices and the application of CPM to synovial joints immediately after TMJ surgery have been completed by Poremba and associates.[26] It was determined that CPM stimulates the regeneration of articular tissue, eliminates adhesions, prevents joint stiffness, reduces pain, and is well tolerated by patients.[26,27] These workers concluded that in order to fully determine the reliability of the findings in their preliminary studies, a formally controlled large-scale, long-term clinical study should be completed.[27]

Today, we have a better understanding of the roles of synovial fluid in diarthrodial joints, namely nutrition, lubrication, and excretion. Movement is necessary within the joint to bring about transportation of the synovial fluid. A two-part study was conducted by the Department of Orthodontics, at The University of Washington School of Dentistry, to examine the effects of CPM on the TMJ after surgery.

The first part of the study addressed the appliance design and fabrication. The second part of the study addressed the appliance, improvement, normal subject evaluation, and apparent clinical trials.[26,27] The investigators point out that, although there are several CPM devices available for the TMJ (Toronto Medical and Walter Lorenz), the majority of physical therapists interviewed by us were not in favor of widespread use. However, there may be special cases such as surgery for ankylosis of the joint when a CPM device may be recommended.

SUMMARY

Today, TMJ arthroscopy seems to be accepted and integrated by more and more oral and maxillofacial surgeons, spurred by the increase in the number of arthroscopy workshops offered as well as by the increase in the training in arthroscopy during residency programs.

Arthroscopy in the diagnosis and management of hypomobility following orthognathic surgery has been reported by Sanders and colleagues.[28] Surgical exposure for maxillofacial fractures may be reduced, and confirmation of reduction may be enhanced through the visualization capability of endoscopy.

The future of arthroscopic surgery belongs to those who have an intense interest in first the basic sciences and in the surgery of the TMJ. New techniques will be introduced and assisted by biomedical and technologic advances. Although one may be capable of performing technically specific procedures, this does not make them therapeutic. It is therefore less important to invent new techniques and more important to improve on existing ones, thus enabling researchers to complete extensive long-term studies that will ultimately benefit us all.

References

1. Hasselbacher P: Joints: Normal structure and function. In Kelly W (ed): Textbook of Internal Medicine. Philadelphia: JB Lippincott, 1989, pp 968–971.
2. Simkin PA: Joints: Structure and function. In Schumacher R (ed): Primer on Rheumatic Diseases. Arthritis Foundation, Atlanta, Georgia, Schumake R 1988, pp 18–23.
3. Howell DS, Manicourt DH: Complex polysaccharides. In Schumacher R (ed): Clinical Rheumatology. Philadelphia: WB Saunders, 1986, pp 51–55.
4. Schmid FR, Ogata RL: The composition and examination of synovial fluid. J Prosthet Dent 18:449, 1967.
5. Toller PA: The synovial apparatus and TMJ function. Br Dent J 3:355, 1961.
6. Yehia SR, Duncan H: Synovial fluid analysis. Clin Orthop 107:11, 1925.
7. Kopp S, Wenneberg B, Clemensson E: Clinical, microscopic and biochemical investigation of synovial fluid for TM joints. Scand J Dent Res 91:33, 1983.
8. Hatton MN, Swann D: Studies on bovine TMJ synovial fluid. J Prosthet Dent 56:635, 1986.
9. Owen DS, Cooke CL, Toone E: Practical synovial fluid examination. Virginia Med Monthly 97:88, 1970.
10. Israel HA: Synovial fluid: Keratin sulfate concentrations with arthroscopically diagnosed osteoarthritis. Presented at the AAOMS Meeting Abstract, New Orleans, 1990.
11. Quinn JH: Identification of prostaglandin E_2 and leukotriene B_4 in the synovial fluid of painful, dysfunctional TMJ's. JOMS 48:968–971, 1990.
12. Bert P: Sur La greffe Animale. C R Acad Sci 61:587, 1865.
13. Dupertius SM: Actual growth of young cartilage transplants in rabbits. Arch Surg 43:32–63, 1941.
14. Hunter W: On the structure and diseases of articulating cartilage. Philos Trans R Soc Lond Scr B 9:267, 1743.
15. Sokoloff L: The remodeling of articular cartilage. Rheumatology 7:11–18, 1982.
16. Grande DA, Pitman MI, Peterson L, Menche D, Klein M: The repair of experimentally produced defects in rabbits articular cartilage by autologous chondrocyte transplantation. J Orthop 7:208–218, 1989.
17. Sokoloff L: Cell biology and the repair of articular cartilage. J Rheum 1:1–10, 1974.
18. Sokoloff L: In vitro culture of skeletal tissues. In Sokoloff L (ed): The Joints and Synovial Fluid, Vol 2. New York: Academic Press, 1978, pp 1–27.
19. Thomas M, Grande DA, Haug R: Development of an in vitro temporomandibular joint cartilage analog. (Submitted for publication.) 1991.
20. Kent JN, Misiek DJ: Biomaterials for cranial, facial, mandibular and TMJ reconstruction. In Fonseca R, Walker R(eds): Oral and Maxillofacial Trauma, Philadelphia: W.B. Saunders Co., 1991, pp 781–1026.
21. Grande DA, Pitman MI: The use of adhesives in chondrocyte surgery: Preliminary studies. Hosp Bone Joint Dis 48:140–148, 1988.
22. Kurita K, Westesson PL, Eriksson L, Sternby NH: Osteoplasty of the mandibular condyle with preservation of the articular soft tissue cover. Oral Surg Oral Med Oral Path 69:661–667, 1990.
23. Pitman MI, Menche D, Song EK, et al: The use of adhesives in chondrocyte transplantation surgery: In vivo studies. Hosp Bone Joint Dis 49:213–220, 1989.
24. Spivak JM, Grande DA, Grelsamer RP, et al: The effect of low level Nd:YAG laser energy on adult canine cartilage. Presented at the 36th Annual Meeting, Orthopedic Research Society, New Orleans, 1990.
25. Indresano AT, Braderick JP, Eckhauser ML: The Nd:YAG Laser Triology. Cleveland, Ohio: Metro Health Medical Center, Case Western Reserve University, 1989.
26. Poremba EP, Moffett BC: The effects of continuous passive motion on the TMJ after surgery. Part I. Oral Surg Oral Med Oral Pathol 67:490–498, 1989.
27. Sebastian MH, Moffett BC: The effects of continuous passive motion on the TMJ after surgery. Part II. Oral Surg Oral Med Oral Pathol 67:644–653, 1989.
28. Sanders B, Kaminishi R, Buoncristiani R, et al: Arthroscopic surgery for treatment of temporomandibular joint hypomobility after mandibular sagittal osteotomy. Oral Surg Oral Med Oral Pathol 69:45–47, 1990.

B. Laser-Assisted Arthroscopy of the Temporomandibular Joint

JON P. BRADRICK, D.D.S.,
THOMAS A. INDRESANO, D.M.D.

The use of arthroscopy in the temporomandibular joint (TMJ) has been limited by technologic advances and the small size of the joint. Laser-assisted arthroscopic surgery (LAS) potentially can solve some of the related problems. Mating of the two technologies can allow tissue manipulation in the confined joint space with minimal instrumentation. Also, coaxial laser fiberoptic introduction can eliminate the need for triangulation. Debridement, coagulation, vaporization, and contraction can potentially be accomplished.

LASER SELECTION

Selection of the appropriate laser for LAS involves consideration of surgical requirements, capabilities, and feasibilities of the various systems available (Table 22-1).

CO_2 Lasers

The CO_2 surgical laser is familiar to many oral and maxillofacial surgeons.[1] Known for its excellent tissue vaporization properties, it would seem to be the ideal laser for LAS. The excellent water absorption of the CO_2 laser's 10,600-nm wavelength facilitates efficient tissue ablation; for this reason, it *cannot* be utilized in TMJ LAS. The CO_2 laser beam cannot be transmitted through traditional fiberoptics. Even if the beam could be delivered through a fiberoptic, it would fail to transit a saline-distended joint space.

Some investigators have experimented with meniscal ablation utilizing open arthrotomy, CO_2 gas–distended joints, and articulated hollow arms with internal mirrors to reflect CO_2 laser beams into joint spaces.[2-4] Early results showed minimal tissue alteration in fibrocartilage away from the area of vaporization; however, subsequent studies with electron microscopy reveal collagen alterations four to five times more distant.[5] The clinical implications of this are unknown.

Advances in optical technology have produced fiberoptics that can transmit CO_2 laser beams. These fibers are constructed of substances such as silver halide crystals or beryllium copper.[6,7] They are currently limited by length, diameter, and efficiency of transmission. The concept that a CO_2 laser beam will fail to affect tissue surrounded by water has been attacked by Isner and colleagues.[8] This group has shown in vitro that "dynamic optical cavities" will allow tissue ablation under as much as 5 mm of fluid with a CO_2 laser. However, despite the advances in CO_2 laser technology, its clinical application in TMJ LAS is remote.

Argon Lasers

The argon laser produces a beam with a wavelength of 488 to 514 nm in the blue-green portion of the visible spectrum. This wavelength is primarily absorbed by hemoglobin. It has found use in retinal detachment surgery and in angioplasty.[9] The beam can be transmitted along simple fiberoptics and through water. Unfortunately, most medical-grade argon lasers have a maximum power output of only 15 watts, which would severely inhibit the laser's effect on fibrocartilage.[10] This laser could be considered suitable for TMJ LAS only if one wishes to selectively affect the vascular (synovial) components of the joint.

Table 22-1. LASER SYSTEMS

Laser	Wavelength (nm)	Maximum Power (Watts)	Fiberoptic	Water Transmissible	Primary Applications
CO_2	10600	100 (CW)	Experimental only	No	Open tissue ablation, cutting
Er:YAG	2940	Kilowatts, ultra-short pulse	Special, zirconium fluoride	No	Open tissue ablation, cutting
Tm-Ho-Cr:Yag	2150	Kilowatts, ultra-short pulse	Special, silica	No	Open tissue ablation, cutting
MULTIYAG	1060 1320 1440	100 50 50 (CW)	Standard, quartz	Yes Yes No(?)	Deep coagulation, hemostasis, cutting
Nd:YAG	1060	100 (CW)	Standard, quartz	Yes	Deep coagulation, hemostasis, some cutting
KTP-532	532	15–20 (CW)	Standard, quartz	Yes	Cutting, ablation, coagulation, hemostasis
Argon	488–514	15 (CW)	Standard, quartz	Yes	Ophthalmology, cardiovascular
Eximer	193–351	Megawatt, 14–20 nsec (pulse)	Standard, quartz (only with higher wavelengths)	Yes	Experimental, possibly radial keratotomy

CW, Continuous wave mode.

Yttrium-Aluminum-Garnet Lasers

The next class of potential lasers has a solid crystal of yttrium-aluminum-garnet (YAG) as the active medium. The wavelengths of these lasers are determined by introducing impurities of rare earth elements (1 to 3%) into the YAG crystal lattice. These "mid-infrared" lasers have beams that are invisible, and are fiberoptic transmissible and produce a maximum of 50 to 100 watts of output power. Depending on the wavelength, they have variable water absorption and will function in continuous wave or pulsed output. Currently the most popular is the neodymium:YAG (Nd:YAG) laser, with a wavelength of 1060 nm. Used mainly in endoscopic surgery, this laser is popular with general surgeons, urologists, and thoracic surgeons.

Three other YAG lasers that are undergoing experimental trials may be applicable to TMJ LAS. The thulium-holmium-chromium (TM-Ho-Cr:YAG) with a wavelength of 2150 nm is transmissible along special silica fibers. A higher water absorption coefficient provides more superficial tissue ablation than the Nd:YAG laser, while retaining adequate tissue coagulation capabilities. Energy output is confined to 1-joule 200-µsec pulses at 3 Hz. This laser can therefore deliver 5000 watts in very small pulses.

The erbium (Er):YAG laser, with a wavelength of 2940 nm, operating in pulse mode only, features even more water absorption of its beam. Because laser beams close to the 3-micron wavelength limit have beams that are not transmissible along standard fiberoptics, the Er:YAG laser must use zirconium fluoride fibers, which are fragile, water-soluble, and toxic.[11,12] The Tm-Ho-Cr and Er:YAG hybrids both have questionable water transmission because their wavelengths have high water absorption. This would make them of negligible use in a fluid-distended joint space.

Another YAG laser deserving of discussion is the MULTIYAG (Aurora Laser, Inc., Edmonton, Alberta, Canada). This is a Nd:YAG laser with three freely selectable wavelengths: 1060 nm, 1320 nm, and 1440 nm. It is a continuous wave output laser capable of producing 100 watts of 1060-nm output and 50 watts at the other two wavelengths. The clinical advantages of three selectable wavelengths that provide a spectrum of tissue interaction from deep coagulation to tissue cutting, all transmitted along a standard quartz fiberoptic, are obvious. Although the 1440-nm setting may result in decreased water transmission within a joint space, the MULTIYAG is deserving of animal trials.[13]

A laser that holds immediate promise for TMJ LAS is the KTP-532 (Laserscope, Santa Clara, CA). This laser is a standard 1060-nm Nd:YAG laser with an output beam directed through a crystal of potassium-titanyl phosphate (KTP). The resulting beam's wavelength is halved to 532 nm and appears emerald green. The beam is transmissible along standard quartz fiberoptics and is not appreciably absorbed by water, enabling it to function in a fluid-filled cavity. Maximum power output is 15 to 20 watts in continuous wave mode. The KTP-532 laser is advertised as being a compromise between the CO_2 and Nd:YAG systems. This laser will cut and coagulate tissue, depending on power output and spot size of the incident beam (i.e., distance between tissue and fiberoptic). It will not cut and vaporize as fast as the CO_2 laser, nor will it coagulate as well as the Nd:YAG. The KTP-532 is employed primarily in urology, otolaryngology, and gynecologic surgery.[14-16] In vitro experiments in our laboratory showed the Nd:YAG laser required approximately 25 times more laser energy (joules) than the KTP-532 to create histologically identical lesions in canine TMJ disc tissue.[17]

Excimer Laser

The final laser system of interest is the Excimer laser. The Excimer produces ultrashort pulses (14 to 20 nsec) of high energy in the ultraviolet spectrum. The active element is a mixture of gaseous halogens and other noble gases that produce wavelengths of 193 to 351 nm, depending on which gases are used. The laser pulse is in the megawatt range, producing photon energy six times greater than that from an Nd:YAG laser and 60 times greater than that from a CO_2 laser. Tissue absorption of ultraviolet light exceeds that of a CO_2 beam by an order of magnitude. The method of tissue destruction is controversial but is believed to be "photo-ablative" and nonthermal. It is possible that tissue is disrupted by the actual breaking of chemical bonds, because of many reactive organic chemical radicals observed in the laser plume. Problems with the Eximer include the following: (1) active element gases are toxic, (2) special fiberoptics are necessary, and (3) there are potential mutagenic results from high-energy ultraviolet radiation.[18]

SAFETY CONSIDERATIONS

Animal experimentation with laser-assisted TMJ arthroscopy has been initiated to explore the feasibility and potential complications of this technique. An early concern was secondary thermal damage to adjacent tissue with laser activation. The tip of a quartz fiberoptic transmitting an Nd:YAG beam may reach temperatures of 400°F during activation.[19] In our experience with the canine TMJ model, radiant heat may be felt over the joint during prolonged, continuous-wave Nd:YAG beam activation under arthroscopic control. When a fiberoptic catheter is directed at joint structures during laser-assisted arthroscopy, bubbles are produced at the fiber tip with laser activation. These bubbles are presumed to be vaporization of saline irrigant within the joint space. Even if the irrigation circuit is functioning perfectly, some of these bubbles will rise within the joint, impacting on the end of the arthroscope and temporarily obscuring the view. Joint space irrigation will eventually remove them.

Ophthalmologists have described corneal endothelial cell damage associated with gas bubbles produced during YAG laser application. They speculated that the bubbles are filled with ionized or heated gases.[20] If the laser interacts with tissue, the gas bubbles may contain other chemical species. Rastegar and co-workers[21] discovered microbubbles containing CO_2, N_2, H_2, and CH_4 when thrombi and atherosclerotic plaques immersed in saline were irradiated with an argon laser. Other investigators have identified gas-phase photoproducts formed during pulse laser irradiation of tissue and blood.[8]

Experiments in our laboratory involving Nd:YAG LAS in conjunction with temperature probes within a joint space were undertaken to define thermal risk. When the temperature probe was within the field of view of the arthroscope, but *not* within the laser beam's path, an analog temperature monitor would instantly go off the scale (>100°C) with laser activation. Continuous joint space irrigation with room-temperature fluids rapidly returned the temperature to normal. If the temperature probe is within the joint space but is not visible within the arthroscope's field of view, a less dramatic temperature elevation with laser activation was noted. This suggests the presence of a significant temperature gradient originating at the tip of the laser fiberoptic, or at beam impact point, that rapidly dissipates over distance.

A tempting solution to this problem is to decrease the temperature of the joint irrigation fluid in an attempt to limit excess heat production during LAS. Laufer and colleagues[22] showed that CO_2 laser damage to tissue was decreased with precooling of the tissue surface. However, Haina and co-workers,[23] comparing maximal coagulation depths of human skin with different lasers, found that coagulation depths *increased* with surface cooling. They postulated that cooling decreased carbonization of the surface, thereby removing a barrier protecting deeper layers. Increased laser energy could now reach these layers, resulting in more extensive coagulation.[23] It is known that attempting to coagulate a bleeding peptic ulcer with an endoscopically guided Nd:YAG laser fiber will be difficult if a large blood vessel below the lesion acts as a heat sink.

A more practical solution to the problems of heat and bubble formation rests with the laser beam itself. If the beam energy is delivered in larger amounts (watts), but in shorter pulses, tissue adjacent to the irradiated zone has time to cool off between pulses, thus preventing excessive adjacent thermal damage. A physical upper limit may result from optical fiber shattering, secondary to inability to transmit large energy pulses.[24]

One other point to be made involving safety concerns about LAS is equipment. The performance of this technique requires a laser. Even with advances in technology, a medical-grade laser is large, difficult to move, and sometimes requires special electrical and water support. The distal ends of the optical fibers require polishing, unless disposable ones are used. Special safety precautions are necessary, such as eye protection and operating room doorway and window covering, to prevent inadvertent beam damage to operating room personnel. However, these precautions do not assume as much importance with LAS, as the beam is contained within the joint space, and safety glasses are not necessary when viewing the video monitor. If one desires to photograph the procedure with a 35-mm camera attached to the arthroscope, the operator must wear the appropriate safety glasses, further complicating an already difficult challenge.

INSTRUMENTATION AND EQUIPMENT

If the laser fiber is introduced through a separate portal and its movements are controlled by triangulation, design alterations of the arthroscope are not necessary. We have found it convenient to blunt the bevel of a 15-gauge spinal needle to function both as an irrigation outflow portal and as a sheath to allow passage of a 600-micron laser fiberoptic (Fig. 22-1). However, the size of LAS usable fiberoptics (400 to 600 microns) has allowed the construction of special "operating laser arthroscopes." Currently, we utilize a specially modified 5-degree, 1.9-mm–diameter Hopkins rod lens arthroscope with a coaxial channel that permits a 400-micron fiberoptic to be directed through an angled sideport.[25] This instrument allows instantaneous delivery of the laser fiber to the field of view, eliminating the need for triangulation and simplifying control of the fiberoptic (Fig. 22-2).

Another arthroscope design, utilized by Ohnishi,[26] involves a straight operating channel for fiberoptic insertion with a bent optical pathway ending with an angled sideport eyepiece. These specially designed arthroscopes require a perforated rubber gasket over the operating channel portal. This is necessary to prevent air from being drawn into the arthroscope, and therefore into the joint space, by the flow of irrigation fluids. The arthroscopist need violate only the joint

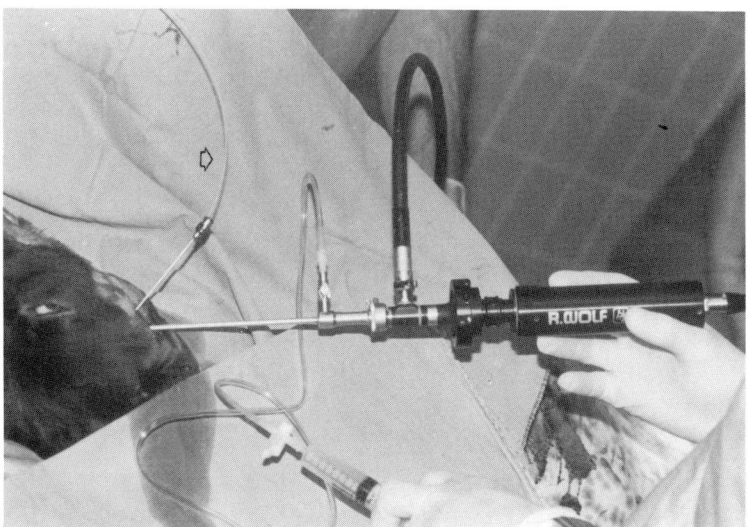

Figure 22–1. Canine temporomandibular joint arthroscopy with a 2.7-mm arthroscope. The laser fiberoptic enters through the irrigation outflow portal (*arrow*).

space with the arthroscope and a small outflow portal when using these special instruments.

Research in TMJ LAS in our laboratory utilized the canine model and has been limited to the Nd:YAG laser.[27] Non-contact coagulation burns and bare fiber contact burns have been produced in disc, capsule, synovial, and cortical bone tissues of the canine TMJ (Fig. 22–3). Second-look TMJ arthroscopy at 1- or 2-week intervals postoperatively revealed contracture healing of the synovial and capsular wounds; however, all fibrocartilaginous and bone wounds remained unaltered (Figs. 22–4 through 22–7).

Histologic staining of acute and chronic wounds revealed definite layers of tissue alteration, consisting of a surface coagulum zone, a thin zone of cavitation, and a deep acidophilic zone (Fig. 22–8). The normal linear, wavy bands of fibrocartilage were coagulated into homogeneous globules. Loss of nuclear architecture was also prominent in these areas. Gross examination of bone wounds histologically and at autopsy revealed no perforations outside the superior joint space. One disturbing finding was condylar marrow fibrosis under an articulating surface contact burn, underscoring the potential for deep tissue injury so characteristic

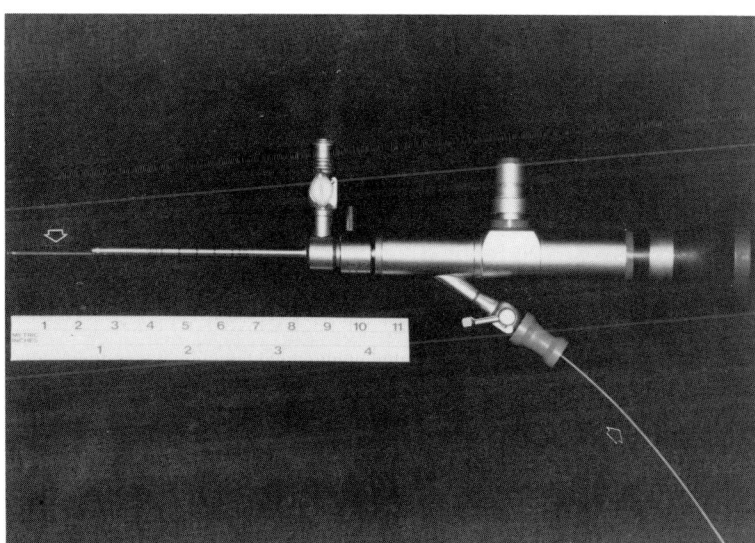

Figure 22–2. Operating 1.9-mm laser arthroscope. The laser fiberoptic enters through the rubber-capped side port and exits coaxially with the working end.

Figure 22–3. Two-week-old noncontact Nd:YAG laser burns of a canine temporomandibular disc. The top lesion demonstrates deep thermal destruction; the bottom lesion demonstrates surface destruction. No inflammatory or healing response can be seen. (Movat's pentachrome stain; magnification × 4.)

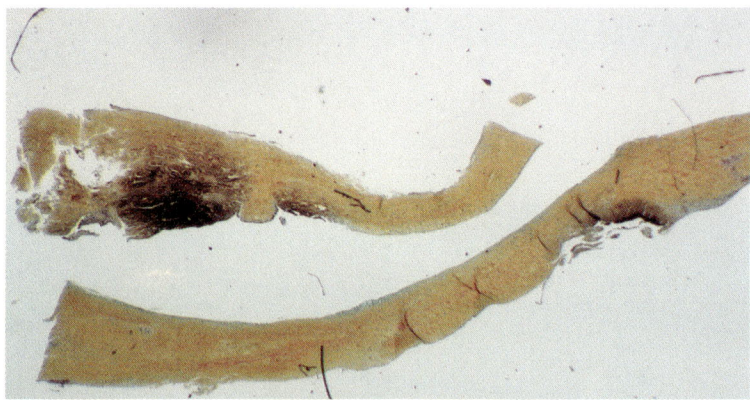

of the Nd:YAG laser (Figs. 22–9 and 22–10).[25]

CONCLUSIONS

The recent acceleration of technologic advances in arthroscopy of small joints and in laser systems makes marriage of the two likely. Increasing capabilities of surgical TMJ arthroscopy can lower the frequency of open arthrotomy. We believe that practitioners of TMJ arthroscopy should refrain from presiding over this marriage without a long courtship.

Well-designed and well-executed animal studies to develop techniques, outline risks, and discover complications should precede human trials. Human protocols must be approved by the surgeon's institutional review board with risk assignment before Federal Drug Administration (FDA) application for Investigational Device Exemption status. Many of the laser systems discussed previously have a slim envelope of FDA application approvals. Transgression outside this system of experimental checks and balances invites legal destruction of the adventurous practitioner.

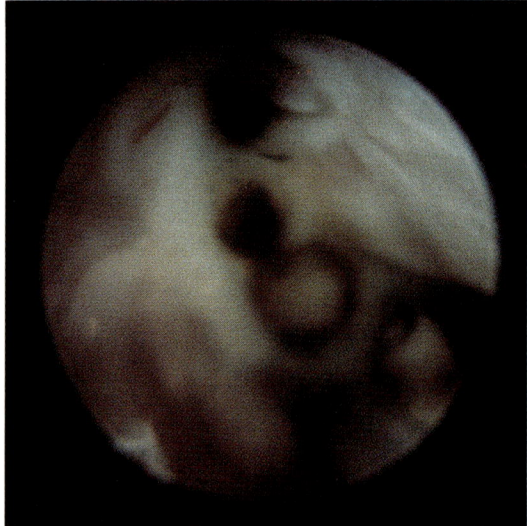

Figure 22–4. Intraoperative arthroscopic photograph of contact Nd:YAG burns of canine temporomandibular medial capsular tissue. Note the small, crater-like depressions (center), which are equal in diameter to the laser fiberoptic (small white cylinder at 5 o'clock). Anterior is to the right; superior is at the top; disc is from 12 to 3 o'clock. The photograph was made through a 1.9-mm operating laser arthroscope.

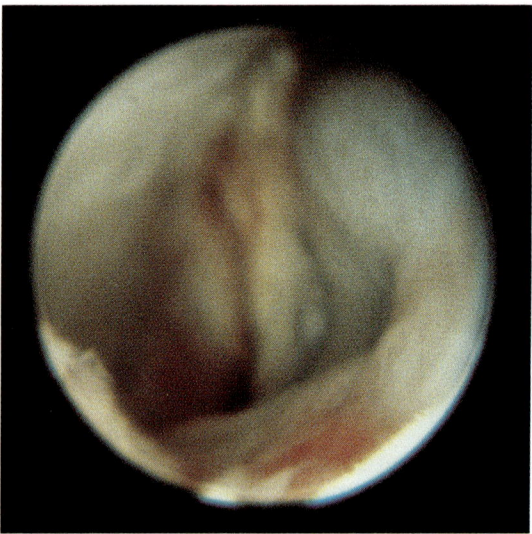

Figure 22–5. Arthroscopic appearance of the lesions in Figure 22–4 after 2 weeks. Note the linear scar band in the medial capsule (center).

B. Laser-Assisted Arthroscopy of the Temporomandibular Joint ■ 333

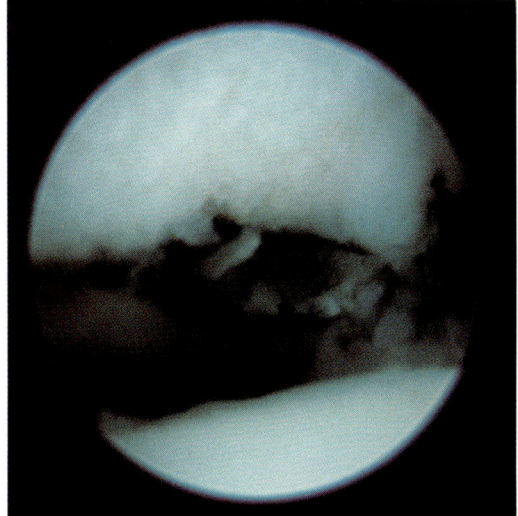

Figure 22–6. Arthroscopic appearance 2 weeks following a contact Nd:YAG laser wound of glenoid fossa cortical bone (center). Disc is from 4 to 7 o'clock.

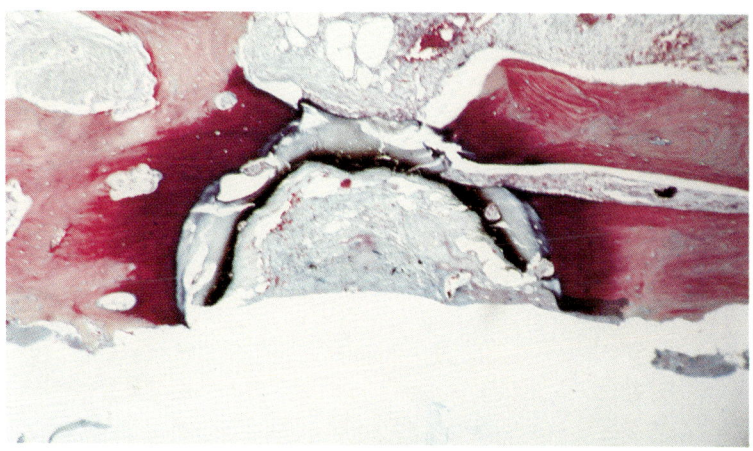

Figure 22–7. Photomicrograph of the lesion in Figure 22–6. Note the differential layering of the wound. (Movat's pentachrome stain; magnification × 20.)

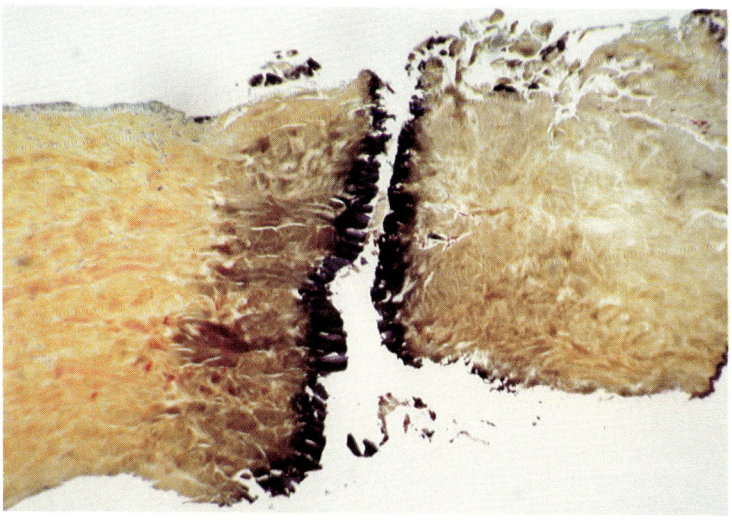

Figure 22–8. Photomicrograph of a 2-week-old contact Nd:YAG burn of a canine temporomandibular disc. (Movat's pentachrome stain; magnification × 15.7.)

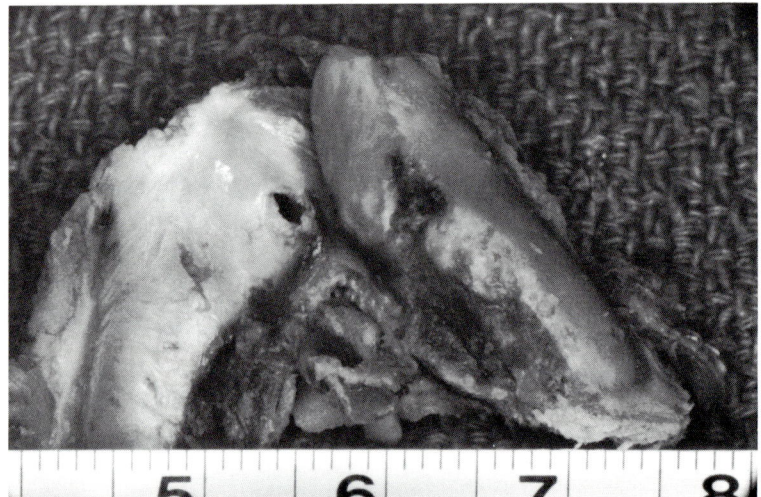

Figure 22–9. Autopsy specimen of a canine temporomandibular joint demonstrating a transmural Nd:YAG burn of the disc (left) and a corresponding lesion on the underlying condylar head (right). Autopsy was performed 2 weeks following burn.

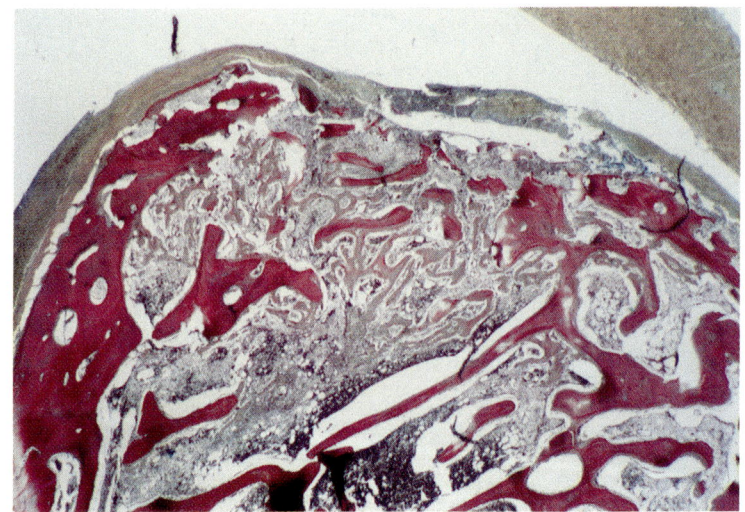

Figure 22–10. Photomicrograph of the condylar head in Figure 22–9 demonstrating a non-contact Nd:YAG burn of the articular surface and underlying marrow fibrosis. (Movat's pentachrome stain; magnification × 4.)

An excellent review by Norton and Norton[28] outlines the intricacies of informed consent, negligence actions, regulatory interaction, product liability, and laser credential approval. Knowledge of the concepts outlined in their article is critical for the success of any practitioner who is considering laser-assisted TMJ arthroscopic surgery.

References

1. Pecaro BC, Garehime WJ: The CO_2 laser in oral and maxillofacial surgery. J Oral Maxillofac Surg 41:725, 1983.
2. Whipple TL, Caspari RB, Meyers JF: Arthroscopic laser meniscectomy in a gas medium. Arthroscopy 1(1):2, 1985.
3. Whipple TL, Caspari RB, Meyers JF: Synovial response to laser-induced carbon ash residue. Lasers Surg Med 3:291, 1984.
4. Philandrianos G: Le laser à gaz carbonique en chirurgie arthroscopique du genou. Presse Med 14:2103, 1985.
5. Whipple TL, Marotta JJ, May TC, et al: Electron microscopy of CO_2 laser induced effects in human fibrocartilage. Lasers Surg Med 7:184, 1987.
6. Zeevi B, Gal D, Wolf N, et al: The use of carbon dioxide laser catheter for atrial septostomy. Am Heart J 116:117, 1988.
7. Baggish MS, Baltoyannis P: Carbon dioxide laser laparoscopy performed with a flexible fiber in humans. Am J Obstet Gynecol 157:1129, 1987.

8. Isner JM, DeJesus SR, Clarke RH, et al: Mechanism of laser ablation in an absorbing fluid field. Lasers Surg Med 8:543, 1988.
9. Kramer JR, Bott-Silverman C, Ratliff NM, et al: Removal of atherosclerotic plaque using multiple short exposures of argon ion laser light. Am Heart J 113:1038, 1987.
10. Metcalf RW, Dixon JA: Use of lasers for arthroscopic meniscectomy: A preliminary report on laboratory investigation. Abstract Presentation, 4th Annual Meeting of the American Society of Laser Medicine and Surgery, Salt Lake City, Utah, 1984.
11. Treat MR, Trokel SL, DeFilippi VJ, et al: Mid-infrared lasers for endoscopic surgery: A new class of surgical lasers. Am Surg 55:81, 1989.
12. Treat MR, Trokel SL, Reynolds D, et al: Preliminary evaluation of a pulsed 2.15-μm laser system for fiberoptic endoscopic surgery. Lasers Surg Med 8:322, 1988.
13. Martiniuk R, Bauer JA, McKean JDS, et al: New long-wavelength Nd:YAG laser at 1.44 μm: Effect on brain. J Neurosurg 70:249, 1989.
14. Levine HL: Endoscopy and the KPT/532 laser for nasal sinus disease. Ann Otol Rhinol Laryngol 98:46, 1989.
15. Shanberg A, Baghdassarian R, Tansey L, et al: KTP 532 laser in treatment of urethral strictures. Urology 32:517, 1988.
16. Daniell JF, Miller W, Tosh R: Initial evaluation of the use of potassium-titanyl-phosphate (KTP/532) laser in gynecologic laparoscopy. Fertil Steril 46:373, 1986.
17. Bradrick JP, Indresano AT: Unpublished data.
18. Cross FW, Bowker TJ: The physical properties of tissue ablation with Eximer lasers. Med Instrum 21:226, 1987.
19. Enderby CE: Laser instrumentation. In Dixon JA (ed): Surgical Applications of Lasers, 2nd Ed. Chicago: Year Book Medical Publishers, 1987, p 69.
20. Böhnke M, Keller C, Winter R: Corneal endothelial cell damage associated with contact to gas bubbles during YAG laser application. Ophthalmic Res 19:357, 1987.
21. Rastegar S, van Gemert MJC, Welch AJ, et al: Laser ablation of discs of agar gel. Phys Med Biol 33:133, 1988.
22. Laufer G, Joachims HZ, Mordechovitz D, et al: Tissue precooling for thermochemical damage reduction during laser surgery. Lasers Surg Med 7:160, 1987.
23. Haina D, Landthaler M, Braun-Fulco O, et al: Comparison of maximum coagulation depth in human skin for different types of medical lasers. Lasers Surg Med 7:355, 1987.
24. Cross FW, Bowker TJ, Brown SG: Arterial healing in the dog after intraluminal delivery of pulsed Nd:YAG laser energy. Br J Surg 74:430, 1987.
25. Indresano AT, Bradrick JP, Eckhauser ML: Use of the laser in arthroscopic animal studies. Presented at the International Symposium on Arthroscopic Surgery for Temporomandibular Disorders, Maui, Hawaii, Dec 8–11, 1989.
26. Ohnishi M: Clinical use of lasers in arthroscopy. Use of the operating arthroscope. Presented at the International Symposium on Arthroscopic Surgery for Temporomandibular Disorders, Maui, Hawaii, Dec 8–11, 1989.
27. Bradrick JP, Eckhauser ML, Indresano AT: Morphologic and histologic changes in canine temporomandibular joint tissues following arthroscopic guided neodymium:YAG laser exposure. J Oral Maxillofac Surg 47:1177, 1989.
28. Norton ML, Norton EV: Medical lasers and the law. Leg Med 1986, p 134.

☐ C. Role of Viscosurgery in Arthroscopy

CHARLES WEISS, M.D.

The ultimate goal of arthroscopy is to restore physicochemical homeostasis to the temporomandibular joint (TMJ). To date, arthroscopy has been shown to be highly effective in relieving pain and mechanical dysfunction in injured or arthritic TMJs. By decreasing the surface area of degenerated cartilage and relieving the mechanical stress resulting from torn or displaced interarticular tissues, the inalterable advance of osteoarthritis of this joint may be slowed significantly. Arthroscopy, however, also inflicts its own damage to the joint surfaces, disrupting delicate synovial membrane linings and injuring joint surfaces. Joint lavage with saline during surgery dilutes and removes the joint surfaces' protective hyaluronan covering, causing further loss of proteoglycans.[1] Synovial inflammation and scuffing of the articular surface result from the diminished macromolecular protection of the articular cartilage and disc surfaces. The late results of these injuries may become apparent as degenerative arthritic change.[2-7]

The application of biologically inert viscoelastic devices (hyaluronan) had eliminated many similar mechanical problems in ophthalmic surgery,[8-13] and new, more highly viscous cross-linked preparations of this material (hylan) may have significant protective and stabilizing functions in the temporomandibular joint.[14, 15] The term viscosurgery[9, 16] was coined by Balazs to indicate surgical procedures in which biologically inert viscoelastic devices in the form of hyaluronan jellies, gels, and solutions can be used as tools* and implants† to minimize trauma associated with arthroscopic procedures and to provide a tissue environment conducive to healing.[9] Sodium hyaluronan's biocompatibility (it is present in all connective tissue matrices of primates) and unique rheologic properties (unmatched by any other natural or synthetic polymer) make it the logical choice for viscosurgery.[2, 4, 14] Noninflammatory sodium hyaluronan has adequate viscoelastic properties for many forms of ophthalmic surgery, but it lacks sufficient viscosity, elasticity, and residence time in tissues for most orthopedic and musculoskeletal uses. A cross-linked form of hyaluronan called hylan has significantly altered rheologic properties with very high viscosity at low shear, very high elasticity at high frequency and molecular weights up to 24 million.[14] Hylans can also be cross-linked to form water soluble gels, membranes, and tubes.

Studies on tendons have shown hylan to reduce adhesion formation significantly while not interfering with tendon healing.[17, 18] Studies in rabbit arthritis models have demonstrated significant slowing in the rate of arthritis development because of increased surface protection.[19] In arthroscopy, hylan devices have been successful in protecting surfaces from instrument damage, in improving visibility and debris control, and in overall facilitation of the surgical procedure.[15, 19]

Through the use of hylan, injury is minimized by maintaining or creating tissue spaces within which the surgeon can safely operate.[15, 19] The mechanical trauma of instruments to cells and tissue surfaces is diminished by the viscoelastic properties of this material. By ensuring separation and lubrication of normally nonadherent tissue surfaces, and by preventing and controlling the movement and activities of sensitive cells, joint homeostasis may be maintained. The viscoelastic nature of these molecules allows them to act as mechanical shock absorbers and lubricants, providing a protective coating for delicate tissues and membranes. The use of this device as a protective lubricating coating during arthroscopic surgery provides a milieu analogous to that of the endogenous fluids bathing the healthy joint surface. Studies have demonstrated the improved technical ease and mechanical protection that these devices can provide during arthroscopic surgery of this small joint.[15] Unlike saline, hyaluronic acid will not pass easily through the synovium. It maintains a buffer space between the instrument and articular cartilage when applied to the surface of the instrument or when injected into the joint during arthroscopy. When the surfaces are traumatized, these molecules can form a protective buffer zone around the injured site—physically excluding inflammatory cells from the area and preventing further injury and tissue breakdown.

References

1. Johnson RG, Herbert MA, Wright S, et al: The response of articular cartilage to the in vivo replacement of synovial fluid with saline. Clin Orthop 174:285, 1983.
2. Balazs EA: The physical properties of synovial fluid and the special role of hyaluronic acid. In Helfet AJ (ed): Disorders of the Knee, Vol 4. Philadelphia: Lippincott, 1982, p 61.
3. Balazs EA, Bloom GD, Swann DA: Fine structure and glycosaminoglycan content of the surface layer of articular cartilage. Fed Proc 25:1813, 1966.
4. Balazs EA, Gibbs DA: The rheological properties and biological function of hyaluronic acid. In Balazs EA (ed): Chemistry and Molecular Biology of the Intercellular Matrix. London: Academic Press, 1970, pp 1241–1254.
5. Dustmann HO, Phul W, Schulitz KP: Knorpelveranderungen beim hemarthros unter besonder berucksichtigung der ruhigstelling. Arch Orthop Trauma Surg 71:148, 1971.
6. Finsterbush A, Friedman B: Early changes in immobilized rabbit's knee joints: A light and electron microscopic study. Clin Orthop 92:305, 1973.
7. Wigren A, Wik O: The influence of hyaluronic acid on immobilized knees. Upsala J Med Sci [Suppl] 16:1, 1974.

---

*Viscosurgical tools are used during surgery to maintain spaces for surgical manipulation, protect surfaces, and manipulate tissues.[14, 16, 19]

†Viscosurgical implants may be used prior to, after, or instead of surgery to exclude blood cells and fibrinogen, decrease adhesion formation, seal surfaces from proteoglycan leakage, and maintain surface separation.[14, 16, 19]

8. Balazs EA, Freeman MI, Kloti R, et al: Hyaluronic acid and replacement of vitreous and aqueous humor. Mod Probl Ophthalmol 10:3, 1972.
9. Balazs EA: Sodium hyaluronate and viscosurgery. In Miller D, Stegmann R (eds): Healon: A Guide to Its Use in Ophthalmic Surgery. New York: John Wiley, 1983, pp 5–28.
10. Edmund J: Vitreous substitute in the treatment of retinal detachment. Limitations and prospects for retinal surgery. Mod Probl Ophthalmol 12:370, 1974.
11. Pape LG, Balazs EA: The use of sodium hyaluronate (Healon) in human anterior segment surgery. Ophthalmology 87:699, 1980.
12. Regnault F, Bregeat P: Treatment of severe cases of retinal detachment with highly viscous hyaluronic acid. Limitations and prospects for retinal surgery. Mod Probl Ophthalmol 12:378, 1974.
13. Schepens CL, Constable IJ: Open-sky vitrectomy: Operative technique and instrumentation. In Freeman HM, Hirose T, Schepens CL (eds): Vitreous Surgery and Advances in Fundus Diagnosis and Treatment. New York: Appleton-Century-Crofts, 1977, pp 465–467.
14. Balazs EA, Leshchiner EA: (1989). Hyaluronan, its crosslinked derivative—hylan—and their medical applications. In Inagaki H, Phillips GO (eds): Cellulosics Utilization: Research and Rewards in Cellulosics. Proceedings of Nisshinbo International Conference on Cellulosics Utilization in the Near Future. New York: Elsevier Applied Science, 1989, pp 233–241.
15. McCain JP, Balazs E, De La Rua H: Preliminary studies on the use of a viscoelastic solution in arthroscopic surgery of the temporomandibular joint. J Oral Maxillofac Surg 17:1–8, 1989.
16. Weiss C, Balazs EA: The physiologic function of hyaluronic acid and the therapeutic role of viscosurgery in the skeletal system. In Jaffee WL, Neuwirth MG (eds): Mediguide to Orthopedics, Vol 4. New York: Delacorte, 1984, pp 1–4.
17. Weiss C, Levy HJ, Denlinger JL, et al: The role of Na-hylan in reducing postsurgical tendon adhesions. Bull Hosp J Dis Orthop Inst 46:9–15, 1986.
18. Weiss C, Suros JM, Michalow A, et al: The role of Na-hylan in reducing postsurgical tendon adhesions: Part 2. Bull Hosp J Dis Orthop Inst 47:31–39, 1987.
19. Weiss C, Balazs EA: Arthroscopic viscosurgery. Arthroscopy 3:138, 1987.

Section VI
Case Reports of Arthroscopic Pathology

Chapter 23

CASE REPORTS OF ARTHROSCOPIC PATHOLOGY

A. Osteoarthritis

KEN-ICHIRO MURAKAMI, D.D.S., PH.D

The patient, a 76-year-old woman, was referred by her dentist with a chief complaint of painful hypomobility of the left temporomandibular joint (TMJ). She gave no history of trauma, clicking, or locking. For the past several months she had noticed a gradually more severe hypomobility with increased pain and crepitation.

Maximal mouth opening was 30 mm, with severe pain. Tenderness on the lateral and posterior aspects of the left TMJ was present. She was missing the lower molar teeth bilaterally.

Screening radiographic examination revealed mild degenerative changes on the left mandibular condyle. Routine laboratory tests were within normal limits, and there were no clinical signs of rheumatoid arthritis.

Oral nonsteroidal anti-inflammatory drugs administered over a 4-week period were ineffective in eliminating symptoms. Two intra-articular steroid injections (betamethasone 2 mg) decreased the joint pain slightly, but painful hypomobility remained.

Diagnostic arthroscopy was performed 3 months after the patient's initial visit, under local anesthesia in the outpatient clinic, and disclosed an extensive perforation of the disc and posterior attachment (Fig. 23–1, Area B). Significant synovitis and inflammatory synovial villi were evident in the posterior pouch (Fig. 23–2B, photograph of Area B in Fig. 23–1), and expansion of the capillary net-

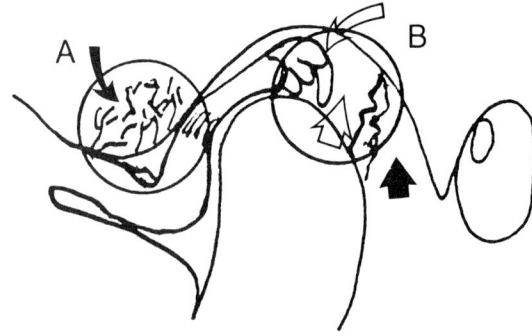

Figure 23–1. Diagrammatic illustration of temporomandibular joint, showing areas of pathology. *A*, Eminence with hyperemia (large solid curved arrow); *B*, posterior synovial pouch with perforation. Large solid straight arrow indicates retrodiscal tissue. Open arrow indicates perforation. Open curved arrow indicates synovial villi.

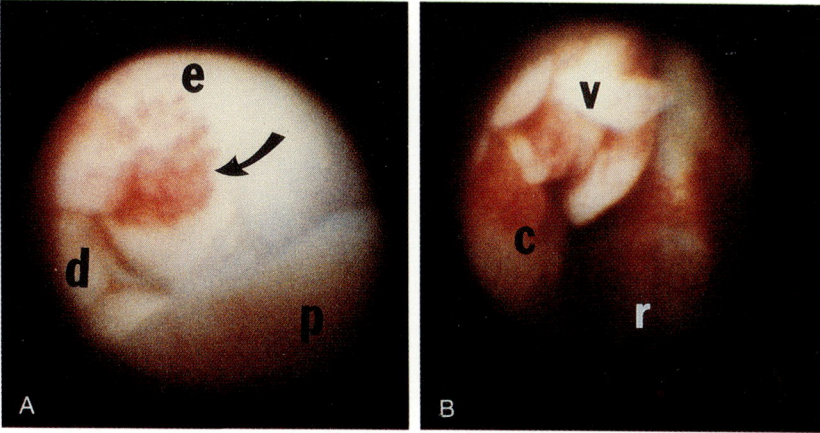

Figure 23–2. *A* and *B,* Arthroscopic photographs of areas *A* and *B,* respectively, in Figure 23–1. Arrow indicates hyperemic capillary network. v = villous synovitis; c = condyle; r = retrodiscal tissue; d = disc; e = eminence; p = posterior attachment.

work from the anterior recess was observed at the apex of the articular eminence (Fig. 23–2A, photograph of Area A in Fig. 23–1). Arthroscopic diagnosis was active osteoarthritis.

Lavage of the upper joint cavity and steroid placement was performed. Pain was decreased postoperatively. Prosthodontic restoration was achieved and the outcome has been assessed as good.

☐ B. Diagnosis and Lavage: Joint Degeneration by "Hyalinization"

SIDNEY L. BRONSTEIN, D.D.S., M.Sc.D.

The patient was a 44-year-old woman who was seen with bilateral pain and tenderness, right greater than left. History revealed that she had a silicone elastomer implant placed in the right temporomandibular joint (TMJ) several years previously. She had been suffering from progressive increase in pain and dysfunction.

Examination revealed a maximal incisal opening (MIO) of 15 mm, with 4+ pain. Range of motion was decreased, with deviation to the right on opening. Bilateral clicking was noted. Radiographic studies showed the right-sided implant, with degenerative bony changes and decreased translation; the left TMJ appeared within normal limits.

The right TMJ was opened and the implant was removed, followed by joint debridement and placement of interpositional temporalis fascia. Arthroscopic examination of the left joint showed an essentially avascular joint (Fig. 23–3). Incipient chondromalacia was also diagnosed. Essentially normal condyle roofing by the disc was seen, but there was slight bilaminar zone redundancy. Lysis and lavage was completed.

This joint is now painless and function is increasing.

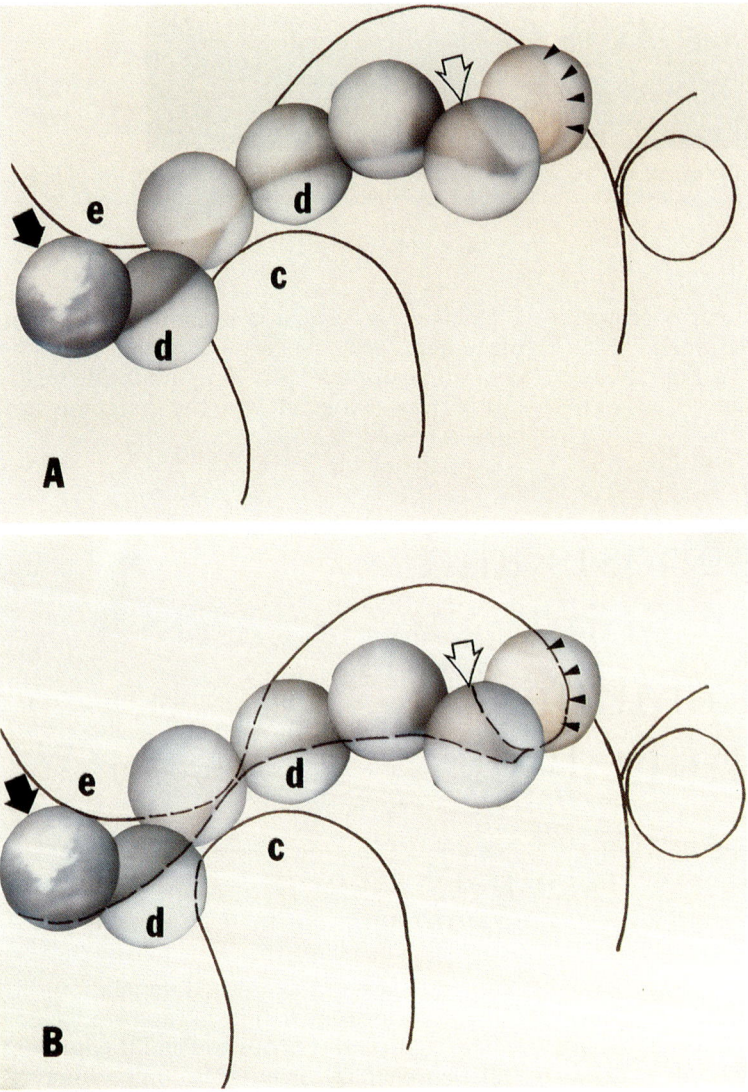

Figure 23–3. *A* and *B*, Composite arthroscopic photographs reveal lack of vascular markings. Chondromalacia is present at the eminence *(solid arrow)*, bilaminar zone redundancy is seen with the closed position *(open arrow)*, and there is bilaminar zone configuration with the open position *(arrowheads)*. c = condyle; d = disc; e = eminence.

C. Lysis, Lavage, and Debridement: Proliferative Fibrosis and Synovitis

SIDNEY L. BRONSTEIN, D.D.S., M.Sc.D.

The patient, a 38-year-old woman, was seen in November of 1988 complaining of constant, gradually increasing facial pain and discomfort, mostly on the left, for the past year. She had had arthroplasty procedures done in April of 1986, consisting of a left disc removal with placement of a temporary silicone elastomer implant and a right disc repair. Tomography was ordered 7 months later because of nagging symptoms and showed degenerative changes on the left and a normal joint on the right. Medications, orthotics, and physical therapy provided variable and temporary relief of symptoms, which were usually exacerbated during stress.

Clinical examination revealed hypomobility, pain, and joint tenderness bilaterally, but more on the left than the right. Magnetic resonance imaging showed degenerative changes bilaterally, mostly on the left, and normal disc position on the right.

Right arthroscopy showed a prominent posterior attachment and a rather normal disc in appearance and position. When the joint was evaluated anteriorly, proliferative tissue was noted at the apex of the eminence, and synovial proliferation was seen in the anterior pouch (Fig. 23-4). The joint was debrided in this area using suction and hand forceps. Pathologic examination was interpreted as nonspecific cartilage and fibrous tissues.

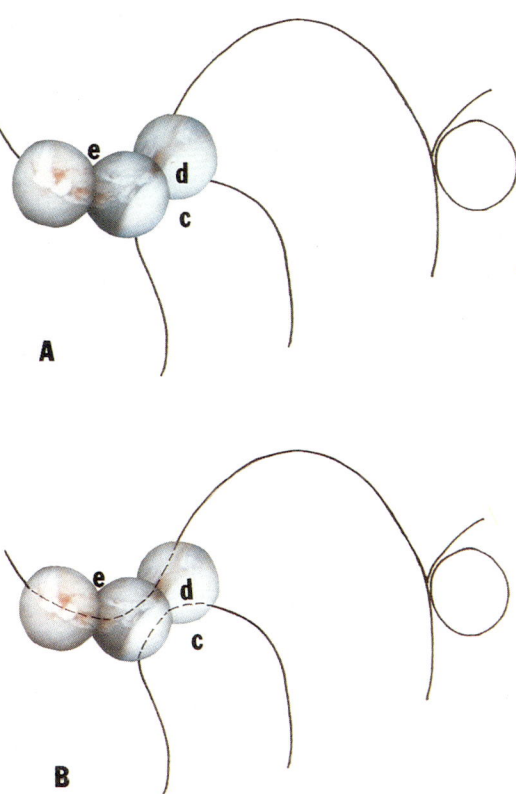

Figure 23–4. *A* and *B*, Composite arthroscopic photographs of the left temporomandibular joint. Proliferative tissue can be seen at the apex of the eminence. c = condyle; d = disc; e = eminence.

☐ D. Lysis, Lavage, and Disc Manipulation: Painful Hypomobility with Disc Displacement and Chondromalacia

SIDNEY L. BRONSTEIN, D.D.S., M.Sc.D.

This 17-year-old female patient presented with bilateral pain, locking, increasing dysfunction, and bilateral joint noises, but especially crepitus in the left temporomandibular joint (TMJ). These symptoms were accompanied by headaches and neck and ear pain.

Symptoms had begun 3 to 4 months previously. Pertinent history includes a fall on the chin 6 years ago. Locking occurred approximately twice daily, finally increasing to a closed lock. No noise had been noted on the right TMJ for the past 2 months. The patient has used an orthotic for 3 weeks, with no change in signs and symptoms. Bruxism has increased recently.

Examination revealed crepitus on the left, a maximal incisal opening (MIO) of 30 mm accompanied by pain, a right laterotrusion of 19 mm, and a left laterotrusion of 5 mm.

Radiography showed an osteophyte on the right condyle, and bilateral posterior condylar positioning and bilateral anterior disc displacement without reduction on the right and with reduction on the left. Disc morphology appeared normal.

Arthroscopy was performed bilaterally. The right TMJ had a disc displaced far anteromedially, which could not be completely reduced by instrumentation. The left side showed anterior disc displacement that was successfully reduced by manipulation. Grade I–II chondromalacia was seen (Fig. 23–5).

The left side has responded well to treatment, but the right side required opening 5 months later. A discopexy procedure was done to reposition the disc more normally and has provided relief of symptoms.

D. Lysis, Lavage, Disc Manipulation: Hypomobility with Disc Displacement Chondromalacia ■ 343

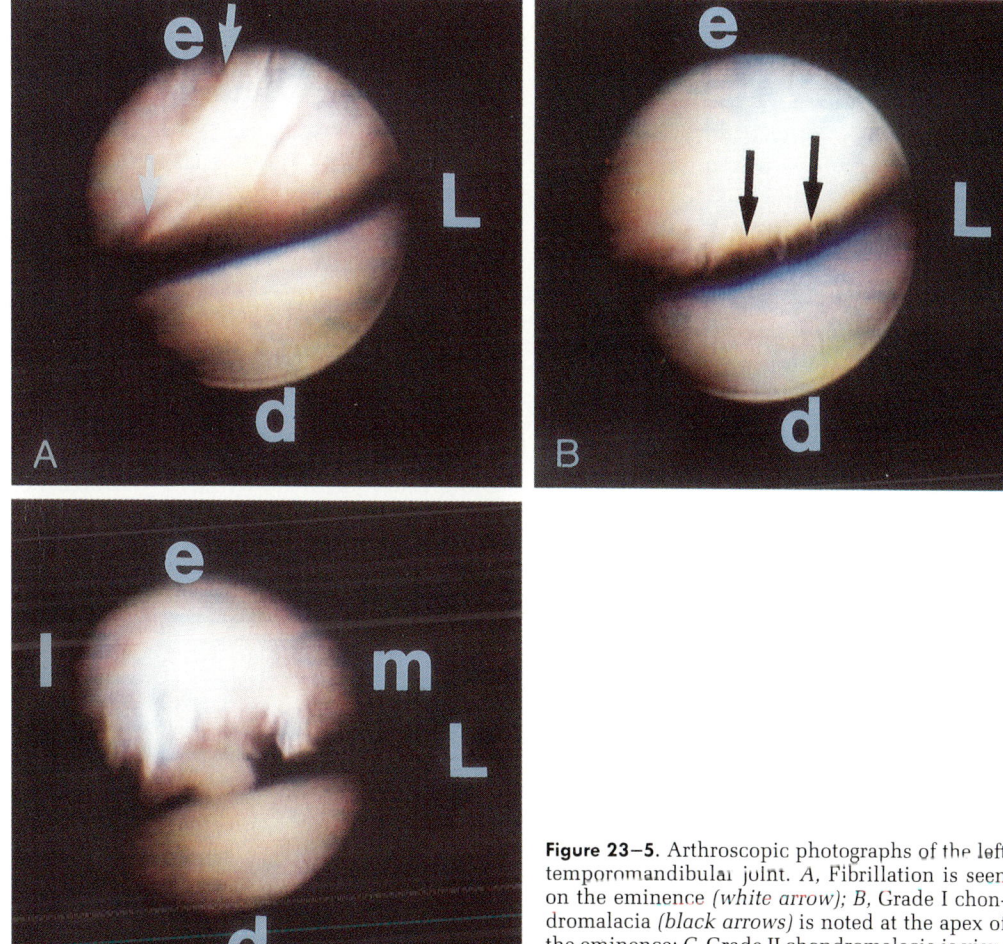

Figure 23–5. Arthroscopic photographs of the left temporomandibular joint. *A*, Fibrillation is seen on the eminence *(white arrow)*; *B*, Grade I chondromalacia *(black arrows)* is noted at the apex of the eminence; *C*, Grade II chondromalacia is visualized further into the anterior synovial pouch. d = disc; e = eminence; l = lateral; m = medial.

E. Diagnostic Arthroscopy: Severe Adhesions and Disc Perforation

SIDNEY L. BRONSTEIN, D.D.S., M.Sc.D.

The patient was a 26-year-old woman; her chief problem was dysfunctional pain on opening, closing, and chewing. This was primarily left-sided and was accompanied by popping and grinding noises. The noises were first noted 6 years ago after an episode of joint dislocation.

The present symptoms began about 6 months prior to the patient's first office visit. She had been using a splint for the past 5 months, without effect.

The only pertinent findings revealed by examination were slight joint tenderness and a maximal incisal opening (MIO) of 30 mm with pain. Right, left, and protrusive excursions were within normal limits. Transcranial radiographic studies showed decreased anterior joint space on the left, with "beaking" of the left condyle. Magnetic resonance imaging diagnosed left anterior disc dislocation without reduction.

Diagnostic arthroscopy was performed on the left side and revealed severe adhesions and fibrosis anteriorly in the inferior space (Fig. 23–6). A perforated disc was seen in the lateral portion of the disc near the junction of the posterior attachment and posterior band (Fig. 23–7). Joint mobility could not be increased with lysis and lavage procedures. Immediate arthrotomy was done, and the disc was removed.

To date, healing is progressing splendidly and function has returned to normal limits, without pain.

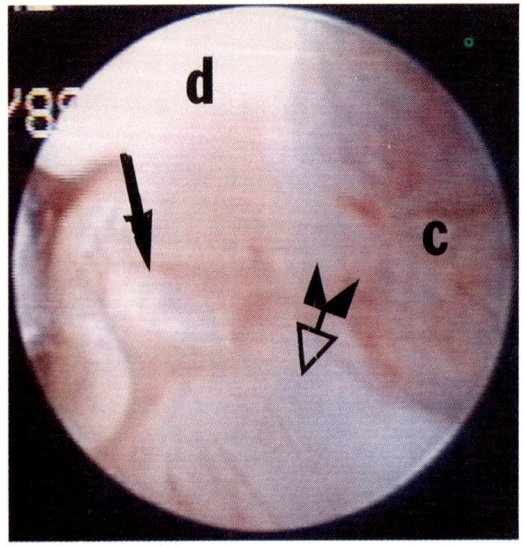

Figure 23–6. A very large well-formed adhesion *(solid arrow)* and capsular fibrosis *(open arrowhead)* are seen in the anterior synovial pouch of the inferior temporomandibular joint space. c = capsule; d = disc.

E. Diagnostic Arthroscopy: Severe Adhesions and Disc Perforation ■ 345

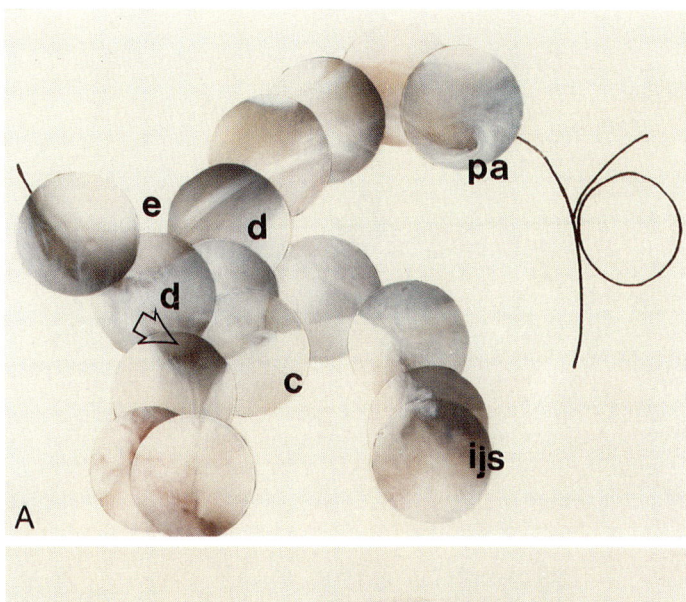

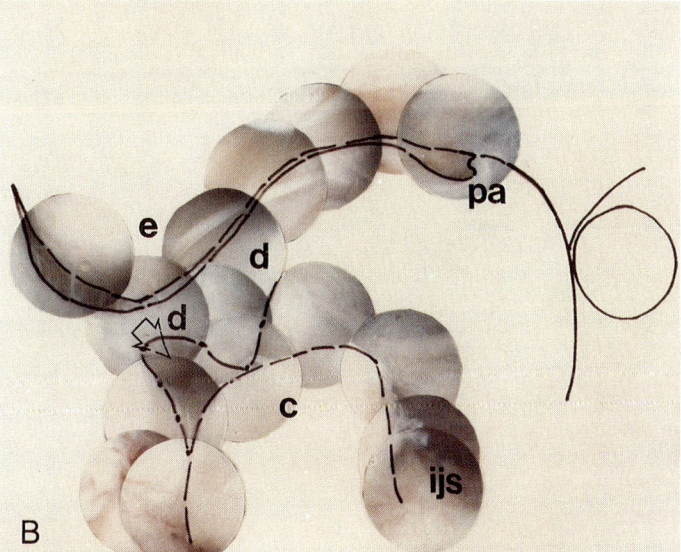

Figure 23–7. *A* and *B*, Composite arthroscopic photographs showing the relationships of the perforation *(arrows)* and the adjacent temporomandibular joint structures. c = condyle; d = disc; e = eminence; ijs = inferior joint space; pa = posterior attachment.

■ APPENDICES

Appendix A
American Association of Oral and Maxillofacial Surgeons Statement on Temporomandibular Joint Arthroscopy

AMERICAN ASSOCIATION OF
ORAL AND MAXILLOFACIAL
SURGEONS POSITION PAPER ON
TMJ ARTHROSCOPY*

I. Preamble

Temporomandibular joint (TMJ) disorders are a major cause of patient pain and dysfunction and an important focus of attention by health care providers. Based on specific criteria, surgical modalities may be the indicated form of treatment for certain TMJ disorders. Recent advances in small joint arthroscopic instrumentation have opened an important new option in the management of TMJ disorders, analogous to the impact of arthroscopic surgery on therapy for large joint (e.g. knee, shoulder, ankle, etc.) disorders. Visualization through arthroscopy has proved to be a valuable addition in the armamentarium of therapeutic approaches to the TMJ. Potentially less invasive than open arthrotomy, arthroscopy offers both diagnostic and therapeutic options in the management of internal derangements and degenerative joint diseases.

II. Definitions

Internal derangement: A disruption within the internal aspects of the TMJ, in which there is displacement of the disc from its normal functional relationship with the mandibular condyle and the articular portion of the tem-

---

*Position paper of the American Association of Oral and Maxillofacial Surgeons provided as a membership service.

poral bone, or alterations in the normal dynamic motion of intracapsular elements leading to joint dysfunction.

Degenerative joint disease (osteoarthritis, arthrosis): A non-inflammatory focal disorder, characterized by progressive deterioration of the articular surfaces within the joint, usually associated with pain and impaired function.

III. Indications for TMJ Arthroscopy

A. Diagnostic arthroscopy

This procedure is indicated for those joint conditions that warrant direct examinations in order to confirm the presence of clinically suspected disease/disorder states that cannot be confirmed by other means of evaluation and where confirmation of the disease will affect the patient's care, or when direct examination will enhance an established diagnosis for purposes of making treatment decisions.

Examples:

1. Unexplained, persistent TMJ pain, unresponsive to medical therapy.
2. Confirmation of other diagnostic findings that could warrant surgical intervention.
3. Biopsy of suspected lesions or diseases.

B. Operative arthroscopy

These procedures are indicated for selected joint conditions that constitute a disability for the patient, are refractory to medical treatment, and require internal structural modifications.

Examples:

1. Internal derangements
2. Hypomobility, secondary to intra-joint adhesions
3. Synovitis
4. Degenerative joint disease
5. Hypermobility, resulting in painful subluxation or dislocation.

IV. Contraindications to Arthroscopy

Contraindications to arthroscopy include skin infection, possible tumor seeding, and medical and other circumstances unique to the patient.

V. Techniques of Operative Arthroscopy

A variety of techniques are used in the arthroscopic management of patients with internal derangements or degenerative joint disease and may involve ablation of adhesions, restoration of disc mobility and position, instillation of medication, and lavage of the joint using the arthroscopic inflow-outflow mechanism. The lavage eliminates microscopic debris and tissue breakdown products which may play a role as a causative factor in the production of pain in the dysfunctional state. Additionally, capsular and discal attachment scarification or plication may be used to help in the reduction of hypermobility.

VI. Guidelines for Patient Care

Arthroscopic procedures are usually performed under general anesthesia, in the operating room, and may be accomplished on an outpatient basis. Overnight stay may be required. In some instances the arthroscopic examination may need to be followed by open arthrotomy to complete the surgical procedure.

VII. Clinical Privileges

The following may serve as guidelines to grant clinical privileges in TMJ arthroscopy, but can be modified to accommodate individual hospital requirements:

A. Board certified or Board eligible oral and maxillofacial surgeon; or surgeons with current privileges in open arthrotomy of the TMJ.

B. Documentation as operating surgeon or first assistant of at least 15 open TMJ arthrotomies.

C. At least 16 hours of didactic and clinical continuing education courses on the subject of TMJ arthroscopy.

D. Documentation of cadaver technique experience.

E. Satisfactorily proctored performance of at least three TMJ arthroscopic procedures.

F. Demonstrated competence in arthroscopic procedures during residency training, substantiated by the residency director, or surgeons with current privileges in TMJ arthroscopic surgery. Compliance with this requirement excludes items B, C, D and E above.

G. Current proficiency and knowledge in TMJ arthroscopic surgery.

VIII. Summary

The American Association of Oral and Maxillofacial Surgeons recognizes the value and acknowledges the use of arthroscopy, when appropriate, in the overall approach to clinical management of the patient with disease or disorder of the TMJ. While no single means of therapy is applicable to all forms of TMJ disease/disorder, arthroscopy has been demonstrated to be useful in selected instances, when consistent with the specific needs of individual patients.

Selected References For Position Paper on TMJ Arthroscopy

This list of selected references is intended only to acknowledge some of the sources of information drawn upon in the preparation of this document. Citation of the reference material is not meant to imply endorsement of any statement contained in the reference material, nor that the list is an exhaustive compilation of information on the topic. Readers should consult other sources to obtain a complete bibliography on the topic.

AAOMS 1984 Criteria Statement for TMJ Meniscus Surgery.

Murakami, K., Matsuki, M., Iizuka, T., and Ono, T., Diagnostic Arthroscopy of the TMJ: Differential Diagnosis in Patients with Limited Jaw Opening. J Craniomandibular Pract. 4:117-26, 1986

Ohnishi, M., Arthroscopy of the Temporomandibular Joint. J. Stomatol Soc. Jpn. 42:202-13, 1975

Sanders, B., Arthroscopic Surgery of the Temporomandibular Joint: Treatment of Internal Derangement with Persistent Closed Lock. Oral Surg. 62:361-72, 1986

Sanders, B., Buoncristiani, R., Diagnostic and Surgical Arthroscopy of the Temporomandibular Joint: Clinical Experience with 137 Procedures over a Two Year Period. J Craniomandibular Pract. 1:202-13, 1987

Johnson, L.L., Arthroscopic Surgery Principles & Practice. Mosby-Third Edition Volumes I & II

Watanabe, M., Arthroscopy of Small Joints. Igaku-Shoin Tokyo, New York

Heffez, L., Blaustein P., Diagnostic Arthroscopy of the Temporomandibular Joint: Part 1: Normal Arthroscopic Findings. Oral Surg., Oral Med., Oral Pathol. 64(6), pp. 653-78 1987 Dec.

Nuelle, P.G., Alpern, M.G., Ufema, J.W., An Arthroscopic Perspective of the Temporomandibular Joint: A Clinical Study. Clin. Orthop. 21(2) pp 110-16 1987 Feb.

Holmlund, A., Hellsing, G., Wredmark, T., Arthroscopy of the Temporomandibular Joint: A Clinical Study. Int. J Oral Maxillofac Surg. 15(6) pp. 715-21 1986 Dec.

Liedberg, J., Westesson, P.L., Diagnostic Accuracy of Upper Compartment Arthroscopy of the Temporomandibular Joint: Correlation with Postmortem Morphology. Oral Surg., Oral Med., Oral Pathol. 62(6) pp. 618-24 1986 Dec.

Hellsing, G., Holmlund, A., TMJ Disorders: A Diagnostic Challenge. J Prosthet. Dent. 1986 Nov. (Review)

Murakami, K., Ono, T., TMJ Arthroscopy by Inferolateral Approach. J Oral Maxillofac Surg. 1986 Aug.

Alpern, M.C., Nuelle, D.G., Ufema, J.W., Direct Parasagittal Computer Tomography and Arthroscopic Surgery of the TMJ. Angle. Orthop. 1986 Apr.

Eriksson, L., Westesson, P.L., Deterioration of Temporary Silicone Implant in the Temporomandibular Joint: A Clinical and Arthroscopic Follow-Up Study. Oral Surg., Oral Med., Oral Pathol. 62(1) pp. 2-6 1986 July

Murakami, K.I., Iizuka T., Matsuki, M., Ono, T., Diagnostic Arthroscopy of the TMJ: Differential Diagnosis in Patients with Limited Jaw Opening. Cranio. 4(2) pp. 117-26 1986 Apr.

Ufema, J.W., Alpern, M.G., Nuelle, P.G., Corrected Parasagittal Direct CT Imaging of the Temporomandibular Joint With Arthroscopic Correlation. Angle. Orthop. 56(2) pp. 102-17 1986 Apr.

Murakami, K., Hoshino, K., Histological Studies on the Inner Surfaces of the Articular Cavities of Human TM Joints with Special Reference to Arthroscopic Observations. Anat. Anz. 1985

Holmlund, A., Hellsing, G., Arthroscopy of the TMJ: An Autopsy Study. Int J Oral Surg. 1985 Apr.

Hellsing, G., Holmlund, A., Nordenram, A., Wredmark, T., Arthroscopy of the TMJ. Examination of 2 Patients with Suspected Disk Derangement. Int J Oral Surg. 1984 Feb.

Murakami, K., Matsumoto, K., Iizuka, T., Suppurative Arthritis of the TMJ. Report of a case with Special Reference to Arthroscopic Observations. J Maxillofac Surg. 1984 Feb.

Murakami, K., Hoshini, K., Regional Anatomical Nomenclature and Arthroscopic Terminology in Human Temporomandibular Joints. Okamimal Folia Anat. Jpn. 58(4-6) pp. 745-60 1982 Mar.

Ohnishi, M., Clinical Application of Arthroscopy in the Temporomandibular Joint Diseases. Bull. Tokyo Med. Dent. Univ. 27(3) pp. 141-50 1980 Sep.

McCain, J.P., Arthroscopy of the Human Temporomandibular Joint. To be published J Oral Maxillofac Surg. 1988 Fall

Appendix B
Patient Consent Form

I hereby authorize Dr. _____ to perform (unilateral, bilateral) arthroscopic examination and arthroscopic surgery of my temporomandibular (jaw) joints. I understand that this procedure is somewhat exploratory in nature and is being done to alleviate my symptoms of pain, noises, and limited motion of my jaw joint(s). I further understand that a regular surgical procedure may still be necessary to correct my joint problem.

I understand that certain complications are inherently possible with this procedure, including, but not limited to the following:

1. Weakness of the nerve allowing wrinkling of the forehead, usually temporary but occasionally permanent.
2. Bleeding within the joint cavity, necessitating opening the joint to control it.
3. Involvement of the ear canal or middle ear from the irrigating procedures, possibly requiring additional treatment.
4. Possible decreased hearing of a temporary nature, but in rare instances permanent.
5. Unsuccessful entry into the joint or inability to accomplish the surgery because of limited movement of the joint.
6. Possibility of requiring joint opening to retrieve a portion of a broken instrument.
7. Possibility of damage to the joint surfaces during arthroscopic examination and surgery; usually of a reversible nature.

I further understand that immediate physical therapy will be necessary and probably continued support and stabilization of my bite will be required.

I authorize photographs and/or videotaping of this procedure for use in continuing education programs.

Witness _____   Patient _____
Date _____   Date _____

I have explained the above surgery, its indications, and its possible complications, risks, extent of procedure, postoperative restrictions, alternatives and placement of incisions (scars) with this patient.

Physician Signature: _____
Date: _____

Appendix C
Diagram of Operating Room Showing Positions of Surgeon and Assisting Personnel and Placement of Equipment Needed for Performing Arthroscopic Procedures

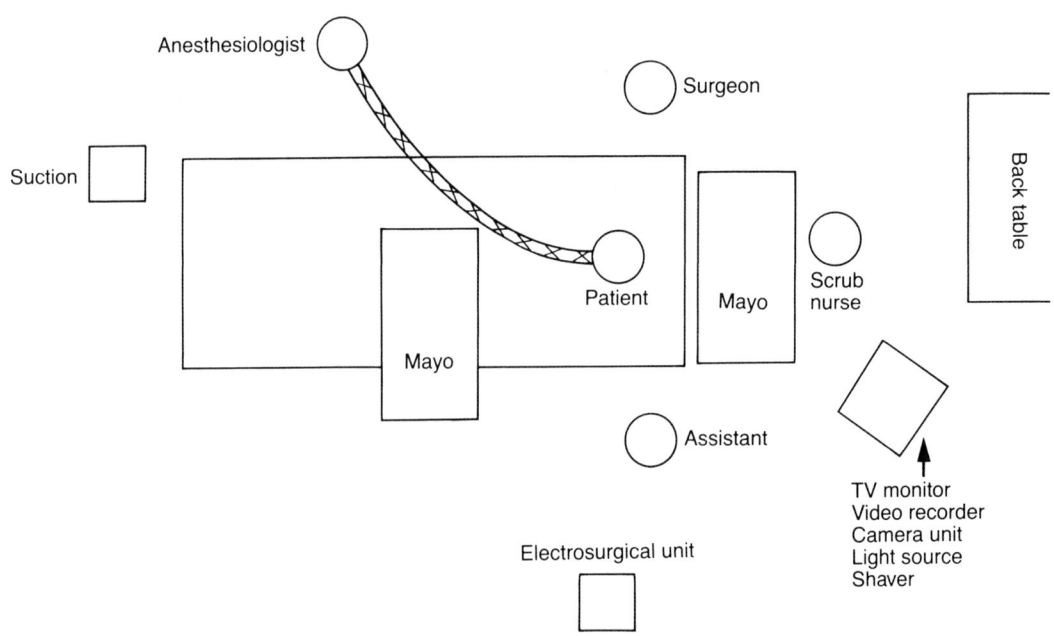

Appendix D

Example of Insurance Claim Form to Be Completed After Providing Therapy for Temporomandibular Joint Disorders

ATTENDING PHYSICIAN'S MEDICAL CLAIM

Patient's Name: _____ Birthdate: _____
Address: _____
Policy Holder's Name: _____
    Insurance Company: _____
    Group Number: _____ Subscriber Number: _____
    Claim Number: _____

Diagnosis (ICD-9-CM Code)

Osteoarthrosis	R	L	715.9	Bruxism			959.9
Degenerative Joint				Myalgia	R	L	959.9
Disease	R	L	715.9	Traumatic	R	L	959.9
Capsulitis	R	L	726.9	Myofascial Pain			
Sprained Capsular				Dysfunction	R	L	729.1
Ligaments	R	L	848.1	Synovitis	R	L	524.6
Disc Displacement	R	L	830.0	Chondromalacia	R	L	524.6
Internal Derangement	R	L	524.6	Surgical opera-			
Lateral Ligament				tion causing			
Prolapse	R	L	524.6	reaction			E878.2
				Other:			

Result of accident? _____ Date: _____

Disability? _____

Place of service: _____

D Example of Insurance Claim Form After Therapy for Temporomandibular Joint Disorders

Treatment	CPT	Fee/Date	Treatment	CPT	Fee/Date
TMJ Consultation/Examination			Coronoidectomy R L	21070	
Comprehensive	90020		Bilateral	21070-50	
Office Visits	90050		Surgery		
Observe Treatment	90050		Disc Removal R L	21060	
Orthosis Impressions	90060		Bilateral	21060-50	
Assistant Surgeon	09980		Fascia Graft	15770	
Surgical Assistant	09966		Prosthetic Joint		
Arthroscopy			Replacement R L	21243	
Diagnostic R L	29800		Bone Graft, Minor	20900	
Synovectomy R L	29804		Bone Graft, Major	20902	
Synovial Biopsy R L			Cartilage Graft;		
Disc Reduction R L			Costochondral	20910	
Sclerotherapy R L			Graft, Ear Cartilage	21235	
Arthrocentesis R L	20600		Disc Removal R L	21060	
Hospital Mgmt.	90200/90270		Bilateral	21060-50	
Orthosis			Arthroplasty R L	21240	
Flat Plane	97700		Bilateral	21240-50	

Total Fee: _____

Signed: _____ ID#: _____ Date: _____

I hereby authorize payment directly to Dr. _____ of the benefits otherwise payable to me, but not to exceed the charge stated above. I understand that I am financially responsible for charges not covered by the authorization. I authorize Dr. _____ to disclose to my insurance agency any and all information with respect to any treatment relative to my person or dependent. I understand that in executing this authorization I waive the right for such information to be privileged.

Date: _____ Signed: _____

                              Witness: _____

Appendix E
Example of Questionnaire to Be Completed by Patient with Temporomandibular Joint Problems

Name _____
Date _____

TMJ Questionnaire

1. Describe the problem in your own words. _____
   _____
   _____
   _____
   _____

2. Describe, in order if possible, any dental or medical treatment you have received for your present jaw problem(s).
   a. Splint _____
   b. Medications _____
   c. Physical therapy _____
   d. Stress counseling _____
   e. Orthodontics _____
   f. Restorative dentistry _____
   g. Surgery _____
   h. Other _____

3. Do you now have any of the following symptoms?

	Location	How Long?
Headaches ___	_____	_____
Neck pain ___	_____	_____
Jaw joint pain ___	_____	_____
Ear: Pain ___	_____	_____
Dizziness ___	_____	_____
Stuffiness ___	_____	_____
Ringing or buzzing ___	_____	_____
Facial pain ___	_____	_____
Pain behind the eyes ___	_____	_____

4. Is the pain:
    Constant? _____
    Burning? _____
    Stabbing? _____
    Aching? _____
    Worse in the afternoon or evening? _____
    Worse in the morning on awakening? _____
    Referred to other areas of the face, head, or neck? _____

5. Does it hurt:
    To eat or chew? _____
    To talk? _____
    To open wide? _____
    To smile, kiss, etc.? _____
    To swallow? _____

6. Does the pain interfere with your:
    Occupation? _____
    Social life? _____
    Family life? _____
    Sleep? _____

7. Please diagram where your pain occurs.

Right   Left

8. Place an "x" along the lines below to show how your pain is today.

Absent	Most Intense

Not Unpleasant	Most Unpleasant

9. Do you now notice or have you ever noticed any noises from your jaw joints?

	Right	Left	On Opening	On Closing
Popping	_____	_____	_____	_____
Clicking	_____	_____	_____	_____
Grating	_____	_____	_____	_____

10. Has your jaw ever "locked"? How often?
    Open _____ _____
    Closed _____ _____
    Was the "locking" associated with a particular event?

11. Can you remember any injury or trauma to your lower jaw? _____
    What kind?
    Motor vehicle accident _____
    Athletic injury _____
    Bodily injury _____
    _____
    Please indicate which area of your jaw was injured.

12. Have you ever had orthodontia (braces)? _____

13. Have you had your wisdom teeth removed? _____

14. Have you ever had long dental appointments or general anesthesia? _____

15. Do you ever clench or grind your teeth? _____
    During the day? _____   At night? _____
    If so, do you associate this with any particular cause? _____

16. Are your jaw muscles often sore and stiff when you awaken in the morning? _____

17. Are your teeth ever sore or sensitive to hot, cold, or chewing? _____

Appendix F
Temporomandibular Joint Clinical Examination Form

Name of Patient _____
Date _____

CLINICAL EXAMINATION FORM

A. Temporomandibular Joint
   1. ROM

Opening	Pain	ROM		Incisor Relation
		R	L	
0	+			Overbite ___ mm
10	+			Overjet ___ mm
20	+			Open Bite ___ mm
30		**Deviation on Open**		Pain Click
		To L		To L To L
40		To R		To R To R
50				Prot. Prot.
		Deviation on Prot.		
60		To L	To R	

   2. Joint sounds
      a. Popping: Hypertranslatory at ___ mm   R ___ L ___
      b. Clicking
          Reciprocal at ___ mm   R ___ L ___
          Nonreciprocal at ___ mm   R ___ L ___
      c. Crepitation   R ___ L ___
      f. Ever occur before accident
      e. First noticed after accident

   3. Joint tenderness: 1+ to 4+
      a. Intracanal   b. Lateral   c. Ever occur
          Right, closed   Right, closed   before accident
          Right, open/closing   Right, open   d. First noticed
          Left, closed   Left, closed   after accident
          Left, open/closing   Left, open

   4. Other pertinent findings
      a. Click eliminated by
          Opening bite?
          Anterior functioning?

CLINICAL EXAMINATION FORM (Continued)
Name of Patient _____

B. Masticatory and Cervical Muscles
Intensity: + to ++++
No pain: (−)
Location: (x)
Referral: →

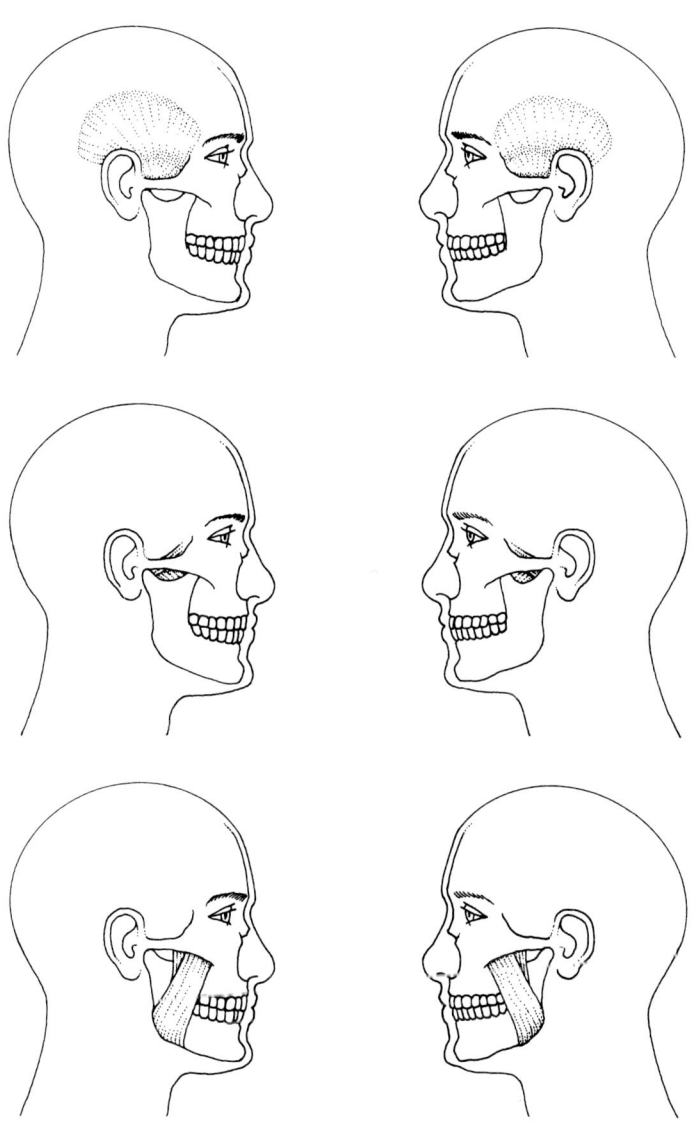

C. Oral Tissues
1. Mucosal lesions _____
2. Swellings _____
3. Periodontal disease _____
4. Alveolar process _____
5. Evidence of cheek- or lip-biting _____

CLINICAL EXAMINATION FORM (Continued)

Name of Patient _____

D. Dentition
1. Caries _____
2. Tooth mobility _____
3. Missing teeth _____
4. Prosthetic replacements _____
5. Impactions _____
6. Supraerupted teeth _____
7. Occlusion
   a. Class I   d. Crossbite
   b. Class II   e. Interferences
   c. Class III f. Prematurities
8. Mandibular displacement from initial tooth contact to full closure
   a. Patient notices   d. Examiner notices
   b. Anterior   e. Posterior
   c. Right lateral   f. Left lateral
9. Attrition

E. Radiographic Examination
1. Teeth and jaws
   Panoramic
2. Temporomandibular Joint
   TCP
   Tomograms
   CT
   Arthrograms
   MRI

F. Summary
Masseter, superficial
    deep
Lateral pterygoid
Temporalis belly:
  Posterior
  Middle
  Anterior
Tendon
SCM:
  Upper
  Lower
Trapezius
Occipital
Suprahyoid
Other

F Temporomandibular Joint Clinical Examination Form ■ 361

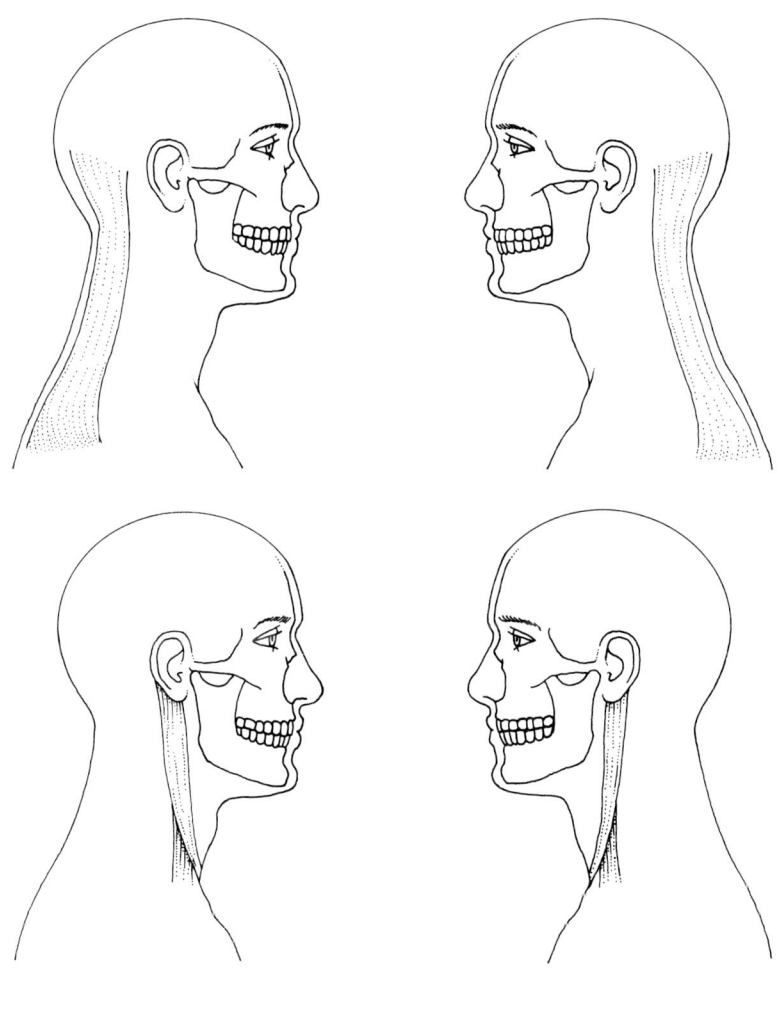

Right　　　　　　　　　　　　　　　Left

CLINICAL EXAMINATION FORM (Continued)

Name of Patient _____

TMJ MANAGEMENT PLAN

Clinical Data
1. History
2. Symptoms:
   Pain
   Dysfunction
   Noises

Diagnostic Imaging
1. Tomograms
2. Arthrograms
3. MRI

Treatment
1. Reconstructive arthroplasty
2. Disc removal arthroplasty
3. Arthroscopy
4. Biopsy
5. Nonsurgical

Admitting Diagnoses
1. Painful hypomobility
   Acute locking
   Chronic locking
   Postsurgical
   Posttraumatic
   Osteoarthrosis (degenerative joint disease)
2. Painful normal mobility with clicking or crepitation
3. Painful dysfunctional hypermobility
4. Painless dysfunctional clicking
5. Undiagnosed radiographic disease requiring biopsy
6. Traumatic capsulitis/myalgia

Appendix G
Patient Information Sheet Regarding Temporomandibular Joint Disease

Disorders of the temporomandibular joint (TMJ) can be classified into the general categories of congenital and developmental disturbances, traumatic injuries, arthritis, tumors, and pain/dysfunction syndrome. These disorders involve the bony and/or soft tissue components of the joint as well as the associated muscles that control the joint. Common symptoms include pain and limitation of movement of the lower jaw, jaw muscle tenderness, and joint noise (clicking, popping, or grating).

For appropriate evaluation of temporomandibular joint disease, many diagnostic measures may be required: (1) a detailed history of the disorder; (2) physical examination of the joint and dental structures, especially the occlusion, or "bite"; (3) x-ray examination, which may include examination of the teeth and supporting structures, routine TMJ x-ray examination, tomographic TMJ examination, and arthrographic examination of the TMJ (this last examination involves the placing of material within the joint space that can be visualized on the x-ray film and that outlines the disc within the joint); (4) diagnostic injections of the joint or associated muscles with local anesthesia; (5) diagnostic plastic bite plates to temporarily and reversibly change the bite; and (6) psychometric testing and/or evaluation and counseling.

Because of the variety of conditions involving the TMJ as well as many unrelated conditions that produce similar signs and symptoms, diagnosis may be very difficult, particularly in cases that have a prominent psychological, stressful, or emotional overlay.

Most TMJ disorders have taken many months or years to develop and patients have been living with the problem; only recently have tests been available to allow us to diagnose these conditions more easily. Neither diagnosis nor therapeutic results can be obtained in a short time, and your commitment to the therapy is necessary.

The initial therapy for many of the conditions involving the TMJ involves the management of the symptoms by such means as medications, physical therapy, occlusal appliances, and modification of deleterious jaw habits, such as clenching. When the acute symptoms have been relieved or controlled and the patient's condition remains stable for a reasonable period of time, additional forms of therapy will be needed or more permanent-type appliances will require fabrication. The permanent forms of therapy may include alterations in occlusion or bite by balancing of the teeth; restorative treatment by crowns, removable prosthetic appliances, or fillings; orthodontia; orthognathic surgery; or a combination of these procedures. These other types of management will not be instituted until some months after the acute symptoms have been controlled and the cause of the condition has been determined.

There are many conditions involving the TMJ, however, that initially or subsequently require surgical management. This involves repositioning of the disc within the joint or reconstruction of the joint and will also require follow-up care using either occlusal or surgical reconstruction of the bite.

The cause of TMJ disease is usually a multifactorial problem requiring the services or input of many of the dental disciplines.

Appendix H
Letter of Pre-determination for Temporomandibular Joint Insurance Coverage*

Re: PATIENT'S NAME:
INSURED'S NAME:
GROUP NUMBER:
SUBSCRIBER NUMBER:

To Whom it May Concern:

I am writing this letter for pre-determination of medical and surgical benefits for the above named patient.

The patient's signs and symptoms are as follows:
Temporomandibular Joint Pain   Jaw Hypermobility
Headaches   Jaw Hypomobility
Joint Noises   Joint Dysfunction

Radiographic examination shows:
Disc Displacement   Osteoarthrosis
Disc Deformity   Bony Hypertrophy

My diagnosis and ICD-9-CM Codes are as follows:
Osteoarthrosis   R L   715.9
Capsulitis   R L   726.9
Internal Derangement   R L   524.6
Synovitis   R L   524.6

My recommended treatment, CPT-4 codes, and estimated fee involved are as follows:

> Bilateral temporomandibular joint arthroscopic surgery with lysis of adhesions, joint lavage, and disc reduction.
> CPT-4 Code 29804 or 29800 $_____

---

*Adapted from Robert Schwartz, D.D.S.

If arthroscopic procedures are not successful, open joint surgery, CPT Code 21240, with an estimated fee of $_____, may be required. If the joint requires surgical opening during the same admission then there is no charge for the arthroscopy.

Outpatient surgery will be performed by myself at _____ Medical Center in _____ with possible admission as an inpatient if open surgery is required. Due to the nature of the surgical procedure, it will be performed under general anesthesia.

Please be good enough to pre-determine benefits for the above patient. If you have any questions or require further information, please feel free to contact me.

Very truly yours,

Appendix I
TMJ Treatment Follow-Up Questionnaire*

PLEASE CIRCLE THE CORRECT RESPONSE WHERE INDICATED:

NAME:
DATE:

1. Do you have any pain now?   YES or NO

   If YES, please answer Questions 2 and 3, otherwise please go directly to Question 4.

2. Please rate your pain by placing an "X" on the line indicating (A) your present pain and (B) your usual pain. Mark each "X" with the corresponding letter:

   _____
   No Pain   Most Intense
                                              Pain Imaginable

3. Please indicate on the drawing those areas where you have pain.

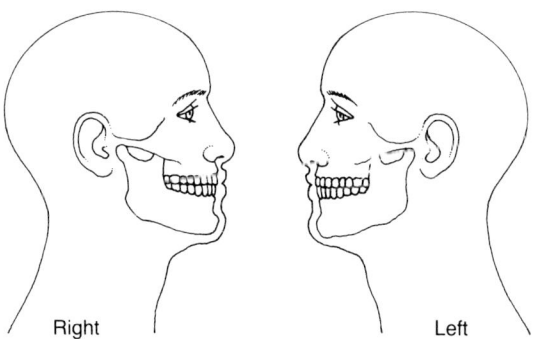

   Right   Left

4. Are you awakened from sleep with pain?   YES or NO
5. Are you aware of clenching or grinding of your teeth? YES or NO

*Courtesy of Dr. F. Dolwick, University of Florida, Gainesville, FL.

6. Is the pain worse on functioning (chewing, talking)?   YES or NO
7. Do you have limited opening?   YES or NO
8. Do you have any dietary limitation related to your jaw problem?   YES or NO
9. Does your jaw make noises on functioning?   YES or NO
10. Have you experienced jaw locking since treatment?   YES or NO
11. How do you feel now compared to the time you were treated here?

   |————————————————|————————————————|
   Worse   Originally   Better

12. Please rate your ability to chew by placing an "X" on the line indicating your present ability to chew.

   |————————————————————————————————|
   No Difficulty   Unable to Chew
   Chewing

13. How can you chew now compared to when you were treated here?

   |————————————————|————————————————|
   Worse   Originally   Better

Appendix J
Postoperative Instructions Following TMJ Arthroscopy

You have opted for arthroscopic surgery of the temporomandibular joint, which is usually performed on an outpatient basis. At the time of discharge from the ambulatory care or day surgery unit, you may have a pressure dressing or a small Band-Aid. Unless otherwise instructed, the pressure dressing may be removed the next day and the Band-Aid changed as needed. Please follow the instructions as outlined below very closely.

DRESSING

There may be several puncture wounds with or without stitches in front of your ear. These are placed for access and washing the joint. The Band-Aid or dressing may be stained with fluid or blood; however, excessive drainage or bleeding is not expected. If observed, you are to contact me or the nearest emergency room facility for evaluation and treatment.

MEDICATIONS

Appropriate antibiotics and pain medications will be prescribed prior to discharge, taking into account your medical history and your special needs. Nonsteroidal medications (e.g., Anaprox, Motrin) are always prescribed following arthroscopy for a period of time, unless contraindicated for whatever reason.

CARE OF WOUNDS

You may discontinue the Band-Aid and shower 48 hours after surgery. Keep the surgical area dry (sponge dry), and a thin film of bacitracin or any other antibiotic ointment may be applied. Blood in the ear can be washed out with diluted vinegar solution(50%) or mineral oil, using a dropper two to three times a day.

DIET

Full liquid diet for 48 hours followed by a soft nonchewed diet (e.g., pasta, cottage cheese) until the office visit, at which time there may be a change. At no point should regular diet be resumed or certain foods tested without a discussion with me.

ORAL HYGIENE

Resume and maintain oral hygiene starting the day after surgery. If restricted by jaw opening, a soft junior tooth brush is recommended.

ACTIVITY

Should not include strenuous activity or high/low impact exercise for a period of 3 months, unless otherwise instructed.

PHYSICAL THERAPY APPOINTMENT

You are required to see the physical therapist for a preoperative visit, followed by active physical therapy commencing 24 to 48 hours after surgery. I believe that physical therapy is an important adjunct in the successful management of your condition and postoperative period. Physical therapy is usually indicated for at least 4 to 6 weeks following surgery. The goals of physical therapy are to reduce swelling and to increase the range of motion of your jaw. Instruction sheets are available for your physical therapist if requested.

DENTAL APPOINTMENT

You are required to schedule an appointment with your dentist 1 to 2 weeks after surgery for evaluation and adjustment of your oral appliance if indicated.

PRECAUTIONS

Pain unrelieved by prescription, elevation of temperature greater than 101° F, or progressive swelling or bleeding is uncommon. If any occur, please contact the office immediately by telephone.

POSTOPERATIVE FINDINGS

The doctor will make every attempt to inform you of the postoperative findings immediately. He/she will often look for a member of your family or friend in the waiting room to discuss the findings. However, it has been my experience that you will best understand the findings at your first postoperative visit. At that time, we can review the video film and discuss what we have seen.

MEDICAL RECORDS

A dictated medical record has been filed at the hospital and my office. A copy of this is usually forwarded to your referring doctor and will be available to you upon request.

OFFICE APPOINTMENT

An appointment should be scheduled with my office at 1 week and 3 weeks after arthroscopic surgery.

Appendix K
Arthroscopic Examination of the TMJ Suggested Recording Sheet

NAME _____ DATE _____

    Right _____   Left _____

Preoperative Diagnosis _____

SUPERIOR JOINT SPACE

Synovium
    A. Fibrillation _____ Anterior Pouch _____ Posterior Pouch _____
    B. Proliferation _____ Anterior Pouch _____ Posterior Pouch _____
    C. Hypervascularity _____ Anterior Pouch _____ Posterior Pouch _____
    D. Adhesions Gross _____ Cobweb _____ Fibrous _____ Ankylosis _____

Retrodiscal Tissue
    A. Hypervascularity _____
    B. Remodeled _____
    C. Redundant _____
    D. Perforation _____

Disc
    A. Displacement
        Roofing _____ % Loss   Open _____ Closed _____
        Anterior _____
        Posterior _____
        Medial _____
        Lateral _____
    B. Quality
        Normal _____
        Loss of Texture and Superficial Sheen _____

Fibrocartilage Lining
    A. Normal _____
    B. Degenerative Changes _____

Bone
    A. Visualized _____
    B. Not Visualized _____
    C. Rough _____
    D. Smooth _____
    E. Spurs _____

Capsule
    A. Fibrous _____
    B. Lateral Impingement _____

Other Findings
    A. Loose Bodies _____   B. Foreign Body _____

Diagnosis

Synovitis   Grade I _____
                    Grade II _____
                    Grade III _____
                    Grade IV _____

Internal Derangement
    A. Displacement with Reduction _____
    B. Displacement without Reduction _____

Degenerative Joint Disease
    A. Osteoarthritis _____   Grade I _____
    B. Chondromalacia _____   Grade II _____
                                                      Grade III _____
                                                      Grade IV _____

Hypermobility _____

TREATMENT RENDERED

Examination using General Anesthesia
    A. Click   Absent _____   Present _____
    B. Range of Motion
        Same _____ Increased _____

Lavage
    A. Normal Saline _____
    B. Lactated Ringer's _____
    C. Sodium Hyaluronate _____

Lysis
    A. Blind _____   Direct Vision _____   Triangulation _____

Medications Injected
    A. Steroid Injection   Intra-Articular _____   Subsynovial _____
    B. Sclerosing Solution Injected into Retrodiscal Tissue _____

Anterior Release
    A. Hand Instruments _____
    B. Cautery _____

Posterior Cauterization
    A. For Relocation of Disc _____
    B. For Hypermobility _____

Synovectomy _____

Arthroplasty
   A. Debridement _____   Osteoplasty _____
   B. Basket Forceps _____
   C. Suction Punch _____
   D. Motorized Shaver _____

INFERIOR JOINT SPACE

Examination   Direct _____   Thru Perforation _____
   A. Findings _____
   B. Procedure Performed _____

Index

Note: Page numbers in *italics* refer to illustrations; numbers followed by t indicate tables.

Acetaminophen, postoperative use of, 307
Achromatic lens systems, 12, *13*
Acidophilic zone, in tissue alteration, 331, *333*
Acquired immune deficiency syndrome, 290, *290*
Acromial impingement syndrome, 249
Acrylic onlays, in disc repositioning, 105, *106*
Activity, postoperative instructions for, 371
Adaptation, of synovial joints, 48–53, *49–52*
Adhesiolysis, case reports in, 341–343
  in joint debridement, 176–177
  in operative arthroscopy, 176–177
Adhesions, case reports in, 344–345, *344–345*
  connective tissue, 45–46, *45*
  fibro-osseous, 242, *242*
  in disc displacement, 126, *127*, 188, *189*, 251, *251*
  in double-contrast arthrography, 126, *127*
  instruments for, 169, *171*
  postoperative evaluation of, 216
Age, treatment outcome and, 77
Aging, defined, 265
AIDS, 290, *290*
Airway obstruction, upper, from arthroscopy, 311–312
Alveolar nerve, inferior, 64, *65*
  injuries to, from arthroscopy, 314
Ambulatory surgery, in arthroscopy, 311
Analgesics, combination semisynthetic narcotic, 306–307, 307t
  non-narcotic, 307–308, 307t
Anatomy. See also *Temporomandibular joint, anatomy of.*
  of retrodiscal tissue, 64–65, *66*
  of synovium, 64–66, *66*
Anesthesia, complications from, 311–312
  postoperative, 306
Angled knife, in arthroscopic surgery, 158
Ankle, arthroscopy of, 2–4
Ankylosing spondylitis, 288
Anterior band release, in disc mobility, 189–190, *190*
Anterior disc displacement, 70–71, *72*, 74
Anterior release, in operative arthroscopy, 177–178, *177*
Anterior repositioning splint, *98*, 99
Anterolateral portal, in endaural arthroscopy, 195, *196–197*
Antibiotics, prophylactic, complications from, 312–313
Anti-inflammatory agents, nonsteroidal, postoperative use of, 309
Apparent field of view, 15–16, *16*
Appointments, postoperative instructions for, 371–372
Arachidonic acid, in inflammation, 43–45, *44*
Arches, dental, *92*
Argon lasers, in arthroscopy, 327

Arrhythmias, from arthroscopy, 312
Arterial complications, from arthroscopy, 316–317
Arteritis, temporal, 287
Arthritis, degenerative. See *Osteoarthritis (degenerative joint disease).*
  of temporomandibular joint, 86–87, 87t
  psoriatic, 288, *289*
  rheumatoid. See *Rheumatoid arthritis.*
Arthrocentesis, in operative arthroscopy, 175–176
Arthrography, complications of, 126
  contraindications for, 119–120, 122t
  diagnostic accuracy of, 133–136, 137t
  equipment for, 120–121, *121*
  findings of, 123–126, *123–126*
  in anterior disc displacement, 97, *97*
  in deformities, 231, *233*
  in hypermobility, 231–232, *232*
  indications for, 119–120, 122t
  techniques for, double-contrast, 122–123, *123–124, 126, 127*, 126–128
    single-contrast, 122, *122–123*, 125, *127*,
    transcranial, 124, *124*
Arthropathy, adaptation in, 48–53, *49–52*
  adhesions in, 45–46, *45*
  biomechanical loading in, 45–46
  classification of, 81, 82t
  degradative enzymes in, 47–48, *48*
  diagnosis of, clinical, 82–85, *83–85*
    differential, 85–87
    symptoms in, 81–82
  inflammation in, 41–45, *42–44*
  nonsurgical management of, case history in, 89
    etiology in, 90–92
    patient interview in, 89–90
    treatment of, 92–96
  nutritional, 37–39, *37*
  of lubrication, 39–41, *40*
  repair and remodeling of, 48–53, *49–52*
  tissue injury in, 47–48, *48*
Arthroscope, early designs of, *2–3*
  illumination of, 18, *19*
  large diameter, 157, *158*
  No. 21, 1–2, *2, 7*
  No. 24, *7*, 8–9
  optical characteristics of, 15–18
  selection of, 18–19
  types of, 12–14
Arthroscopic anatomy. See *Temporomandibular joint, anatomy of.*
Arthroscopic biopsy. See *Biopsy.*
Arthroscopy. See also specific types, e.g., *Endaural arthroscopy*; and specific diseases.
  complications of. See *Complications.*
  continuing education in, 10

Arthroscopy *(Continued)*
  guidelines for, in clinical practice, 229–234
    in hospital credentialing, 228–229
  history of, 1–10
  laboratory scenes in, *8–9*
  operative. See *Operative arthroscopy.*
  pharmacologic management after, 305–309
  position paper on, 347–350
  recording sheet for, 373–375
  research in, 10–11, 325
  staging criteria for, 229, 230t–231t
Articular cartilage, degenerative changes in, 270, *270*
  nutritional impairment of, 37–39, *37*
  research in, 324
  structure and function of, 28–34
Articular disc, lubrication of, *21*, 23–25
Articular eminence, 58–60, *61*
Articular surface, in osteoarthrosis, 261–265, *265– 266*, 267
Articulated teaching attachments, 162, *163*
Asepsis, in arthroscopic procedures, 230, *231*
Atrophy, subcutaneous fat, from arthroscopy, 320–321, *321*
Auditory canal, external, anterior wall of, 194, *195*
Auriculotemporal nerve injury, from arthroscopy, 315
Auscultation, presurgical evaluation of, 295
Autoimmune deficiency syndrome, 290, *290*
Autologous cartilage analog, research in, 324–325, *325*

Banana knife, in arthroscopic surgery, 158
Basket forceps, in arthroscopic surgery, 159
  in biopsy, 200, *201*
"Beaking," in sagittal tomography, 252, *254*
Behçet's syndrome, 289
Biologic lubrication, 23, *24*
  joint, impairment of, 39–41, *40*
Biomechanical loading, 45–46, 252
Biopsy, arthroscopic, 199–202, *200–201*
  forceps in, 159, *161*
  in diagnostic arthroscopy, 166, *167*, 176
  in operative arthroscopy, 176
  synovial, in rheumatoid arthritis, 278–279
Bleeding, from arthroscopy, 317
Bone file, in arthroscopic surgery, 159
Branchial arch, 56, *58*
Burns, from laser arthroscopy, 331, *332–333*

Camera, for intra-articular photography, 162, *162*
Cannula, in operative arthroscopy, 168–169, *169, 177*
Capsular stretch (CS), in pain relief, 256
Capsule. See also *Fibrosis, capsular; Lateral capsule.*
  functions of, 61–63, *63*
  herniation of, 192, *192*
Capsulitis, postoperative, 320
Carbon dioxide lasers, in arthroscopy, 327
Cartilage, articular, degenerative changes in, 270, *270*
  nutritional impairment of, 37–39, *37*
  research in, 324
  structure and function of, 28–34
Cartilage shaver, in arthroscopic surgery, 160, *160*
Cartilaginous canal, 197, *198*
Case reports, in chondromalacia, 342–343, *343*
  in diagnostic arthroscopy, 178–179, 344, *345*

Case reports *(Continued)*
  in hyalinization, 339–340, *340*
  in hypermobility, 184
  in hypomobility, 179–184, *181–183, 185*
  in joint debridement, 184
  in lavage, 339–343
  in lysis, 341–343
  in osteoarthritis, 338–339, *338–339*
  in post-arthrotomy patients, 216–217
  in temporomandibular disorders, 89
  in trauma, 184–196
Cauterization, in stabilization, 206, *206*
Cautery tips, in electrosurgery, 204–205, *205*
Cavitation zone, in tissue alteration, 331, *333*
Cells, of articular cartilage, 29
Central nervous system injuries, from arthroscopy, 314
Character generator, in arthroscopic surgery, 163, *168*
Chondromalacia, case reports in, 342–343, *343*
  cycles of, 259–260, *260*
  etiology of, 270–271
  in hyalinization, 339–340, *340*
  in osteoarthritis, 258–259
  of articular surface, 186, *187*
  pain in, 271
  pathogenesis of, 269–270
  progressive stages of, 271–273, 272t, *272–274*
  treatment of, 273–275
Chondromatosis, synovial, 243–249, 244t–245t, *245–247*
Clicking, of temporomandibular joint, 70–71, 74
Clinical examination form, 359–363
Clinical practice, arthroscopy guidelines for, 229–234
  privileges in, 349
"Closed lock," in disc displacement, 251, *252*
CO_2 lasers, in arthroscopy, 327
Coagulation, joint adhesiolysis and, 176
Cold, postoperative application of, 297
Collagen, of articular cartilage, 29–31, *30*
Color monitors, in arthroscopic surgery, 163
Color video printers, in arthroscopic surgery, 163 *164*
Complications, anesthetic, 311–312
  classification of, 310–311, *311*
  infections as, 312–313
  inflammatory, 320–321
  injuries as, cutaneous thermal, 320, *321*
    neurologic, *313*, 313–315, 315t
    otologic, 318–320, *319*
    vascular, 316–317, *316*
  of arthrography, 126
  of instrument failure, 317–318, 318t, *318*
Computed tomography, diagnostic accuracy of, 133–136, 137t
  imaging with, 118, *120*, 128, *128–129*
  in disc displacement, 106–109, *110*
  in synovial chondromatosis, 244–245, *245*
Condylar head, 58, *60*
Condylar joint debridement, 184, *186*
Condylar marrow fibrosis, in tissue alteration, 331–332, *334*
Condylar remodeling, 256, *257*
Condylar resorption, lateral, 253, *255*
Condylar translation, 72, *73*
Connective tissue disease(s), adhesions in, 45–46, *45*
  ankylosing spondylitis as, 288
  Behçet's syndrome as, 289
  dermatomyositis as, 286–287
  gout as, 288–289, *289*
  juvenile rheumatoid arthritis as, 291, *291*

Connective tissue disease(s) *(Continued)*
  lupus erythematosus as, 283–284, *285*
  Lyme disease as, 290
  mixed, 284
  polymyalgia rheumatica as, 287
  polymyositis as, 286–287
  pseudogout as, 288–289
  psoriatic arthritis as, 288, *289*
  Reiter's syndrome as, 288
  rheumatoid arthritis as, 276–283
  systemic inflammatory, AIDS-related, 290, *290*
  Sjögren's syndrome as, 284–285, *287*
  Takayasu's arteritis as, 287–288
  temporal arteritis as, 287
Consent form, patient, 351
Continuing education, in arthroscopy, 10
Continuous passive motion (CPM), research in, 325–326
Contraction, muscle, in temporomandibular disorders, 90
Cranial nerve injuries, from arthroscopy, *313*, 314–315, 315t
CS (capsular stretch), in pain relief, 256
Curette, ring, in arthroscopic surgery, 158–159
Cutaneous thermal injuries, 320, *321*

Debridement, joint, adhesiolysis in, 176–177
  case reports in, 184, 341
  condylar, 184, *186*
  of knee, 2, *4*, 8
Degenerative joint disease. See *Osteoarthritis (degenerative joint disease)*.
Degradation, cycle of, in osteoarthritis, 50, *50*
  in tissue injury, 47–48, *48*
Dental appointment, postoperative instructions for, 371
Dental arches, *92*
Depth of field, 17
Derangements, internal. See *Internal derangements*.
Dermatomyositis, 286–287
Diagnostic arthroscopy. See also *Arthropathy, diagnosis of*.
  case reports in, 178–179, 339–340, 344, *345*
  indications for, 348
  procedures in, 165–166, 165t
Diagnostic block, 84–85, *85*
Diet, postoperative instructions for, 371
Direction of view, 19
Disc, articular, 21, 23–25
  displacement of, adhesions in, 126, *127*, 188, *189*, 251, *251*
  anatomy of, 249–256
  anterior, 70–71, *72*, 74
  arthrography in, 97, *97*, 124, 125, *125*, 126
  case reports in, 342–343
  deformities in, 117, *117*, 232, *234*
  diagnosis of, 251–252, *252*
  hypomobility secondary to, 85–86, 86t
  imaging of, 116–117, *117*, 117t, *118*
    magnetic resonance, *131*, 132–133, *134*, *136*
  impingement stages in, 249, *250*, 250t
  longitudinal studies of, 110–111
  pathophysiology of, 249–256
  progression of, 109–111
  subjective symptoms in, 109t

Disc *(Continued)*
  tomography in, 106–109, *110*
  treatment modalities for, 97–98, *98*, 100t
  mobility of, case reports in, 342–343
    in displacement, 188, *189*
    increasing, 188–192
  morphology of, in prognosis, 231–232
  reduction of, joint adhesiolysis and, 176
  repositioning of, long-term results of, 105–109
    onlays in, 100–109, *101*–*102*, 103t—104t
    post-treatment arthrography in, 102–104, 103t–104t
  splints in, 98–100, *98*, 100t–101t
  stabilization of, cauterization in, 206, *206*
    suturing in, 207–212, *207*–*212*
  surgery on, in post-arthrotomy patients, 215–217
  suturing devices for, in arthroscopic surgery, 160, *161*
Discectomy, 217, *217*–*221*
Disco-osseous bands, in intracapsular fibrosis, 237–238, *238*
Documentation, in operative arthroscopy, 162–164
Double contrast arthrography, 122–123, *123*–*124*, 126, *127*, 126–128
Double-portal technique, in operative arthroscopy, 175, *175*
Draping, guidelines for, 230, *231*
  in operating room protocol, 155, *157*, 169, *172*
Dressings, postoperative instructions for, 370
Drugs, postoperative instructions for, 370
Dyonics suction punch, in arthroscopic surgery, 159

Education, continuing, in arthroscopy, 10
Elbow, arthroscopy of, 4
Electrical stimulation, postoperative application of, 297, *300*
Electrosurgery, fluids in, 203–204
  history of, 203
  lasers in, 205
  principles of, 203
  uses of, 204–205
Endaural arthroscopy, advantages of, 197–198, 198t
  approaches to, 192–193
  rationale of, 193–195
Endoscopy, of knee, 8.
Entoglenoid process, 60, *62*
Entrance pupil, in objective lens systems, 14–15
Enzymes, synovial, in osteoarthritis, 25–26
Equipment, arthrographic, 120–121, *121*
Erbium:YAG laser, in arthroscopy, 328–329
Exercises, therapeutic, in rehabilitation, 301, *302*–*303*
Eximer laser, in arthroscopy, 329
Exit pupil diameter, in objective lens systems, 17–18
External auditory canal, anterior wall of, 194, *195*
  laceration of, from arthroscopy, 319
External otitis, from arthroscopy, 315–316
Eye relief, 17, *17*

Fat atrophy, subcutaneous, from arthroscopy, 320–321, *321*
Fiberoptics, *13*, 13–14, 330–331, *331*
Fibrocartilage, architecture of, 31–32, *32*–*33*

Fibro-osseous adhesions, in intracapsular fibrosis, 242, *242*
Fibrosis, capsular, fibrous thickening in, 51, *51*
  in post-arthrotomy patient, 178, *178–180*, 218, *219–221*
  of soft tissues, 237, *237*
  condylar marrow, in tissue alteration, 331–332, *334*
  interosseous, 241–242, *242*
  intracapsular, bands in, 236–238, *236–238*
    fibro-osseous adhesions in, 242, *242*
    osseous adhesions in, 242, *242*
    pseudowalls in, 238–241, *239–241*
Fibrosynovial bands, in intracapsular fibrosis, 236–237, *237*
Field of view, defined, 15–16, *16*
Field-widening lens, 15
First assistant, in arthroscopic surgery, 159
Fistula, arteriovenous, from arthroscopy, 316–317
Flat occlusal maxillary splint, 99, *99*
Fluids, in electrosurgery, 203–204.
  synovial, composition of, 21–23, *23*
    enzymes of, in osteoarthritis, 25–26
    intimal layer of, 20–21, *22*
    research in, 323
Follow-up questionnaire, 368–369
Forceps, in arthroscopic surgery, 159, *161*
Function, postoperative evaluation of, 216

Generator, character, in arthroscopic surgery, 163, *168*
Glucocorticoids, postoperative use of, 306, 306t
Golden retriever, in arthroscopic surgery, 159
Gout, 288–289, *289*
Gradient index optics, 12–13, *13*
Grasping forceps, in arthroscopic surgery, 159, *161*
Gross anatomy, of temporomandibular joint, 140–141, *141, 142*
Growth factors, inflammation and, 46

"Half-blind" technique, of arthroscopic biopsy, 200–201, *201*
Hand instruments, for arthroscopic surgery, 158–159
Hard tissue, after disc repositioning, 106–109, *110*
  chondromalacia of, 258–259, 269–275
  osteoarthrosis of, 72–74, *74*, 258–269
Heat, postoperative application of, 297
Hemorrhagic synovitis, 184, *185*
Hemostasis, in electrosurgery, 204, *204*
Herniation, capsular, 192, *192*
History, patient, presurgical evaluation of, 295
Home program, in rehabilitation, 302, *302–303*
Hospital credentialing, arthroscopy guidelines for, 228–229
Hyaline cartilage, architecture of, 31–32, *32–33*
Hyalinization, case reports in, 339–340, *340*
Hyaluronan, in normal synovial fluid, 21–22 *23*
  in viscosurgery, 335–336
  postoperative use of, 306
Hyaluronate, sodium, in normal synovial fluid, 21–22 *23*
Hypermobility, arthrography in, 231–232, *232*
  case reports in, 184
  diagnosis of, 86, 87t
  sclerosing solutions in, 206

Hypertrophic articular tubercles, 253, *255*
Hypomobility, case reports in, 179–184, *181–183*, *185* 342–343
  electrosurgery in, 204, *204*
  in anterior disc displacement, 85–86, 86t

Ideal occlusion, 90–91
Illumination, of arthroscopes, 18, *19*
Imaging, anatomy in, 115, *115–116*
  clinical examination in, 117–118
  diagnostic accuracy of, 133–136, 137t
  in disk displacement, 116–117, *117*, 117t, *118*
  methods of, arthrographic, 118–128
    magnetic resonance, 129–133, *130–136*, 130t
    plain film radiographic, 118, *119*
    radionuclide, 136–137, *137*
    selection of, 137–138
    tomographic, 118, *120*, 128
  post-treatment, 133, *136*
Impingement, in disc displacement, 249, *250*, 250t
  in patellofemoral joint, 2, *4*
Implants, Proplast, 223–226, *223–226*
Index optics, gradient, 12–13, *13*
Infection, from arthroscopy, 312–313
Inferior alveolar nerves, 64, *65*
  injuries to, from arthroscopy, 314
Inferolateral approach, to endaural arthroscopy, 192–193
Inflammation, etiology of, 91
  from arthroscopy, 320–321
  growth factors and, 46
  nonsteroidal agents in, 309
  physiology of, 41–45, *42–44*
  tumor necrosis factor in, 46
Infraorbital nerve injuries, from arthroscopy, 314
Instrumentation, failure of, 317–318, 318t, *318*
  hand, 158–159
  motorized, 160, *160*
  preparation of, 313
  suggestions for, 156
  techniques of, 160–161
Insurance, claim form for, 353–355
  letter of pre-determination for, 366–367
Intermediate space, arthroscopic anatomy of, 145, 147, *146–147*
Internal derangements, arthroscopic surgery in, 78–79, 167
  defined, 266–267, 347–348
  remodeling in, 75–76
  stages in, 70–74, *71–74*
  studies of, anatomic, 74–75
    longitudinal, 76–77
  treatment of, 77–78
Interosseous fibrosis, 241–242, *242*
Intimal layer, of synovial membrane, 20–21, *22*
Intra-articular bleeding, from arthroscopy, 317
Intra-articular injections, in rheumatoid arthritis, 280
Intra-articular photography, camera for, 162, *162*
Intracapsular fibrosis, bands in, 236–238, *236–238*
  fibro-osseous adhesions in, 242, *242*
  osseous adhesions in, 242, *242*
  pseudowalls in, 238–241, *239–241*

Joint cavity, lower, *142*, 149
  upper, arthroscopic anatomy of, 142, *142*
    visual fields in, 148–149, *149*
Joint debridement, adhesiolysis in, 176–177
  case reports in, 184, 341
  condylar, 184, *186*
  of knee, 2, *4*, 8
Joint mobilization, 297–302, *301*
Juvenile rheumatoid arthritis, 291, *291*

Knee joint, arthroscopy of, 2, *4*
  endoscopy of, 8
Knives, in arthroscopic surgery, 158
KTP-532 laser, in arthroscopy, 329

Laboratory scenes, in arthroscopy, 8–9
Laceration, of external auditory canal, 319
Laser-assisted arthroscopy, in electrosurgery, 205
  instrumentation in, 330–332, *331*
  laser selection in, 327–329, 328t
  research in, 325
  safety of, 329–330
Lateral capsule, in operative arthroscopy, 178
  prolapse of, 252, *253*
  release of, in disc mobility, 191
Lateral condylar resorption, 253, *255*
Lateral eminence release (LER), in pain relief, 256
Lateral pterygoid muscle, 63, *64–65*
Lateral spaces, in endaural arthroscopy, 193, *194*
Lavage, case reports in, 339–343
  in rheumatoid arthritis, 279–280
  joint adhesiolysis and, 176–177
Lens endoscope systems, achromatic, 12, *13*
  design of, 14–15, *14*
  gradient index, 12–13, *13*
LER (lateral eminence release) in pain relief, 256
Letter of pre-determination, for insurance coverage, 366–367
Lingual nerves, anatomy of, 64, *65*
  injuries to, from arthroscopy, 314
Lipoxygenases, in inflammation, 44–45
"Lipping," in sagittal tomography, 252, *254*
Loading, biomechanical, 45–46, 252
Local anesthesia, postoperative use of, 306
Locking, acute closed, 72, *73*
  in disc displacement, 71–72, 74
Longitudinal studies, of disc displacement, 110–111
  of internal derangement, 76–77
Loop principle, in electrosurgery, 203
Lower joint cavity, *142*, 149
Lubrication, biologic, 23, *24*
  joint, impairment of, 39–41, *40*
Lupus erythematosus, systemic (SLE), 283–284, *285*
Lyme disease, 290
Lysis of adhesions, case reports in, 341–343
  in joint debridement, 176–177
  in operative arthroscopy, 176–177

Macrotrauma, acute joint, operative arthroscopy in, 168
Magnetic resonance imaging, in disc displacement, 252, *253*
  technique of, 129–133, *130–136*, 130t
Mandible manipulator, in arthroscopic surgery, 160, *161*
Mayo stand setup, in arthroscopic surgery, 155–156
Meckel's cartilage, 56, *57*
Medical records, postoperative instructions for, 372
Medications, for arthroscopic surgery, 156
  postoperative instructions for, 370
Meniscus, 60–61
Metallic onlays, in disc repositioning, 105, *107*
Metalloproteinases, in tissue injury, 47–48
Microscopy, scanning electron, of articular surface, 261–265, *265–266*, 267
Microtrauma, in chondromalacia, 270–271
  operative arthroscopy in, 168
Mixed connective tissue disease, 284
Mobility, disc, case reports in, 342–343
  in displacement, 188, *189*
  increasing, 188–192
Monitors, video, 163, 169, *172*
Monopolar cautery tip, in electrosurgery, 204, *205*
Motorized instruments, in arthroscopic surgery, 160, *160*
MRI. See *Magnetic resonance imaging.*
MULTIYAG laser, in arthroscopy, 329
Myalgia, in temporomandibular disorders, 90

Narcotic analgesics, combination semisynthetic, 306–307, 307t
Needles, positioning of, 172, *173–174*
  spinal, in arthroscopic surgery, 158
Neurologic injuries, from arthroscopy, 64, *313*, 313–315, 315t
Neuromuscular examination, presurgical, 295
Noises, in temporomandibular arthropathy, 81–82
Non-narcotic analgesics, postoperative use of, 307–308, 307t
Nonsteroidal anti-inflammatory agents, post-operative use of, 309
Nutritional impairment, of articular cartilage, 37–39, *37*

Objective lens systems, 14–15, *14*
Obstruction, upper airway, from arthroscopy, 311–312
Occlusal adjustment, 92, *92*
Occlusal splint, 98, *99*, 99t
Occlusion, diagnosis of, 89–96
  etiology of, 90–91
  factors in, 78
  permanent changes of, *95*, 105–106, *108–109*
  treatment of, 92–96
Open surgery, in rheumatoid arthritis, 280
Operative arthroscopy, biopsy in, 176
  case reports in, 178–186
  documentation in, 162–164
  indications for, 166–168, 348
  instrumentation in, 157–161

Operative arthroscopy *(Continued)*
　Mayo stand setup for, 155–156
　　medications in, 156
　　operating rooms for, 155, *155*, *352*
　　procedures in, 175–178
　　techniques in, 168–175, 348
Optics, gradient index, 12–13, *13*
Oral hygiene, postoperative instructions for, 371
Orthoses, 92–95
Osseous adhesions, in intracapsular fibrosis, 242, *242*
Osteoarthritis (degenerative joint disease), 232, *234*, 348
　case reports in, 338–339, *338–339*
　degradation cycle in, 50, *50*
　etiology of, 91–92
　synovial enzymes in, 25–26
Osteoarthrosis, articular surface in, 261–265, *265–266*, 267
　defined, 265–266
　histopathology of, 261, *263–264*
　initial changes in, 259–261, *259–264*
　of hard tissue, 72–74, *74*, 258–269
　of temporomandibular joint, 49, *49*
　primary, 91
　secondary, 91–92
Otitis media, from arthroscopy, 315–316
Otologic injuries, from arthroscopy, 318–320, *319*
Outflow needle, 173, *174*

Pain, in chondromalacia, 271
　in temporomandibular disorders, 81
Palpation, presurgical evaluation of, 295
Parafunction, in temporomandibular disorders, 91
Patellofemoral joint impingement, 2, *4*
Patient(s), care guidelines for, 349
　consent form for, 351
　information sheet for, 364–365
　interviewing of, 89–90. See also *Post-arthrotomy patients*.
　postoperative instructions for, 370–372
　questionnaire for, 356–358
Penfield neurosurgical dissector, 169, *171*
Perforations, case reports in, 344–345, *344–345*
　in disc displacement, 126, *126*
　of tympanic membrane, 319
Peripheral nerve injuries, from arthroscopy, 314
Pharmacologic management, after arthroscopy, 305–309
Photography, intra-articular camera for, 162, *162*
Physical therapy, educational role of, 296
　in temporomandibular disorders, 95–96
　postoperative instructions for, 371
Plain film radiography, 118, *119*
Polymyalgia rheumatica, 287
Polymyositis, 286–287
Post-arthrotomy fibrosis, 178, *178–180*
Post-arthrotomy patients, arthroscopic procedures for, 215–226
　symptoms of, 214, 214t
Posterior synovial pouch, upper, arthroscopic anatomy of, 142–145, *143–145*
Postoperative capsulitis, 320
Postoperative instructions, 370–372
Postoperative period, evaluation during, 297
　pharmacologic management in, 306–309

Post-treatment imaging, 133, *136*
Posture, presurgical evaluation of, 295
Precautions, postoperative instructions for, 371
Presurgical evaluation, 294–296
Pre-treatment questionnaire, 356–358
Primary osteoarthrosis, 91
Printers, color video, in arthroscopic surgery, 163, *164*
Probe, in arthroscopic surgery, 158
Prophylactic antibiotics, complications from, 312–313
Proplast implants, 223–226, *223–226*
Prostaglandins, in inflammation, 43–45, *44*
Prosthodontic repositioning, 95, 105–106, *108–109*
Proteinases, in tissue injury, 47–48
Proteoglycans, in articular cartilage, 31, *31*
　in tissue injury, 48, *48*
Protrusive splint, for disc displacement, 97–98, *98*
Pseudogout, 288–289
Pseudowalls, in intracapsular fibrosis, 238–241, *239–241*
Psoriatic arthritis, 288, *289*
Psychological factors, treatment outcome and, 78
Punch forceps, in arthroscopic surgery, 159

Quality of life, temporomandibular joint and, 67–69
Questionnaire, follow-up, 368–369
　pre-treatment, 356–358

Radiography, in disc displacement, *110*, 111, 111t, *112*, 113t
　in rheumatoid arthritis, 277
Radionuclide imaging, 136–137, *137*
Range of motion, in temporomandibular arthropathy, 82
Real field of view, 15–19, *16–19*
Recording sheet, for arthroscopic examination, 373–375
Reflection arthroscopic prisms, 16–17, *16*
Rehabilitation, evaluation in, postoperative, 297
　presurgical, 294–296
　goals of, 297–304
　home program in, 302, *302–303*
　of soft tissue, 297, *301*
　physical therapist in, 296
　postoperative, immediate considerations in, 297
　　treatment modalities in, 297–302, 298t–300t
　preoperative, 296
　therapeutic exercises in, 301, *302–303*
Reiter's syndrome, 288
Release, lateral capsule, in disc mobility, 191
Remodeling, condylar, 256, *257*
　defined, 265
　in internal derangement, 75–76
　of hard tissue, 72–74, *74*, 260, *261*
　of synovial joints, 48–53, *49–52*
Repositioning, disc, long-term results of, 105–109
　onlays in, 100–109, *101–102*, 103t–104t
　post-treatment arthrography in, 102–104, 103t–104t
　splints for, 94–95, *94–95*
Research, in arthroscopy, 10–11, 325
　in articular cartilage, 324
　in autologous cartilage analog, 324–325, *325*
　in continuous passive motion, 325–326

Research *(Continued)*
 in laser arthroscopy, 325
 in synovial apparatus and fluid, 323
 in viscosurgery, 325
Resection, synovial, in rheumatoid arthritis, 280, *280*
Retrodiscal tissue, functional anatomy of, 64–65, *66*
Retrograde knife, in arthroscopic surgery, 158
Rheumatoid arthritis, diagnosis of, 276–279, *277–279*, 282–283
 inflammation in, 42, *43*
 juvenile, 291, *291*
 pathogenesis of, 276
 treatment of, 279–280
Ring curette, in arthroscopic surgery, 158–159
Rod lenses, 7, *7*, 12
Roofing, postoperative evaluation of, 216
Rotational displacement, 116
Rotational splints, 93–94, *93*

Safety, of laser-assisted arthroscopy, 329–330
Salicylates, postoperative use of, 307
Scanning electron microscopy (SEM), of articular surface, 261–265, *265–266*, 267
Scanning parameters, in magnetic resonance imaging, 130–131, 130t
Scissors, in arthroscopic surgery, 159
 in disc mobility, 190–191
Sclerosing solutions, in hypermobility, 206
Sclerosis, joint adhesiolysis and, 176
Secondary osteoarthrosis, 91–92
Semisynthetic narcotic analgesics, combination, 306–307, 307t
Serine proteinases, in tissue injury, 48
Sex, treatment outcome and, 77
Shaver, cartilage, in arthroscopic surgery, 160, *160*
Shoulder joint, acromial impingement affecting, 249
 arthroscopy of, 2
Sideways displacement, 116
Silicon elastomer implants, *61*
Single-contrast arthrography, 122–123, *123–124*, *126*, *127*, 126–128
Single portal technique, *169*, 170, *170*, 175
Site, surgical, preparation of, 313
Sjögren's syndrome, 284–285, *287*
SLE (systemic lupus erythematosus), 283–284, *285*
Sociocultural background, treatment outcome and, 77
Sociomedical orientation, treatment outcome and, 77
Sodium hyaluronate, in normal synovial fluid, 21–22, *23*
 postoperative use of, 306
Soft tissue, capsular fibrosis of, 237, *237*
 interosseous fibrosis of, 241–242, *242*
 intracapsular fibrosis of, 235–243
 rehabilitation of, 297, *301*
 surgery on, in post-arthrotomy patients, 215–217
 synovial chondromatosis of, 243–249, 244t
Sphenomandibular ligament, 61
Spinal needles, in arthroscopic surgery, 158
Spine, presurgical evaluation of, 296
Splint therapy, in disc displacement, 96–98
 in occlusal disorders, 92–95
Spondylitis, ankylosing, 288
Stabilization, of disc, cauterization in, 206, *206*
 suturing in, 207–212, *207–212*
Staging criteria, in clinical practice, 229, 230t–231t

Sterilization, of instruments, 160–161
Still video recording, in arthroscopic surgery, 163
Still's disease, 291
Subcutaneous fat atrophy, from arthroscopy, 320–321, *321*
Subintimal injections, 206–207, *207*
Suction punch, in arthroscopic surgery, 159, *159*
Superior head, 63, *63*, *65*
Superior posterolateral approach, to endaural arthroscopy, 192–193, 195, *196–197*
Supplies, in arthroscopic surgery, 156
Surgery, ambulatory, 311
 arthroscopic. See *Operative arthroscopy.*
 open, in rheumatoid arthritis, 280
 site preparation for, 313
Suturing, in arthroscopic surgery, 160
 in disc stabilization, 207–212, *207–212*
 post-arthrotomy, 215, *215*
 postoperative evaluation of, 216
Switching sticks, in arthroscopic surgery, 158
Synovial biopsy, in rheumatoid arthritis, 278–279
Synovial chondromatosis, 243–249, 244t–245t, *245–247*
Synovial pouch, lower anterior, 150–153, *151–152*
 upper posterior, 142–145, *143–144*
Synovial recess, upper anterior, *142*, 147–148, *148*, *143–145*
Synovial resection, in rheumatoid arthritis, 280, *280*
Synovitis, hemorrhagic, 184, *185*
 subintimal injections in, 206–207, *207*
Synovium, anatomy of, 64–66, *66*
 fluid in, composition of, 21–23, *23*
 enzymes of, in osteoarthritis, 25–26
 intimal layer of, 20–21, *22*
 postoperative evaluation of, 216
 research in, 323
Systemic inflammatory arthritides. See *Connective tissue disease(s), systemic inflammatory.*
Systemic lupus erythematosus (SLE), 283–284, *285*

Takayasu's arteritis, 287–288
Temporal arteritis, 287
Temporal bone, 56–57, *59*
Temporomandibular drape, in arthroscopic surgery, 155, *157*, 169, *172*
Temporomandibular joint. See also *Arthropathy; Arthroscopy.*
 anatomy of, arthroscopic, 141–152
 components of, 58–67
 distinctive features of, 56–58
 gross, 140–141, *141*, *142*
 in imaging, 116, *116*
 arthroscopic biopsy of, 199–202, *200–201*
 fields of view oriented to, 195, *196*
 mobilization of, 297–302, *301*
 presurgical evaluation of, 295–296
 role of, in quality of life, 67–69
 vascular supply of, 67, *68*
Therapeutic exercises, in rehabilitation, 301, *302–303*
Thermal injuries, cutaneous, 320, *321*
Thulium-holmium-chromium laser, in arthroscopy, 328
Tissue. See *Connective tissue disease(s); Hard tissue; Soft tissue.*
Tissue biopsy. See *Biopsy.*

Tomography, computed, diagnostic accuracy of, 133–136, 137t
  imaging with, 118, *120*, 128, *128–129*
  in disc displacement, 106–109, *110*
  in synovial chondromatosis, 244–245, *245*
Tragal-lateral canthus, 171, *172*
Transcranial arthrography, 124, *124*
Trauma, case reports in, 184–196
  in chondromalacia, 270–271
Triangulation technique, of arthroscopic biopsy, 200–201, *201*
Tropocollagen molecules, *30*, 30–31
Tumor necrosis factor, inflammation and, 46
Tympanic membrane perforation, 319

Upper airway obstruction, from arthroscopy, 311–312
Upper anterior synovial recess, *142*, 147–148, *148*, *143–145*

Upper joint cavity, arthroscopic anatomy of, 142, *142*
  visual fields in, 148–149, *149*
Upper posterior synovial pouch, 142–145, *143–144*

Vascular injuries, from arthroscopy, 316–317, *316*
Vascular supply, of temporomandibular joint, 67, *68*
Venous bleeding, from arthroscopy, 317
Video equipment, in arthroscopic surgery, 163, 169, *172*
Vignetting, in arthroscopy, 18
Viscosurgery, in arthroscopy, 325, 335–336

Wound care, postoperative instructions for, 370

Yttrium-aluminum-garnet (YAG) laser, in arthroscopy, 328–329

Zone of cavitation, in tissue alteration, 331, *333*